Biosensors Based on Nanomaterials and Nanodevices

Nanomaterials and Their Applications

Series Editor: M. Meyyappan

Biosensors Based on Nanomaterials and Nanodevices

Edited by
Jun Li • Nianqiang Wu

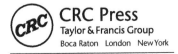

CRC Press
Taylor & Francis Group
Boca Raton   London   New York

CRC Press is an imprint of the
Taylor & Francis Group, an **informa** business

CRC Press
Taylor & Francis Group
6000 Broken Sound Parkway NW, Suite 300
Boca Raton, FL 33487-2742

First issued in paperback 2017

Version Date: 20130725

ISBN 13: 978-1-4665-5151-0 (hbk)
ISBN 13: 978-1-138-07325-8 (bk)

Library of Congress Cataloging-in-Publication Data

Biosensors based on nanomaterials and nanodevices / editors, Jun Li, Nianqiang Wu.
      pages cm -- (Nanomaterials and their applications)
   Includes bibliographical references and index.
   ISBN 978-1-4665-5151-0 (hardback)
   1. Biosensors--Materials. 2. Nanostructured materials. I. Li, Jun, 1966 May 21- editor of compilation. II. Wu, Nianqiang, editor of compilation.

R857.B54B5538 2014
610.28--dc23   2013027289

Visit the Taylor & Francis Web site at
http://www.taylorandfrancis.com

and the CRC Press Web site at
http://www.crcpress.com

Contents

Section III Magnetic Nanoparticles for Biosensing and Cancer Treatment

Section IV Biosensors Based on Thermal Properties

Editors

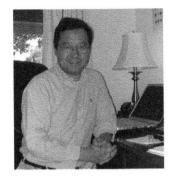

Jun Li earned a PhD in chemistry at Princeton University in 1995. He then served as a postdoctoral research associate at Cornell University from 1994 to 1997. He currently serves as a professor in the Department of Chemistry, Kansas State University, Manhattan, Kansas.

Dr. Li has been engaged in research on nanosciences and nanotechnology through his career with Molecular Imaging Co. (1997–1998), the Institute of Materials Research and Engineering (Singapore, 1998–2000), NASA Ames Research Center (2000–2007), and Kansas State University (2007–present). He has published 120 peer-reviewed papers/book chapters and is a coinventor of 15 patent applications. His research work in nanotechnology has been highlighted in over 40 public news reports. He received the first annual Nano50 Award from NASA Tech Briefs in the Innovator category in 2005. He has also been serving as an associate editor for *IEEE Transactions on Nanotechnology* since 2007.

Dr. Li's research interests include integrating nanomaterials, particularly carbon nanotubes and semiconductor nanowires, into functional devices including on-chip interconnects, thermal interface materials, solar cells, supercapacitors, lithium–ion batteries, nanoelectrode array–based ultrasensitive biosensors, electrical neural interface, and nanodielectrophoretic chips for capture and detection of bacterial or viral particles.

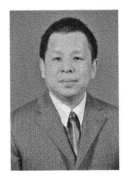

Nianqiang (Nick) Wu currently serves as an associate professor in the Department of Mechanical and Aerospace Engineering at West Virginia University, Morgantown, West Virginia. He earned a PhD in materials science and engineering at Zhejiang University, China, in 1997, and was a postdoctoral fellow at the University of Pittsburgh from 1999 to 2001. Afterward he directed the Keck Surface Science Center at Northwestern University, Evanston, Illinois. He then joined WVNano Initiative and the Department of Mechanical and Aerospace Engineering at West Virginia University in 2005. He currently serves as the secretary of the sensor division in the Electrochemical Society and on the advisory board of *Interface*, the home journal of the Electrochemical Society. He has organized several symposia on biosensors and solar fuels, holds four patents/disclosures, and has published 3 book chapters and more than 110 journal papers.

Dr. Wu's research interests include low-dimension nanomaterials, chemical sensors and biosensors, photocatalysts and photoelectrochemical cells, and electrochemical devices for energy conversion and storage. He strives to develop nanostructures for sensor applications, to study the charge transfer, energy transfer, and mass transport at the nanoscale in sensing materials and devices, and to develop lab-on-chip devices for point-of-care diagnosis.

Contributors

Zoraida P. Aguilar
Zystein, LLC
Fayetteville, Arkansas

Noppadol Aroonyadet
Department of Electrical
    Engineering—Electrophysics
University of Southern California
Los Angeles, California

Prabhu U. Arumugam
Department of Mechanical Engineering
Louisiana Tech University
Ruston, Louisiana

Vikas Berry
Department of Chemical Engineering
Kansas State University
Manhattan, Kansas

Stefan Bossmann
Department of Chemistry
Kansas State University
Manhattan, Kansas

John A. Carlisle
Advanced Diamond Technologies, Inc.
Romeoville, Illinois

Fanqing (Frank) Chen
Division of Life Sciences
Lawrence Berkeley National Laboratory
Berkeley, California

Viktor Chikan
Department of Chemistry
Kansas State University
Manhattan, Kansas

Ana Paula Craig
Department of Agricultural and Biological
    Engineering
Purdue University
West Lafayette, Indiana

and

Federal University of Minas Gerais
Belo Horizonte, Brazil

Liming Dai
Department of Macromolecular Science
    and Engineering
Case Western Reserve University
Cleveland, Ohio

Raj Kumar Dani
Department of Chemistry
Kansas State University
Manhattan, Kansas

Jeremy Dawson
Lane Department of Computer Science and
    Electrical Engineering
West Virginia University
Morgantown, West Virginia

Dan Du
School of Mechanical and Materials
    Engineering
Washington State University
Pullman, Washington

Feng Du
Department of Macromolecular Science
    and Engineering
Case Western Reserve University
Cleveland, Ohio

Chunhai Fan
Shanghai Institute of Applied Physics
Chinese Academy of Sciences
Shanghai, People's Republic of China

Chun Xian Guo
Institute for Clean Energy and Advanced
    Materials
Southwest University
Chongqing, People's Republic of China

Liang-Hong Guo
State Key Laboratory of Environmental
    Chemistry and Ecotoxicology
Research Centre for Eco-Environmental
    Science
Chinese Academy of Sciences
Beijing, People's Republic of China

Bashar Hamza
Lane Department of Computer Science and
    Electrical Engineering
West Virginia University
Morgantown, West Virginia

Shijiang He
Shanghai Institute of Applied Physics
Chinese Academy of Sciences
Shanghai, People's Republic of China

Yan Hong
Department of Mechanical, Materials, and
    Aerospace Engineering
University of Central Florida
Orlando, Florida

Lawrence Hornak
Lane Department of Computer Science and
    Electrical Engineering
West Virginia University
Morgantown, West Virginia

Rongfu Huang
State Key Laboratory of Environmental
    Chemistry and Ecotoxicology
Research Centre for Eco-Environmental
    Science
Chinese Academy of Sciences
Beijing, People's Republic of China

Joseph Irudayaraj
Department of Agricultural and Biological
    Engineering
Purdue University
West Lafayette, Indiana

Fumiaki Ishikawa
Department of Electrical
    Engineering—Electrophysics
University of Southern California
Los Angeles, California

Ulhas S. Kadam
Department of Agricultural and Biological
    Engineering
Purdue University
West Lafayette, Indiana

Anand Kadiyala
Lane Department of Computer Science and
    Electrical Engineering
West Virginia University
Morgantown, West Virginia

Seunghyun Lee
Department of Agricultural and Biological
    Engineering
Purdue University
West Lafayette, Indiana

Chang Ming Li
Chongqing Key Lab for Advanced
    Materials and Clean Energy of
    Technologies
Southwest University
Chongqing, People's Republic of China

Jun Li
Department of Chemistry
Kansas State University
Manhattan, Kansas

Ming Li
Department of Mechanical and Aerospace
    Engineering
West Virginia University
Morgantown, West Virginia

Xiang Li
Lane Department of Computer Science and
    Electrical Engineering
West Virginia University
Morgantown, West Virginia

Yuehe Lin
School of Mechanical and Materials
    Engineering
Washington State University
Pullman, Washington

and

Physical Sciences Division
Pacific Northwest National Laboratory
Richland, Washington

Gang Logan Liu
Micro and Nanotechnology Laboratory
Department of Electrical and Computer
    Engineering
University of Illinois at
    Urbana-Champaign
Urbana, Illinois

Yuxin Liu
Lane Department of Computer Science and
    Electrical Engineering
West Virginia University
Morgantown, West Virginia

Dongling Ma
Énergie Matériaux et Télécommunications
Institut National de la Recherche
    Scientifique
Varennes, Quebec, Canada

Liyuan Ma
Department of Mechanical, Materials, and
    Aerospace Engineering
University of Central Florida
Orlando, Florida

Timothy E. McKnight
Measurement Science and Systems
    Engineering Division
Oak Ridge National Laboratory
Oak Ridge, Tennessee

Anatoli Melechko
Department of Materials Science and
    Engineering
North Carolina State University
Raleigh, North Carolina

Shu Rui Ng
Institute for Clean Energy and Advanced
    Materials
Southwest University
Chongqing, People's Republic of China

Ryan Pearce
Department of Materials Science and
    Engineering
North Carolina State University
Raleigh, North Carolina

Hao Pei
Shanghai Institute of Applied Physics
Chinese Academy of Sciences
Shanghai, People's Republic of China

Shabnam Siddiqui
Advanced Diamond Technologies, Inc.
Romeoville, Illinois

Maurya Srungarapu
Lane Department of Computer Science and
    Electrical Engineering
West Virginia University
Morgantown, West Virginia

Ming Su
Department of Mechanical, Materials, and
    Aerospace Engineering
University of Central Florida
Orlando, Florida

Zhiwen Tang
Physical Sciences Division
Pacific Northwest National Laboratory
Richland, Washington

Chaoming Wang
Department of Mechanical, Materials, and
    Aerospace Engineering
University of Central Florida
Orlando, Florida

Xiaoli Wang
Department of Electrical
    Engineering—Electrophysics
University of Southern California
Los Angeles, California

Nianqiang (Nick) Wu
Department of Mechanical and Aerospace
   Engineering
West Virginia University
Morgantown, West Virginia

Hongjun Zeng
Advanced Diamond Technologies, Inc.
Romeoville, Illinois

Pingping Zhang
Life Sciences Division
Lawrence Berkeley National Laboratory
Berkeley, California

Haiguang Zhao
Énergie Matériaux et Télécommunications
Institut National de la Recherche
   Scientifique
Varennes, Quebec, Canada

Wenwei Zheng
Department of Electrical and Computer
   Engineering
University of California, San Diego
San Diego, California

Chongwu Zhou
Department of Electrical
   Engineering—Electrophysics
University of Southern California
Los Angeles, California

Lin Zhu
Kent Hale Smith Laboratories
Department of Macromolecular Science
   and Engineering
Case Western Reserve University
Cleveland, Ohio

1

Opportunities and Challenges of Biosensors Based on Nanomaterials and Nanodevices

Jun Li and Nianqiang (Nick) Wu

CONTENTS

1.1 Introduction

The last two decades have witnessed the explosion of nanoscience and nanotechnology. Particularly, the establishment of the National Nanotechnology Initiative (NNI) at the end of the last century has greatly stimulated research in this new field [1–5]. The research efforts have produced a plethora of methods for the synthesis, characterization, computer simulating, theoretical modeling, manufacturing, and applications of nanomaterials that have at least one dimension on the nanoscale (1–100 nm). Nanomaterials with the length scale lying between that of molecules and conventional continuum materials (over microns) are in a unique state of matter [6]. They present fundamentally different physical and chemical properties and usually exhibit size- and shape-dependent interactions with electrons, photons, electromagnetic fields, etc. [7,8].

Since the size of nanomaterials is comparable to that of biomolecules, there is a great potential to probe and manipulate biological systems from the molecular level up to macroscopic tissues using nanomaterials and nanodevices [9]. This provides ample opportunities to identify the molecular origins of diseases, to develop more selective therapies, to enable health monitoring and early disease diagnosis, and to establish the knowledge base for biocompatible prosthetics and regenerative medicine [9–12]. In spite of a lot of challenges, the integration of artificial nanomaterials with natural biological systems has achieved significant accomplishments, leading to the rapid development of various nanodevices used for biomedical studies from the molecular and subcellular level to tissue engineering. This book presents the recent progress in the applications of a broad spectrum of nanomaterials in biosensors and biomedical devices based on their unique optical, electrical, magnetic, and thermal properties.

1.2 Principles of Biosensors

Biosensors are the devices or materials that respond selectively to biological targets (or analytes) via a specific molecular recognition probe (typically based on biological materials), and convert the biological recognition event into a sensing signal via a proper transducer. They can be directly used to detect and quantify specific analytes. International Union of Pure and Applied Chemistry (IUPAC) defines a biosensor as "a device that uses specific biochemical reactions mediated by isolated enzymes, immunosystems, tissues, organelles or whole cells to detect chemical compounds usually by electrical, thermal or optical signals" [13]. The scope of the biosensors in this book is broader, as schematically illustrated in Figure 1.1. A biosensor generally consists of at least two components: (1) a molecular recognition probe that selectively interacts with biological materials, such as DNA, aptamer, antibody, ligand, enzyme, microorganism, cell, and tissue; and (2) a physicochemical transducer that converts the selective biological interaction into the physical signal based on the optical, electrical, magnetic, and thermal properties of the transducer materials. The selectivity of a biosensor mostly relies on the specificity of the molecular recognition probe derived from the biological materials. However, the sensitivity and the limit of detection of a biosensor strongly depend on the physicochemical properties of the transducer, which can be improved by the utilization of proper materials and/or the design of new device architectures. Thus, nanomaterials and nanodevices play significant roles in signal transduction.

As compared to conventional analytical instruments, biosensors are portable, miniaturized devices that are ideal for the rapid and high-throughput measurement of analytes and can even provide real-time information [14,15]. The development of biosensors has been accelerated by the increasing demands on simple, rapid, cost-effective, and portable screening methods for the qualitative and quantitative determination of analytes relevant to medical research, clinical diagnosis/treatment, environment and food safety monitoring,

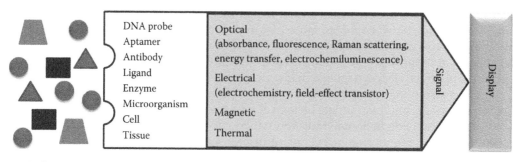

| Analyte | Molecular recognition probe | Signal transducer |

FIGURE 1.1
Schematic of the components of a biosensor.

agricultural inspections, industrial quality control, and biosecurity investigations. The development of a biosensor requires interdisciplinary collaboration involving chemistry, physics, materials science, engineering, as well as the life sciences.

1.3 Functionalization of Nanomaterials and Immobilization of Biomolecules

The molecular recognition probe in a biosensor is normally a biomolecule or other biological material that needs to be attached to the surface of a transducer. The bioactivity of the molecular recognition probe is strongly dependent on the immobilization method [16]. For example, the direct adsorption of an enzyme on a planar inorganic surface may cause the denaturation of the enzyme. In contrast, trapping the enzyme on the nanostructures can retain its bioactivity [16]. In addition, the sensitivity of a biosensor is affected by the immobilization method. Therefore, the immobilization of molecular recognition probes on the surface of a transducer is an important step in the construction of biosensors.

Effective strategies, including physical, covalent, and bioaffinity immobilization, have been developed, which are summarized in review articles [11,14,16] and detailed in relevant chapters. Direct adsorption of the molecular recognition probes on a large area of a flat solid surface of bulk materials not only limits the number of immobilized molecules but also does harm to the activity of biomolecules. Hence, physical immobilization is typically applied to special nanoparticles (NPs) or porous nanostructures. For example, single-stranded DNA can be simply immobilized on the surface of graphene oxide sheets via physical adsorption. Covalent linkage is a commonly used immobilization method, which enables the long-term stability of immobilized biomolecules. A flexible linker molecule is typically employed between the transducer and the molecular recognition probe in order to reduce the steric hindrance by the solid surface and to ensure that the molecular recognition probe remains the same biological activity as those in the bulk solution. The small size and large surface curvature of nanomaterials have been found to significantly reduce the steric effects compared to micro- or macro-transducers. The third immobilization method is to use biochemical affinity reactions. In particular, bioaffinity immobilization is widely used for the attachment of proteins on the transducer. The commonly used bioaffinity pairs include antibody–antigen interaction, receptor–antagonist/agonist, oligonucleotide duplex, affinity-capture ligand system, DNA-directed systems, etc. [14].

In addition, the surface of the transducers may be further passivated with some antiadsorption agents to reduce the nonspecific binding of biological analytes and biofouling by other components in the biological matrices. This needs particular attention for biosensors based on nanomaterials and nanodevices, due to their high specific surface area. Some nanomaterials (such as quantum dots (QDs) plasmonic NPs, and magnetic NPs) require a protective coating or capping agents to avoid their reaction with the solution or the leaking of toxic contents into the sample or body. Ideally, it is highly demanded in nanomedicine to combine multiple functions such as drug delivery/release, antibiofouling, specific recognition, high-contrast imaging, and therapeutic treatment into each single NP [11,17,18]. The functionalization strategies strongly depend on the surface chemical properties of the employed nanomaterials. The details are discussed under each individual chapter.

1.4 Application of Nanomaterials and Nanostructures in Biosensors

Nanomaterials generally refer to materials with at least one of their geometric dimensions falling between 1 and 100 nm. Nanomaterials and nanodevices are much more attractive as transducers than traditional micro- and macrocounterparts. First, as the particle size is reduced, the surface-to-volume dramatically increases. As a result, the interaction of the analytes with the NP-based transducer is much stronger, which causes a larger change in the physical properties of the transducers, generating a stronger signal response. Second, the nanoscale dimension of the transducer is comparable with that of biomolecules, which provides the capability of directly interacting with single molecules. Third, the new physical properties, such as the enhanced fluorescence yield of QDs and surface-enhanced Raman scattering (SERS) by plasmonic NPs, can greatly amplify the signal, leading to dramatically improved sensitivity. Fourth, the size reduction also benefits cost-saving, detection-speed improvement, sample-volume reduction, as well as increase in the degree of multiplexing degree increase, which are not achievable with conventional micro- and macrobiosensors.

Depending on the nature of the nanomaterials, different chemical and physical properties are utilized for biosensing, which will be discussed in later chapters. Here, we selectively present some representative nanomaterials according to the dimension.

Zero-dimensional (0D) nanomaterials: These are the materials whose sizes in all three dimensions are confined to the nanoscale. Important 0D nanomaterials include semiconductor nanocrystals (NCs) or QDs, metal NPs, magnetic NPs, polymer NPs, and phase-change NPs. 0D nanomaterials have a high specific surface area, in which a large number of atoms is exposed at the outer surface. In particular, they show a strong quantum confinement or other size-dependent properties. For example, the fluorescence emission of QDs can be tuned by tailoring the particle size. Multiplexed detection can be realized with a series of QDs of different sizes under the excitation of a single-wavelength light source. In addition, the surface plasmon resonance (SPR) of metallic NPs depends on the particle size and the surrounding medium, which provides great flexibility for developing colorimetric sensors. Furthermore, since their size is comparable to that of biomolecules, gold NPs can act as the electron-transfer relays in electrochemical sensors. Also, gold NPs can replace organic dye molecules to serve as the energy acceptors in fluorescent sensors based on energy transfer.

One-dimensional (1D) nanomaterials: These materials have two of their dimensions confined to the nanoscale, while the third dimension may extend to tens of microns or even longer. The elongated structure makes them appear as nanofibers, nanowires, or nanorods. The 1D nanomaterials covered in this book include carbon nanotubes (CNTs), vertically aligned carbon nanofibers (VACNFs), and semiconductor nanowires (SNWs). The longitudinal electron transport property of 1D nanomaterials is attractive for biosensors. 1D nanomaterials can effectively promote electron transfer in electrochemical sensors. In field-effect transistor (FET) sensors, the small diameter and large length make 1D nanomaterials highly sensitive to modulation to the electrical resistance by biological events that occur at the surface.

Two-dimensional (2D) nanomaterials: The ultrathin films, with two of the three dimensions orthogonal to the third one and extended from the nanoscale to micro- and macroscales, form 2D nanomaterials. Graphene and graphene oxide are representative 2D nanomaterials that have received extensive interests recently. They can be either deposited on solid substrates or freely suspended in solution. Graphene and graphene oxide have been explored in optical, electronic, and electrochemical biosensors. Since graphene has an extremely high surface area, an excellent electric conductivity, and a high mechanical strength, it is a promising support for enzymes and other molecular recognition probes in electrochemical sensors. Unlike graphene, graphene oxide is highly water-soluble and has an optical bandgap, which makes it a unique fluorophore for bioimaging and biosensing. Compared to QDs such as CdTe and PbS, graphene oxide does not contain any toxic element. Its fluorescence band can be tuned by the ratio of the sp^2/sp^3 carbon atoms. Graphene oxide can act not only as an energy donor (fluorophore) but also as an energy acceptor (quencher) in fluorescent sensors based on nonradiative energy transfer.

Three-dimensional (3D) nanostructures: 3D nanostructures can be made either by an assembly of NPs and nanofibers, or by creating a nanoscale feature in 3D space. Even though the dimensions of the assembly may be in the micro- or macroscale, the interior nanostructure endows interesting properties. One example is the 3D photonic crystals, which can be used to manipulate light for biosensing. Another example is the nanocrystalline diamond, whose intrinsic properties are significantly different from those of large diamond particles.

1.5 Biosensing Mechanisms and Organization of the Book

Biosensors are constructed based on the specific mechanism that transduces the biological binding/interaction events into physical signals. Figure 1.1 illustrates the optical, electrical, magnetic, and thermal mechanisms that are addressed in this book. According to the signal transduction mechanisms, the contents of this book are organized in four sections as follows.

1.5.1 Section I: Optical Biosensors

Optical methods based on the interactions of materials with light have received extensive attention due to the convenience, reliability, and high sensitivity. This book starts with the description of the synthesis and characterization of QDs and their optical properties (absorption and photoluminescence), as shown in Chapter 2 by Ma et al. The stability of QDs is particularly emphasized. Subsequently, the applications of QDs in *in vitro* and *in vivo* bioimaging are presented in Chapter 3 by Aguilar. Also, the functionalization and bioconjugation of QDs are described in detail in this chapter. Next, Li and Wu have introduced the fundamental theory and applications of fluorescence spectroscopy, with an emphasis on the new strategies for fluorescent biosensors based on energy transfer and electron transfer, as shown in Chapter 4. The optical biosensors based on fluorescence emission and quenching by graphene are illustrated by Lin et al. in Chapter 5. After a comprehensive description of fluorescent sensors, this book deals with other types of optical biosensors. The fundamental principles of SERS are described by Chen and Liu in Chapter 6. In particular, various plasmonic nanostructures are introduced for SERS biosensing. The research progress in *in vivo* biodetection using SERS is then reviewed in Chapter 7 by Irudayaraj et al. In addition, the theory and fabrication of photonic crystals (PhCs) provides another avenue for biosensing, as described in Chapter 8 by the Dawson and Hornak group. Lastly, Guo et al.

introduce electrochemiluminescence (ECL) biosensors in Chapter 9, where photoemission is generated by an electrochemical reaction triggered with proper electropotentials. In particular, this chapter highlights the enhancement of ECL by various nanomaterials. It also links optical methods with electrical methods in the next section.

1.5.2 Section II: Electrical Biosensors

The electrical methods are attractive since the signal can be directly recorded using modern electronics for multiplex portable systems. This book gives a thorough review of carbon materials, such as diamond, CNTs, graphene, and graphene oxide. Chapter 10 by Arumugam et al. summarizes the label-free electrochemical biosensors based on nanocrystalline diamond films. In Chapter 11, Du et al. describe electrochemical biosensors based on the unique electrical, thermal, and mechanical properties of CNTs. Chapter 12 by Pearce et al. reviews the unique structure of vertically aligned carbon nanofibers (CNFs) interfacing with living systems in applications such as cellular transfection, neural interfacing, and biosensing. Chapter 13 by Li et al. discusses graphene-based electrochemical biosensors. Furthermore, the intrinsic electronic properties of graphene also provide new concepts of bioelectronics for biomolecular and cellular detection, which is discussed in Chapter 14 by Vikas Berry. In Chapter 15, Ishikawa et al. highlight field-effect transistor biosensors using semiconductor nanowires. This method features miniaturization and high sensitivity by interfacing nanoelectronics with biomolecules.

1.5.3 Section III: Magnetic Nanoparticles for Biosensing and Cancer Treatment

The critical step following disease diagnoses is therapeutic treatments. In Chapter 16, Chikan and Bossmann illustrate the principles and application potentials of magnetic NPs for cancer detection and hyperthermia treatment with a controlled magnetic field. This adds the active intervention function to biosensing using the unique superparamagnetic properties of nanomaterials.

1.5.4 Section IV: Biosensors Based on Thermal Properties

In Chapter 17, Su et al. described a biosensing method based on a new type of sensing label, solid–liquid phase-change NPs. Multiplexed detection can be achieved by such NPs, with different melting points measured with differential scanning calorimetry.

1.6 Device Integration

While the main foci of this book are on the illustration of the principles and the demonstration of the feasibilities of biosensors based on nanomaterials and nanodevices, it is important to point out that the integration of these biosensors into a user-friendly system is critical to achieving portability, automation, and applicability to real-world samples. Microfluidics provides an effective means to integrate biosensors with the functional components for sample preparation, reagent delivery, and data acquisition. The achievements and potentials of microfluidic lab-on-chip (LOC) technologies are highlighted in Chapter 18 by Liu et al.

1.7 Remarks on Challenges and Future Opportunities

This book highlights the exciting progress in developing biosensors based on nanomaterials and nanodevices. These research achievements have demonstrated the great potentials of nanotechnology-based methods. In research labs, these methods have already been routinely employed to provide new insights in the biological sciences and the fundamental principles of medicine. Taking them further for clinical diagnostics and medical treatments is still at the infant stage. It requires the collective efforts from the physical and life sciences, clinical research, engineering development, and manufacturing industry. The authors of the book chapters include scientists from academia, national labs, and industry, which represent the perspective views of the different sectors toward future nanomedicine. We foresee that a rapid development in this field will result in high-impact healthcare technologies in the near future. One exciting example has been demonstrated in the development of next-generation DNA-sequencing technologies. Today, commercial systems are available that have reduced the price for mapping the full human genome by nearly four orders of magnitude and shortened the time from years to a few weeks [19,20]. Nanodevices including nanopores and nanogaps have been actively explored as one of the key sensing components that can differentiate nucleotides during DNA translocation as one of the next-generation gene-sequencing technologies [21]. More nanobiosensors are expected to follow this example and be used to tap into core biological and biomedical problems.

References

1. Roco MC, Williams RS, Alivisatos P. Nanotechnology research directions: IWGN workshop report–vision for nanotechnology R&D in the next decade. National Science and Technology Council, Committee on Technology, Interagency Working Group on Nanoscience, Engineering and Technology (IWGN), 1999.
2. National Nanotechnology Initiative. The initiative and its implementation plan. National Science and Technology Council, Committee on Technology, Subcommittee on Nanoscale Science, Engineering and Technology, 2000.
3. National Research Council. *Small Wonders, Endless Frontiers: A Review of the National Nanotechnology Initiative.* Washington, DC: The National Academies Press, 2002.
4. The National Nanotechnology Initiative: Strategic Plan. National Science and Technology Council, Committee on Technology, Subcommittee on Nanoscale Science, Engineering and Technology, 2004.
5. Roco MC. Science and technology integration for increased human potential and societal outcomes. In: *Coevolution of Human Potential and Converging Technologies.* New York: The New York Academy of Sciences, 2004. pp. 1–16.
6. Whitesides G, Alivisatos P. Chapter 1. Fundamental scientific issues for nanotechnology. In: Roco MC, Williams RS, Alivisatos P, eds. Nanotechnology research directions: IWGN workshop report–vision for nanotechnology R&D in the next decade: National Science and Technology Council, Committee on Technology, Interagency Working Group on Nanoscience, Engineering and Technology (IWGN), 1999.
7. Klabunde KJ, ed. *Nanoscale Materials in Chemistry.* New York: John Wiley & Sons, 2001.
8. Klabunde KJ, Richards RM, eds. *Nanoscale Materials in Chemistry.* Hoboken, NJ: John Wiley & Sons, 2009.
9. Whitesides GM. Nanoscience, nanotechnology, and chemistry. *Small* 2005; 1 (2):172–179.

10. Vogel V, Baird B. Nanobiotechnology: Report of the national nanotechnology initiative workshop. In: *National Science and Technology Council CoT*, Subcommittee on Nanoscale Science, Engineering and Technology, ed., 2003.
11. Ferrari M. Cancer nanotechnology: Opportunities and challenges. *Nature Reviews Cancer* 2005; 5:161–171.
12. Khang D, Carpenter J, Chun YW, Pareta R, Webster TJ. Nanotechnology for regenerative medicine. *Biomedical Microdevices* 2008; 12 (4):575–587.
13. http://goldbook.iupac.org
14. Thévenot DR, Toth K, Durst RA, Wilson GS. Electrochemical biosensors: Recommended definitions and classification. *Biosensors and Bioelectronics* 2001; 16 (1–2):121–131.
15. Patel PD. (Bio)sensors for measurement of analytes implicated in food safety: A review. *TrAC Trends in Analytical Chemistry* 2002; 21 (2):96–115.
16. Moyano DF, Rotello VM. Nano meets biology: Structure and function at the nanoparticle Interface. *Langmuir* 2011; 27 (17):10376–10385.
17. Farrell D, Alper J, Ptak K, Panaro NJ, Grodzinski P, Barker AD. Recent advances from the national cancer institute alliance for nanotechnology in cancer. *ACS Nano* 2010; 4 (2):589–594.
18. Gao J, Gu H, Xu B. Multifunctional magnetic nanoparticles: Design, synthesis, and biomedical applications. *Accounts of Chemical Research* 2009; 42 (8):1097–1107.
19. Mardis ER. Next-generation DNA sequencing methods. In: *Annual Review of Genomics and Human Genetics*, Palo Alto, CA. 2008; 9:387–402.
20. Shendure J, Ji HL. Next-generation DNA sequencing. *Nature Biotechnology* 2008; 26 (10):1135–1145.
21. Branton D, Deamer DW, Marziali A, Bayley H, Benner SA, Butler T, Di Ventra M et al. The potential and challenges of nanopore sequencing. *Nature Biotechnology* 2008; 26 (10):1146–1153.

Section I

Optical Biosensors

2

Synthesis and Characterization of Quantum Dots

Haiguang Zhao and Dongling Ma

CONTENTS

2.1 Introduction

Semiconductor quantum dots (QDs) are fluorescent nanocrystals (NCs) normally smaller than 20 nm in diameter [1]. Typically, they are composed of an inorganic core, made up of a few hundred to a few thousand atoms, surrounded by an organic outer layer of surfactant molecules (ligands). Bulk semiconductors are characterized by a composition-dependent bandgap (Figure 2.1a), which is the minimum energy required to excite an electron from the valence band into the conduction band. With the absorption of a photon of energy greater than the bandgap energy, the excitation of an electron leaves an orbital hole in the valence band to form an electron–hole pair (i.e., exciton). The relaxation of the excited electron back to the valence band may be accompanied by the emission of a photon, a process

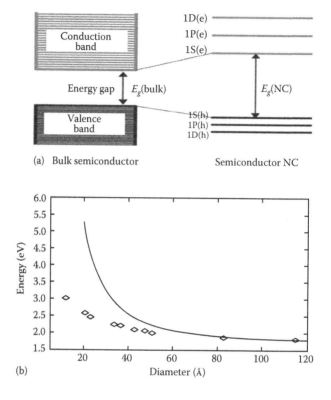

FIGURE 2.1

(a) A bulk semiconductor (left) has continuous conduction and valence energy bands separated by a fixed energy gap, E_g, while a semiconductor NC (right) is characterized by discrete atomic-like states and an NC-size dependent energy gap. (Adapted with permission from McGuire, J.A., Joo, J., Pietryga, J.M., Schaller, R.D., and Klimov, V.I., *Acc. Chem. Res.*, 41, 1810–1819. Copyright 2008 American Chemical Society.) (b) Transition energy between highest occupied molecular orbital and lowest unoccupied molecular orbital of CdSe crystallites as a function of size (diamonds) compared with the prediction of the effective mass approximation (solid line). (Adapted with permission from Murray, C.B., Norris, D.J., and Bawendi, M.G., *J. Am. Chem. Soc.*, 115, 8706–8715. Copyright 1993 American Chemical Society.)

known as radiative recombination. The exciton has a finite size defined by the exciton Bohr radius. When the size of a semiconductor NC is smaller than the Bohr radius, charge carriers become spatially confined and energy levels are quantized, with values directly related to the QD size (Figure 2.1a and b) [1–4]. In the case of quantum confinement, QDs show a size-dependent bandgap, as described in Equation 2.1 [2]:

$$E = E_g + \left(\frac{\hbar^2 \pi^2}{2R^2} \right) \left(\frac{1}{m_e} + \frac{1}{m_h} \right) - \frac{1.8e^2}{\varepsilon R} \tag{2.1}$$

where

E_g is the bandgap energy of the corresponding bulk material
$\hbar$ is the Planck constant
m_e and m_h are the effective masses of the electron and hole, respectively
e is the charge of an electron
R and ε are the radius and the dielectric constant of QDs, respectively

It leads to a unique size-dependent absorption and emission behavior of semiconductor NCs [5–13]. For example, as shown in Figure 2.2a, the emission wavelength of CdSe QDs (bulk E_g, 1.76 eV) can be tuned throughout the visible range by adjusting the QD size [11]. Together with composition control, the emission of QDs can span essentially from the entire visible region to the near infrared (NIR) spectral range up to a few thousand nanometers (Figure 2.2b).

It is worthwhile to make a comparison between QDs and conventional fluorophores. In marked contrast to most conventional fluorophores, QDs have significantly broader absorption and much narrower emission spectra (Figure 2.3a) [14]. Another advantage of QDs is that they have a higher quantum yield (QY, the ratio of photons absorbed to photons emitted) than most organic dyes, which enables a more sensitive detection of analytes in low-concentration solutions [5]. QDs also show much higher photostability, which is advantageous for the long-term, real-time monitoring and tracking of biospecies and bioactivities (Figure 2.3b) [5,15]. Last but not the least, the long fluorescence lifetime of QDs, typically on the order of several tens of nanoseconds (even as long as several microseconds for NIR QDs [16]), allows one to distinguish the emission of QDs from background autofluorescence in cells (Figure 2.3c), which leads to a high signal-to-noise ratio, important for the use of QDs as efficient biolabels [17–23]. To summarize, QDs have great potential to become a new generation of fluorophores for highly demanding applications.

In vivo optical bioimaging prefers the use of fluorophores, whose excitation and emission lights are least absorbed and scattered by biological fluids and tissues (water, hemoglobin, and lipids) [24,25]. Based on this consideration, NIR ranges of 700–900 and 1200–1600 nm have been theoretically predicted and partially experimentally confirmed as the two best spectral windows for bioimaging [24,25]. Although organic NIR dyes are being employed for *in vivo* optical imaging [26,27], their emission wavelengths are limited to below 950 nm [28,29]. Not to mention most of them have the susceptibility to photobleaching [28,29]. It is thus highly desirable to develop more flexible and robust NIR-labeling agents. Over the last 10 years, research interest in NIR-emitting QDs has grown rapidly all over the world. They demonstrate broader absorption, greater tunability in the emission wavelength, higher QY, and better photostability compared to organic dyes. Owing to these beneficial properties, they hold great potential for live-cell imaging, for tracking the movement of molecules within a single cell and for deep-tissue imaging [24,29,30].

2.2 Classification of QDs

The most common QDs are binary semiconductor compounds. Depending on chemical components, they can be classified as II–VI, III–V, and IV–VI semiconductors. Examples of II–VI QDs are cadmium sulfide (CdS), cadmium selenide (CdSe), cadmium telluride (CdTe), zinc selenide (ZnSe), and mercury sulfide (HgS) QDs [31–33]. Indium phosphide (InP) and indium arsenide (InAs) are typical III–V QDs [9,10]. IV–VI QDs comprise IV and VI elements with lead sulfide (PbS), lead selenide (PbSe), and lead telluride (PbTe) being examples [8,34,35]. QDs composed of a single element (such as silicon [Si]) or ternary elements with two of them in either the cation or anion site (such as CdS_xSe_{1-x}, $Zn_xCd_{1-x}S$, and PbS_xSe_{1-x}) have also been reported [36–40].

QDs can also be classified as ultraviolet (UV)-emitting QDs, visible-emitting QDs, and NIR-emitting QDs, depending on their emission wavelengths. Typical examples of

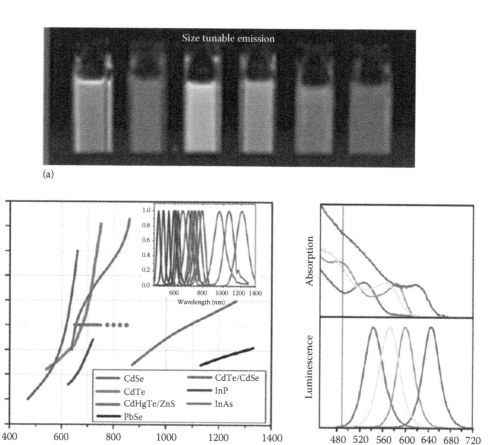

FIGURE 2.2
(See color insert.) (a) Size tunable photoluminescence (PL) image for CdSe QDs under UV lamp irradiation. (Adapted with permission from Zlateva, G., Zhelev, Z., Bakalova, R., and Kanno, I., *Inorg. Chem.*, 46, 6212–6214. Copyright 2007 American Chemical Society.) (b) Emission maxima and sizes of QDs of different composition. (From Bruchez, M., Moronne, M., Gin, P., Weiss, S., and Alivisatos, A.P., *Science*, 281, 2013–2016, 1998. Reprinted with permission of AAAS; Adapted with permission from Yu, W.W., Falkner, J.C., Shih, B.S., and Colvin, V.L., *Chem. Mater.*, 16, 3318–3322. Copyright 2004 American Chemical Society; Reprinted with permission from Guzelian, A., Banin, U., Kadavanich, A.V., Peng, X., and Alivisatos, A.P., *Appl. Phys. Lett.*, 69, 1432–1434. Copyright 1996, American Institute of Physics; Adapted with permission from Guzelian, A., Katari, J.E.B., Kadavanich, A.V., Banin, U., Hamad, K., Juban, E., and Alivisatos, A.P., *J. Phys. Chem.*, 100, 7212–7219. Copyright 1996 American Chemical Society; Adapted with permission from Yu, W.W., Wang, Y.A., and Peng, X., *Chem. Mater.*, 15, 4300–4308. Copyright 2003 American Chemical Society; Adapted with permission from Tsay, J.M., Pflughoefft, M., Bentolila, L.A., and Weiss, S., *J. Am. Chem. Soc.*, 126, 1926–1927. Copyright 2004 American Chemical Society.) Inset: representative emission spectra for some materials. (c) Absorption (upper curves) and emission (lower curves) spectra of four CdSe/ZnS QDs samples. The blue vertical line indicates the 488-nm line of an argon-ion laser, which can be used to efficiently excite all QDs simultaneously. (From Michalet, X., Pinaud, F.F., Bentolila, L.A., Tsay, J.M., Doose, S., Li, J.J., Sundaresan, G., Wu, A.M., Gambhir, S.S., and Weiss, S., *Science*, 307, 538–544, 2005. Reprinted with permission of AAAS; Adapted with permission from Gerion, D., Pinaud, F., Williams, S.C., Parak, W.J., Zanchet, D., Weiss, S., and Alivisatos, A.P., *J. Phys. Chem. B*, 105, 8861–8871. Copyright 2001 American Chemical Society.)

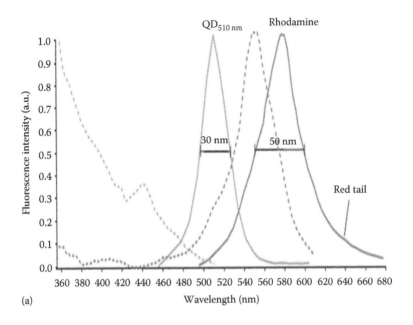

(a)

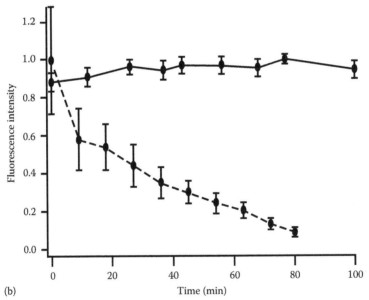

(b)

FIGURE 2.3

(a) The excitation spectrum (broken lines) of a QD (light gray) is very broad, whereas that of an organic dye (rhodamine, gray) is narrow. The emission spectrum (unbroken lines) is narrower for a QD (light gray) than for organic dyes (rhodamine, gray). Values indicate the full spectral width at half-maximum intensity (FWHM value). (Reprinted from *Trends Cell Biol.*, 14, Jaiswal, J.K. and Simon, S.M., Potentials and pitfalls of fluorescent quantum dots for biological imaging, 497–504, Copyright 2004, with permission from Elsevier.) (b) Graph representing the variation of fluorescence intensity of one cell of the rhodamine green dextran–injected embryo (dotted line) and of one cell of the QD-injected embryo (solid line). (From Dubertret, B., Skourides, P., Norris, D.J., Noireaux, V., Brivanlou, A.H., and Libchaber, A., *Science*, 298, 1759–1762, 2002. Reprinted with permission of AAAS.) Time-resolved confocal image of a fixed 3T3 cell.

(continued)

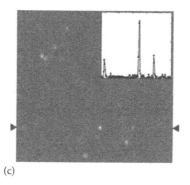

(c)

FIGURE 2.3 (continued)
(c) Gated image constructed from only photons that arrived 35–65 ns after the laser pulse. The image was taken with a laser intensity of 0.1 kW cm² and 25 ms integration time per pixel. The scale bar is 5 mm. The inset shows the cross section along the same horizontal line (indicated by the black arrows) for (c). (Adapted from Dahan, M., Laurence, T., Pinaud, F., Chemla, D.S., Alivisatos, A.P., Sauer, M., and Weiss, S., Time-gated biological imaging by use of colloidal quantum dots, *Opt. Lett.*, 26, 825–827, 2001. With permission of Optical Society of America; From Dubertret, B., Skourides, P., Norris, D.J., Noireaux, V., Brivanlou, A.H., and Libchaber, A., *Science*, 298, 1759–1762, 2002. Reprinted with permission of AAAS.)

NIR-emitting QDs are lead chalcogenide QDs, which include PbS, PbSe, and PbTe, with emission wavelength tuned over a broad NIR wavelength range [8,34,35].

An extremely promising type of QDs, derived from the aforementioned simple structures, are core-shell QDs, which consist of core QDs covered by the shell of a different semiconductor material. Depending on the relative alignment of conduction- and valence-band edges of core and shell semiconductors, the core-shell heterostructure can be denominated as type-I, reverse type-I, and type-II (Figure 2.4a) [41–45]. In the type-I structure, the bandgap of the core is smaller than that of the shell and both band edges of the core are located in the bandgap of the shell. Because of that, electrons and holes are confined in the core (Figure 2.4b). Reverse type-I is exactly the opposite of type-I. In the type-II structure, either the conduction-band edge or the valence-band edge of the shell is located in the bandgap of the core (Figure 2.4a). The band alignment causes the spatial separation of the electrons and holes into different regions (core or shell, Figure 2.4b) [43]. A special case is called *quasi*-type-II. In this case, one type of carrier is delocalized over the entire core-shell structure, while the other type is confined in the core (Figure 2.4b) [43]. It is because in certain type-I core-shell QDs, one type of carriers is not strictly confined. The most extensively studied core-shell systems are type-I QDs, including CdSe/ZnS and PbS/CdS [7,16]. In type-II systems, CdS/ZnSe and CdTe/CdSe QDs have been studied [42,44]. A special example of *quasi*-type-II core-shell QDs is PbSe/CdSe, which indeed shows the type-I band alignment [43].

2.3 Synthesis of QDs

The synthesis routes for QDs have been well developed, beginning in the 1980s and extending to today. Synthesis methods of colloidal QDs can be divided into two categories: wet-chemical synthesis and gas- (or vapor-) phase deposition. Synthesis has

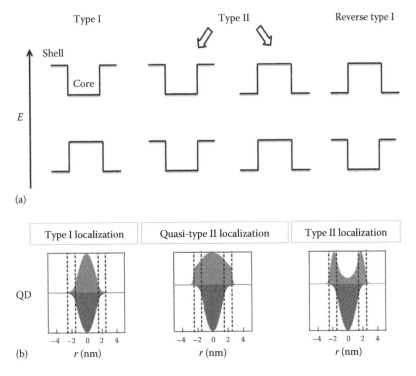

FIGURE 2.4
(a) Schematic representation of the energy-level alignment in different core-shell systems. The lower and upper edges of the rectangles correspond to the positions of the valence band and conduction band edge of the core (center) and shell materials, respectively. (b) Electron and hole wave function of core-shell QDs. In type-I, electron and hole are confined in the same region (either core or shell); in type-II, they are spatially separated. In a *quasi*-type-II, one carrier is fully delocalized over the entire volume and one is localized in one region. (Adapted with permission from De Geyter, B., Justo, Y., Moreels, I., Lambert, K., Smet, P.F., Van Thourhout, D., Houtepen, A.J., Grodzinska, D., de Mello Donega, C., Meijerink, A., Vanmaekelbergh, D., and Hens, Z., *ACS Nano*, 5, 58–66. Copyright 2010 American Chemical Society.)

focused on producing QDs with better size and shape control and higher optical quality. Other factors, such as yield and green chemistry, have also been taken into consideration.

2.3.1 Wet-Chemical Synthesis

The synthesis of QDs has been conducted in both organic and aqueous phases. The most typical way to synthesize high-quality colloidal QDs is based on the thermal decomposition of organometallic precursors in an organic solvent. As reported by La Mer and Dinegar [46], the production of monodisperse colloidal NCs requires a temporally discrete nucleation stage followed by slower controlled growth on the existing nuclei (Figure 2.5a). The NCs can become very uniform if the percentage of NC growth during the nucleation period is small, compared with subsequent growth [47]. Following this principle, monodispersed QDs, including II–VI, III–V, and IV–VI semiconductors, have been synthesized by varying the reaction parameters such as reaction temperature, molar ratios of precursors, concentration, reaction time, etc. The typical reaction setup is shown in Figure 2.5b. Meanwhile, QDs have been synthesized using many other approaches, such

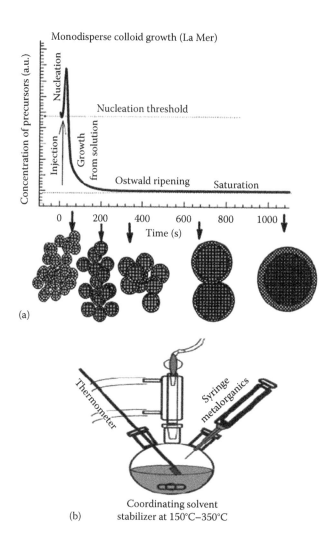

(a)

(b)

FIGURE 2.5

(a) Cartoon depicting the stages of nucleation and growth for the preparation of monodisperse NCs in the framework of the La Mer model. As NCs grow with time, a size series of NCs may be isolated by periodically removing aliquots from the reaction vessel. (b) Representation of the simple synthetic apparatus employed in the preparation of monodisperse NC samples. (Adapted with permission from Murray, C.B. and Kagan, C.R., *Annu. Rev. Mater. Sci.*, 30, 545–610. Copyright 2000 Annual Review.)

as electrochemical [48] and microwave irradiation techniques [49–52]. Nonetheless, those with high QY are almost exclusively synthesized by a high-temperature organometallic route using the popular hot-injection method [34]. As an example of early II–VI QD synthesis [31], CdO, trioctylphosphine oxide (TOPO), hexylphosphonic acid (HPA), and tetradecylphosphonic acid (TDPA) were loaded in a three-neck flask. At about 300°C, a reddish CdO powder was dissolved and generated a colorless homogeneous solution. After the formation of the complex, an injection of selenium dissolved in tributylphosphine (TBP) at 250°C–300°C generated high-quality CdSe NCs. The tunable particle sizes of CdSe QDs in the range of 2–8 nm can be obtained by changing the growth temperature and reaction time. Another example is the organometallic synthesis of NIR-emitting PbS QDs [34]. Typical details of synthesis are described as follows. First, a certain amount of PbO dissolved in oleic acid (OA) was purged with nitrogen gas flow and heated in a reaction flask to 150°C. Stock solutions of bis(trimethylsilyl) sulfide ((TMS)$_2$S) and octadecene (ODE) were then added to the flask and mixed under vigorous stirring, where PbS NCs nucleated quickly. The temperature was maintained at 100°C for the growth of NCs. Different sizes of QDs can be simply obtained by varying the reaction time. This synthetic approach is able to produce PbS NCs with peak emission ranging from about 800 to 2000 nm, as well as narrow emission peak. The hot-injection method has also been applied to the preparation of other QDs, such as CdS and PbSe [8,31].

In general, it is highly desirable to have reproducible methods to obtain highly monodisperse QDs with excellent optical properties through high-yield and large-scale synthesis. Recently, microwave-assisted synthesis has been used to synthesize colloidal UV–visible–emitting QDs (such as CdSe and InP) having a narrow size distribution and excellent optical properties with very short reaction time [49,50]. As an example, the synthesis of CdSe [49] is carried out by using trioctyl phosphine selenide (TOPSe) as the Se^{2-} source and cadmium stearate as the Cd^{2+} source in decane under ambient conditions. The size of CdSe QDs can be tuned by changing the reaction temperature and time.

On the other hand, for biological applications, QDs are required to have good water solubility and colloidal stability. Nowadays, several methods have been employed to synthesize water-soluble QDs. One approach is the direct synthesis of QDs in water [54–56]. For example, in an aqueous synthesis route of PbS QDs [54], a soluble Pb^{2+} salt, usually perchlorate or nitrate, is prepared first. Then, the S^{2-} source (H$_2$S or Na$_2$S) is added in the presence of thiols, which act as ligands to provide both size and shape control as well as aid in the dispersion of QDs. In general, this approach leads to QDs with broad size distribution, low QY, and broad emission. Moreover, the as-synthesized water-soluble QDs show very poor stability due to the sensitivity of the QD surface to oxygen. Ligand exchange, based on the concept of transferring high-quality QDs originally prepared in an organic phase into water via changing surface capping agents from hydrophobic to hydrophilic ones, appears to be a better approach [57,58]. Over the past decade, this approach has been widely used as an efficient way to move QDs from an organic phase into water. For example, PbS QDs were transferred from an organic solvent into an aqueous solution by replacing the oleate-capping ligands with (1-mercaptoundec-11-yl) tetra (ethylene glycol) [58]. The aqueous dispersion is stable over days at physiological pH. The maximum QY of PbS QDs that can be achieved by this method is 26% in a buffer solution [58].

The drawback of the ligand exchange method is that the stripping of the original surface ligands from QD surfaces leads to a decrease of the QY after water transfer [57,58]. To avoid ligand stripping and thereby keep the high QY of organometallically prepared QDs, the method of amphiphilic polymer encapsulation has recently been investigated [59–62]. This approach will not disturb the original capping ligands on the QD surface. Instead, multiple hydrophobic chains of the amphiphilic polymer can have numerous interactions with the native hydrophobic ligands on the QD surface, thus helping "fix" the ligands on the surface. On the other hand, the hydrophilic end groups of the amphiphilic polymer endow the QDs with good water-solubility and even biocompatibility, depending on the nature of the end groups. This approach has indeed been successfully applied to UV–visible–emitting QDs, such as CdSe/ZnS and CdSe/CdS, and NIR-emitting QDs, such as PbS and PbS/CdS [59–63]. As an example, water-soluble NIR-emitting PbS QDs were achieved by performing the following procedures: PbS QDs capped with oleylamine were first synthesized by the hot-injection approach in an organic phase [64]. Then, the PbS QDs were mixed with the amphiphilic polymer poly(maleic anhydride-alt-1-octadecene)-co-poly(ethylene glycol) (PMAO–PEG) in chloroform and stirred. After that, air-free water was added to the chloroform solution [61,62]. Chloroform was then gradually removed by evaporation. In this case, the PEG group of the amphiphilic polymer is also expected to improve the biocompatibility and ease of bioconjugation of the QDs.

2.3.2 Gas- or Vapor-Phase Deposition

Semiconductor QDs can also be formed via deposition from the vapor phase onto appropriate substrates in molecular beam epitaxy (MBE), metal organic chemical vapor deposition (MOCVD), or pulsed laser deposition (PLD) reactors [65–67]. PLD is a cold-wall processing technique, which excites only a small area on the target by the focused laser beam. It can produce QDs with high chemical purity and controlled stoichiometry.

In PLD, the size distribution of QDs can be controlled by varying the parameters such as target-to-substrate distance, laser fluence, and background gas pressure. For example, PLD has been used to produce PbS QDs with peak emission tunable in the wide NIR region (Figure 2.6) [67]. The average size of these PbS QDs can be fairly controlled from 2.5 to 8.5 nm by adjusting the number of laser ablation pulses.

2.3.3 Synthesis of Core-Shell QDs

The properties of QDs capped by organic ligands are sensitive to the variation of their surface status due to their high surface-to-volume ratio [7]. Surface defects serve as "trap states" for electrons or holes, preventing their radiative recombination that leads to the considerable decrease of fluorescence QY. Recent studies have revealed that a core-shell

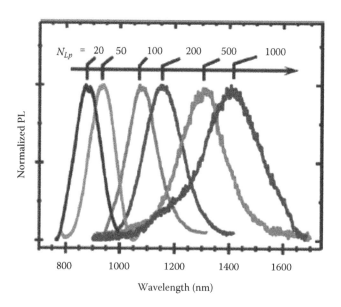

FIGURE 2.6
PL spectra of PbS QDs PLD-deposited at laser ablation pulses ranging from 20 to 1000. (With kind permission from Springer Science + Business Media: *J. Nanopart. Res.*, Tailoring the photoluminescence of PbS-nanoparticles layers deposited by means of the pulsed laser ablation technique, 13, 2011, 2269–2274, Ka, I., Ma, D., and El Khakani, M.A.)

structure can stabilize and maximize the fluorescence of core QDs [68–71]. A robust, larger-bandgap inorganic shell (in the type-I structure) not only passivates surface atoms but also buries the core semiconductor in a potential energy well, thus concentrating the charge carriers in the NC core and keeping them away from their surrounding environment [69–71]. As a result, surface defect states, trap sites, and environmental factors will have diminished impact on the optical property of QDs [69–74].

The core-shell QDs have most commonly been achieved in a two-step procedure [45]: initial synthesis of core NCs, followed by a purification step, and subsequent shell growth. Via this approach, many core-shell QDs, such as CdSe/ZnS, CdSe/CdS, CdS/HgS, CdSe/ ZnTe, and InP/ZnS, have been synthesized [61,73,75–77]. A representative example for visible-emitting QDs is the use of diethylzinc (Zn precursor) and hexamethyldisilathiane (S precursor) for the synthesis of ZnS-overcoated CdSe QDs [73]. The reaction flask containing CdSe QDs dispersed in TOPO/TOP was heated under N_2 atmosphere. The temperature at which the precursors were added ranged from 140°C to 220°C, depending on the size of the CdSe cores. When the desired temperature was reached, the Zn and S precursors were added dropwise to the vigorously stirred reaction mixture over a period of 5–10 min. After the addition was complete, the mixture was cooled to 90°C and left stirring for several hours. In order to prevent the homogeneous nucleation of the shell material and the uncontrolled ripening of the core NCs, the temperature for the shell growth is generally lower than that used for the core NC synthesis ($T_2 < T_1$). Typically, only a small number of monolayers (1–5) of the shell material are deposited on the cores. ZnS is one of the most important shell materials used for overcoating various II–VI and III–V semiconductor QDs. The optical property of as-synthesized core-shell QDs has been enhanced compared to that of pure QDs. For example, the QY of InP QDs increases from 10%–22% to 60% with the deposition of a thin ZnS shell [78]. In the earlier synthesis, the core size remains essentially constant during the overcoating process. A similar approach has also been explored for synthesizing NIR-emitting core-shell QDs, such as PbSe-PbS [74].

Another approach for producing the core-shell-structured QDs is the successive ionic layer adsorption and reaction (SILAR) method, which is based on the formation of one monolayer shell by alternating the injections of cationic and anionic precursors [79]. As an example, for the synthesis of CdSe/CdS core-shell QDs, the CdSe NCs in hexane were mixed with ODE and octadecylamine (ODA) in a three-neck flask [79]. After the removal of hexane and air under vacuum, the mixture was heated to 240°C in argon for the shell growth. The Cd precursor solution was injected first, followed by the same mole of the S precursor. The SILAR technique has also been used for the growth of other core-shell colloidal QDs, such as CdTe/CdSe [80]. In general, compared to the two-step approach for synthesizing core-shell QDs, the shell thickness can be better controlled via the SILAR technique.

Recently, a relatively less used approach, cation exchange, has been reported for the growth of a wider bandgap material onto lead chalcogenide QDs [68]. In contrast to the aforementioned common approaches, only the precursor of the cationic constituent of a shell material was introduced during the shell formation process and the shell growth proceeds through the gradual replacement of core cations by newly introduced cations in solution and the anion sublattice remains basically undisturbed [68]. As a result, the shell grows at the expense of core NCs, that is, the shell growth is accompanied by the decrease of the lead chalcogenide core size. For example, PbS/CdS QDs have been synthesized via a cation exchange method [16,68]. In general, the PbS QDs were firstly synthesized [81]. After purification, the PbS QDs were dispersed in toluene. In a separate flask, a CdO/OA

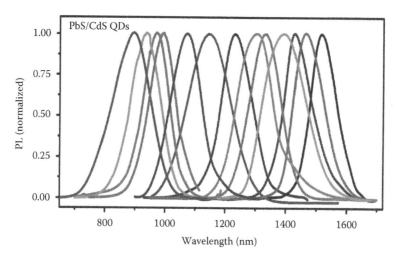

FIGURE 2.7
PL spectra of PbS/CdS QDs synthesized via cation exchange approach. (From Zhao, H., Chaker, M., Wu, N., and Ma, D., *J. Mater. Chem.*, 21, 8898–8904, Copyright 2011. Adapted with permission of The Royal Society of Chemistry.)

mixture was heated to 255°C under N_2 in ODE. The clear solution was cooled to 155°C under vacuum. PbS QDs dispersed in toluene were heated to 100°C immediately. The Cd/OA mixture was then injected into the PbS dispersion. The core size of the PbS/CdS QDs can be tuned by varying the reaction temperature and time. As shown in Figure 2.7, the as-synthesized PbS/CdS core-shell QDs show the PL emission covering the whole NIR region with quite a narrow PL peak width [16].

Similar to the synthesis of "un-coated" QDs, recently, microwave irradiation has also been used to synthesize core-shell-structured QDs [52]. For example, water-soluble CdSe/ZnS core-shell QDs have been synthesized via microwave-assisted synthesis with emission maxima ranging from 511 to 596 nm. The as-synthesized QDs possess a high degree of crystallinity, high QY, and a narrow PL peak width, and have demonstrated stability in an aqueous buffer [52].

2.4 Characterization of QDs

Characterization methods for the structure (such as size distribution and core-shell morphology), optical properties (such as absorption, PL, and QY), and stability (such as colloidal stability and photostability) of QDs will be presented as follows.

2.4.1 Structure Characterization

2.4.1.1 Morphology

Structure characterization is essential for QDs. It helps to disclose structural details, gain the understanding of interesting properties, and guide the further exploration of QDs. Many tools, such as scanning tunneling microscopy (STM), scanning electron microscopy (SEM), transmission electron microscopy (TEM), and atomic force microscopy (AFM), have been used to characterize the structure of QDs. TEM is a very popular and powerful tool to image QDs, with high-resolution TEM being able to reveal structure details down to ~0.1 nm. The shape of QDs can be directly observed by TEM and the average size and size distribution of QDs can be obtained from TEM-image analysis. As shown in Figure 2.8a, TEM measurements indicate that the PbS QDs have average size of around 6 nm in diameter with a very narrow distribution [64]. The high-resolution TEM image suggests that the NCs are highly crystallized (Figure 2.8a). The lattice fringes match well with the {200} planes of pure PbS [64].

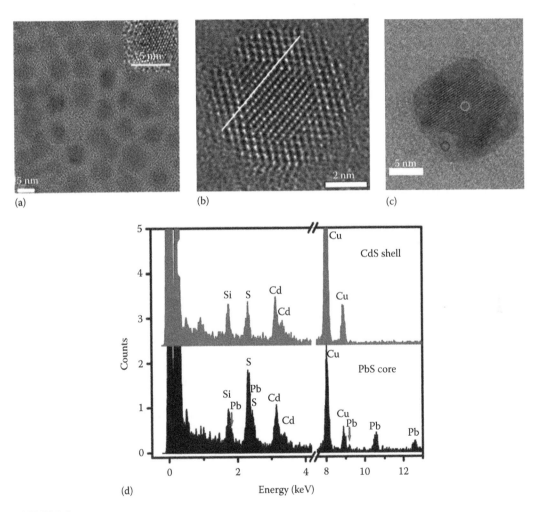

FIGURE 2.8
(a) High magnification TEM image of PbS QDs. Inset of (a) is the high resolution TEM image of a single PbS QD. (Adapted with permission from Zhao, H., Chaker, M., and Ma, D., *J. Phys. Chem. C*, 113, 6497–6504. Copyright 2009 American Chemical Society.) (b) High-resolution TEM image of a PbTe/CdTe core-shell QD in the ⟨110⟩ direction. (Adapted with permission from Lambert, K., De Geyter, B., Moreels, I., and Hens, Z., *Chem. Mater.*, 21, 778–780. Copyright 2009 American Chemical Society.) (c) TEM image of a PbS/CdS QD. (From Zhao, H., Chaker, M., Wu, N., and Ma, D., *J. Mater. Chem.*, 21, 8898–8904, 2011. Adapted with permission of The Royal Society of Chemistry.) (d) EDX spectra from the core (gray circle) and shell (black circle) of the PbS/CdS QD.

2.4.1.2 Chemical Composition

The chemical composition of QDs can be determined by, for example, energy dispersive x-ray spectrometry (EDX), x-ray photoelectron spectroscopy (XPS), and x-ray fluorescence spectroscopy. Inductively coupled plasma optical emission spectrometry (ICP-OES) can also be used to characterize the chemical composition of QDs. For instance, Cademartiri et al. have used XPS and ICP-OES to identify that the atomic ratio Pb/S is between 1.3 and 1.5 for PbS QDs produced by the diffusion-controlled organometallic approach [83]. In addition, they found that the charge balance of QDs is provided by Cl⁻ ions adsorbed on the surface of Pb-rich QDs, as confirmed by XPS and EDX [83].

2.4.1.3 Crystalline Structures

The crystalline structures of QDs can be determined by x-ray powder diffraction (XRD) [16,81,83]. By measuring and analyzing their diffraction pattern, the crystallite phase of QDs can be identified. Furthermore, the average size and the size distribution of crystallites can be estimated via the Debye–Scherrer equation [84,85]:

$$D = \frac{0.9\lambda}{\beta \cos \theta} \tag{2.2}$$

where
  D is the QD diameter
  λ is the wavelength of light
  β is the full width at the maximum of the peak in radians
  θ is the Bragg angle

2.4.1.4 Core-Shell Structure Characterization

Most basic characterization techniques for QDs, such as TEM, XRD, or XPS, can also be applied to core-shell QDs [45]. As mentioned earlier, except for those prepared by the cation exchange approach, the overall diameter of QDs will increase after shell deposition as compared to initial core QDs, while the core size remains relatively unchanged. The shell thickness of QDs can thus be estimated by TEM by comparing the observed size before and after shell deposition. The observed size difference is also considered to be the most direct proof of successful shell growth.

However, for the lead chalcogenide core-shell QDs synthesized via the cation exchange approach, their overall diameter does not show any significant change during the core-shell structure formation process [16,68]. In addition, it is also challenging to observe the core-and-shell boundary for thin-shell QDs [68]. As a result, it is hard to estimate the core size and the shell thickness from TEM in this case. For the cation-exchange–prepared core-shell QDs with a thick shell (in general > 1.5 nm), the core-shell structure can be identified and the average shell thickness can be estimated based on their high-resolution TEM images (Figure 2.8b and c). In particular, TEM coupled with EDX can give valuable insight into the composition of obtained core-shell structures [16]. As shown in Figure 2.8c and d, point EDS analysis was applied to a PbS/CdS core-shell QD with nonuniform shell thickness [16]. Although both Pb and Cd are present in the core (indicated by a gray circle), Pb is absent in the shell region (indicated by a black circle), strongly suggesting that the shell is made of CdS, instead of the ternary $Pb_xCd_{1-x}S$ alloy (Figure 2.8d) [16]. Another technique that can be used to identify the core-shell–structured NCs is XPS with tunable synchrotron radiation, which has been used to convincingly prove the core-shell structure of $NaYF_4$-$NaGdF_4$ NCs [86]. This approach can be extended to core-shell QDs, although so far there has not been any related report for core-shell QDs yet.

2.4.2 Capping Agents

As-synthesized colloidal QDs are normally capped by ligands, which can control the size and shape of QDs during their synthesis and also increase the colloidal stability of QDs in the solution. In addition, the presence of these capping agents improves the optical property of QDs by surface-defect passivation. In general, the QDs capped with hydrophobic ligands (such as TOPO, TOP, OA, and oleylamine) can disperse well in an organic phase [16,73,79,81,83], while those capped with hydrophilic ligands (e.g., 3-mercaptopropionic acid) can disperse in water [5,6].

The initial surface-capping agents used for QD synthesis can be exchanged during the post-synthesis treatment either for the purpose of phase transfer or for further surface functionalization [57,58,87]. For example, the oleylamine ligands on the surface of PbS QDs can be replaced by OA by adding an excess amount of OA to the QD solution [87]. After precipitation with ethanol and centrifugation, the QDs can be redispersed in solution. The excess OA could be removed by further purification.

Capping agents on a QD surface can be identified by Fourier transform infrared spectroscopy, XPS, and nuclear magnetic resonance spectroscopy (NMR) [87,88]. For example, NMR measurements show that the PbS QDs are capped solely by oleylamine, even when TOP is simultaneously employed during synthesis [87].

2.4.3 Optical Properties

2.4.3.1 Absorption and Steady-State PL

Due to the quantum confinement effect, QDs show size-dependent absorption and emission. Thus, the variation of absorption and PL peak position can be achieved by tuning the size of QDs [2]. Figure 2.9 clearly shows this behavior of UV–visible-emitting CdS, CdSe, and CdTe QDs [89]. A similar phenomenon has been reported for NIR-emitting PbS QDs, as shown in Figure 2.10 [83]. Conversely, the average size of QDs can be estimated from their absorption peak using the following equation [85,89]:

$$CdS: D = (-6.6521 \times 10^{-8})\lambda^3 + (1.9957 \times 10^{-4})\lambda^2 - (9.2352 \times 10^{-2})\lambda + 13.29 \qquad (2.3)$$

$$CdSe: D = (1.6122 \times 10^{-9})\lambda^4 - (2.6575 \times 10^{-6})\lambda^3 + (1.6242 \times 10^{-3})\lambda^2 - (0.4277)\lambda + 41.57 \quad (2.4)$$

$$CdTe: D = (9.8127 \times 10^{-7})\lambda^3 - (1.7147 \times 10^{-3})\lambda^2 + (1.0064)\lambda - 194.84 \qquad (2.5)$$

$$PbS: \frac{1239}{\lambda} = 0.41 + \frac{3.84}{D^2} + \frac{1.7}{D} \qquad (2.6)$$

where
  D (nm) is the average size of QDs in a given sample
  λ (nm) is the wavelength of the first excitonic absorption peak of the corresponding sample

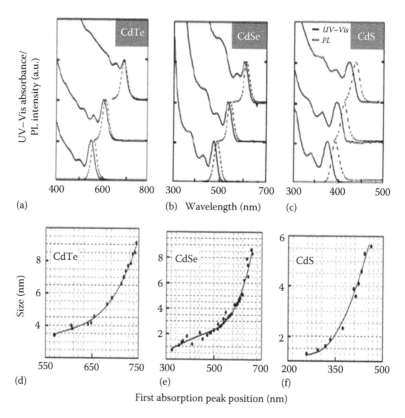

(a)   (b)   Wavelength (nm)   (c)

(d)   (e)   (f)

First absorption peak position (nm)

FIGURE 2.9
UV–visible and PL spectra of the representative NC samples of CdTe (a), CdSe (b) and CdS (c). Sizing curves for CdTe (d), CdSe (e), and CdS (f) NCs. (Adapted with permission from Yu, W.W., Qu, L., Guo, W., and Peng, X., *Chem. Mater.*, 15, 2854–2860. Copyright 2003 American Chemical Society.)

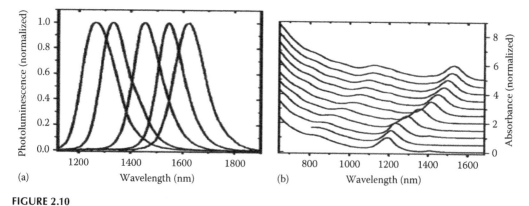

(a)   (b)

FIGURE 2.10
(a) PL of PbS QDs during growth. (b) Absorption of PbS QDs during growth (the small features at 1200 and 1400 nm are artifacts). (Adapted with permission from Cademartiri, L., Bertolotti, J., Sapienza, R., Wiersma, D.S., Kitaev, V., and Ozin, G.A., *J. Phys. Chem. B*, 110, 671–673. Copyright 2006 American Chemical Society.)

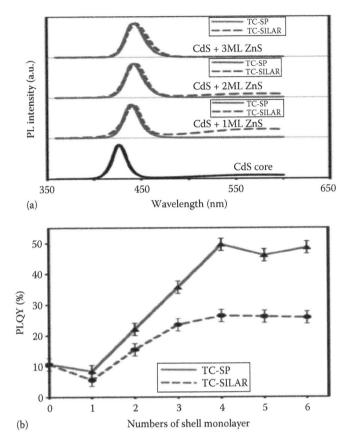

FIGURE 2.11
(a) PL properties of the CdS/ZnS core-shell NCs in comparison to the initial core NCs. (b) CdS/ZnS core-shell NCs grown by TC-SP and TC-SILAR are shown. (Adapted with permission from Chen, D.A., Zhao, F., Qi, H., Rutherford, M., and Peng, X.G., *Chem. Mater.*, 22, 1437–1444. Copyright 2010 American Chemical Society.)

Thessing et al. have further used the absorption and PL peak width to evaluate the size distribution of QDs [90].

In addition to indicating the size distribution of QDs, PL spectra also yield the information of surface states and provide the guide for the optimal synthesis of QDs. As shown in Figure 2.11a, the core-shell CdS/ZnS NCs synthesized by thermal-cycling–coupled SILAR (TC-SILAR) showed substantial trap emission located on the longer-wavelength side of the PL spectra, if the shell thickness was less than three monolayers [91]. In stark contrast, though from the same batch of core NCs (Figure 2.11a, bottom plot), the core-shell NCs synthesized via "thermal-cycling–coupled single precursor" (TC-SP) showed a complete elimination of the trap emission even if only one monolayer of the shell was in place. The PL QY of the core-shell CdS/ZnS QDs showed a significant increase as a function of ZnS shell thickness due to the improved surface passivation and strongly depends on the thickness of the shell (Figure 2.11b) [91].

Absorption spectra of QDs, either dispersed in a solvent or in the powder form, can be acquired with a UV–visible–NIR spectrophotometer. Fluorescence spectra can be taken with a fluorescence system using either a lamp or laser as an excitation source.

The fluorescence QY (Φ), an important index for evaluating the QD quality, can be estimated from the absorption and PL spectra of QDs. The most common method for recording Φ is the comparative method of Williams et al. [92], which involves the use of well-characterized standard samples with known Φ values. Basically, solutions of the standard and test QD samples, with identical absorbance at the same excitation wavelength can be assumed to be absorbing the same number of photons. Hence, a simple ratio of the integrated fluorescence intensities of the two solutions recorded under identical conditions will yield the ratio of their Φ values. As Φ for the standard sample is known, it is trivial to calculate Φ for the test sample. Then the absolute QY value can be obtained using a standard sample that has a known fluorescence QY value as a reference, according to the following equation:

$$\frac{\Phi_x}{\Phi_{st}} = \left(\frac{Grad_x}{Grad_{st}} \right) \times \left(\frac{\eta_x^2}{\eta_{st}^2} \right) \qquad (2.7)$$

where
the subscripts st x denote the standard and unknown samples, respectively
Φ is the fluorescence QY
Grad is the gradient from the plot of integrated fluorescence intensity *versus* absorbance
η is the refractive index of the solvents used for the measurements

Another method does not rely on making comparisons with standard materials, but aims to directly determine the absolute number of absorbed and emitted photons using an integrating sphere [93]. Both methods have been used to evaluate the QY of QDs. For PbS QDs, the reference sample is typically IR-125 or IR-26 [16,87,94]. Both methods confirm that PbS QDs show PL QY between 20% and 80% depending on their size [81,94]. For UV–visible–emitting QDs, various reference samples have been used. The measured QY is in the range of 30%–60% for CdSe/ZnS QDs and 60%–80% for CdSe/CdS QDs [73,95,96].

2.4.3.2 Transient Absorption and Dynamic PL

In addition to steady-state optical measurements, dynamic measurements of absorption and PL can help to further understand the optical property of QDs. A powerful technique for studying the electronic states of QDs is ultrafast pump-probe spectroscopy [97]. The effect of size, surface passivation, and pump intensity on the variation of the lifetime of the excited states of simple QDs has been investigated. Recently, studies have been extended to more complex nanostructures, such as 1D structures and core-shell QDs [97]. For example, Wheeler et al. have studied the ultrafast dynamics of both PbS and PbS/CdS QD solutions using ultrafast pump-probe spectroscopy [97]. Figure 2.12 is a plot of the transient time-decay profiles (in ps) for these QDs following an excitation wavelength of 750 nm (maintained at a pulse energy of 100 nJ/pulse) and a probe wavelength of 600 nm. Strong, broad transient signals were observed from 600 to 750 nm following an initial excitation wavelength of 750 nm. The lifetime of the transient absorption feature was independent of the wavelength and was fit to decays of 8.2 and 98 ps for the PbS QDs versus 6.3 and 79 ps for the PbS/CdS QDs. The relatively faster decay of the PbS/CdS QDs was found to be due to the decreased density of the trap states via the surface passivation of the parent PbS material.

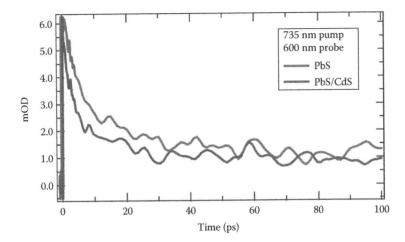

FIGURE 2.12
Transient absorption relaxation traces of PbS and PbS/CdS at a probe wavelength of 600 nm following a 750 nm, 200 nJ/pulse pump. (With kind permission from Springer Science+Business Media: *Sci. China Chem.*, Ultrafast exciton relaxation dynamics of PbS and core/shell PbS/CdS quantum dots, 54, 2011, 2009–2015, Wheeler, D.A., Fitzmorris, B.C., Zhao, H., Ma, D., and Zhang, J.Z.)

The fluorescence lifetime (i.e., the lifetime of electron–hole pairs) of QDs has also been studied [98]. There are two complementary techniques, based either on frequency domain or time domain, with the latter being most commonly used. In the frequency domain approach, a sample is excited by a modulated source of light. The fluorescence is modulated and phase-shifted from the excitation curve, from which the lifetime can be calculated. In the time-domain approach, a short pulse of light excites a sample, and the subsequent fluorescence emission is recorded as a function of time. The time-domain lifetime measurement can be done in a multichannel scaler (MCS) mode or time-correlated single-photon counting (TCSPC) mode, depending on the value of the lifetime [16,98]. The decay signals can be fitted according to the following equation:

$$I(t) = \sum_{i=1}^{n} a_i \exp\left(\frac{-t}{\tau_i}\right) \tag{2.8}$$

where
τ_i is the lifetime associated with the ith component
I is the PL intensity
t is the time
a_i represents the amplitude of the ith component at $t=0$
n is the number of decay components

Depending on the semiconductor material, surface states, and surrounding environment, QDs could show a single lifetime or multiple lifetimes. CdS QDs have been shown to have three components of lifetime, in the range of several ns to several tens of ns [99]. The value and number of lifetimes of QDs can help to understand the mechanism of many processes, such as energy-transfer and charge-transfer processes [88,100]. Recently, both the transient-absorption and time-resolved PL spectroscopic techniques have been used to investigate the carrier multiplication in QDs (also named multiple exciton generation) [4,101,102].

2.4.4 Stability

2.4.4.1 Structural Stability

The structural stability of QDs is very sensitive to the change in their environment due to their small size. The obvious variation in the average size and size distribution, surface states, and capping ligands, caused by environmental changes, can largely affect the optical property of QDs [16,60,90]. For example, it was found that directly setting monodispersed QDs in an organic solvent at a relatively high temperature inevitably led to the Ostwald ripening of QDs in the cases of CdSe and PbS QDs, giving rise to broader-, double-, or even multiple-size distributions confirmed by their TEM images [16,90].

Another tool to monitor the change in the structure of QDs is PL or absorption spectra [60,103]. In one study, freshly prepared PbSe QDs were kept at room temperature for 2 months. It was found that the emission peak wavelength blue-shifted around 114 nm due to the effective size decrease of the PbSe core caused by surface oxidation [103]. Another example is that the stability of PbS QDs can be detected by the absorption spectra. As shown in Figure 2.13a, the as-synthesized large PbS NCs showed an 88 nm blue-shift in their excitonic peak in the 6 days' ambient storage. In big contrast, small PbS QDs showed no blue-shift during the ambient storage, indicating that smaller-sized QDs show a better stability as compared to larger-sized QDs. Furthermore, XPS was used to test the surface-structure change of QDs by measuring the binding energy of core-level electrons [60]. As shown in Figure 2.13c and d, a PbS QD film was annealed at 90°C in air for 10 min to accelerate the aging process. The large dots have more surface oxidation compared to small dots, which accounts for the larger shift of the absorption peaks of larger-sized QDs [104].

2.4.4.2 Colloidal Stability

Colloidal stability is required in most applications. It denotes whether QDs can resist flocculation or aggregation and whether they exhibit a long shelf life. The hydrodynamic size of colloidal QDs can be characterized by dynamic light scattering. If QDs are aggregated, the dynamic size of QDs will largely increase. For example, both Zhao et al. and Cornacchio et al. reported that the aggregation of thiolate-capped PbS NCs in water was due to the oxidation of thiol-capping groups via dynamic light scattering [54,105]. Since the PL of QDs is very sensitive to the aggregation of QDs, one can also check the colloidal stability of QDs by fluorescence spectra [57]. For example, it has been found that poly(acrylic acid)-capped PbS QDs gradually experienced a decrease in QY, accompanied by the blue-shift of both absorption and emission bands due to the aggregation of QDs [57]. PMAO–PEG–encapsulated PbS/CdS QDs, on the other hand, have been reported to be very stable in water without any sign of QD aggregation with time, as supported by the absence of any variations of the PL spectra [61,62].

A high salt concentration normally leads to the aggregation of QDs due to the decrease of the electrostatic repulsion among QDs [106]. Interestingly, polymer-encapsulated PbS/CdS core-shell QDs show very good colloidal stability against salt concentration [62]. Whatever the shell thickness (0.2–2.1 nm), the PL intensity of the QDs in a buffer does not change with the addition of NaCl, even at a concentration as high as 300 mM. The good dispersion of these QDs at a high salt concentration was further confirmed by their TEM images [62].

2.4.4.3 Photostability

For practical applications, QDs should show very good photostability. Unfortunately, the surface of QDs is very sensitive to high-intensity light [103,107]. Both surface oxidation and

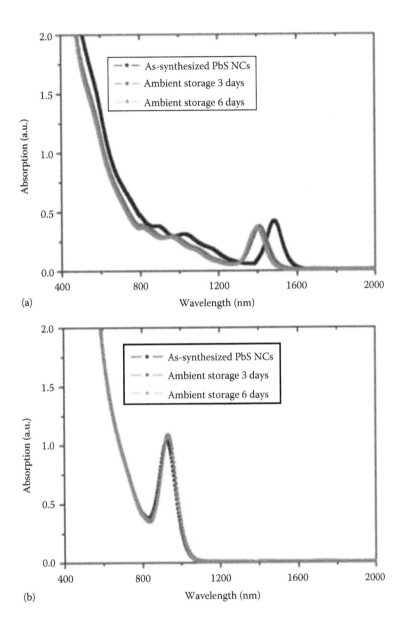

FIGURE 2.13
(See color insert.) Comparison of oxidation characteristics of large (a, c) and small (b, d) PbS NCs. Absorption change of (a) large PbS NCs and (b) small PbS NCs stored in octane solution in ambient for 0 day (black), 3 days (red), and 6 days (cyan); XPS S 2p spectra of as-fabricated film (black), film annealed in air at 90°C for 10 min (red), and annealed for 90 min (cyan) of large PbS NCs (c) and small PbS NCs (d). We use peaks at binding energy of 160.8 eV for PbS, 162.0 eV for S–C in ethanedithiol, 163.7 eV for S–S in oxidation products of ethanedithiol, 165.4 eV for PbSO$_3$, and 167.8 eV for PbSO$_4$. (Adapted with permission from Tang, J., Brzozowski, L., Barkhouse, D.A.R., Wang, X., Debnath, R., Wolowiec, R., Palmiano, E., Levina, L., Pattantyus-Abraham, A.G., Jamakosmanovic, D., and Sargent, E.H., *ACS Nano*, 4, 869–878. Copyright 2010 American Chemical Society.)

(continued)

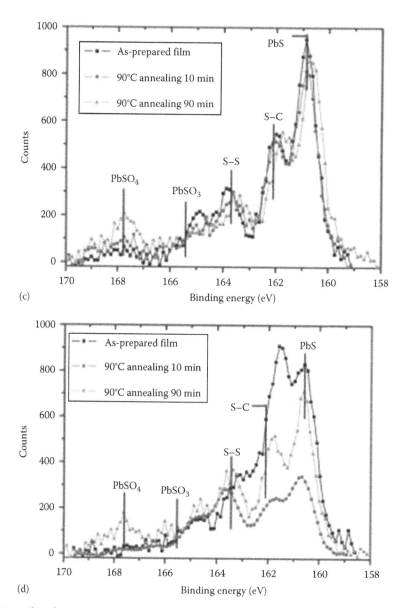

FIGURE 2.13 (continued)
(See color insert.) Comparison of oxidation characteristics of large (a, c) and small (b, d) PbS NCs. Absorption change of (a) large PbS NCs and (b) small PbS NCs stored in octane solution in ambient for 0 day (black), 3 days (red), and 6 days (cyan); XPS S 2p spectra of as-fabricated film (black), film annealed in air at 90°C for 10 min (red), and annealed for 90 min (cyan) of large PbS NCs (c) and small PbS NCs (d). We use peaks at binding energy of 160.8 eV for PbS, 162.0 eV for S–C in ethanedithiol, 163.7 eV for S–S in oxidation products of ethanedithiol, 165.4 eV for PbSO$_3$, and 167.8 eV for PbSO$_4$. (Adapted with permission from Tang, J., Brzozowski, L., Barkhouse, D.A.R., Wang, X., Debnath, R., Wolowiec, R., Palmiano, E., Levina, L., Pattantyus-Abraham, A.G., Jamakosmanovic, D., and Sargent, E.H., *ACS Nano*, 4, 869–878. Copyright 2010 American Chemical Society.)

ligand-etching process of QDs can be accelerated by irradiation, which leads to a decrease in the PL intensity [103,107]. The photostability of QDs dispersed in different solvents or QDs in film can be tested using a UV lamp or laser by following their PL spectra variation with respect to illumination time. In addition, the oxidation or ligand etching of QDs can be measured by XPS [107]. For example, Ma et al. have reported that a strong lamp can cause the ligand desorption from PbS QDs, thus degrading their PL [61]. The introduction of dangling bonds from the ligand etching was confirmed by XPS.

In contrast, PbS/CdS QDs do not exhibit any considerable PL-peak broadening or shift during the irradiation period of 2 h, suggesting that there is no detectable photooxidation or etching of PbS cores [62]. The amplitude of the variation of the PL intensity, however, differs among samples of different shell thicknesses. A PbS/CdS QD with the thickest shell is the most stable. The differences in the photostability of the samples with different shell thicknesses are quite possible due to the amplitude of the exciton wave function at the outer interface of the shell [108].

2.5 Future Directions and Challenges

Current techniques have enabled the synthesis of a high optical quality of QDs and an in-depth characterization, allowing a good understanding of QDs. Some aspects still need to be further improved or explored. In synthesis, it is highly desirable to develop a reproducible method to achieve a high-yield and large-scale synthesis of QDs with good quality. The microwave approach has proved to yield certain high-quality QDs with relatively large quantities in a short period. This technique should be extended to a wide range of QDs and the synthesis should also be further amplified by using a larger-volume microwave reactor, more compatible with industry settings. As for stability, although it has been improved by applying the core-shell strategy, QDs are still sensitive to oxygen under certain circumstances, which could lead to the dramatic degradation of their optical properties. To make QDs with excellent stability against their environment change is of high importance. It will open the door for QDs to many real-world applications, such as the application of QDs to a complicated system like blood. In addition, toxicity is an important factor to consider before QDs can be put into practical use. The toxicity of QDs is affected by many parameters, such as chemical composition, size, shape, aggregation status, surface coating, and dose [109–111]. Although some types of QDs can be presently prepared with tight size- and shape-control and various surface chemistries, and demonstrate no obvious toxicity in a short period [109–111], their long-term toxicity needs to be thoroughly investigated and systematically evaluated at the molecular, *in vitro*, and *in vivo* levels.

References

1. Alivisatos, P. 1996. Semiconductor clusters, nanocrystals, and quantum dots. *Science* 271:933–937.
2. Brus, L. E. 1984. Electron-electron and electron-hole interactions in small semiconductor crystallites—The size dependence of the lowest excited electronic state. *Journal of Chemical Physics* 80:4403–4409.

3. McGuire, J. A., Joo, J., Pietryga, J. M., Schaller, R. D., and Klimov, V. I. 2008. New aspects of carrier multiplication in semiconductor nanocrystals. *Accounts of Chemical Research* 41:1810–1819.
4. Murray, C. B., Norris, D. J., and Bawendi, M. G. 1993. Synthesis and characterization of nearly monodisperse CdE (E=Sulfur, Selenium, Tellurium) semiconductor nanocrystallites. *Journal of the American Chemical Society* 115:8706–8715.
5. Michalet, X., Pinaud, F. F., Bentolila, L. A., Tsay, J. M., Doose, S., Li, J. J., Sundaresan, G., Wu, A. M., Gambhir, S. S., and Weiss. S. 2005. Quantum dots for live cells, in vivo imaging, and diagnostics. *Science* 307:538–544.
6. Bruchez, M., Moronne, M., Gin, P., Weiss, S., and Alivisatos, A. P. 1998. Semiconductor nanocrystals as fluorescent biological labels. *Science* 281:2013–2016.
7. Gerion, D., Pinaud, F., Williams, S. C., Parak, W. J., Zanchet, D., Weiss, S., and Alivisatos, A. P. 2001. Synthesis and properties of biocompatible water-soluble silica-coated CdSe/ZnS semiconductor quantum dots. *The Journal of Physical Chemistry B* 105:8861–8871.
8. Yu, W. W., Falkner, J. C., Shih, B. S., and Colvin, V. L. 2004. Preparation and characterization of monodisperse PbSe semiconductor nanocrystals in a noncoordinating solvent. *Chemistry of Materials* 16:3318–3322.
9. Guzelian, A., Banin, U., Kadavanich, A. V., Peng, X., and Alivisatos, A. P. 1996. Colloidal chemical synthesis and characterization of InAs nanocrystal quantum dots. *Applied Physics Letters* 69:1432–1434.
10. Guzelian, A., Katari, J. E. B., Kadavanich, A. V., Banin, U., Hamad, K., Juban, E., and Alivisatos, A. P. 1996. Synthesis of size-selected, surface-passivated InP nanocrystals. *The Journal of Physical Chemistry* 100:7212–7219.
11. Zlateva, G., Zhelev, Z., Bakalova, R., and Kanno, I. 2007. Precise size control and synchronized synthesis of six colors of CdSe quantum dots in a slow-increasing temperature gradient. *Inorganic Chemistry* 46:6212–6214.
12. Yu, W. W., Wang, Y. A., and Peng, X. 2003. Formation and stability of size-, shape-, and structure-controlled CdTe nanocrystals: ligand effects on monomers and nanocrystals. *Chemistry of Materials* 15:4300–4308.
13. Tsay, J. M., Pflughoefft, M., Bentolila, L. A., and Weiss, S. 2004. Hybrid approach to the synthesis of highly luminescent CdTe/ZnSandCdHgTe/ZnS nanocrystals. *Journal of the American Chemical Society* 126:1926–1927.
14. Jaiswal J. K. and Simon S. M. 2004. Potentials and pitfalls of fluorescent quantum dots for biological imaging. *Trends in Cell Biology* 14:497–504.
15. Dubertret, B., Skourides, P., Norris, D. J., Noireaux,V., Brivanlou, A. H., and Libchaber, A. 2002. In vivo imaging of quantum dots encapsulated in phospholipid micelles. *Science* 298:1759–1762.
16. Zhao, H., Chaker, M., Wu, N., and Ma, D. 2011. Towards controlled synthesis and better understanding of highly luminescent PbS/CdS core/shell quantum dots. *Journal of Materials Chemistry* 21:8898–8904.
17. Nirmal, M., Dabbousi, B. O., Bawendi, M. G., Macklin, J. J., Trautman, J. K., Harris, T. D., and Brus, L. E. 1996. Fluorescence intermittency in single cadmium selenide nanocrystals. *Nature* 383:802–804.
18. Hennig, S., van de Linde, S., Heilemann, M., and Sauer, M. 2009. Quantum dot triexciton imaging with three-dimensional subdiffraction resolution. *Nano Letters* 9:2466–2470.
19. Rogach, L., Eychmüller, A., Hickey, S. G., and Kershaw, S. V. 2007. Infrared-emitting colloidal nanocrystals: Synthesis, assembly, spectroscopy, and applications. *Small* 3:536–557.
20. Joo, J., Na, H. B., Yu, T., Yu, J. H., Kim, Y. W., Wu, F., Zhang, J. Z., and Hyeon, T. 2003. Generalized and facile synthesis of semiconducting metal sulfide nanocrystals. *Journal of the American Chemical Society* 125:11100–11105.
21. Peng, X., Manna, L., Yang, W. D., Wickham, J., Scher, E., Kadavanich, A., and Alivisatos, A. P. 2000. Shape control of CdSe nanocrystals. *Nature* 404:59–61.
22. Weissleder, R. 2001. Progress continues in the development of smaller, more penetrable probes for biological imaging. *Nature Biotechnology* 19:316–317.

23. Dahan, M., Laurence, T., Pinaud, F., Chemla, D. S., Alivisatos, A. P., Sauer, M., and Weiss, S. 2001. Time-gated biological imaging by use of colloidal quantum dots. *Optics Letters* 26:825–827.

24. He, Y. and Wang, R. 2004. Dynamic optical clearing effect of tissue impregnated with hyper-osmotic agents and studied with optical coherence tomography. *Journal of Biomedical Optics* 9:200–206.

25. Gao, X., Yang, L., Petros, J. A., Marshall, F. F., Simons, J. W., and Nie, S. 2005. In vivo molecular and cellular imaging with quantum dots. *Current Opinion in Biotechnology* 16:63–72.

26. Hintersteiner, M., Enz, A., Frey, P., Jaton, A. L., Kinzy, W., Kneuer, R., Neumann, U. et al. 2005. In vivo detection of amyloid-β deposits by near-infrared imaging using an oxazine-derivative probe. *Nature Biotechnology* 23:577–583.

27. Zaheer, A., Lenkinski, R. E., Mahmood, A., Jones, A. G., Cantley, L. C., and Frangioni, J. V. 2001. In vivo near-infrared fluorescence imaging of osteoblastic activity. *Nature Biotechnology* 19:1148–1154.

28. Alivisatos, P., Gu, W. W., and Larabell, C. 2005. Quantum dots as cellular probes. *Annual Review of Biomedical Engineering* 7:55–76.

29. Hyun, B. B., Chen, H., Rey, D. A., Wise, F. W., and Batt, C. A. 2007. Near-infrared fluorescence imaging with water-soluble lead salt quantum dots. *The Journal of Physical Chemistry B* 111:5726–5730.

30. Aswathy, R. G., Yoshida, Y., Maekawa, T., and Kumar, D. S. 2010. Near-infrared quantum dots for deep tissue imaging. *Analytical and Bioanalytical Chemistry* 397:1417–1435.

31. Peng, Z. A. and Peng, X. 2001. Formation of high-quality CdTe, CdSe, and CdS nanocrystals using CdO as precursor. *Journal of the American Chemical Society* 123:183–184.

32. Deng, Z., Lie, F. L., Shen, S., Ghosh, I., Mansuripur, M., and Muscat, A. J. 2009. Water based route to ligand selective synthesis of ZnSe and Cd-doped ZnSe quantum dots with tunable ultraviolet A to blue photoluminescence. *Langmuir* 25:434–442.

33. Borchert, H., Dorfs, D., McGinley, C., Adam, S., Möller, T., Weller, H., and Eychmüller, A. 2003. Photoemission study of onion like quantum dot quantum well and double quantum well nano-crystals of CdS and HgS. *The Journal of Physical Chemistry B* 107:7486–7491.

34. Hines, M. A. and Scholes, G. D. 2003. Colloidal PbS nanocrystals with size-tunable near-infra-red emission: observation of post-synthesis self-narrowing of the particle size distribution. *Advanced Materials* 15:1844–1849.

35. Lu, W. G., Fang, J. Y., Stokes, K. L., and Lin, J. 2004. Shape evolution and self assembly of mono-disperse PbTe nanocrystals. *Journal of the American Chemical Society* 126:11798–11799.

36. Ma, X. Y., Yan, Z. J., Yuan, B. H., and Li, B. J. 2005. The light-emitting properties of Ge nanocrys-tals grown by pulsed laser deposition. *Nanotechnology* 16:832–835.

37. Zaknoon, B. and Bahir, G. 2008. Study of single silicon quantum dots' band gap and single-electron charging energies by room temperature scanning tunneling microscopy. *Nano Letters* 8:1689–1694.

38. Swafford, L. A., Weigand, L. A., Bowers, M. J., McBride, J. R., Rapaport, J. L., Watt, T. L., Dixit, S. K., Feldman, L. C., and Rosenthal, S. J. 2006. Homogenously alloyed CdS_xSe_{1-x} nanocrystals: synthesis, characterization, and composition/size-dependent band gap. *Journal of the American Chemical Society* 128:12299–12306.

39. Zhong, X., Feng, Y., Knoll, W., and Han, M. 2003. Alloyed $Zn_xCd_{1-x}S$ nanocrystals with highly narrow luminescence spectra width. *Journal of the American Chemical Society* 125:13559–13563.

40. Akhtar, J., Afzaal, M., Banski, M., Podhorodecki, A., Syperek, M., Misiewicz, J. Bangert, U. et al. 2011. Controlled synthesis of tuned band gap nanodimensional alloys of PbS_xSe_{1-x}. *Journal of the American Chemical Society* 133:5602–5609.

41. Tytus, M., Krasnyj, J., Jacak, W., Chuchmala, A., Donderowicz, W., and Jacak, L. 2008. Differences between photoluminescence spectra of type-I and type-II quantum dots. *Journal of Physics: Conference Series* 104:012011–012014.

42. Kim, S., Fisher, B., Eisler, H. J., and Bawendi, M. 2003. Type-II quantum dots: CdTe/CdSe(core/shell) and CdSe/ZnTe(core/shell) heterostructures. *Journal of the American Chemical Society* 125:11466–11467.

43. De Geyter, B., Justo, Y., Moreels, I., Lambert, K., Smet, P. F., Van Thourhout, D., Houtepen, A. J. et al. 2010. The different nature of band edge absorption and emission in colloidal PbSe/CdSe core/shell quantum dots. *ACS Nano* 5:58–66.

44. Ivanov, S. A., Piryatinski, A., Nanda, J., Tretiak, S., Zavadil, K., Walalce, W. O., Werder, D., and Klimov, V. I. 2007. Type-II core/shell CdS/ZnSe nanocrystals: Synthesis, electronic structures, and spectroscopic properties. *Journal of the American Chemical Society* 129:11708–11719.

45. Reiss, P., Protiére, M., and Li, L. 2009. Core/shell semiconductor nanocrystals. *Small* 5:154–168.

46. La Mer, V. K. and Dinegar, R. H. 1950. Theory, production and mechanism of formation of monodispersed hydrosols. *Journal of the American Chemical Society* 72:4847–4854.

47. Reiss, H. 1951. The growth of uniform colloidal dispersions. *Journal of Chemical Physics* 19:482–487.

48. Yang, Y. J., He, L. Y., and Zhang, Q. F. 2005. A cyclic voltammetric synthesis of PbS nanoparticles. *Electrochemistry Communications* 7:361–364.

49. Aaron, L. W. and Geoffrey, F. S. 2009. Selective microwave absorption by trioctyl phosphine selenide: Does it play a role in producing multiple sized quantum dots in a single reaction? *Chemistry of Materials* 21:2770–2776.

50. Gerbec, J. A., Magana, D., Washington, A., and Strouse, G. F. 2005. Microwave-enhanced reaction rates for nanoparticle synthesis. *Journal of the American Chemical Society* 127:15791–15800.

51. Li, L., Qian, H., and Ren, J. 2005. Rapid synthesis of highly luminescent CdTe nanocrystals in the aqueous phase by microwave irradiation with controllable temperature. *Chemical Communications* 4:528–530.

52. Roy, M. D., Herzing, A. A., De Paoli Lacerda, S. H., and Becker, M. L. 2008. Emission-tunable microwave synthesis of highly luminescent water soluble CdSe/ZnS quantum dots. *Chemical Communications* 18:2106–2108.

53. Murray, C. B. and Kagan, C. R. 2000. Synthesis and characterization of monodisperse nanocrystals and close-packed nanocrystal assemblies. *Annual Review of Materials Science* 30:545–610.

54. Zhao, X. S., Gorelikov, I., Musikhin, S., Cauchi, S., Sukhovatkin, V., Sargent, E. H., and Kumacheva, E. 2005. Synthesis and optical properties of thiol-stabilized PbS nanocrystals. *Langmuir* 21:1086–109047.

55. Hennequin, B., Turyanska, L., Ben, T., Beltran, A. M., Molina, S. I., Li, M., Mann, S., Patane, A., and Thomas,N. R. 2008. Aqueous near-infrared fluorescent composites based on apoferritin-encapsulated PbS quantum dots. *Advanced Materials* 20:3592–3596.

56. Turyanska, L., Bradshaw, T. D., Sharpe, J., Li, M., Mann, S., Thomas, N. R., and Patane, A. 2009. The biocompatibility of apoferritin-encapsulated PbS quantum dots. *Small* 15:1738–1741.

57. Lin, W., Fritz, K., Guerin, G., Bardajee, G. R., Hinds, S., Sukhovatkin, V., Sargent, E. H., Scholes, G. D., and Winnik, M. A. 2008. Highly luminescent lead sulfide nanocrystals in organic solvents and water through ligand exchange with poly(acrylic acid). *Langmuir* 24:8215–8219.

58. Hinds, S., Myrskog, S., Levina, L., Koleilat, G., Yang, J., Kelley, S. O., and Sargent, E. H. 2007. NIR-emitting colloidal quantum dots having 26% luminescence quantum yield in buffer solution. *Journal of the American Chemical Society* 129:7218–7219.

59. Yu, W. W., Chang, E., Falkner, J. C., Zhang, J., Al-Somali, A. M., Sayes, C. M., Johns, J., Drezek, R., and Colvin, V. L. 2007. Forming biocompatible and nonaggregated nanocrystals in water using amphiphilic polymers. *Journal of the American Chemical Society* 129:2871–2879.

60. Zhao, H., Wang, D., Chaker, M., and Ma, D. 2011. Photoluminescence effect of different types of surface ligands on the structure and optical property of water-soluble PbS quantum dots encapsulated by amphiphilic polymers. *The Journal of Physical Chemistry C* 115:1620–1626.

61. Zhao, H., Wang, D., Zhang, T., Chaker, M., and Ma, D. 2010. Two-step synthesis of high-quality water-soluble near-infrared emitting quantum dots via amphiphilic polymers. *Chemical Communications* 46:5301–5303.

62. Zhao, H., Chaker, M., and Ma, D. 2011. Effect of CdS shell thickness on the optical properties of water-soluble amphiphilic polymer encapsulated PbS/CdS quantum dots. *Journal of Materials Chemistry* 21:17483–17491.

63. Di Corato, R., Quarta, A., Piacenza, P., Ragusa, A., Figuerola, A., Buonsanti, R., Cingolani, R., Manna,L., and Pellegrino, T. 2008. Water solubilization of hydrophobic nanocrystals by means of poly(maleic anhydride-alt-1-octadecene). *Journal of Materials Chemistry* 18:1991–1996.

64. Zhao, H., Chaker, M., and Ma, D. 2009. Bimodal photoluminescence during the growth of PbS quantum dots. *The Journal of Physical Chemistry C* 113:6497–6504.

65. Dashiell, M. W., Denker, U., Müller, C., Costantini, G., Manzano, C., Kern, K., and Schmidt, O. G. 2002. Photoluminescence of ultrasmall Ge quantum dots grown by molecular beam epitaxy at low temperatures. *Applied Physic Letters* 80:1279–1281.

66. El-Emawy, A. A., Birudavolu, S., Wong, P. S., Jiang, Y. B., Xu, H., Huang, S., and Huffaker, D. L. 2003. Formation trends in quantum dot growth using metalorganic chemical vapor deposition. *Journal of Applied Physics* 93:3529–3534.

67. Ka, I., Ma, D., and El Khakani, M. A. 2011. Tailoring the photoluminescence of PbS-nanoparticles layers deposited by means of the pulsed laser ablation technique. *Journal of Nanoparticle Research* 13:2269–2274.

68. Pietryga, J. M., Werder, D. J., Williams, D. J., Casson, J. L., Schaller, R. D., Klimov, V. I., and Hollingsworth, J. A. 2008. Utilizing the lability of lead selenide to produce heterostructured nanocrystals with bright, stable infrared emission. *Journal of the American Chemical Society* 130:4879–4885.

69. Peng, X., Schlamp, M. C., Kadavanich, A. V., and Alivisatos, A. P. 1997. Epitaxial growth of highly luminescent CdSe/CdS core/shell nanocrystals with photostability and electronic accessibility. *Journal of the American Chemical Society* 119:7019–7029.

70. Aharoni, A., Mokari, T., Popov, I., and Banin, U. 2006. Synthesis of InAs/CdSe/ZnSe core/shell1/shell2 structures with bright and stable near-infrared fluorescence. *Journal of the American Chemical Society* 128:257–264.

71. Smith, M. and Nie, S. 2009. Semiconductor nanocrystals: structure, properties, and band gap engineering. *Accounts of Chemical Research* 43:190–200.

72. McBride, J., Treadway, J., Feldman, L. C., Pennycook, S. J., and Rosenthal, S. J. 2006. Structural basis for near unity quantum yield core/shell nanostructures. *Nano Letters* 6:1496–1501.

73. Dabbousi, B. O., Rodriguez-Viejo, J., Mikulec, F. V., Heine, J. R., Mattoussi, H., Ober, R., Jensen K. F., and Bawendi M. G. 1997. (CdSe)ZnS core-shell quantum dots: Synthesis and optical and structural characterization of a size series of highly luminescent materials. *The Journal of Physical Chemistry B* 101:9463–9475.

74. Brumer, M., Kigel, A., Amirav, L., Sashchiuk, A., Solomesch, O., Tessler, N., and Lifshitz, E. 2005. PbSe/PbS and PbSe/PbSexS1–x core/shell nanocrystals. *Advanced Functional Materials* 15:1111–1116.

75. Mews, A., Eychmüller, A., Giersig, M., Schooss, D., and Weller, H. 1994. Preparation, characterization, and photophysics of the quantum dot quantum well system cadmium sulfide/mercury sulfide/cadmium sulfide. *The Journal of Physical Chemistry* 98:934–941.

76. Chen, C. Y., Cheng, C. T., Lai, C. W., Hu, Y. H., Chou, P. T., Chou, Y. H., and Chiu, H. T. 2005. Type-II CdSe/CdTe/ZnTe (core–shell–shell) quantum dots with cascade band edges: The separation of electron (at CdSe) and hole (at ZnTe) by the CdTe layer. *Small* 1:1215–1220.

77. Wang, C. H., Chen, C. W., Chen, Y. T., Wei, C. M., Chen, Y. F., Lai, C. W., Ho, M. L., Chou, P. T., and Hofmann, M. 2010. Surface plasmon enhanced energy transfer between type I CdSe/ZnS and type II CdSe/ZnTe quantum dots. *Applied Physics Letters* 96:071906.

78. Xu, S., Ziegler, J., and Nann, T. 2008. Rapid synthesis of highly luminescent InP and InP/ZnS nanocrystals. *Journal of Materials Chemistry* 18:2653–2656.

79. Li, J. J., Wang, Y. A., Guo, W. Z., Keay, J. C., Mishima, T. D., Johnson, M. B., and Peng, X. G. 2003. Large-scale synthesis of nearly monodisperse CdSe/CdS core/shell nanocrystals using air-stable reagents via successive ion layer adsorption and reaction. *Journal of the American Chemical Society* 125:12567–12575.

80. Chin, P. T. K., de Mello Donega, C., van Bavel, S. S., Meskers, S. C. J., Sommerdijk, N. A. J. M., and Janssen, R. A. J. 2007. Highly luminescent CdTe/CdSe colloidal heteronanocrystals with temperature-dependent emission color. *Journal of the American Chemical Society* 129:14880–14886.

81. Zhao, H., Zhang, T., Chaker, M., and Ma, D. 2010. Ligand and precursor effects on the synthesis and optical properties of PbS quantum dots. *Journal of Nanoscience and Nanotechnology* 10:4897–4905.

82. Lambert, K., De Geyter, B., Moreels, I., and Hens, Z. 2009. PbTe/CdTe core/shell particles by cation exchange, a HR-TEM Study. *Chemistry of Materials* 21:778–780.

83. Cademartiri, L., Bertolotti, J., Sapienza, R., Wiersma, D. S., Kitaev, V., and Ozin, G. A., 2006. Multigram scale, solventless, and diffusion-controlled route to highly monodisperse PbS nanocrystals. *The Journal of Physical Chemistry B* 110:671–673.

84. Klug, H. P. and Alexander, L. E. 1959. *X-Ray Diffraction Procedures*. John Wiley & Sons: New York.

85. Cademartiri, L., Montanari, E., Calestani, G., Migliori, A., Guagliardi, A., and Ozin, G. A. 2006. Size-dependent extinction coefficients of PbS quantum dots. *Journal of the American Chemical Society* 128:10337–10346.

86. Abel, K. A., Boyer, J. C., and van Veggel, F. C. J. M. 2009. Hard proof of the $NaYF_4/NaGdF_4$ nanocrystal core/shell structure. *Journal of the American Chemical Society* 131:14644–14645.

87. Moreels, I., Justo, Y., De Geyter, B., Haustraete, K., Martins, J. C., and Hens, Z. 2011. Size-tunable, bright, and stable PbS quantum dots: a surface chemistry study. *ACS Nano* 5:2004–2012.

88. Wang, D. F., Baral, J. K., Zhao, H. G., Gonfa, B. A., Truong, V., Khakani, M. A. E., Izquierdo, R., and Ma, D. 2011. Controlled fabrication of PbS quantum-dot/carbon-nanotube nanoarchitecture and its significant contribution to near-infrared photon-to-current conversion. *Advanced Functional Materials* 21:4010–4018.

89. Yu, W. W., Qu, L., Guo, W., and Peng, X. 2003. Experimental determination of the extinction coefficient of CdTe, CdSe, and CdS nanocrystals. *Chemistry of Materials* 15:2854–2860.

90. Thessing, J., Qian, J. H., Chen, H. Y., Pradhan, N., and Peng, X. 2007. Interparticle influence on size/size distribution evolution of nanocrystals. *Journal of the American Chemical Society* 129:2736–2737.

91. Chen, D. A., Zhao, F., Qi, H., Rutherford, M., and Peng, X. G. 2010. Bright and stable purple/blue emitting CdS/ZnS core/shell nanocrystals grown by thermal cycling using a single-source precursor. *Chemistry of Materials* 22:1437–1444.

92. Williams, A. T. R., Winfield, S. A., and Miller, J. N. 1983. Relative fluorescence quantum yields using a computer controlled luminescence spectrometer. *Analyst* 108:1067–1071.

93. de Mello, J. C., Wittmann, H. F., and Friend, R. H. 1997. An improved experimental determination of external photoluminescence quantum efficiency. *Advanced Materials* 9:230–232.

94. Semonin, O. E., Johnson, J. C., Luther, J. M., Midgett, A. G., Nozik, A. J., and Beard, M. C. 2010. Absolute photoluminescence quantum yields of IR-26 dye, PbS, and PbSe quantum dots. *The Journal of Physical Chemistry Letters* 1:2445–2450.

95. Jun, S. and Jang, E. 2005. Interfused semiconductor nanocrystals: Brilliant blue photoluminescence and electroluminescence. *Chemical Communications* 36:4616–4618.

96. Pan, D. C., Wang, Q., Jiang, S. C., Ji, X. L., and An, L. J. 2005. Synthesis of extremely small CdSe and highly luminescent CdSe/CdS core-shell nanocrystals via a novel two-phase thermal approach. *Advanced Materials* 17:176–178.

97. Wheeler, D. A., Fitzmorris, B. C., Zhao, H., Ma, D., and Zhang J. Z. 2011. Ultrafast exciton relaxation dynamics of PbS and core/shell PbS/CdS quantum dots. *Science China Chemistry* 54:2009–2015.

98. Wang, X., Qu, L., Zhang, J., Peng, X., and Xiao, M. 2003. Surface-related emission in highly luminescent CdSe quantum dots. *Nano Letters* 3(8):1103–1106.

99. Sadhu, S. and Patra, A. 2012. Lattice strain controls the carrier relaxation dynamics in $Cd_xZn_{1-x}S$ alloy quantum dots. *The Journal of Physical Chemistry C* 116:15167–15173.

100. Shafran, E., Mangum, B. D., and Gerton, J. M. 2010. Energy transfer from an individual quantum dot to a carbon nanotube. *Nano Letters* 10:4049–4054.

101. Schaller, R. D., Petruska, M. A., and Klimov, V. I. 2005. Effect of electronic structure on carrier multiplication efficiency: Comparative study of PbSe and CdSe nanocrystals. *Applied Physics Letters* 87:253102.

102. Semonin, O. E., Luther, J. M., Choi, S., Chen, H. Y., Gao, J., Nozik, A. J., and Beard, M. C. 2011. Peak external photocurrent quantum efficiency exceeding 100% via meg in a quantum dot solar cell. *Science* 334:1530–1533.
103. Stouwdam, W., Shan, J., vanVeggel, F. C. J. M., Pattantyus-Abraham, A. G., Young, J. F., and Raudsepp, M. 2007. Photostability of colloidal PbSe and PbSe/PbS core/shell nanocrystals in solution and in the solid state. *The Journal of Physical Chemistry C* 111:1086–1092.
104. Tang, J., Brzozowski, L., Barkhouse, D. A. R., Wang, X., Debnath, R., Wolowiec, R., Palmiano, E. et al. 2010. Quantum dot photovoltaics in the extreme quantum confinement regime: The surface- chemical origins of exceptional air- and light-stability. *ACS Nano* 4:869–878.
105. Cornacchio, A. L. P. and Jones, N. D. 2006. Thiolate-capped PbS nanocrystals in water: sensitivity to O_2, pH and concentration, an alternate pathway for crystal growth and a top-down synthesis. *Journal of Materials Chemistry* 16:1171–1177.
106. Koole, R., Liljeroth, P., Donega, C. M., Vanmaekelbergh, D., and Meijerink, A. 2006. Electronic coupling and exciton energy transfer in CdTe quantum-dot molecules. *Journal of the American Chemical Society* 128:10436–10441.
107. Zhang, T., Zhao, H., Riabinina, D., Chaker, M., and Ma, D. 2010. Concentration-dependent photoinduced photoluminescence enhancement in colloidal PbS quantum dot solution. *The Journal of Physical Chemistry C* 114:10153–10159.
108. Blaudeck, T., Zenkevich, E. I., Cichos, F., and von Borczyskowski, C. 2008. Probing wave functions at semiconductor quantum-dot surfaces by NON-FRET photoluminescence quenching. *The Journal of Physical Chemistry C* 112:20251–20257.
109. Derfus, A., Chan, W. C. W., and Bhatia, S. N. 2004. Probing the cytotoxicity of semiconductor quantum dots. *Nano Letters* 4:11–18.
110. Kirchner, C., Liedl, T., Kudera, S., Pellegrino, T., Javier, A., Gaub, H., Stölzle, S., Fertig, N., and Parak, W. 2005. Cytotoxity of colloidal CdSe and CdSe/ZnS nanoparticles. *Nano Letters* 5:331–338.
111. Hardman. R. A. 2006. Toxicologic review of quantum dots: Toxicity depends on physicochemical and environmental factors. *Environmental Health Perspectives* 114:165–172.

3

Quantum Dots for Bioimaging

Zoraida P. Aguilar

CONTENTS

3.1 Introduction

Nanomaterials exhibit unique size-tunable as well as shape-dependent physicochemical properties that do not resemble those of bulk materials. Recent advances in nanomaterials open new avenues to develop various novel biosensors. These nanomaterial-based biosensors, nanobiosensors, make use of the electrochemical and optical properties of nanomaterials. These nanobiosensors are expected to demonstrate an improved limit of detection, sensitivity, ease of use, portability, low cost, and selectivity.[1–3] The size of nanomaterials that is comparable to the dimensions of biomolecular probes and to biological analytes make them excellent components of biosensors.[4–10]

Among the most versatile nanomaterials are those which are called quantum dots (QDs). QDs are semiconductor nanomaterials with diameters ranging between 2 and 10 nm that are characterized by a broadband excitation wavelength and narrow emission wavelength. They emit size-dependent bright fluorescence that is very resistant to photobleaching. These unique properties make QDs a new class of fluorescent imaging labels for *in vitro* and *in vivo* biological applications.

QDs are usually synthesized in an organic medium making them purely hydrophobic. To make the QDs hydrophilic and biocompatible, they have to be converted to the water-soluble form. This conversion may be accomplished through the use of coating materials such as thiol-containing compounds or amphiphilic polymers with hydrophilic functional groups that make them water-soluble. The hydrophilic QDs usually have functional groups on the surface that can be covalently linked with biomolecules such as proteins, peptides, nucleic acids, or small-molecule ligands. Once these biomolecules are attached to QDs (QD-biomolecules), they can be used as biological labels for molecular and cellular imaging.

A QD nanobiosensor may use a solid surface called the capture platform (Figure 3.1). This capture platform may be a lab-on-a-chip, glass, silicon wafer, polymer, or other solid material that is coated with a capture receptor or capture probe. The capture probe is a biomolecule that specifically recognizes and collects the biological molecule of interest called the analyte. The capture probe can be a protein such as an antibody that captures a protein (antigen) in an immunoassay. The capture probe can also be a single strand of DNA that captures the analyte which is a complementary DNA in a DNA-assay. In the solid-phase nanobiosensor depicted in Figure 3.1, the detection probe is attached to a QD making it a QD-nanobiosensor. This sensor can be used to detect a biomolecule (DNA, protein, peptide, etc.), a whole cell, a virus, a microorganism, or a tissue.

In this chapter, the various fluorescence-imaging applications of QDs will be discussed. These applications will mainly focus on fluorescence imaging in protein immunoassays, DNA assays, whole-cell imaging *in vitro*, and *in vivo* animal imaging. Collectively, these various biomolecule-imaging applications will be called QD-based fluorescence-imaging nanobiosensors or simply QD nanobiosensors.

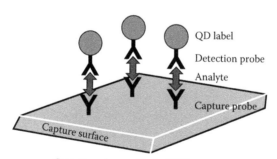

Capture probe = antibody, DNA, receptor
Analyte = protein, DNA, peptide, whole cell, virus, bacteria
Detection probe = antibody, DNA, receptor
Label for signal = QD

FIGURE 3.1
Schematic diagrams of QD-based nanobiosensor for a protein, DNA, peptide, whole cell, or whole organism.

3.2 Surface Modification of QDs for Nanobiosensors

The nanotechnology industry is receiving a lot of attention in the development of novel sensing systems, as well as in the enhancement of the performance of bioanalytical assays.[11–13] Current advances in materials science and synthetic chemistry have made it possible to produce high-quality quantum dots, and other nanomaterials[14,15] that are currently being used for the development of biosensors.[4,5,8–10,12,16–18] These nanomaterials offer significant advantages, which include (1) unique size-tunable properties, (2) a large surface-to-volume ratio, (3) lower energy consumption, (4) miniaturization, and (5) low cost.

A number of nanomaterials (NMs) for biosensing systems are getting more attention due to their size- and shape-dependent physical, chemical, and electrochemical properties.[19] An analyte detection binding event (i.e., an antibody–antigen interaction or a complementary DNA hybridization) occurring on the NMs' surface may have a significant effect on the NMs' optical (change of the light absorption/emission) or electrochemical properties (oxidation/reduction current), offering novel alternatives for biosensing. Enormous attention and interest are focused on inorganic semiconductor QDs composed of group II–VI elements (i.e., CdSe, ZnSe, CdTe, etc.).[20] According to Chan's group, "In comparison with organic dyes (such as rhodamine), QDs are highly fluorescent, 20 times brighter and 100 times more stable against photobleaching, and one third as wide in spectral line width."[21] With these characteristics, QDs present an enormous potential for fluorescence-imaging detection.

The most unique property of QDs for fluorescence imaging is the very small number of QDs required to acquire a signal. This property termed "blinking" or "flickering" is a phenomenon that is due to the presence of a small number of QDs.[21,22] QD blinking demonstrates that single QDs can be observed that may be in a monolayer condition, which is indicative of a sensitivity limit of one QD per target analyte. This property is made more versatile by the availability of QDs in a theoretically unlimited number of well-separated colors that are all excitable by a single wavelength, which can simplify image acquisition for multiple analytes during confocal microscopy.[21–23]

One of the most important aspects of QD application for fluorescence imaging is surface modification. A proper surface modification of QDs with different biomolecules offers great potential for attachment to various bioreceptors that can be used for analyte recognition (Figure 3.2). This indicates that the applications of QDs for biosensor development are strongly related to their properties that are controlled by the mode of synthesis, which is responsible for the quality of the resulting QDs and the post-synthesis modifications, both chemical and biological. The preparation of QDs and other NMs for biological applications, either in colloidal solutions or grown on solid substrates, has been extensively reviewed.[24] Not only is it possible to vary their size, shape, and composition, these can be tailored for specific binding affinities to different biomolecules through surface modification and meticulous nanoscale engineering. A QD-nanobiosensor can be specifically designed for the detection of cancer biomarkers, HER2 (human epidermal growth factor receptor 2). HER2 is encoded by the gene ERBB2 and is colocalized with the gene GRB7 that is associated with breast, testicular germ cell, gastric, and esophageal tumors.[25,26] The HER2 proteins have been found to form clusters on cell membranes that may be responsible for tumor formation.[25] Several studies have been published on the QD-based fluorescence imaging of HER2-bearing cancer cells using.[5,10,27]

For a QD to be effective in bioimaging applications, selective binding to a cell or tissue surface that can involve the adsorption of the nanoparticle to the proteins on the cell surface must occur.[28–30] However, proteins randomly bind to QDs, and this can be influenced

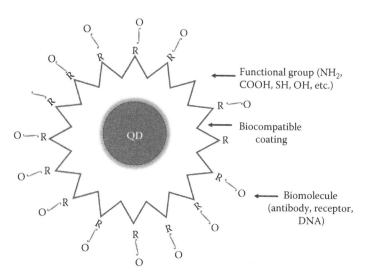

FIGURE 3.2
Schematic diagram of a QD that can be modified with different biomolecules for specific imaging biosensor applications.

by the properties of the nanoparticles, the biomolecule, the cell surfaces, as well as the environment surrounding the nanoparticles and the biological entities. In the presence of neutral groups such as CH_3- and polyethylene glycol (PEG) on the surface of the nanomaterials, low protein binding is observed, indicating that such groups have a low affinity for proteins. In the case of basic or acidic groups on NM surfaces, two mechanisms of protein binding occur: specific and nonspecific binding. To control the binding process and to quantify binding, specific binding is the mechanism of choice. Nonspecific binding is the choice for quick and qualitative QD-based imaging processes.

Specific binding: In a specific-binding interaction, the QD surface has to be modified so that only the target proteins or analyte will be recognized, which is the basic concept involved in a nanobiosensor. This process is made possible through QD surface modification that involves the attachment of specific receptors that target the proteins or analyte of interest; these analytes may be found on the surface of a particular cell or on tissues or organs. For example, a breast cancer cell may express certain proteins more extensively than a normal cell. One example of such a protein is the human epidermal receptor called HER2. Hence, a QD that is specifically engineered for imaging a breast cancer cell will be modified with a receptor for HER2 (i.e., antibody against HER2 or anti-HER2).

Nonspecific binding: During a nonspecific binding interaction, random binding between the QDs and proteins or any other components on the cell surfaces occurs.[31] In these processes, the charge on the surface of the QD and the overall charge on the exposed portion of the protein or the cell control the binding event. For instance, a positive QD surface can bind to an exposed negative portion of a protein surface or a negative cell surface. It is also possible for hydrophobic interactions to lead to nonspecific binding of the biomaterials to the QD and vice versa.

In either of these two binding processes, the orientation of proteins as they adsorb on the QD surface plays an important role in the stability of the binding. Both of these mechanisms can be used to bind the QD to small or large protein molecules as wells as cells, DNA, viruses, microorganisms, or tissues and organs. In either case, the surface modification of the QD has to be carried out to make it biocompatible.

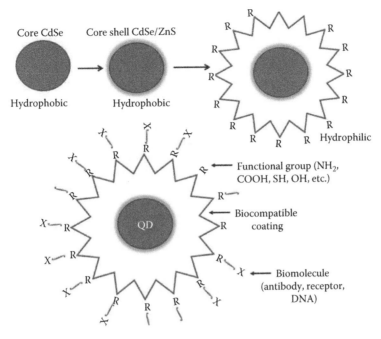

FIGURE 3.3
Schematic of converting hydrophobic QDs to hydrophilic QDs for fluorescence imaging.

The surface modification of the QD surface involves prior conversion from the organic-soluble form into the water-soluble form. Most NMs including QDs[32] are synthesized utilizing long-chain ligands such as oleic acid (C18) to control nucleation and particle growth. The QDs have to be converted into the water-soluble form by replacing the hydrophobic surface ligands with amphiphilic ligands through (1) ligand exchange with simple thiol-containing molecules[21,33,34] or more sophisticated ones such as oligomeric phosphines,[35] peptides,[36] and dendrons[37]; (2) encapsulation by a layer of amphiphilic diblock[38–41] or tri-block copolymers,[38] silanization,[42–45] polymer shells,[46] phospholipid micelles,[47,48] or amphiphilic polysaccharides[49]; and (3) a combinations of layers of different molecules.[32,43,50–53] All these strategies for surface modification result in water-soluble nanostructures.

For fluorescent tagging or labeling, it is important to have water-soluble QDs with stable physical and optical properties, which are not affected by environmental factors. The various methods of surface modifications that convert QDs from the hydrophobic into the hydrophilic form, allowing biocompatibility and the attachment of medically relevant molecules for nanobiosensor applications are discussed below (Figure 3.3).

3.2.1 Ligand Exchange

Ligand exchange is one of the methods by which the surfaces of QDs are modified to make them water-soluble in preparation for nanobiosensor development. A ligand can be an ion, atom, molecule, or functional group forming a complex with QDs that results in an interface between the core QDs or core/shell and the surroundings (Figure 3.3). Ligands are important for the various applications of QDs that involve interactions between the NM and its surroundings. Some ligands for nanomaterial ligand exchange include hexanethiol, dodecanethiol, octadecanethiol, trioctylphosphine, trioctylphosphine oxide, perfluorated lauric acid, oleic acid, didodecylamine, trioctyl aluminum, and a mixture of dodecanethiol and trioctylphosphine. The thiols and oleic acid increase the air stability,[54] while other ligands precipitate nanoparticles (perfluorated lauric acid and the mixture of dodecanethiol and trioctylphosphine). Ligand exchange can be accomplished by

- Dissolving the QDs in a solution containing the new ligand[21,55,56]
- Using a phase-transfer approach, where water-soluble particles are transferred to an organic phase (or vice versa) by adding a suitable ligand that acts as a phase-transfer agent such as mercapto acids that have been used to transfer CdTe QDs from an organic phase to an aqueous phase.[53,57,58]

Ligand exchange alters the solubility or even the electrophoretic mobility of QDs. However, it should be noted that ligand exchange has serious effects on the QD properties, especially their luminescence/fluorescence properties. This means that electrons in QDs that absorb energy from light can relax back to their ground state through luminescence, and the efficiency of this process crucially depends on the QDs' surface. Surface defects in the nanocrystal structure can act as a temporary trap for electrons preventing their radiative recombination.[32] Alternation between ion trapping and untrapping results in intermittent fluorescence (blinking) that is visible at the single-molecule level.[59,60] This process reduces the overall quantum yield, QY, which is the ratio of the emitted to the absorbed photons. To minimize or prevent these occurrences, as well as to protect surface atoms from oxidation and other chemical reactions, a shell consisting of a few atomic layers of a material with a larger bandgap is grown on top of the nanocrystal core. The shell can enhance photostability by several orders of magnitude compared with conventional dyes[50] and result in a QY close to 90%.[61] The ligands, which can passivate the trap states, can affect the luminescence efficiency of the semiconductor QDs; the change in luminescence can be used to monitor the ligand–QD interaction.[32]

Bifunctional ligands that contain one functional group that attaches at the QD surface and a second group that is exposed to the surroundings is one way to engineer very versatile QDs. This is demonstrated by the use of thiols that make CdSe QDs adsorb at gold surfaces or by polymeric materials such as PEG that carry either a carboxyl, amine, hydroxyl, or a combination of these functional groups (Figure 3.1). In a biosensor, the functional groups on the QDs are attached to probes, which provide affinity to a specific analyte. One such QD was prepared through encapsulation with an amphiphilic polymer upon which a pH-sensitive squaraine dye was conjugated.[62] In this structure, the CdSe/ZnS nanocrystal may either fluoresce or undergo fluorescence resonance energy transfer (FRET) to the squaraine dye. The FRET efficiency results from the dye's absorption profile that is controlled by pH while the ratio of the QD to dye emission is a measure of the pH of the environment.

3.2.1.1 Thiols for Ligand Exchange

Various thiols such as monothiols,[63–65] dithiothreitol,[33] bidentate thiols,[64,66] silanes/silanols,[42,64,66] oligomeric phosphines,[35,64] amine box dendrimers,[37,64,66] and amphiphilic saccharides[49,64] are used to prepare NMs for medical applications. For example, CdSe nanocrystals were coated with hydrophilic deprotonated thiol (thiolate) ligands and used in a pseudo–steady-state titration. These were used to determine the precipitation pH of nanocrystals coated by electron-donating ligands[67] in comparison with CdTe coated with the same types of ligands. The results showed that the ligands were removed from the surface due to protonation in a relatively low pH range, between 2 and 7 depending on the size.

The instability of QDs that are converted into the water-soluble form through thiol ligand exchange, has been solved by the direct adsorption of bifunctional ligands on the nanocrystal surface,[21] and by surface coating with a silica layer.[42] The direct adsorption of bifunctional ligands on the QD surface is carried out with both organic-soluble and water-soluble functional groups. The organic-soluble group orients towards the hydrophobic QDs, while the hydrophilic group projects away from the organic-soluble region toward the aqueous solution, resulting in water-soluble NMs.

Mercaptoacetic acid is used to make QDs water-soluble through the sulfur affinity to Zn atoms, while the carboxylic acid group is hydrophilic and reactive to biomolecules.[21] The surface modification process causes the fluorescence quantum yields to drop below 10% after water–solubilization,[68] and mercaptoacetic acid on the QD surface desorbs, leading to the aggregation and precipitation of the QDs. In a modification of this method, the attachment involves electrostatic interactions[52] and the use of dithiothreitol.[33]

Method for ligand exchange

This method was used to prepare water-soluble CdSe/CdS/ZnS QDs for imaging applications:[69]

1. Use acetone to precipitate organic soluble CdSe/CdS/ZnS QDs two times to remove free octadecylamine (ODA).

2. Disperse the purified QDs in chloroform and add 40 mg of polyethylene imine (PEI, MW 10 kDa) to 0.5 nmol of CdSe/CdS/ZnS QDs in chloroform.

3. Shake the mixture at room temperature for 2 h and evaporate the solvent under argon. This yields a QD film.

4. Dissolve the QD film with ultra-pure water (18 MΩ).

5. Centrifuge at 6000 g for 10 min, leading to a clear supernatant solution and white residue.

6. Dialyze the supernatant (MW cutoff = 50 kDa) against water or borate buffer solution (10 mM, pH 7.4) with at least three exchanges over 24 h to remove other impurities.

7. Store at 2°C–8°C until use.

3.2.2 Encapsulation of Nanomaterials

Encapsulation of QDs can be performed using polymer shells,[46] amphiphilic diblock or tri-block copolymers,[38] silica shells,[42,43] or phospholipid micelles.[47] Encapsulation can be used to introduce new functional groups on the QD surface such as carboxylic acids, amines, or hydroxides. Such functional groups can serve in the attachment of different biomolecules for nanobiosensor applications.

3.2.2.1 *Encapsulation with Silane*

Silane encapsulation of QDs leads to additional advantages. The silanized QDs remain stable over a wide range of pH, and eliminate the release of undesirable heavy elements. Additionally, the siloxane shell gives extra stability to the nanostructures. Silanization can be carried out by condensing alkoxysilanes either in acid or base medium, following the Stöber process,[45] which results in highly fluorescent silica-coated QDs. Yang et al.[70]

employed the reverse microemulsion method to coat CdTe nanocrystals with silica to avoid silane self-condensation. Various organosilanes in toluene are used to treat nanocrystals to carry out the multifunctionalization of semiconductor QDs.[71] One silane reagent, 3-mercaptopropyltrimethoxysilane, is used to displace the triocytlphosphine (TOPO) molecules and form a silica/siloxane shell on the QD surface by the introduction of a base and the hydrolysis of the silanol groups. Polymerization of the silanol groups prevents aggregation, making the QDs soluble in intermediate polar solvents, such as methanol and dimethyl sulfoxide. Further reaction with bifunctional methoxy compounds (i.e., aminopropyl trimethoxysilane) is used to convert the particles in the water-soluble form. The polymerized siloxane-coated QDs are more stable against aggregation compared with those formed with mercaptoacetic acid.

3.2.2.2 Polymer Coating

Water-soluble polymer-coated nanocrystals have been applied in biological studies.[72–76] The amphiphilic polymer-shell coating makes these NMs hydrophilic. Polymer coating of QDs is achieved by the reaction of the amphiphilic polymer, bis(6-aminohexyl)amine with surfactant-protected molecules that results in the cross-linking of the polymer chains around the nanoparticle that renders them water-soluble.[46] It has also been demonstrated that biomolecules and phospholipid micelles can be covalently linked with semiconductor QDs.

A series of PEG-terminated dihydrolipoic acids (DHLA–PEG) have been used as capping substrates.[66,77] These were produced from thioctic acid and polyethylene glycols (PEGs) simple esterification schemes, followed by the reduction of the 1,2-dithiolane. The exchange reaction of trioctylphosphine (TOP)/TOPO-capped QDs with these substrates led to water-soluble QDs that were stable over time in a broad pH range, from weakly acidic to basic conditions (pH 5–12). However, these could not be used for specific applications because of the lack of functional end groups for easy conjugation techniques. This was solved by Uyeda's group (74) that studied the design and synthesis of ligands functionalized with a biotin end group. They designed ligands with a central tetraethylene glycol (TEG) section, a dithiol terminal group for attachment on the QD surface, and a biotin at the end of the QD surface—which allowed for avidin–biotin binding that was useful for the attachment of proteins and other biomolecules on the QD surface.

Chitosan, a polysaccharide consisting of randomly distributed β-(1–4)-linked D-glucosamine (deacetylated unit) and N-acetyl-D-glucosamine (acetylated unit) provides a natural, biocompatible, cationic, and hydrophilic polymer coating that is suitable for the affinity purification of proteins and magnetic bioseparation.[78] Dextran, a polysaccharide, has also been applied in coating NMs.

A coating method for the biosensor application of QDs involves the use of different cyclodextrins.[79,80] The hydrophobic pockets of the polysaccharide interact with the aliphatic chains of the TOPO present on the QD surface, wherein the immobilized cyclodextrins retain their capability of engaging molecular recognition. This phenomenon and the observed fluorescence changes during analyte–binding make this method very promising for possible sensor applications.[80] Similar to this approach is the use of calixarenes, which are similar organic cyclic systems[81,82] that preserve the emission intensity of the QDs and their small diameter. Calixarenes are cyclic oligomers formed from the hydroxyalkylation of phenol and an aldehyde. These could be functionalized with sugars or peptides to allow biological applications of the resulting coated QDs.[81]

Here, we highlight the method for the amphiphilic polymer-coating of nanomaterials, which is adopted from Hessel's paper.[83]

Synthesis of the amphiphilic polymer

1. Use a capped, single-neck round-bottom flask, for 100 mL of anhydrous tetrahydrofuran (THF), 15 mmol dodecylamine (about 3.45 mL), and poly(isobutylene-*alt*-maleic anhydride) (20 mmol of monomer units, 3.084 g) are added sequentially to form a turbid white solution.

2. Sonicate for 1 min to dissolve the remaining solids.

3. Heat the mixture to 60°C for 3 h with vigorous stirring for 15 min after which the mixture becomes clear. This indicates that the polymer is dissolved in THF through covalent coupling to the hydrophobic dodecylamine molecules.

4. Bring the temperature down to room temperature (RT).

5. Decrease the volume down to 20 mL using a rotary evaporator.

6. Bring the temperature of the clear solution to 60°C with constant stirring for 12 h, to allow complete coupling between the polymer and dodecylamine.

7. Bring down to room temperature and dry the remaining solvent with a rotary evaporator. At the end of this process, a pale yellow, solid amphiphilic polymer is left in the flask.

8. Transfer the flask containing the polymer to a nitrogen-filled glovebox (<0.1 ppm O_2).

9. Add 25 mL of anhydrous $CHCl_3$ to give a monomer unit concentration of 0.8 M.

10. Leave the amphiphilic polymer solution in a glass vial in the glovebox until use.

Coating the QDs with polymer[83]

1. In a 50 mL round-bottom flask, mix the amphiphilic polymer stock solution (0.8 M monomer units in $CHCl_3$, 53 µL), and alkyl-Si QDs at 3.0 mg/mL in anhydrous $CHCl_3$, 0.40 mL, and anhydrous $CHCl_3$ (2.55 mL). You may use other nanoparticles as well.

2. Vortex the mixture and stir with a magnetic stirrer for 15 min at room temperature.

3. Remove the solvent by rotary evaporation to yield a yellow Si-polymer film on the inner wall of the flask.

4. Add an aqueous sodium borate buffer (SBB) (50 mM borate, 2.0 mL, pH 12) and stir for 15 min at room temperature to disperse the Si-polymer.

5. Add 13.0 mL of DI water to dilute the nanomaterials.

6. Pass the suspension through a 0.2 µm-pore syringe filter (Corning, PES membrane), followed by a 0.1 µm-pore syringe filter (Whatman, inorganic membrane).

7. Place the filtered nanocrystal solution in an ultracentrifugation filter (Amicon Ultra, regenerated cellulose membrane, 50 kDa molecular weight cutoff) and centrifuge at 4000× g for 4 min at RT.

8. Discard the colorless filtrate and retain the concentrated NMs solution above the membrane.

9. Dilute the QDs solution with 15.0 mL of sterile-filtered phosphate-buffered saline (PBS, 150 mM, pH 7.4).

10. Repeat the ultracentrifugation two more times using PBS to dilute the retained QDs solution.

11. Store the final aqueous QDs solution in a glass tube under ambient conditions until use.

12. Characterize the amphiphilic polymer-coated QDs.

3.3 Bioconjugation

The immobilization of capture probes in QD nanobiosensors requires strategies that will protect the integrity of the QD and the probes, thereby keeping them active. The bioactivity of the probes in the QD-bound stage is maintained through proper immobilization strategies that involve the control of orientation to keep the active conformation of the biomolecules. The active conformation of the biomolecules controls the stability and reproducibility of signals.[5,10,84–87] Nonspecific adsorption of biomolecules such as proteins,[88–90] DNA,[31,84,85,89,91] whole cells,[9,10,31,85,89,92,93] and microorganisms adsorb on the QD surfaces can cause the inactivation of the targeting biomolecules.[31,94,95] This process can be circumvented with the use of a linker, which provides a small distance between the capture surface and the target analyte.[96–99] A covalent attachment is generally preferred over adsorption because of the possibility to control the binding orientation between the QD and the capture probe.[93,100] Additionally, QDs like other NMs, possess a high surface-to-volume ratio with a porous network structure that alleviates surface fouling effects that can lead to the enhanced retention of bioactivity. This results in a large amount of captured biological molecules (e.g., enzyme, antibody, cell, and DNA) that are immobilized on the active surface of the QD-bound probes, leading to an intense response signal.[100]

3.3.1 Direct Adsorption

Direct adsorption is one of the ways by which QDs can be modified for imaging applications. Direct adsorption had been used in developing nanomaterial-based biosensors for the detection of DNA,[101,102] proteins,[93,103–106] whole cells,[10,31,102,107,108] and parts of cells.[31,106,109]

The group of Ehrenberg determined the time course of protein adsorption through the incubation of -COOH-functionalized nanoparticles in serum.[106] Protein adsorption on the nanoparticle surface was shown to take seconds and reached a plateau in less than 5 min. A constant amount of protein was adsorbed in less than 5 min indicating rapid adsorption compared with cellular binding. This relative speed was also reported in the literature, demonstrating adsorption rate constants on the order of seconds[105] compared to the time scale of at least a few more minutes for attachment to cell surfaces.

Studies have shown that nanoparticles adsorb to proteins on the surface of endothelial cells.[106] Quantification exhibited that high-binding nanoparticles were maximally coated in seconds to minutes, which indicated that proteins on cell surfaces can mediate cell association. The cellular association was not dependent on the identity of the adsorbed proteins, which indicated that during adsorption, there is no need for specific binding to any particular cellular receptor. These results demonstrated that nanoparticle-surface chemistry mediated the protein adsorption during nonspecific interactions, which account for a large portion of the nanoparticle-binding to endothelial cell surfaces. Their results also indicated that carboxyl-based surface chemistry, which are covalently modified with bioreceptors, reduced the nonspecific protein-binding of the nanoparticles on the cells.[106] Nonspecific adsorption was observed the least from positively charged lysine, followed by the neutral groups, CH_3, and cysteine, and the greatest from PEG.

The direct adsorption of biomolecules on nanomaterials is fast and easy to perform following conventional adsorption techniques.[103] Adsorption results from hydrophobic interaction or electrostatic interaction between the biomolecules and the nanoparticle surface. It has been used for the detection of specific nucleic acid (NA) sequences that has important applications in medical research and diagnosis.[11,18,19,85,91,110–113] In most cases, specific sequences are identified through the hybridization of an immobilized probe that is complementary to the target NA after the latter has been modified with a covalently linked fluorescent or enzyme label.[11,85,89,91,110,114]

3.3.2 Covalent Binding

The alternative way to avoid the instability and inactivation of biomolecules is to covalently bind to QD surfaces.[4,5,9,10,92,96,115] Low-molecular bifunctional linkers, which have the anchor groups for their attachment to NM surfaces and the functional groups for their covalent coupling to the target biomolecules, have been extensively used in the generation of covalent-tethered conjugates of biomolecules with various NMs.[116] Anchor groups such as thiols, disulfides, or phosphine ligands are often used for the binding of the bifunctional linkers to QDs such as CdS, CdSe, and other NMs.[117] Various terminal functional groups such as amine, active ester, and maleimide groups are commonly used to covalently couple biological compounds by means of carbodiimide-mediated esterification and amidation reactions or through reactions with thiol groups.[116]

The covalent conjugation of biomolecules to nanomaterials may be done following conventional bioconjugation techniques with a slight modification.[118] These methods are useful for the conjugation of proteins, oligonucleotides,[119] or other molecules to various types of functionalized nanomaterials[4,5,11,19,120–122] that are used for the detection of cells,[10,31,115,123] proteins,[93] DNA,[4,5,11,121,124] and microorganisms. There are two methods to conjugate biomolecules to NMs: (1) the one-step method and (2) the two-step method. These methods are described next.

3.3.2.1 One-Step Conjugation

The following step-by-step protocol is recommended for the one-step conjugation protocol.[4,5,10,92,96] Conjugating a protein or DNA or other molecules to NMs must be optimized for each type of biomolecule. An NM-to-biomolecule molar ratio of 1:1–1:50 is recommended depending upon the need of the studies as well as the stability of the NMs. Low molar ratios are recommended for expensive biomolecules.

Chemicals

1. 1–1.25 nmol of QDs with carboxyl groups (QD-COOH) on the surface that are dispersed in 100–125 μL of deionized (DI) water.
2. Freshly prepared solution containing 1 mg of *N*-ethyl-*N*′-dimethylaminopropyl-carbodiimide (EDC) in 0.5 mL of buffer A.
3. Buffer A: 1.5 mL of 0.01 M H_3BO_3, pH 5.5.
4. Buffer B: 0.1 mL of 1 M glycine or 1 M lysine.
5. Buffer C: 3 mL 0.01 M of 0.01 M H_3BO_3, pH 7.2.
6. Biomolecules (protein, DNA, etc.) in 0.01 M H_3BO_3 (or PBS), pH 7.0–7.4. If the biomolecule is in a different buffer and/or contains glycerol, these must be removed through dialysis, ultracentrifugation, or spin filtration to replace the buffer with H_3BO_3.

Method

1. Transfer 1–1.25 nmol of the QD-COOH into a low-protein-binding centrifuge tube.
2. Place 300 μL of buffer A and vortex.
3. Add the appropriate amount of biomolecule from the stock solution (a 10 mg/mL stock solution is advised but dilute solutions are usable except that the reagents will also be diluted so the reaction may take longer) to have a QD:protein ratio between 1:1 and 1:50 and mix well. The QD:biomolecule ratio has to be optimized to prevent precipitation/aggregation.
4. Add 50 μL of the fresh EDC solution and mix well.
5. React at room temperature for 1–2 h, with constant gentle shaking.
6. Add 10 μL of buffer B and react for another 15 min.
7. Purification can be accomplished with dialysis, ultracentrifugation, or spin filtration.
8. Wash three times with buffer C.
9. Reconstitute with buffer C to 4 μM QD, or as desired. This will be the QD–biomolecule.
11. Prepare a 1%–1.5% agarose gel at 100 V for 30–40 min with the original QD and the QD–biomolecule to verify the conjugation efficiency.
12. Store the QD–biomolecule conjugates at 2°C–8°C until use. Use of a low-percent (0.02%–0.05%) sodium azide can prevent contamination. Keep the QD–biomolecule conjugates at 2°C–8°C for 1–3 months depending upon the aseptic conditions during the conjugation process. The shelf-life has to be optimized and established.

3.3.2.2 Two-Step Conjugation

Some QD conjugations with biomolecules require a two-step process to maintain colloidal stability in the aqueous solution.[125] Conjugating a protein, DNA, or other molecules to QDs must be optimized for each type of biomolecule and each type of QD. A QD-to-biomolecule molar ratio of 1:1–1:50 is recommended depending upon the need of the studies. Low molar ratios are recommended for larger and expensive biomolecules. It is recommended that all parameters be optimized on a case-to-case basis.

Chemicals

1. 1–1.25 nmol of QDs (QD-COOH) in 100–125 μL of ultrapure water.
2. 2 mg of *N*-ethyl-*N*′-dimethylaminopropyl-carbodiimide (EDC) in 0.5 mL buffer A.
3. 1 mg of NHS (sulfo-*N*-hydroxysuccinimide).
4. Buffer A consists of 1.5 mL of 0.01 M H_3BO_3, pH 5.5.
5. Buffer B consists of 2 mL of 0.01 M H_3BO_3, pH 8.5.
6. Buffer C contains 0.1 mL of 1 M glycine or 1 M lysine.
7. Buffer D contains 3 mL of 0.01 M of 0.01M H_3BO_3, pH 7.2.
8. Biomolecules (protein, DNA, etc.) in 0.01M H_3BO_3 (or PBS), pH 7.0 to 7.4. If the biomolecule is in a different buffer, and/or contains glycerol and other preservatives, these must be purified through dialysis, ultracentrifugation, or spin filtration to replace the buffer with H_3BO_3.

Method

1. Transfer 1–1.25 nmol of the QDs-COOH into a low-protein-binding tube.
2. Combine the 2 mg of EDC and 1 mg of NHS and add 1 mL Buffer D.
3. Transfer 300 µL of buffer A to the QDs tube and mix well.
4. Add 80 µL of fresh EDC/NHS solution and mix well.
5. Incubate with shaking for 5–20 min then add 500 µL of buffer B.
6. Add the appropriate amount of biomolecule (that may be a protein such as an antibody or bovine serum albumin, BSA) from the stock solution (a 10 mg/mL stock solution is advised but dilute solutions are usable except that the reagents will also be diluted so the reaction may take longer) and mix well.
7. React at room temperature for 1–2 h with gentle shaking.
8. Add 10 µL of buffer C and react for another 15 min.
9. Remove all excess reagents by dialysis, ultracentrifugation, or spin filtration.
10. Purify by washing three times with buffer D.
11. Reconstitute with buffer D to 4 µM QD or as desired.
12. Run the original unconjugated QD and the QD–biomolecule in 1%–1.5% agarose gel at 100 V for 30–40 min to verify the conjugation efficiency.
13. Keep the purified QD–biomolecule conjugates at 4°C until use.

Although these protocols may be applied to various types of QDs with carboxyl groups on the surface, the conditions for each type of QD may vary. Thus, for each type of QD and for each type of biomolecule, the conditions for conjugation must be optimized.

Figure 3.4 is an example of a 1.5% agarose gel electrophoresis of QDs with carboxyl groups on the surface, thereby allowing them to migrate toward the positive electrode. The right lane contains the unconjugated QDs and the left lane contains the QD–BSA conjugate. The results indicate the retardation of migration toward the positive pole after conjugation, which is expected as the surface of the QD gets covered with the proteins. Both the QD and QD–BSA show a slight tailing on the gel, which is indicative of the insignificant particle size distribution of the QDs.

3.3.3 Quantification of Biomolecules Loaded on QDs

Surface modification of QDs is one of the preliminary steps in the preparation of nanobiosensors. Complete coverage of the QD surface with the biomolecules and the blocking agent is essential, to eliminate the nonspecific adsorption of analytes on the QD. Thus, it is very important to know the amount of bioreceptors on the surface of QDs before the capture of the analyte of interest. The number of immobilized bioreceptors on the QD surface is directly proportional to the amount of analyte that binds with the capture probe. To quantify the amount of analyte captured by the nanobiosensor, a calibration curve is used as a standard for each nanobiosensor.

In protein immunoassays, the capture probe that is immobilized on the QD surface can be an antibody, a hapten, or an immunogen. Taking a protein immunoassay for the detection of an antigen as a model, the conjugation of the detector antibody to the QD is the first step in the preparation of this type of nanobiosensors. To generate the heterogeneous QD–nanobiosensor depicted in Figure 3.1, the capture probes are first immobilized

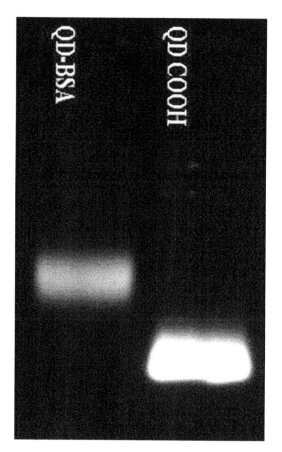

FIGURE 3.4
Agarose gel electrophoresis of QD with and without conjugated BSA.

on a solid substrate.[5,9,10,86,91–92,96] This is followed by exposure to the analyte source or the sample containing the analyte of interest. The assay is completed by exposure to the QD–biomolecule that was engineered in the previous section. The following is a description of the entire sandwich-type immunoassay for the detection of the well-studied mouse IgG that will be used as the model analyte.

Chemicals

1. 1–1.25 nmol of QDs with carboxyl groups (QD-COOH) on the surface in 100–125 mL of deionized water.
2. 2 mg of *N*-ethyl-*N'*-dimethylaminopropyl-carbodiimide (EDC) in 0.5 mL of buffer A.
3. 1 mg of NHS (sulfo-*N*-hydroxysuccinimide).
4. Buffer A: 1.5 mL of 0.01 M H_3BO_3, pH 5.5.
5. Buffer B: 2 mL of 0.01 M H_3BO_3, pH 8.5.
6. Buffer C: 0.1 mL of 1 M glycine or 1 M lysine.
7. Buffer D: 3 mL 0.01 M of 0.01 M H_3BO_3, pH 7.2.

8. Goat antimouse IgG (GAM) in 0.01 M H_3BO_3 (or PBS), pH 7.0–7.4. If the GAM is in a different buffer and/or contains glycerol, these must be removed through dialysis, ultracentrifugation, or spin filtration to replace the buffer with H_3BO_3.

9. Donkey antigoat IgG-HRP (DAG-HRP), 20 µg/mL in 0.01 M H_3BO_3 (or PBS), pH 7.0.

10. TMB-tetramethylbenzidene.

11. Blocking buffer.

Method for quantifying the number of immobilized antibodies (Ab) on the QDs surface
Preparation of the antibody-modified QD:

1. Pipet 1 nmol of the QD-COOH into a low-protein-binding centrifuge tube. If the QD-COOH is dilute, concentrate (by ultracentrifugation) down to 4 uM.

2. In a separate tube, mix the 2 mg of EDC and 1 mg of NHS and add 1 mL Buffer D.

3. Add 300 µL of buffer A to the QD-COOH and vortex to mix well.

4. Add 80 µL of the fresh EDC/NHS solution and vortex to mix well.

5. Incubate with shaking for 5–20 min.

6. Add 500 µL of buffer B and mix well.

7. Prepare a 4 mM anti-BSA solution in water. Quantify the Ab by taking the OD at 280 nm (Ab280).

8. Add 20 nmol (5 µL) of the anti-BSA to create a 1QD:20 Ab ratio and mix well. (Lower or higher QD-to-Ab ratio may also be used depending upon the stability of the resulting antibody-modified QD. This has to be optimized on a case-to-case basis depending upon the nature and the size of the QD).

9. React at room temperature for 1–2 h with constant gentle shaking.

10. Add 10 µL of buffer C and react for another 15 min.

11. Purify by ultracentrifugation and save the supernatant for leftover Ab quantification (Sup280).

12. Wash three times with buffer D.

13. Take 20–100 µL of the QD-anti-BSA and 80–100 µL of buffer D.

14. Reconstitute with buffer D to get the desired concentration.

15. Run the original QD-COOH and the QD-anti-BSA in 1%–1.5% agarose gel at 100 V for 30–40 min to verify the conjugation efficiency. The QD-anti-BSA (QD-Ab) should migrate slower than the QD-COOH.

To quantify the number of Ab per QD:

1. Take the absorbance of the supernatant at 280 nm (Sup280).

2. Take the absorbance of 4 µL of water in 10 µL of buffer C in 500 µL buffer B+ 80 µL EDC/NHS+ 300 µL of buffer A(Solv280).

3. Prepare a calibration curve of Ab at 280 nm using 1, 2, 4,8, 10, 20, and 50 nM Ab in water.

4. Calculate the absorptivity constant (α) of Ab using

$$A = \alpha\, bC$$

where
  A is the absorbance at 280
  b is the path length
  C is the nM concentration of Ab.

5. Calculate the concentration of Ab on the QD-Ab as follows:

$$C \text{ of Ab on QD} \sim Ab = \frac{[Ab280 - (Sup280 + Solv280)]}{\alpha\, b}$$

6. Calculate the number of Ab per QD as follows:

$$\text{Nanomole Ab per QD} = \frac{C \text{ of Ab on QD} - Ab \times 5\,\mu L}{1 \text{ nmol QD}}$$

3.4 Bioimaging Applications

The size-dependent optical and electrochemical properties of QDs offer various signal transduction modes, including simultaneous approaches (optical and electrochemical) that are not available with other materials.[4,5,11,12,115,126,129–131] The range of potential applications of nanobiosensors depends on the QD properties, the biomolecules to detect, as well as the type of sample to be analyzed. Nanobiosensors can be used for the detection of DNA, protein, bacteria, virus, and cell analysis using fluorescence imaging.[4,5,9,82,115,122,129,132–135]

Conventional colorimetric methods that use organic dyes for imaging applications have been in existence for a long time.[136,137] These have been used for DNA, proteins, bacteria, virus, cells, and other biomolecules.[2,137–141] These have been coupled with polymerase chain reaction (PCR), HPLC, ELISA, and other assays. In combination with molecular fluorophore, these assays offer a high sensitivity of detection, but they suffer from several drawbacks that include complex handling procedures, easy contamination, high cost, and lack of portability.[4,11,96,120–122,142–144] Hence, QDs offer simple detection alternatives that are more sensitive, more stable, and more reproducible and have recently also dominated the literature.[9,92] QDs are extensively used in fluorescent biosensors even though they are toxic.

3.4.1 Immunoassay

QDs have been reported for the imaging of proteins in immunoassays.[4,65,82,96,132,135,145,146] Mouse IgG was used as a model protein in the development of a QD-based fluorescence immunoassay for proteins[96] on a solid platform. The capture antibody was covalently immobilized on the silanized glass slide. The mouse IgG was captured on the antibody-modified silanized microscope glass slide. To complete the assay, the capture slide was exposed to QD-conjugated goat antimouse IgG. In Figure 3.4, the red dots indicate that the mouse IgG was captured on a glass slide and labeled in a sandwich-type complex consisting of rabbit antimouse IgG + mouse IgG + QD-goat antimouse IgG. The results showed that the mouse IgG protein was successfully captured and imaged using QD–goat anti-mouse

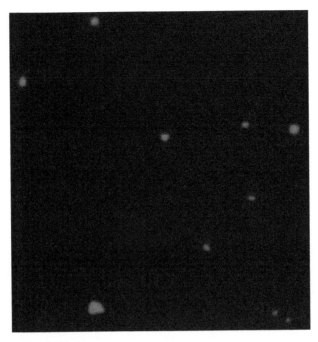

FIGURE 3.5
QD-based fluorescence imaging sensor for mouse IgG proteins.

IgG conjugates. The proteins appeared as bright red-colored dots under a UV-illuminated microscope (Figure 3.5). The QD-based fluorescent detection of the protein mouse IgG was stable at 4°C even after a couple of weeks. This system demonstrated the use of QDs for the protein-imaging sensor application. These results were very promising for applications in clinical diagnosis, environmental monitoring, food analysis, and biological applications.

3.4.2 DNA Assay

In a separate study, total internal reflection fluorescence microscopy (TIRFM) was combined with fluorescent quantum dot (QD)–labeling, into an ultrasensitive single-molecule detection (SMD) method for the quantification of DNA.[102] In this chapter, the capture DNA that was immobilized on a silanized coverslip was used to detect the target DNA (tDNA) after the QD-labeled DNA probe was hybridized with the tDNA. The images of the QD-labeled hybridized DNA were recorded with a highly sensitive CCD. The captured tDNA was quantified by counting the bright spots on the images and later compared against a calibration curve that gave an LOD of 10 pM. The parameters that affected the signal included image acquisition, fluorescence probe, substrate preparation, noise elimination from solutions and glass coverslips, and nonspecific adsorption/binding of solution-phase detection probes. Lia's method is also applicable for quantifying messenger RNA (mRNA) in cells.

The QD-based detection of the hybridization and cleavage of DNA was reported by Willner and coworkers.[120] DNA/QD conjugates were initially hybridized with the complementary Texas Red–labeled DNA. The addition of DNase I resulted in the cleavage of DNA and the partial recovery of the fluorescence emission of QDs. The previous studies used organic dyes as quenchers, which have promoted the development of biosensing. Au NPs have been demonstrated to be more efficient quenchers than conventional organic dyes.

The nonradiative quenching of QD emission by Au NPs is due to long-distance dipole–metal interactions that extend significantly beyond the classical Förster distance (~6 nm). The quenching efficiency strongly depends on the particle size and the quenching constant increases with an increase in the Au NP size, because the absorption cross section of Au NPs is the main parameter affecting the energy transfer efficiency. The assembly with QDs as the donor and the Au NP as the acceptor is extremely attractive for bioassays.

3.4.3 Whole-Cell Imaging *In Vitro*

Several QD-based fluorescence whole-cell imaging sensors that offer rapid, reproducible, accurate, and long-term cell staining system were recently reported.[4,5,9,38,92,115,147–149] Xu and his group developed a fluorescence QD–based cell imaging system on a glass slide (Figure 3.6).[10] The solid-phase QD-based imaging sensor involved the capture of whole cells

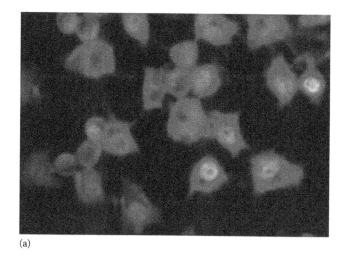

(a)

(b)

FIGURE 3.6
(See color insert.) QD-fluorescence imaging sensors for breast cancer cell line SK-BR3 (under white light, (a)) that appeared red with greenish nucleus that was stained with DAPI under UV light (b).

with highly specific antibodies (Ab) against the overexpressed cell-membrane proteins. The capture antibodies against the cell-membrane proteins were covalently immobilized on silanized-glass microscope slides. After immobilization on the silanized-glass slide, the whole cells were exposed to a second antibody against epithelial cell adhesion molecule (EpCAM) proteins that are found on the surface of the cells. The complete assay is a sandwich-type assay. To complete the sensor, QD-labeled antibodies against the anti-EpCAM were exposed to the assay complex. To detect the signal, QDs (attached to the EpCAM or to another antibody against the anti-EpCAM) emitting at 620 nm giving a red color rendered the cells as bright red circular objects under a UV-illuminated microscope (Figure 3.6). The cells were stained with DAPI (4′,6-diamidino-2-phenylindole) to differentiate the nucleus (seen as bluish green) from the membrane proteins. The QD-based fluorescent whole-cell imaging sensor exhibited brighter signals compared with those using the organic dye. About 5000 cells were detected using about 1 pmol of QD in an unoptimized system. This QD-based whole-cell fluorescent imaging biosensor showed great promise for application in clinical diagnosis, food analysis, environmental monitoring, and other biological/biomedical applications.

Novel composite NMs, such as QD–carbon nanotubes and QD–graphene oxides, are among the emerging NMs that are efficient candidates for fluorescent biosensors. Applications of graphene oxide have been reported for biosensors because of its facile surface modification, high mechanical strength, good water-dispersibility, and photoluminescence.[150] Aside from the advantageous planar structure that facilitates electron and energy transportation, graphene oxide is also the ideal support for nanoparticle loading. Jung and coworkers reported a graphene oxide–based immunobiosensor for rotavirus pathogen detection with high sensitivity and selectivity. This sensor was based on the photoluminescence quenching of graphene oxides through the FRET process induced by the Au NPs. In this study, the antibody-modified graphene oxides could recognize the pathogen due to the specific antigen–antibody interaction showing a detection limit of 10^5 pfu/mL, which was comparable with that of the conventional ELISA technique. In another study, carbon nanotubes were demonstrated to be efficient fluorescence quenchers in biosensors.[119] The carbon nanotubes' high stability and mechanical strength allow their use in a stringent detection environment.

3.4.4 *In Vivo* Animal Imaging

The upsurge of molecular-imaging instruments enabled the characterization of the molecular status of tumors and cancer within living animals.[16] Deep-tissue multiphoton microscopy is used to image cells in three dimensions with high sensitivity plus high spatial and temporal resolution but the tissue penetration of light is low while conventional fluorophores have insufficient brightness or stability for effective visualization. The use of QDs for live-cell and live-animal imaging overcomes these issues. Research abound on the use of QDs for live-animal imaging, particularly in the near-infrared and infrared regions that present superior brightness and a deeper penetration of the skin and tissue allowing detection in deep sites.[16] QDs have exhibited long-term stability and brightness that facilitate detection *in vivo* and long-term use. QDs can be used to label live mammalian cells through functionalization with specific probes, allowing up to 2 billion QDs to be delivered to the nucleus of a single cell without altering function or viability. QD-labeled cells have been used in embryogenesis,[151] cancer metastasis,[152] and stem-cell therapy[153] with multiplexing for multiple markers. QD-labeled B16 melanoma cells injected into the tail veins of mice were found in the lung, liver, and spleen,[152] enabling the tracking of the distribution of the B16 melanoma cells with single-cell sensitivity. QD-labeled dendritic cells were studied to track their migration after injection into mice foot pads.[154] This was very important in understanding the use of dendritic cell-based vaccination, which also allowed the imaging of the cells as well as real-time longitudinal studies without frequent animal sacrifice for improved experimental control, reduced cost, and diminished animal suffering. QDs conjugated with luciferase facilitated the live-animal imaging[155] with enhanced sensitivity in small animals. All these QD-based animal-imaging studies allowed the visualization at deep sites in tissues while eliminating the effect of tissue autofluorescence. QDs have also been demonstrated for tracking antibodies in *in vivo* experiments.[16]

3.5 Applications

Today, a few *in vitro* diagnostic products using NMs have penetrated the market with an estimated $0.78 billion in sales for 2004,[156] with projected sales of $9.5 billion dollars in 2013.[163] NMs are used for novel sensors and *in vitro* tests, which offer the following advantages: improve the sensitivity of existing tests; allow for point-of-care applications, or to develop new diagnostic test platforms. The platforms include DNA nanobiosensors[127,128] that provide powerful tools for the rapid and sensitive determination of pathogens, diseases, genetic disorders, drug screening, and other *in vitro* diagnostic applications.[157] One such nanobiosensor is an ultrasensitive single-molecule detection (SMD) method for the quantification of DNA coupled with total internal reflection fluorescence microscopy (TIRFM).[102] For this sensor, a silanized coverslip was used to immobilize the capture DNA. The capture surface was blocked with ethanolamine and bovine serum albumin. The capture DNA was next exposed to the target DNA (tDNA) and signal detection was carried out with a QD-labeled DNA probe that was complementary to the tDNA. Using TIRFM, fluorescent images of the QD-based sandwich-DNA hybridization assay were taken with a highly sensitive CCD. The tDNA was quantified by counting the bright spots on the images showing 1×10^{-14} mol/L limit of detection for the imaging sensor.[102]

QDs are used as protein immunosensors because they exhibit a higher surface area–to-volume ratio that provides a larger active surface area for higher detection sensitivity. Properly functionalized QDs allow surface engineering for a variety of architectures on the surface that consists of biomolecules such as enzymes or antibodies for biorecognition events. Since proteins (e.g., enzymes, peptides, and antigens) have dimensions that are comparable to QDs, it is possible that biomolecule–QD systems may provide new materials for a new generation of biosensors with excellent prospects for interfacing biological recognition events with signal transduction, giving high sensitivity.

QDs have been reported for the fluorescence-imaging detection of proteins, cells, and other biological molecules in different substrates.[4,5,9,10,16,38,40,92,96,148,149] These biosensors proved to be superior to conventional organic dye-based fluorescence imaging. One of these studies used mouse IgG as the model analyte. The process used the covalent attachment of the capture antibody that was used to capture the analyte. The assay was completed with QD-Ab against the mouse IgG where the QD emits at 620 nm. The captured proteins appeared as bright red fluorescent images under a fluorescence microscope. This QD-based fluorescence-imaging sensor for mouse IgG was stable at 4°C for more than 2 weeks.

The growing applications of NMs have indicated new prospects for exploring living cells for the evaluation of chemical species in specific organelles. The exploitation of the unique properties of these NMs indicates a possible ultrasensitive nanoscale detection of a cell and its components. This requires a proper interfacing of biological recognition probes with the surface-modified NMs such as QDs, which can provide excellent solutions to meet biointerfacing requirements, owing to their tailorable physical and chemical properties by varying size, composition, and shape at the nanoscale.[3,158,159] NPs are very effective in the sensing of whole cells that include human cells and bacterial cells for *in vitro* diagnosis because of their nanoscale dimensions.

Semiconductor QDs have been used to detect whole cancer cells that overexpress HER2, a surface-coating protein that is found in breast cancer cell lines such as SKBR3.[4,9,10,92,115] Studies have used carboxyl-functionalized CdSe/ZnS emitting at 620 nm and/or 530 nm that were covalently conjugated with antibodies against HER2. When exposed to suspended or adherent SKBR3 cells *in vitro*, the QD-labeled probes adhered to the cells. Adherent cells were immediately inspected under the microscope while suspended cells were mounted on glass slides before taking microscope images using a UV-light source. The studies indicated that the fluorescent cancer cells were detected more easily and over a longer time frame than the cells that were stained with antibodies conjugated with the organic dye. A method for whole-cell QD-based fluorescent imaging is discussed next.

3.5.1 Procedure for QD-Based Detection of Breast Cancer Cells

A breast cancer cell imaging sensor using QDs has been reported.[10] The QD-fluorescence imaging sensor used a silanized glass slide as the solid capture surface. The following procedure uses human breast cancer cell lines (SK-BR3) that overexpress HER2[160,161] as a model for the development of the QD-based whole-cell imaging sensor.

Cell culture

1. The SK-BR3 cells from ATCC (Manassas, VA) are grown in RPMI-1640 medium, with 10% fetal bovine serum (FBS) and 1% streptomycin/penicillin antibiotics. These are incubated at 37°C with 5% CO_2 in a cell culture incubator. Every three days the medium is replaced.
2. Harvest the cells at about 80%–90% confluence by adding 1 mL of trypsin for digestion and detachment from the flask.
3. Wash the cells with 1 mL 1× DPBS buffer two times. Establish the cell count and use right after harvest.

Prepare the silanized glass slides

1. Soak the glass slide in 10% KOH (overnight).
2. Soak in 40% (3-aminopropyl) triethoxysilane for 2 h at RT.
3. Wash thoroughly with deionized (DI) water and dry with nitrogen gas.
4. On the silanized glass slide place 100–500 μL of 0.2 M EDC (ethyl-aminopropyl-carbodiimide hydrochloride) containing 5 μg of anti-HER2/neu antibody that are freshly prepared to generate the Ab-modified slide (slide-Ab).
5. Incubate at 4°C overnight, then wash thoroughly with autoclaved DI water.
6. Expose this slide to SK-BR3 cells for 30–60 min at room temperature to form the slide-Ab+SK-BR3.
7. Wash the capture slide thoroughly with 1× DPBS, pH 7.4.

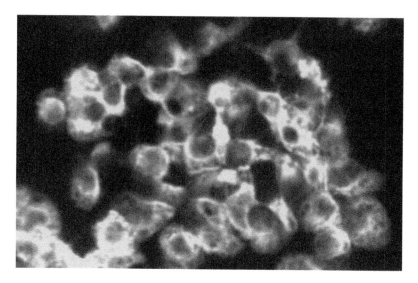

FIGURE 3.7
SK-BR3 cells captured on an antibody modified silanized glass slide and then exposed to QD-anti HER2.

8. Expose the slide-Ab+SK-BR3 to anti-EpCAM-QD, and incubate for 30–60 min at 37°C with 5% CO_2. This forms the slide-Ab+SK-BR3+anti-EpCAM-QD.

9. Wash thoroughly with 1× DPBS, pH 7.4.

10. Detect the cells under a fluorescence microscope (Figure 3.7).

The SK-BR3 cells captured on the glass slide are labeled with the QD-labeled antibody against epithelial cell adhesion molecules (anti-EpCAM-QD), which are abundant on the cell surface. Figure 3.6 shows a digital photograph of slide-Ab + SK-BR3 + anti-EpCAM-QD cells captured on the silanized antibody-modified glass slide. The cells were captured through the HER2 proteins and detected through the EpCAM cell-membrane proteins.

3.6 Executive Summary and Future Perspective

The early developments and advances in QDs as new materials in nanotechnology have enabled important shifts in imaging biosensors. QDs in fluorescence bioimaging promise enhanced sensitivity, shorter turn-around time, and possibly cost-effectiveness. In spite of pending regulatory, safety, and intellectual property issues, and the technologies themselves still needing further optimization, QDs are very promising in transforming the field of bioimaging.

The use of QDs as components of imaging biosensors utilizes their unique physicochemical properties that open up new possibilities for the improvement of the sensing performance. The new area of QDs nanoimaging biosensors involves interaction among material sciences, engineering, physics, chemistry, and biology at the nanoscale. Utilizing the unique absorption and emission properties, the area of QDs nanoimaging sensors is quite promising especially in areas that could not be accomplished by conventional bulk materials.

The semiconductor QDs have emerged as novel fluorescent labels in biosensing and imaging, and are proving to be excellent substitutes to the conventional organic fluorophores. This is a consequence of the great advantages of the QDs over the conventional organic dyes. Semiconductor QDs exhibit broad excitation profiles, narrow and symmetric emission spectra, high photostability and high quantum efficiency with excellent multiplex detection capability.[42,142] Unlike conventional organic dyes, inorganic QDs with different emission wavelengths can be excited by a single excitation source allowing for multiplex detection capabilities. The need for the simultaneous detection of more targets in a single assay drives the development of inorganic nanocrystal-based fluorescent imaging to replace organic fluorophores.[21,132,133,135,162]

To date, most of the research on QD-imaging fluorescence biosensors is proof-of-concept work that demonstrated the advantages. In the future, more efforts need to be made to move the proof-of-concept studies to the applications of QD-imaging fluorescence biosensors to the real-world samples. Future developments will focus on the integration of nanostructured sensors with microfluidics to form lab-on-chip devices. Additionally, studies need to concentrate on the integration of the nanostructured sensors with signal-processing instruments to build portable devices for the onsite measurement of analytes to meet the need for an ontime (real-time) monitoring of the targets of interest for a rapid assessment of risks. In the future, QD-imaging fluorescence biosensors are projected as portable point-of-care device that has an increasing demand as the cost of healthcare rises worldwide.

References

1. Velasco, M. N. Optical biosensors for probing at the cellular level: A review of recent progress and future prospects. *Semin Cell Dev Biol* 2009, *20*, 27–33.
2. Fan, X., White, I. M., Shopova, S. I., Zhu, H., Suter, J. D., Sun, Y. Sensitive optical biosensors for unlabeled targets: A review. *Anal Chim Acta* 2008, *620*, 8–26.
3. Khanna, V. K. New-generation nano-engineered biosensors, enabling nanotechnologies and nanomaterials. *Sens Rev* 2008, *28*, 39–45.
4. Aguilar, Z., Aguilar, Y., Xu, H., Jones, B., Dixon, J., Xu, H., Wang, A. Nanomaterials in medicine. *ECS Trans* 2010, *33*, 69–74.
5. Aguilar, Z., Xu, H., Jones, B., Dixon, J., Wang, A. Semi conductor quantum dots for cell imaging. *MRS Proceedings* 2010, *1237*, 1237-TT1206-1201.
6. Dyadyusha, L., Yin, H., Jaiswal, S., Brown, T., Baumberg, J., Booye, F., Melvin, T. Quenching of CdSe quantum dot emission, a new approach for biosensing. *Chem Commun* 2005, 3201–3203.
7. Neely, A., Perry, C., Varisli, B., Singh, A., Arbneshi, T., Senapati, D., Kalluri, J., Ray, P. Ultrasensitive and highly selective detection of Alzheimer's disease biomarker using two-photon Rayleigh scattering properties of gold nanoparticle. *ACS Nano* 2009, *3*, 2834–2840.
8. Vaseashta, A., Dimova-Malinovska, D. Nanostructured and nanoscale devices, sensors and detectors. *Sci Technol Adv Mat* 2005, *6*, 312–318.
9. Xu, H., Aguilar, Z., Dixon, J., Jones, B., Wang, A., Wei, H. Breast cancer cell imaging using semiconductor quantum dots. *ECS Trans* 2009, *25*, 69–77.
10. Xu, H., Aguilar, Z., Wei, H., Wang, A. Development of semiconductor nanomaterial whole cell imaging sensor on silanized microscope slides. *Front Biosci* 2011, *E3*, 1013–1024.
11. Merkoci, A. Nanoparticles-based strategies for DNA, protein and cell sensors. *Biosens Bioelectron* 2010, *26*, 1164–1177.
12. Wang, J. Nanomaterial-based electrochemical biosensors. *Analyst* 2005, *130*, 421–426.

13. Yun, Y., Eteshola, E., Bhattacharya, A., Dong, Z., Shim, J., Conforti, L., Kim, D., Schulz, M., Ahn, C., Watts, N. Tiny medicine: Nanomaterial-based biosensors. *Sensors* 2009, *9*, 9275–9299.

14. Hu, L., Kim, H., Lee, J., Peumans, P., Cui, Y. Scalable coating and properties of transparent, flexible, silver nanowire electrodes. *ACS Nano* 2010, *4*, 2955–2963.

15. Xianmao, L., Yavuz, M., Tuan, H., Korgel, B., Xia, Y. Ultrathin gold nanowires can be obtained by reducing polymeric strands of oleylamine-AuCl complexes formed via aurophilic interaction. *J Am Chem Soc* 2008, *130*, 8900–8901.

16. Byers, R., Hitchman, E. Quantum dots brighten biological imaging. *Prog Histochem Cytochem* 2011, *45*, 201–237.

17. Jaiswal, J., Mattoussi, H., Mauro, J., Simon, S. Long-term multiple color imaging of live cells using quantum dot bioconjugates. *Nat Biotechnol* 2003, *21*, 47–51.

18. Liu, J., Lu, Y. A colorimetric lead biosensor using DNAzyme-directed assembly of gold nanoparticles. *J Am Chem Soc* 2003, *125*, 6642–6643.

19. Rosi, N., Mirkin, C. Nanostructures in biodiagnostics. *Chem Rev* 2005, *105*, 1547–1562.

20. Murphy, S. Interpretation of Boulder Creek Phosphorous Data. June 15, 2002 [cited September 3, 2002].

21. Chan, C., Nie, S. Quantum dot bioconjugates for ultrasensitive nonisotopic detection. *Science* 1998, *281*, 2016–2018.

22. Xiao, Y., Barker, P. Semiconductor nanocrystal probes for human metaphase chromosomes. *Nucleic Acids Res* 2004, *32*, e28.

23. Lacoste, T., Michalet, X., Pinaud, F., Chemla, D., Alivisatos, A., Weiss, S. Ultrahigh-resolution multicolor colocalization of single fluorescent probes. *Proc Natl Acad Sci USA* 2000, *97*, 9461.

24. Parak, W., Gerion, D., Pellegrino, T., Zanchet, D., Micheel, C., Williams, S., Boudreau, R., Le Gros, M., Larabell, C., Alivisatos, A. Biological applications of colloidal nanocrystals. *Nanotechnology* 2003, *14*, R15–R27.

25. Kaufmann, R., Muller, P., Hildebrand, G., Hausmann, M., Cremer, C. Analysis of Her2/neu membrane protein clusters in different types of breast cancer cells using localization microscopy. *J Microsc* 2011, *242*, 46–54.

26. Coussens, L., Yang-Feng, T. L., Liao, Y. C., Chen, E., Gray, A., McGrath, J., Seeburg, P. H., Libermann, T. A., Schlessinger, J., Francke, U. Tyrosine kinase receptor with extensive homology to EGF receptor shares chromosomal location with neu oncogene. *Science* 1985, *230*, 1132–1139.

27. Tada, H., Higuchi, H., Wanatabe, T. M., Ohuchi, N. In vivo real-time tracking of single quantum dots conjugated with monoclonal anti-HER2 antibody in tumors of mice. *Cancer Res* 2007, *67*, 1138–1144.

28. Onoda, G., Liniger, E. Experimental determination of the random-parking limit in two dimensions. *Phys Rev A* 1986, *33*, 715–716.

29. Su, T., Lu, J., Thomas, R., Cui, Z., Penfold, J. The conformational structure of bovine serum albumin layers adsorbed at the silica-water interface. *J Phys Chem B* 1998, *102*, 8100–8808.

30. Tilton, R., Robertson, C., Gast, A. Lateral diffusion of bovine serum albumin adsorbed at the solid-liquid interface. *J Colloid Interface Sci* 1990, *137*, 192–203.

31. Aguilar, Z., Xu, H., Dixon, J., Wang, A. Blocking non-specific uptake of engineered nanomaterials. *ECS Trans* 2010, *25*, 37–48.

32. Michalet, X., Pinaud, F., Bentolila, L., Tsay, J., Doose, S., Li, J., Sundaresan, G., Wu, A., Gambhir, S., Weiss, S. Quantum dots for live cells, in vivo imaging, and diagnostics. *Science* 2005, *307*, 538–544.

33. Pathak, S., Choi, S., Arnheim, N., Thompson, M. Hydroxylated quantum dots as luminescent probes for in situ hybridization. *J Am Chem Soc* 2001, *123*, 4103–4104.

34. W.C.W. Chan, S. M. N. Quantum dot bioconjugates for ultrasensitive nonisotopic detection. *Science* 1998, *281*, 2016–2018.

35. Kim, S., Bawendi, M. Oligomeric ligands for luminescent and stable nanocrystal quantum dots. *J Am Chem Soc* 2003, *125*, 14652–14653.

36. Pinaud, F., King, D., Moore, H., Weiss, S. Bioactivation and cell targeting of semiconductor CdSe/ZnS nanocrystals with phytochelatin-related peptides. *J Am Chem Soc* 2004, *126*, 6115–6123.
37. Guo, W., Li, J., Wang, Y., Peng, X. Conjugation chemistry and bioapplications of semiconductor box nanocrystals prepared via dendrimer bridging. *Chem Mater* 2003, *15*, 3125–3133.
38. Gao, X., Cui, Y., Levenson, R., Chung, L., Nie, S. In vivo cancer targeting and imaging with semiconductor quantum dots. *Nat Biotechnol* 2004, *22*, 969–976.
39. Wu, X., Liu, H., Liu, J., Haley, K., Treadway, J., Larson, J., Ge, N., Peale, F., Bruchez, M. Immunofluorescent labeling of cancer marker Her2 and other cellular targets with semiconductor quantum dots. *Nat Biotechnol* 2003, *21*, 41–46.
40. Ballou, B., Lagerholm, B., Ernst, L., Bruchez, M., Waggoner, A. Noninvasive imaging of quantum dots in mice. *Bioconj Chem* 2004, *15*, 79–86.
41. Alexandridis, P., Tsianou, M. Block copolymer-directed metal nanoparticle morphogenesis and organization. *Eur Polymer J*, 2011, *47*, 569–583.
42. Bruchez Jr., M., Moronne, M., Gin, P., Weiss, S., Alivisatos, A. Semiconductor nanocrystals as fluorescent biological labels. *Science* 1998, *281*, 2013–2015.
43. Gerion, D., Pinaud, F., Williams, S., Parak, W., Zanchet, D., Weiss, S., Alivisatos, A. Synthesis and properties of biocompatible water-soluble silica-coated CdSe/ZnS semiconductor quantum dots. *J Phys Chem B* 2001, *105*, 8861–8871.
44. Gao, X., Chan, C., Nie, S. Quantum-dot nanocrystals for ultrasensitive biological labeling and multicolor optical encoding. *J Biomed Opt* 2002, *7*, 532–537.
45. Parak, W., Gerion, D., Zanchet, D., Woerz, A., Pellegrino, R., Micheel, C., Williams, S. et al. Conjugation of DNA to silanized colloidal semiconductor nanocrystalline quantum dots. *Chem Mater* 2002, *14*, 2113–2119.
46. Pellegrino, T., Manna, L., Kudera, S., Liedl, T., Koktysh, D., Rogach, A., Keller, S., Radler, J., Natile, G., Parak, W. Hydrophobic nanocrystals coated with an amphiphilic polymer shell: A general route to water soluble nanocrystals. *Nano Lett* 2004, *4*, 703–707.
47. Dubertret, B., Skourides, P., Norris, D., Noireaux, V., Brivanlou, A., Libchaber, A. In vivo imaging of quantum dots encapsulated in phospholipids micelles. *Science* 2002, *298*, 1759–1762.
48. Goldman, E., Anderson, G., PT, T., Mattoussi, H., Charles, P., Mauro, J. Conjugation of luminescent quantum dots with antibodies using an engineered adaptor protein to provide new reagents for fluoroimmunoassays. *Anal Chem* 2002, *74*, 841–847.
49. Osaki, F., Kanamori, T., Sando, S., Sera, T., Aoyama, Y. A quantum dot conjugated sugar ball and its cellular uptake on the size effects of endocytosis in the subviral region. *J Am Chem Soc* 2004, *126*, 6520–6521.
50. Sukhanova, A., Devey, J., Venteo, L., Kaplan, H., Artemyev, M., Oleinikov, V., Klinov, D., Pluot, M., Cohen, J., Nabiev, I. Biocompatible fluorescent nanocrystals for immunolabeling of membrane proteins and cells. *Anal Biochem* 2004, *324*, 60–67.
51. Matsuzaki, H., Dong, S., Loi, H., Di, X., Liu, G. Y., Hubbell, E., Law, J. et al. Genotyping over 100,000 SNPs on a pair of oligonucleotide arrays. *Nature Methods* 2004, *1*, 109–111.
52. Mattoussi, H., Mauro, J., Goldman, E., Anderson, G., Sundar, V., Bawendi, M. Self-assembly of CdSe-ZnS quantum dot bioconjugates using an engineered recombinant protein. *J Am Chem Soc* 2000, *122*, 12142–12150.
53. Wuister, S. F., Swart, I., van Driel, F., Hickey, S. G., Donega, C. D. Highly luminescent water-soluble CdTe quantum dots. *Nano Lett* 2003, *3*, 503–507.
54. Kanninen, P., Johans, C., Merta, J., Kontturi, K. Influence of ligand structure on the stability and oxidation of copper nanoparticles. *J Colloid Interface Sci* 2008, *318*, 88–95.
55. Lambert, K., Wittebrood, L., Moreels, I., Deresmes, D., Grandidier, B., Hens, Z., L Langmuir-Blodgett monolayers of InP quantum dots with short chain ligands. *J Colloid and Interface Sci* 2006, *300*, 597–602.
56. Zhang, C., O'Brien, S., Balogh, L. Comparison and stability of CdSe nanocrystals covered with amphiphilic poly(amidoamine) dendrimers. *J Phys Chem B* 2002, *106*, 10316–10321.

57. Gaponik, N., Talapin, D. V., Rogach, A. L., Eychmuller, A., Weller, H. Efficient phase transfer of luminescent thiol-capped nanocrystals: From water to nonpolar organic solvents. *Nano Lett* 2002, *2*, 803–806.

58. Sondi, I., Siiman, O., Koester, S., Matijevic, E. Preparation of aminodextran-CdS nanoparticle complexes and biologically active antibodyaminodextran-CdS nanoparticle conjugates. *Langmuir* 2000, *16*, 3107–3118.

59. Nirmal, M., Dabbousi, B. O., Bawendi, M. G., Macklin, J. J., Trautman, J. K., Harris, T. D., Brus, L. E. Fluorescence intermittency in single cadmium selenide nanocrystals. *Nature* 1996, *383*, 802.

60. Banin, U., Bruchez, M., Alivisatos, A. P., Ha, T., Weiss, S., Chemla, D. S. Evidence for a thermal contribution to emission intermittency in single CdSe/CdS core/shell nanocrystals. *J Chem Phys* 1998, *110*, 1195–1201.

61. Reiss, P., Bleuse, J., Pron, A. Highly luminescent CdSe/ZnSe core/shell nanocrystals of low size dispersion. *Nano Lett* 2002, *2*, 781–784.

62. Snee, P., Somers, R., Nair, G., Zimmer, J., Bawendi, M., Nocera, D. A ratiometric CdSe/ZnS nanocrystal pH sensor. *J Am Chem Soc* 2006, *128*, 13320–133221.

63. Mitchell, G., Mirkin, C., Letsinger, R. Programmed assembly of DNA functionalized quantum dots. *J Am Chem Soc* 1999, *121*, 8122–8123.

64. Murray, C., Norris, D., Bawendi, M. Synthesis and characterization of nearly monodisperse CdE (E = sulfur, selenium, tellurium) semiconductor nanocrystallites. *JACS* 1993, *115*, 8706–8715.

65. Willard, D., Carillo, L., Jung, J., van Orden, A. CdSe-ZnS quantum dots as resonance energy transfer donors in a model protein-protein binding assay. *Nano Lett* 2001, *1*, 469–474

66. Uyeda, H., Medintz, I., Jaiswal, J., Simon, S., Mattoussi, H. Synthesis of compact multidentate ligands to prepare stable hydrophilic quantum dot fluorophores. *J Am Chem Soc* 2005, *127*, 3870–3878.

67. Aldana, J., Lavelle, N., Wang, Y., Peng, X. Size-dependent dissociation pH of thiolate ligands from cadmium chalcogenide nanocrystals. *J Am Chem Soc* 2005, *127*, 2496–2504.

68. Chan, C. PhD Thesis: Semiconductor Quantum dots for Ultrasensitive Biological Detection and Imaging, Type, Indiana University, Bloomington, IN, 2001.

69. Duan, H., Nie, S. Cell-penetrating quantum dots based on multivalent and endosome-disrupting surface coatings. *J Am Chem Soc* 2007, *129*(11): 3333–3338.

70. Yang, Y., Gao, M. Preparation of fluorescent SiO_2 particles with single CdTe nanocrystal cores by the reverse microemulsion method. *Adv Mater* 2005, *17*, 2354–2357.

71. Zhu, M.-Q., Chang, E., Sun, J., Drezek, R. Surface modification and functionalization of semiconductor quantum dots through reactive coating of silanes in toluene. *J Mater Chem* 2007, *17*, 800–805.

72. Sun, Y., Rollins, H. Preparation of polymer-protected semiconductor. *Chem Phys Lett* 1998, *288*, 585–588.

73. Fahmi, A., Oertel, U., V, S., Froeck, C., Stamm, M. Ring and disk-like CdSe nanoparticles stabilized with copolymers. *Macromol Rapid Commun* 2003, *24*, 625–629.

74. Wisher, A., Bronstein, I., Chechik, V. Thiolated PAMAM dendrimer-coated CdSe/ZnSe nanoparticles as protein transfection agents. *Chem Commun* 2006, *15*, 1637–1639.

75. Xu, J., Wang, J., Mitchell, M., Mukherjee, P., Jeffries-EL, M., Petrich, J., Lin, Z. Organic-inorganic nanocomposites prepared by grafting conjugated polymers onto quantum dots. *J Am Chem Soc* 2007, *129*, 12828.

76. Skaff, H., Sill, K., Emrick, T. Quantum dots tailored with poly(para-phenylene vinylene). *J Am Chem Soc* 2004, *126*(36), 11322–11325.

77. Susumu, K., Uyeda, H., Medintz, I., Mattoussi, H. Design of biotin-functionalized luminescent quantum dots. *J Biomed Biotechnol* 2007, *2007*, 1–7.

78. Gupta, A., Naregalkar, R., Vaidya, V., Gupta, M. Recent advances on surface engineering of magnetic iron oxide nanoparticles and their biomedical applications. *Nanomedicine* 2007, *2*, 23–39.

79. Feng, J., Ding, S. Y., Tucker, M. P., Himmel, M. E., Kim, Y. H., Zhang, S. B., Keyes, B. M., Rumbles, G. Cyclodextrin driven hydrophobic/hydrophilic transformation of semiconductor nanoparticles. *Appl Phys Lett* 2005, *86*, 033108.

80. Palaniappan, K., Hackney, S. A., Liu, J. Supramolecular control of complexation-induced fluorescence change of water-soluble, b-cyclodextrin-modified CdS quantum dots. *Chem Commun* 2004, 2704–2705.

81. Jin, T., Fujii, F., Sakata, H., Tamura, M., Kinjo, M. Calixarene-coated water-soluble CdSe-ZnS semiconductor quantum dots that are highly fluorescent and stable in aqueous solution. *Chem Commun* 2005, 2829–2831.

82. Jin, T., Fujii, F., Sakata, H., Tamura, M., Kinjo, M. Amphiphilic psulfonatocalix[4]arene-coated quantum dots for the optical detection of the neurotransmitter acetylcholine. *Chem Commun* 2005, 4300–4302.

83. Hessel, C. M., Rasch, M. R., Hueso, J. L., Goodfellow, B., Akhavan, V. A., Puvanakrishnan, P., Tunnel, J. W., Korgel, B. A. Alkyl passivation and amphiphilic polymer coating of silicon nanocrystals for diagnostic imaging. *Small* 2010, *6*, 2026–2034.

84. Aguilar, Z. P. Development of self-contained microelectrochemical bioassay platforms for small volumes, PhD Dissertation, University of Arkansas, Fayetteville, AR, 2002.

85. Aguilar, Z. P. Small volume detection of *Plasmodium falciparum* CSP gene using a 50-μm diameter cavity with self-contained electrochemistry. *Anal Chem* 2006, *78*, 1122–1129.

86. Fakunle, E. S., Aguilar, Z. P., Fritsch, I. Evaluation of screen printed gold on low temperature co-fired ceramics as a substrate for Immobilization of electrochemical Immunoassay. *Langmuir* 2006, *22*, 10844–10853.

87. Richarsdson, J. R., Aguilar, Z. P., Kaval, N., Andria, S., Shtoyko, T., Seliskar, C. J., Heineman, W. R. Optical and electrochemical evaluation of colloidal Au nanoparticle-ITO hybrid optically transparent electrode and their applications to attenuated total reflection spectroelectrochemistry. *Electrochim Acta* 2003, *48*, 4291–4299.

88. Aguilar, Z. P., Sirisena, M. Development of automated amperometric detection of antibodies against *Bacillus anthracis* protective antigen. *Anal Bioanal Chem* 2007, *389*, 507–515.

89. Aguilar, Z. P., Van Nguyen, C., Sirisena, M., Gertsch, J., Arumugam, P., Spencer, D., Wansapura, C., Aguilar, Y., Homesley, J. In *Chemical Sensors 7 and MEMS/NEMS 7*, Hesketh, P., Hunter, G., Akbar, S. et al., Eds., ECS Transactions: Pennington, NJ, 2006, Vol. 3, pp. 125–137.

90. Aguilar, Z. P., Vandaveer, W. R., Fritsch, I. Self-contained microelectrochemical immunoassay for small volumes using mouse IgG as a model system. *Anal Chem* 2002, *74*, 3321–3329.

91. Aguilar, Z. P., Fritsch, I. F. Immobilized Enzyme Linked DNA-hybridization Assay with Electrochemical Detection for *Cryptosporidium parvum* hsp70 mRNA. *Anal Chem* 2003, *75*, 3890–3897.

92. Xu, H., Aguilar, Z., Waldron, J., Wei, H., Wang, Y. *Application of Semiconductor Quantum Dots for Breast Cancer Cell Sensing, 2009 Biomedical Engineering and Informatics.* IEEE Computer Society BMEI 2009, Tianjin, China, Vol. 1, pp. 516–520.

93. Chu, X., Duan, D., Shen, G., Yu, R. Amperometric glucose biosensor based on electrodeposition of platinum nanoparticles onto covalently immobilized carbon nanotube electrode. *Talanta* 2007, *71*, 2040–2047.

94. Buijs, J., Norde, W. Changes in the secondary structure of adsorbed IgG and F(ab')2 studied by FTIR. *Langmuir* 1996, *12*, 1605–1613.

95. Soderquist, M. E., Walton, A. G. Structural changes in proteins adsorbed on polymer surfaces. *J Colloid Interface Sci* 1980, *75*, 386–397.

96. Xu, H., Aguilar, Z., Wang, Y. Quantum dot-based sensors for proteins. *ECS Trans* 2010, *25*, 1–10.

97. Aguilar, Z., Sirisena, M., Gertsch, J., Pacsial-Ong, E., Narasimhan, P., Wansapura, C., Kuzmicheva, G. et al. Development of self-contained microelectrochemical array assays for whole organisms. *ECS Trans* 2008, *16*, 165–176.

98. Aguilar, Z., Sirisena, M. Development of automated amperometric detection of antibodies against *Bacillus anthracis* protective antigen. *Anal Bioanal Chem* 2007, *389*, 507–515.

99. Zull, J. E., Reed-Mundell, J., Lee, Y. W., Vezenov, D., Ziats, N. P., Anderson, J. M., Sukenik, C. N. Problems and approaches in covalent attachment of peptide and proteins to inorganic surfaces for biosensor applications. *J Ind Microbiol* 1994, *13*, 137–143.

100. Wu, N., Li, H., Eds. One-dimensional nanostructures for chemical sensors and biosensors. *Handbook of Nanoceramics and Their Based Nanodevices.* American Scientific Publishers: Valencia, CA, 2009.

101. Fujiwara, M., Yamamoto, F., Okamoto, K., Shiokawa, K., Nomura, R. Adsorption of duplex DNA on Mesoporous Silicas: Possibility of inclusion of DNA into their mesopores. *Anal Chem* 2005, *77*, 8138–8145.

102. Li, L., Li, X., Li, L., Wang, J., Jin, W. Ultrasensitive DNA assay based on single-molecule detection coupled with fluorescent quantum dot-labeling and its application to determination of messenger RNA. *Anal Chim Acta* 2011, *685*, 52–57.

103. Wang, W., Chen, C., Qian, M., Zhao, X. Aptamer biosensor for protein detection using gold nanoparticles. *Anal Biochem* 2008, *373*, 213–219.

104. Topoglidis, E. A., Cass, E., Gilardi, G., Sadeghi, S., Beaumont, N., and Durrant, J.R. Protein adsorption on nanocrystalline TiO2 films: An immobilization strategy for bioanalytical devices. *Anal Chem* 1998, *70*, 5111–5113.

105. Docoslis, A., Wu, W., Giese, R., van Oss, C. Measurements of the kinetic constants of protein adsorption onto silica particles. *Colloids Surf B Biointerfaces* 1999, *13*, 83–104.

106. Ehrenberg, M., Friedman, A., Finkelstein, J., Oberdorster, G., McGrath, J. The influence of protein adsorption on nanoparticle association with cultured endothelial cells. *Biomaterials* 2009, *30*, 603–610.

107. Wang, M., Mi, C., Wang, W., Liu, C., Wu, Y., Xu, Z., Mao, C., Xu, S. Immunolabeling and NIR-excited fluorescent imaging of HELA cells by using NaYF4:Yb, Er upconversion nanoparticles. *ACS Nano* 2009, *3*, 1580–1586.

108. Xu, H., Aguilar, Z. P., Yang, L., Kuang, M., Duan, H., Xiong, Y., Wei, H., Wang, A. Y. Antibody conjugated magnetic iron oxide nanoparticles for cancer cell separation in fresh whole blood. *Biomaterials* 2011, *32*, 9758–9765.

109. Herr, J. K., Smith, J. E., Medley, C. D., Shangguan, D., Tan, W. Aptamer-conjugated nanoparticles for selective collection and detection of cancer cells. *Anal Chem* 2007, *78*, 2918–2924.

110. Bauemner, A. J., Humiston, M. C., Montagna, R. A., Durst, R. A. Detection of viable oocysts of *Cryptosporidium parvum* following nucleic acid sequence based amplification. *Anal Chem* 2001, *73*, 1176–1180.

111. He, W., Yang, Q., Liu, Z., Yu, X., Xu, D. DNA array biosensor based on electrochemical hybridization and detection. *Anal Lett* 2005, *38*, 2567–2578.

112. Kerman, K., Kobayashi, M., Tamiya, E. Recent trends in electrochemical DNA biosensor technology. *Meas Sci Technol* 2004, *15*, R1–R11.

113. Wang, J., Fernandes, J. R., Kubota, L. T. Polishable and renewable DNA hybridization biosensors. *Anal Chem* 1998, *70*, 3699–3702.

114. Ivnitski, D., Abdel-Hamid, I., Atanasov, P., Wilkins, E. Biosensors for detection of pathogenic bacteria. *Biosens Bioelectron* 1999, *14*, 599–624.

115. Su, H., Xu, H., Gao, S., Dixon, J., ZP, A., Wang, A., Xu, J., Wang, J. Microwave synthesis of nearly monodisperse core/multishell quantum dots with cell imaging applications. *Nanoscale Res Lett* 2010, *5*, 625–630.

116. Niemeyer, C. Nanoparticles, proteins, and nucleic acids: Biotechnology meets materials science *Angew Chem Int Ed* 2001, *40*, 4128–4158.

117. Katz, E., Willner, I. Integrated biomolecule hybrid systems: Synthesis, properties, and applications. *Angew Chem Intl Ed* 2004, *43*, 6042–6108.

118. Hermanson, G. T. In *Bioconjugate Techniques*, Academic Press, Inc.: San Diego, CA, 1996, pp. 169–173.

119. Yang, R., Jin, J., Chen, Y., Shao, N., Kang, H., Xiao, Z., Tang, Z., Wu, Y., Zhu, Z., Tan, W. Carbon nanotube-quenched fluorescent oligonucleotides: Probes that fluoresce upon hybridization. *J Am Chem Soc* 2008, *130*, 8351–8358.

120. Gill, R., Willner, I., Shweky, I., Banin, U. Fluorescence resonance energy transfer in CdSe/ZnS-DNA conjugates: Probing hybridization and DNA cleavage. *J Phys Chem B* 2005, *109*, 23715–23719.
121. Clapp, A., Medintz, I., Mauro, J., Fisher, B., Bawendi, M., Mattoussi, H. Fluorescence resonance energy transfer between quantum dot donors and dye-labeled protein acceptors. *J Am Chem Soc* 2004, *126*, 301–310.
122. Dennis, A., Bao, G. Quantum dot-fluorescent protein pairs as novel fluorescence resonance energy transfer probes. *Nano Lett* 2008, *8*, 1439–1445.
123. Yang, L., Cao, Z., Sajja, H., Mao, H., Wang, L., Geng, H., Xu, H., Jiang, T., Wood, W., Nie, S., Wang, A. Development of receptor targeted iron oxide nanoparticles for efficient drug delivery and tumor imaging. *J Biomed Nanotech* 2008, *4*, 1–11.
124. Du, P., Li, H., Mei, Z., Liu, S. Electrochemical DNA biosensor for the detection of DNA hybridization with the amplification of Au nanoparticles and CdS nanoparticles. *Bioelectrochemistry* 2009, *75*, 37–43.
125. Ehrenberg, M., McGrath, J. Binding between particles and proteins in extracts: Implications for microrheology and toxicity. *Acta Biomater* 2005, *1*, 305–315.
126. Merkoci, A. Elecrochemical biosensing with nanoparticles. *FEBS J* 2007, *274*, 310–316.
127. Merkoci, A., Aldavert, M., Tarrasón, G., Eritja, R., Alegret, S. Toward an ICPMS-linked DNA assay based on gold nanoparticles immunoconnected through peptide sequences. *Anal Chem* 2005, *77*, 6500–6503.
128. Wang, J. Nanoparticle-based electrochemical DNA detection. *Anal Chim Acta* 2003, *500*, 247–257.
129. Surendiran, A., Sandhiya, S., Pradhan, S. C., Adithan, C. Novel applications of nanotechnology in medicine. *Indian J Med Res* 2009, *130*, 689–701.
130. Ambrosi, A., Castaneda, M., Killard, A., Smyth, M., Alegret, S., Merkoci, A. Double-codified gold anolabels for enhanced immunoanalysis. *Anal Chem* 2007, *79*, 5232–5240.
131. Dabbousi, B. O., Rodríguez-Viejo, J., Mikulec, F. V., Heine, J. R., Mattoussi, H., Ober, R., Jensen, K. J., Bawendi, M. G. (CdSe)ZnS core–shell quantum dots: Synthesis and characterization of a size series of highly luminescent nanocrystallites. *J Phys Chem B* 1997, *101*, 9463–9475.
132. Cai, W., Shin, D., Chen, K., Gheysens, O., Cao, Q., Wang, S. X., Gambhir, S. S., Chen, X. Peptide-labeled near-infrared quantum dots for imaging tumor vasculature in living subjects. *Nano Lett* 2006, *6*, 669–676.
133. Geiber, D., Charbonnière, L. J., Ziessel, R. F., Butlin, N. G., Löhmannsröben, H., Hildebrandt, N. Quantum dot biosensors for ultrasensitive multiplexed diagnostics. *Angew Chem Int Ed* 2010, *49*, 1–6.
134. Han, M., Gao, X., SU, J., Nie, S. Quantum dot tagged microbead for multiplexed coding of biomolecules. *Nat Biotechnol* 2001, *19*, 631–635.
135. Lidke, D. S., Nagy, P., Heintzmann, R., Arndt-Jovin, D. J., Post, J. N., Grecco, H. E., Jares-Erijman, E. A., Jovin, T. M. Quantum dot ligands provide new insights into erbB/HER receptor-mediated signal transduction. *Nat Biotechnol* 2004, *22*, 198–203.
136. Resch-Genger, U., Grabolle, M., Cavaliere-Jaricot, S., Nitschke, R., Nann, T. Quantum dots versus organic dyes as fluorescent labels. *Nat Methods* 2008, *5*, 763–775.
137. Chuang, H., Macuch, P., Tabacco, M. B. Optical sensors for detection of bacteria. 1. General concepts and initial development. *Anal Chem* 2001, *73*, 462–466.
138. Chaplin, M. F. In *Molecular Biology and Biotechnology*, 4th edn., Royal Society of Chemistry, Cambridge, U.K., 2000.
139. Deisingh, A. Biosensors for Microbial Detection. 2003 [cited 2005]. Available from: http://www.sfam.org.uk. (Accessed June 7, 2012).
140. Vurek, G. G. In *Handbook of Chemical and Biological Sensors*, Taylor, R. F., Schultz, J. S., Eds., Institute of Physics Publishing, Bristol, CT, 1996, pp. 399–417.
141. Watts, H. J., Lowe, C. R. Optical biosensor for monitoring microbial cells. *Anal Chem* 1994, *66*, 2465–2470.

142. Medintz, I., Clapp, A., Mattoussi, H., Goldman, E., Fisher, B., Mauro, J. Self-assembled nanoscale biosensors based on quantum dot FRET donors. *Nat Mater* 2003, *2*, 630–638.

143. Roy, R., Hohng, S., Ha, T. A practical guide to single-molecule FRET. *Nat Method* 2008, *5*, 507–516.

144. Li, J., Zhao, X., Zhao, Y., Gu, Z. Quantum-dot-coated encoded silica colloidal crystals beads for multiplex coding. *Chem Commun* 2009, 2329–2331.

145. Somers, R., Bawendi, M., Nocera, D. CdSe nanocrystal based chem-/bio- sensors. *Chem Soc Rev* 2007, *36*, 579–591.

146. Wolcott, A., Gerion, D., Visconte, M., Sun, J., Schwartzberg, A., Chen, S., Zhang, J. Z. Silica-coated CdTe quantum dots functionalized with thiols for bioconjugation of IgG proteins. *J Phys Chem B* 2006, *110*, 5779–5789.

147. Parak, W. J., Pellegrino, T., Plank, C. Labeling of cells with quantum dots. *Nanotechnology* 2005, *16*, R9–R25.

148. Smith, A. M., Duan, H., Mohs, A. M. Bioconjugated quantum dots for in vivo molecular and cellular imaging. *Adv Drug Deliv Revs* 2008, *60*.

149. Smith, A. M., Gao, X., Nie, S. Quantum dot nanocrystals for in vivo molecular and cellular imaging. *Photochem Photobiol* 2004, *80*, 377–385.

150. Jung, J., Cheon, D., Liu, F., Lee, K., Seo, T. A graphene oxide based immuno-biosensor for pathogen detection. *Angew Chem Int Ed* 2010, *49*, 1–5.

151. Murasawa, S., Kawamoto, A., Horii, M., Nakamori, S., Asahara, T. Niche-dependent translineage commitment of endothelial progenitor cells, not cell fusion in general, into myocardial lineage cells. *Arterioscler Thromb Vasc Biol* 2005, *25*, 1388–1394.

152. Voura, E. B., Jaiswal, J. K., Mattoussi, H., Simon, S. M. Tracking metastatic tumor cell extravasation with quantum dot nanocrystals and fluorescence emission-scanning microscopy. *Nat Med* 2004, *10*, 993–998.

153. Slotkin, J. R., Chakrabarti, L., Dai, H. N., Carney, R. S., Hirata, T., Bregman, B. S., Gallicano, G. I., Corbin, J. G., Haydar, T. F. In vivo quantum dot labeling of mammalian stem and progenitor cells. *Dev Dyn* 2007, *236*, 3393–3401.

154. Noh, Y. W., Lim, Y. T., Chung, B. H. Noninvasive imaging of dendritic cell migration into lymph nodes using near-infrared fluorescent semiconductor nanocrystals. *FASEB* 2008, *22*, 3908–3918.

155. So, M. K., Xu, C., Loening, A. M., Gambhir, S. S., Rao, J. Self-illuminating quantum dot conjugates for in vivo imaging. *Nat Biotechnol* 2006, *24*, 339–343.

156. Wagner, W., Dullaart, A., Bock, A. K., Zweck, A. The emerging nanomedicine landscape. *Nat Biotechnol* 2006, *24*, 1211–1217.

157. Mao, X., Liu, G. Nanomaterial based electrochemical DNA biosensors and bioassays. *J Biomed Nanotechnol* 2008, *4*, 419–431.

158. Hu, J., Li, L., Yang, W., Manna, L., Wang, L., Alivisatos, A. P. Linearly polarized emission from colloidal semiconductor quantum rods. *Science* 2001, *292*, 2060–2063.

159. Peng, X., Manna, L., Yang, W., Wickham, J., Scher, E., Kadavanich, A., Alivisatos, A. P. Shape control of CdSe nanocrystals. *Nature* 2000, *404*, 59–61.

160. Merlin, J., Barberi-Heyob, M., Bachmann, N. In vitro comparative evaluation of trastuzumab (Herceptin (R)) combined with paclitaxel (Taxol (R)) or docetaxel (Taxotere (R)) in HER2-expressing human breast cancer cell lines. *Ann Oncol* 2002, *13*, 1743.

161. Menendez, J., Vellon, L., Mehmi, I., Oza, B., Ropero, S., Colomer, R., Lupu, R. Inhibition of fatty acid synthase (FAS) suppresses HER2/neu (erbB-2) oncogene overexpression in cancer cells. *Proc Natl Acad Sci USA* 2004, *101*, 10715.

162. Freeman, R., Tali Finder, T., Bahshi, L., Willner, I. β-Cyclodextrin-modified CdSe/ZnS quantum dots for sensing and chiroselective analysis. *Nano Lett* 2009, *9*, 2073–2076.

163. Biologic Imaging Reagents, BCC Research, http://www.bccresearch.com/market-research/biotechnology/biologic-imaging-reagents-bio064a.html (Accessed September 3, 2013).

4

Fluorescent Sensors Based on Energy Transfer and Charge Transfer

Ming Li and Nianqiang (Nick) Wu

CONTENTS

4.1 Introduction

Fluorescence spectroscopy has been developed as one of the most common tools in a wide range of fields such as sensing and biomedical diagnostics [1]. Fluorescence sensing has a lot of advantages including high sensitivity, excellent selectivity, availability of versatile fluorophores, etc. Fluorescence sensing requires a change in the spectral response to the analyte, for example, changes in the intensity, lifetime, anisotropy, and excitation or emission spectrum. When a fluorophore, a donor, is placed in close proximity to another fluorophore (or a nanoparticle), an acceptor, the donor and the acceptor will interact with each other if certain requirements are met, leading to either energy transfer or charge transfer from the donor to the acceptor. This will alter the intensity of at least one of the fluorophores in this donor–acceptor system, enabling a unique type of fluorescent sensor. One typical example is a Förster (or fluorescence) resonance energy transfer (FRET) sensor [2], which is a spectroscopic technique capable of measuring the analyte concentration or the distances between the donor and the acceptor.

In conventional FRET sensors, either organic dye molecules or fluorescent biomolecules act as the donor or the acceptor. In the past two decades, nanomaterials such as inorganic quantum dots, gold nanoparticles, and graphene emerged, which has brought new opportunities for the development of fluorescent sensors based on energy transfer and charge transfer.

This chapter will introduce the theories of energy transfer and charge transfer. It will describe the strategies for the construction of fluorescent sensors based on either energy transfer or charge transfer. An emphasis will be placed on the incorporation of nanomaterials and nanostructures into such fluorescent sensors. It will also review the applications of such fluorescent sensors in environmental monitoring, biomedical diagnostics, and optical imaging.

4.2 Principle of Charge Transfer and Resonance Energy Transfer

4.2.1 Charge Transfer

Charge transfer typically takes place when the electronic wavefunctions of the donor are coupled to the acceptor [3]. The charge transfer can be categorized into electron exchange (called Dexter interaction), intramolecular photoinduced electron transfer (PET), and interfacial electron transfer. These mechanisms are not mutually exclusive, may occur simultaneously. In the Dexter interaction, a double exchange of electrons occurs *via* the overlap of the wavefunctions of electronic clouds in the donor and the acceptor [4]. An electron is transferred from the highest occupied molecular orbital (HOMO) of the excited donor to the HOMO of the acceptor; simultaneously an electron is transferred from the lowest unoccupied molecular orbital (LUMO) of the acceptor to the LUMO of the donor (Figure 4.1a). The overlap extent of the wavefunctions of electron clouds plays an important role in the rate constant of electron transfer. Since the electron density decreases exponentially with distance from the nuclei, the rate constant (k_{CT}) of electron transfer is described by [4,5]

$$k_{CT}(r) = \frac{2\pi}{h} V_0^2 J_D \exp\left(\frac{-2r}{L}\right)$$

(4.1)

where

h is the Planck's constant

V_0 is the electronic coupling matrix between the donor and the acceptor, at contact distance

J_D is the overlap integral of the wavefunctions of the electron clouds of the donor and the acceptor

r is the distance from the donor to the acceptor

L is the effective Bohr radius of orbitals

Equation 4.1 shows that the electron transfer rate exponentially decreases with increasing distance, indicating that the electron transfer is much more efficient at very short distances. This is due to the small size of electron clouds (2 Å).

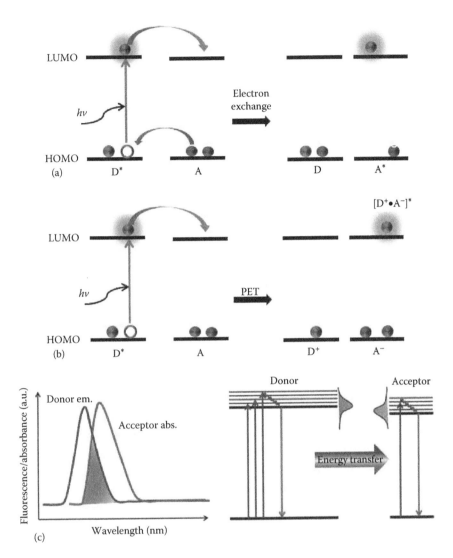

FIGURE 4.1
Schematic for (a) Dexter interaction, (b) photoinduced electron transfer process, and (c) energy transfer.

In addition to the Dexter interaction, PET is another type of electron transfer (Figure 4.1b). In PET, a complex is usually formed between the electron donor and the acceptor [6–9]. The excited complex can return to the ground state from the excited state without the emission of a photon, and the extra electron is eventually returned to the electron donor. In general, the PET process exhibits many similar properties to the Dexter process. A classical theory to rationalize the interfacial electron transfer process at the solid/liquid (or solid) interface has been described by Rudolph Marcus, which was awarded the 1992 Nobel Prize in Chemistry [10]. This theory has been extended to describe the electron transfer from a single donating state to a continuum of accepting states, such as those in the conduction band of a semiconductor [11]. This theory describes the dependence of electron transfer rate on the free energy driving force for systems of organic dye/semiconductor nanocrystal donors coupled to various semiconductors. According to the Marcus theory, the electron transfer rate, k_{CT}, is expressed as [11,12]

$$k_{CT} = \frac{2\pi}{h}|H_{AB}|^2 \frac{1}{\sqrt{4\pi W k_b T}} \exp\left[-\frac{(W+\Delta G^\circ)^2}{4W k_b T}\right]$$

(4.2)

where

h is the reduced Planck's constant
$|H_{AB}|$ is the electronic coupling between the initial and final states
k_b is the Boltzmann's constant
W is the system's reorganizational energy
ΔG° is the total Gibbs free energy change for the electron transfer reaction
T is the absolute temperature

4.2.2 Resonance Energy Transfer

4.2.2.1 *Förster Resonance Energy Transfer*

FRET represents the nonradiative energy transfer through the dipole–dipole interaction between the donor and the acceptor, as shown in Figure 4.1c [13–16]. Energy transfer in the FRET process does not undergo the emission of a photon from the fluorescent donor and readsorption by the acceptor. The donor molecules typically emit at a shorter wavelength that overlaps with the absorption spectrum of the acceptor; and the acceptor does not necessarily fluoresce. The theory of FRET has been described by the classic quantum mechanical model. Assuming the donor–acceptor as an isolated system, neglecting electron exchange interaction (at a large distance) and only considering the Coulomb coupling, the rate of energy transfer (k_T) in FRET is given by [16,17]

$$k_T = \frac{Q_D \kappa^2}{\tau_D r^6}\left(\frac{9000(\ln 10)}{128\pi^5 N n^4}\right)\int_0^\infty F_D(\lambda)\varepsilon_A(\lambda)\lambda^4\, d\lambda = \frac{1}{\tau_D}\frac{R_0^6}{r^6}$$

(4.3)

$$R_0^6 = \frac{9000(\ln 10)Q_D \kappa^2}{128\pi^5 N n^4}\int_0^\infty F_D(\lambda)\varepsilon_A(\lambda)\lambda^4\, d\lambda$$

(4.4)

where

Q_D is the quantum yield of the donor in the absence of the acceptor
κ^2 is a factor describing the relative orientation in space of the transition dipoles of the donor and the acceptor
τ_D is the lifetime of the donor in the absence of the acceptor
r is the distance between the donor and the acceptor
N is the Avogadro's number
n is the refractive index of the medium
$F_D(\lambda)$ the corrected fluorescence intensity of the donor in the wavelength range from λ to $\lambda+\Delta\lambda$ with the total intensity normalized to unity
$\varepsilon_A(\lambda)$ is the corrected extinction coefficient of the acceptor in the wavelength range from λ to $\lambda+\Delta\lambda$ with the total intensity normalized to unity

The integral, $\int_0^\infty F_D(\lambda)\varepsilon_A(\lambda)\lambda^4 d\lambda$, represents the spectral overlap of the normalized fluorescence spectrum of the donor and the extinction spectrum of the acceptor. R_0 is a very important parameter describing the FRET process, which is equal to the donor–acceptor distance at an energy transfer efficiency of 50%.

The energy transfer efficiency (E) in the FRET process follows [5]

$$E = \frac{k_T(r)}{\tau_D^{-1} + k_T(r)} \tag{4.5}$$

Substituting Equation 4.3 into Equation 4.5 yields

$$E = \frac{R_0^6}{R_0^6 + r^6} \tag{4.6}$$

This equation shows that the energy transfer efficiency is strongly dependent on the donor–acceptor distance when the distance is near the Förster distance (R_0). In addition, the energy transfer efficiency can also be measured using the relative fluorescence intensity or lifetime in the absence and presence of the acceptor:

$$E = 1 - \frac{F_{DA}}{F_D} = 1 - \frac{\tau_{DA}}{\tau_D} \tag{4.7}$$

where

F_D and τ_D are the relative fluorescence intensity and the lifetime in the absence of the acceptor

F_{DA} and τ_{DA} are the relative fluorescence intensity and the lifetime in the presence of the acceptor

It is worth noting that Equations 4.3 through 4.7 are only suitable for the case where one donor species interacts with one acceptor. When one donor interacts with several acceptors in close proximity simultaneously, Equation 4.6 needs to be modified to account for the presence of these complex interactions, which is expressed as [16]

$$E = \frac{xR_0^6}{xR_0^6 + r^6} \tag{4.8}$$

where x is the number of acceptor molecules interacting with one donor. In particular, the donor and the acceptor are treated as dipoles in the interaction space. If nanomaterials or biomolecules are used as the donor or the acceptor, these species have a finite size and are relatively larger compared with the organic dyes, which leads to a deviation from these equations to some extent.

4.2.2.2 Nanosurface Energy Transfer

FRET has been widely used as a spectroscopic technique capable of measuring the analyte concentration or the distances between two sites on a biomacromolecule. Conventional FRET systems employ the fluorescent organic dye as the energy donor, and fluorescent (or nonfluorescent) organic dye as the energy acceptor. In the classical FRET process, the efficient energy transfer distance ranges from 3 to 8 nm, which is typically the size of a protein or the thickness of a cellular membrane. Nevertheless, the limited detectable distance cannot meet the requirements in case the extending detectable distance is being sought in the resonance energy transfer–based applications. Recently, Au nanoparticles (NPs) and graphene oxide (GO) have emerged as alternatives to the organic dye molecules in the energy transfer systems [18–22]. These novel quenchers circumvent the limitation of small detection distances, which forms nanosurface energy transfer (NSET) systems [23,24]. As aforementioned, the FRET process physically originates from the weak electromagnetic coupling of two dipoles. The Fermi golden rule in the dipole approximation relates the energy transfer rate to a product of the interaction elements of the donor (F_D) and the acceptor (F_A), $k_T \approx F_D \cdot F_A$ [25], that is, $F \approx 1/r^3$ for single dipoles; $F \approx 1/r$ for a two-dimensional dipole array; and $F =$ constant for a three-dimensional dipole array. Therefore, $k_T \approx 1/r^6$ is applied to the FRET system, which consists of two single dipoles.

Nevertheless, in case of the metallic planar surface, the energy transfer rate follows [23]

$$k_T = 0.225 \frac{c^3}{\omega_D^2 \omega_F k_F r^4} \frac{\Phi_D}{\tau_D} = \frac{1}{\tau_D} \left(\frac{R_0}{r} \right)^4 \tag{4.9}$$

$$R_0 = \left(0.225 \frac{c^3 \Phi_D}{\omega_D^2 \omega_F k_F} \right)^{1/4} \tag{4.10}$$

where

ω_D is the angular frequency for the donor
ω_F is the angular frequency for the bulk metal
k_F is the Fermi wavevector for the bulk metal
r is the separation distance
Φ_D and τ_D are the quantum yield and the lifetime of the donor in the absence of the acceptor
R_0 is the Förster critical distance at the energy transfer efficiency of 50%

The energy transfer efficiency in NSET can be expressed as a function of the separation distance (r):

$$E = \frac{R_0^4}{R_0^4 + r^4} \tag{4.11}$$

Experimental results have demonstrated that small Au NPs (<3 nm in diameter), Au films, two-dimensional carbon films, and graphene act as the quenchers, following the NSET mechanism [23–28]. These techniques based on the NSET mechanism allow for the detection of the interactions between biological macromolecules with the dynamic distance beyond the conventional detection distance (~ 6 nm) in the FRET spectroscopic ruler.

4.2.2.3 Chemiluminescence Resonance Energy Transfer

Both FRET and NSET require the simultaneous external excitation of both the donor and the acceptor. In contrast, chemiluminescence resonance energy transfer (CRET) does not need an external excitation source [29,30]. CRET occurs *via* the specific oxidation of luminescent substrates during the chemiluminescence reaction. The energy generated by chemiluminescence or bioluminescence can initiate the excitation of the donor, and simultaneously transfers the energy to the acceptor. This is especially useful to *in vivo* study because the internal light source for activating the CRET can avoid the strong absorption by the issues, which mitigates the background interference over the bioassay. It should be noted that CRET is a nonradiative dipole–dipole energy transfer process, similar to FRET or NSET. Therefore, the basic theory and the derived equations in FRET and NSET are suitable for the CRET process.

4.3 Design Strategies of Fluorescent Sensors

The donor and the acceptor can use different materials, which results in different fluorescent sensors based on energy transfer and charge transfer, as shown in Table 4.1. In conventional FRET systems, organic dyes are widely employed. Organic dyes, however, suffer from photobleaching, limited brightness, short lifetimes, narrow excitation spectra, etc. Novel fluorescent inorganic nanoparticles such as semiconducting quantum dots (QDs), Ag clusters, Au NPs, graphene, or GO are emerging for fluorescent sensing applications, which bring new features and improved performances [31–36].

By deliberate design, the fluorescence of donors (or acceptors) can be either turned off or turned on. In some cases, it is difficult or even impossible to control the fluorophore concentration at each site, especially when the probes are used in the cell, because the local probe concentration changes continually due to diffusion and/or photobleaching. In order to overcome this shortcoming, the wavelength-ratiometric design strategy is used to construct fluorescent sensors. By using the ratio between the emission intensities at two different wavelengths as the analytical signal, the effect of factors such as photobleaching, sensor concentration, and the fluctuation of excitation sources can be minimized.

In general, the fluorescent sensing architecture varies depending on the specific applications, and numerous different configurations of fluorescent sensors can be found in the literature [37]. This chapter gives several typical design strategies for fluorescent sensors, as shown in Figure 4.2. These sensing platforms are principally based on the electronic interaction or energy transfer upon the introduction of analytes, which causes the quantitative variation of the signals in response to the analyte (Figure 4.2a). External stimulus

TABLE 4.1

Typical Fluorescent Sensors Constructed by Different Materials

Donor	Acceptor	Mechanism	Distance-Dependent Efficiency
Organic dye	Organic dye	FRET	$E \propto r^{-6}$
Quantum dots	Organic dye	FRET	$E \propto r^{-6}$
Organic dye	Au particle	NSET	$E \propto r^{-4}$
Quantum dots	Au particle	NSET	$E \propto r^{-4}$
Organic dye	Graphene oxide or graphene	NSET	$E \propto r^{-4}$
Graphene oxide	Au particle	NSET	$E \propto r^{-4}$
Organic dye	Metal ions	Electron transfer	$E \propto e^{-r}$
Graphene oxide	Metal ions	Electron transfer	$E \propto e^{-r}$

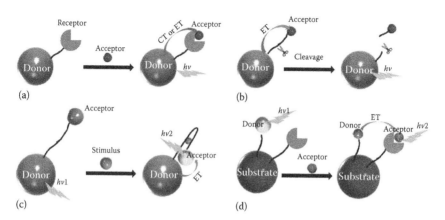

FIGURE 4.2
Representative sensing schemes of fluorescent sensors. (a) Fluorescent sensors in which the binding of acceptor (or analyte) results in the charge transfer or energy transfer, and subsequently FRET "switch on." (b) Fluorescent sensors in which external stimulus induces the cleavage of the donor–acceptor pair, and subsequently FRET "switch off." (c) Fluorescent sensors based on the induced close proximity of the donor to the acceptor by the binding of analyte, and then FRET "switch on." (d) Fluorescent sensors in which energy transfer occurs from the surface grafted donor on substrates (i.e., nanomaterials) to the bonded analyte (acceptor).

or additives results in the dissociation of the donor–acceptor pair, and then the FRETs "switch off" so that the fluorescence is recovered (Figure 4.2b). Another design strategy is the induced proximity of the donor to the acceptor by the addition of an external stimulus or analyte (Figure 4.2c), which enables the fluorescence enhancement of the acceptor (or donor) due to the energy transfer. In *in vivo* biological study, the design strategy shown in Figure 4.2d is typically used, in which fluorescent donors are firstly labeled to biomacromolecules (i.e., protein, tissue, lipid, membrane). Physiological activities cause the binding of the acceptor (or analyte), leading to energy transfer between the donor and the acceptor.

4.4 Applications of Energy Transfer–Based Fluorescent Sensors

Fluorescent sensors have become fascinating tools for biological studies *in vitro* and even *in vivo*, enabling a wide range of applications, with high sensitivity and spatial resolution. In particular, the introduction of nanomaterials (NMs) into fluorescent sensors has improved the sensing performances such as sensitivity and multiplexed detection capability.

4.4.1 Quantification of Analytes

Fluorescent NPs are often employed as the energy donor while the energy acceptor can be NPs, organic dyes, and even analytes [38,39]. Mattoussi et al. have demonstrated a FRET-based TNT sensor using a hybrid QD–antibody assembly [40]. In this sensor, the anti-TNT specific antibody fragments, appended with an oligohistidine sequence, are bound onto the surface of CdSe–ZnS QDs. A dye-labeled TNT analogue prebound in the binding/recognition site quenches the fluorescence of QDs *via* proximity-induced FRET. When TNT displaces the dye-labeled analogue, FRET is eliminated, leading to a

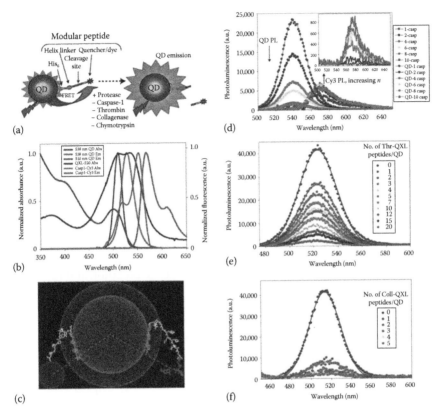

FIGURE 4.3
(See color insert.) (a) Schematic illustration of the QD–peptide assembly. (b) Absorption and emission spectra of dyes and QDs: Cy3 dye and QXL-520 dark quencher. (c) Model structure of the QD–peptide conjugates. (d) Deconvoluted fluorescence spectra of the assembling with an increasing number of Casp1–Cy3 per 538 nm QD. The inset shows the Cy3 PL contribution due to direct excitation from the equivalent amount of free Casp1–Cy3 peptide. (e) Fluorescence spectra for an increasing ratio of Thr–QXL per 522 nm QD. (f) Titration of 510 nm QDs with an increasing number of Coll–QXL. (Reproduced from Medintz, I. L. et al., *Nat. Mater.*, 5, 581, 2006.)

concentration-dependent recovery of the fluorescence. This sensor exhibited high sensitivity for the TNT detection in both aqueous and solid samples. In addition, the high specificity of this sensor was confirmed by comparing the fluorescence recovery in the coexistence of TNT with its three analogues. Furthermore, they have designed a series of nanoscale sensing assemblies consisting of QD–peptide conjugates capable of specifically detecting the activities of proteolytic enzymes (Figure 4.3) [41].

QDs have size-tunable absorption and emission wavelengths, narrow and symmetric emission bands, and broad excitation spectra. These superior properties allow QDs with different emission wavelengths to be excited at a single excitation source in contrast with organic dyes [42]. The use of QDs as the donors enables the FRET sensor to detect multiple analytes simultaneously. Hildebrandt et al. have reported a homogeneous assay format for the simultaneous detection of five different bioanalytes [43]. In their work, terbium complexes (LTCs) were used as the energy donor and five different-sized QDs with emissions at 529, 565, 604, 653, and 712 nm, as the acceptors. Initially, LTCs and QDs emit luminescence with decay times on the orders of millisecond and nanosecond, respectively. After LTC-labeled streptavidin (LS) binds to biotinylated QDs with different antibodies,

FRET occurs from the LTCs to the QDs, which results in the luminescence quenching of LTCs and the appearance of a long-lived QD luminescence with a decay time of milliseconds. Thus, time-gated detection can lead to the suppression of the nanosecond luminescence; and the millisecond luminescence of QDs at the varying emission wavelengths can be used for the measurement of analytes. This design leads to a sensitivity approximately 40–240 fold higher than a well-established homogeneous immunoassay– FRET pair. More importantly, this approach can be easily extended to the practical diagnostic assays of biological analytes *via* the RNA-, DNA-, aptamer-, peptide-, or protein-based recognition. In a multiplexed assay, QDs with different emission wavelengths can act as not only the acceptors but also the energy donors. Mattoussi et al. have developed a multiplexed fluorescent immunoassay, in which four different QDs were used as the energy donors [44,45]. This sensor was employed for the simultaneous detection of cholera toxin, ricin, shiga-like toxin 1, and staphylococcal enterotoxin B in the single well of a microliter plate. A large number of studies have shown that FRET is efficient to detect a wide range of analytes such as heavy-metal ions, small molecules, and biomacromolecules.

There are two ways to lower the limit of detection (LOD) of fluorescent sensors, including (1) enhancing the fluorescence intensity of the donor or the acceptor, and (2) increasing the energy transfer efficiency. It has been demonstrated that encoding nano-/microbeads with multiple QDs or organic dyes is an efficient strategy to achieve high fluorescence intensity [42,46,47]. In addition, surface plasmon resonance (SPR) can efficiently enhance the fluorescence of QDs or dyes, strongly depending on the geometric parameters of periodic metal structures [48–52]. Similar to the surface-enhanced Raman scattering, the enhancement of fluorescence by SPR occurs in the "hot spot" with the concentrated electromagnetic field. The SPR-enhanced fluorescence spectroscopy can greatly improve the sensitivity of sensors. For example, Chou et al. have developed a three-dimensional plasmonic antenna array for the enhanced fluorescent immunoassay of IgG, in which the LOD was reduced from 0.9 nM to 300 *a*M, compared to a similar assay performed on the glass plate [53]. In addition, the plasmonic field can modify the energy transfer rate in the FRET process by changing the excitation, radiative and nonradiative decay rates [54,55]. The effects of SPR on the energy transfer depend on the size and the shape of plasmonic materials as well as the distance between the donor and the acceptor [56]. A fundamental understanding of the interaction between SPR and FRET will aid in the design of high-performance FRET-based fluorescent sensors.

Au NPs have been explored as the acceptor in the energy transfer–based fluorescent sensors [57,58]. Strouse et al. have found that energy transfer follows the NSET mechanism when small Au NPs (~1.5 nm) are used as the quencher of the organic dye [23]. Lee et al. have reported the fluorescence quenching of the QDs by the Au NPs with different sizes from 1.1 to 4.9 nm [59]. The energy transfer efficiency increases with increasing particle size. The authors have studied the underlying mechanism of energy transfer from the QD to the Au NP (Figure 4.4) [17]. Both the single-stranded DNA–conjugated QDs and the Au NPs exist in a single assay. Due to the repulsion of the mismatched single-stranded DNA on each type of NP, the QD and the Au NP are separated far away. In this case, the QDs emit strong fluorescence under light excitation. When Hg(II) ions are present in the assay, DNA hybridization occurs *via* the sandwich of Hg(II) ions in the mismatched base pairs. As a result, the QDs are linked to the Au NPs *via* the double-stranded DNA, which enables the energy transfer, leading to the fluorescence quenching of the QD. The gap between the QD and the Au NP can be tuned by the number of base pairs in DNA. Our results show that both the 15- and 80 nm–sized Au NPs exhibit strong SPR. Both the Au NPs quench the fluorescence of the QD *via* the FRET mechanism. In contrast, the 3 nm–sized Au NP has

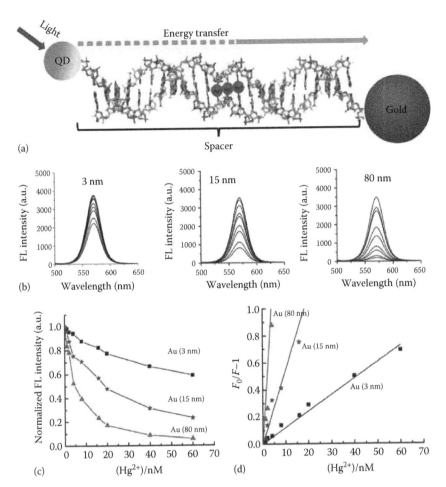

FIGURE 4.4
(a) Illustration of the quantum dot (donor)-DNA-Au nanoparticle (acceptor) ensemble in the presence of Hg(II) ions. (b) Fluorescence emission spectra of the solutions containing the DNA-quantum dots and the different sized Au nanoparticles after addition of various Hg(II) ion concentration (0–60 nM). (c) Normalized fluorescence emission intensity as a function of the Hg(II) ion concentration. (d) Stern–Volmer plots showing the quenching efficiencies by the Au nanoparticles. (Reproduced from Li, M. et al., *J. Phys. Chem. Lett.,* 2, 2125, 2011.)

negligible SPR, which quenches the fluorescence of the QD *via* the NSET mechanism. The NSET sensors exhibit an LOD of 0.4 and 1.2 ppb toward Hg(II) ions in the buffer solution and in river water, respectively [60]. Ray group has also demonstrated that the NSET sensor is able to detect Hg^{2+} in drinking water, river water, and solid samples [61]. In addition, a fluorescent sensor has used the NSET mechanism to detect Hepatitis C virus RNA [62].

The Au NPs have distinct advantages as the acceptors in the energy transfer–based sensors [31]: (1) high fluorescence-quenching efficiency, (2) tunable SPR absorption, (3) stable optical property, and (4) ease of labeling for biocompatible applications. Besides Au NPs, two-dimensional amorphous carbon, graphene, and GO are excellent quenchers with high quenching efficiency, following the NSET mechanism [63–65].

In both FRET and NSET discussed earlier, an external light source is required to excite the donor. However, tissues in humans and animals have strong absorption at shorter excitation wavelengths, leading to background interference in many biological applications. CRET or bioluminescence resonance energy transfer (BRET) allows the direct excitation of the donor by the energy generated *via* chemical reaction without the excitation of external light. Willner et al. have developed CRET sensors for the detection of metal ions and DNA [66–68]. In their sensor, the active hemin-G-quadruplex DNAzyme acted as the functional component to catalyze the generation of chemiluminescence. The ATP–aptamer or the Hg^{2+}–DNA subunits/hemin-G-quadruplex DNAzyme structures were bounded to the QDs. The oxidation of luminol by H_2O_2, yielded luminescence at 420 nm, which enabled the excitation of QDs, by energy transfer from luminol. Graphene has been used as an energy acceptor in CRET sensors. Due to the oxygen-containing functional groups on the edge of chemically derived graphene or graphene oxide (GO), antibodies and other biomolecules could easily be conjugated onto graphene or GO by carbodiimide chemistry. Recently, Park et al. have developed a graphene-based CRET platform for an immunoassay of C-reactive protein (CRP) [69]. Anti-CRP antibody was covalently conjugated to graphene nanosheets for the capture of the CRP biomarker. In this assay, the oxidation of luminol by H_2O_2 yielded chemiluminescence in the presence of horseradish peroxidase. The chemiluminescence was quenched by graphene *via* the CRET process. This CRET sensor has achieved a LOD as low as 0.93 ng/mL toward CRP in human serum.

4.4.2 Spectroscopic Ruler

In addition to quantitative analysis, FRET and NSET sensors are used to monitor the distance between the biological sites or the donor–acceptor pairs *in vitro* and *in vivo* studies. It is well-known that FRET follows the r^{-6} distance dependence; and the characteristic Förster distance R_0 is about 6 nm, which is typically in the dimensional scale of biomolecules such as protein and cellular membrane. Previous studies have demonstrated that FRET is an excellent technique to measure the distances between the sites of interest in proteins [70]. The two sites are labeled with the donor and the acceptor, respectively. The energy transfer efficiency is calculated by comparing the intensity of the donor in the presence and absence of the acceptor. Mattoussi et al. have introduced a FRET-based modeling technique for determining the orientation and the position of a maltose-binding protein (MBP) [16]. Six different single-cysteine MBP mutants on the protein surface were labeled with Rhodamine red dye. Also, the QDs were conjugated onto Rhodamine red-labeled-MBP protein assemblies. The distance from each of the six different Rhodamine red-acceptor MBP locations to the center of the energy-donating QDs can be determined from the FRET efficiency. It was found that some of the MBP mutants quenched the emission of the donor while the other MBP mutants had no quenching. Thus, the orientation of MBP mutants could be determined with the aid of the MBP crystallographic coordinates and the least-squares approach. As mentioned earlier, the use of the LTC–QD systems could achieve ultrasensitive multiplexed diagnostics. Following this discovery, Hildebrandt et al. further demonstrated that the LTC–QD pairs could be used as the multiplexed FRET molecular rulers [71]. The resulting FRET spectroscopic ruler was able to measure a large FRET distance ($R_0 \sim 11$ nm).

As mentioned previously, the use of Au NPs as the acceptor in the energy transfer system results in the NSET mechanism, which enables a larger detection distance (more than 30 nm). Ray et al. have reported a NSET ruler using the popcorn-shaped Au NPs as the energy acceptor [72]. This NSET ruler has been used to monitor the photothermal response during the photothermal therapy of human prostate cancer cells. This nanoruler was very sensitive to small changes in the dye–particle distance, and exhibited an efficient detection distance of more than 30 nm, three times larger than that of the conventional FRET ruler. Furthermore, single-molecule FRET and NSET spectroscopic rulers are powerful techniques that are able to reveal the dynamical information on biological systems [73,74]. They can be used to detect the real-time conformational change and the molecular interaction during biological processes through observing the on–off blinking of the fluorescence intensity. It is worth noting that FRET and NSET spectroscopic rulers are efficient to reveal the distance change but not efficient to provide the absolute distance because of the non-distance-related FRET change.

4.4.3 Bioimaging

Fluorescence imaging is an important technique for biomedical applications due to its high sensitivity and spatial resolution. With the assistance of confocal fluorescence microscopy, one can obtain the detailed information on the cellular interaction and dynamics. The fluorescent probes used for *in vitro* and *in vivo* imaging, require: (1) a high quantum efficiency of emission, (2) a suitable excitation/emission wavelength to minimize the noise background, (3) high photostability, and (4) fitting into both a confocal microscopy and a whole-body optical imaging system [75]. Since Chapter 3 deals with the conventional fluorescence imaging with nanomaterial labels, this chapter is only focused on the energy transfer–based fluorescence imaging.

In order to monitor the physiological condition, Bao et al. have developed a ratiometric pH sensor by conjugating the pH-sensitive fluorescent protein (mOrange) to the QDs (Figure 4.5) [76]. The FRET process occurs from the pH-sensitive fluorescent proteins to the QDs; and the pH value modulates the acceptor-to-donor emission ratio. To demonstrate the ability of the FRET-based pH sensors to image the intracellular pH change temporally and spatially, the cultured Hela cells were incubated with the QD-fluorescent protein nanoprobes. It was found that the pH variation altered the ratiometric fluorescence intensity of the fluorescent proteins and the QDs through the FRET interaction. That is, the FRET efficiency was high when the pH value was neutral in the extracellular environment and early endosome. The FRET efficiency was reduced as the endosome matured and the endosomal pH decreased, which reduced the emission from mOrange and simultaneously recovered the fluorescence of the QD. Any probe that escapes the endosome regains its elevated FRET efficiency in the pH-neutral cytoplasm. The use of QDs in the sensor enabled the high contrast and photostability in comparison with the organic fluorophores.

Similarly, both NSET and CRET are capable of *in vitro* and *in vivo* bioimaging. For example, Rao et al. have developed a strategy for multiplexed *in vivo* imaging based on the BRET from *R. reniformis luciferase* (Luc8) to QDs without the need of an external excitation (Figure 4.6) [77]. Different-sized QDs with fluorescence emission at 650, 655, 705, and 800 nm, were conjugated with Luc8 (QD605-Luc8, QD655-Luc8, QD705-Luc8, and QD800-Luc8), in which the fluorescence of all the QDs can be excited by a light at 480 nm. The bioluminescence emission of QDs in the QD–Luc8 conjugates was observed upon addition of coelenterazine because Luc8 emitted at 480 nm. The energy transfers from Luc8 to all the QDs used, leading to the simultaneous excitation of all the QDs. The bioluminescence emission of each QD–Luc8 conjugate can be distinguished from each other whether it was alone or in a mixture.

Upconversion luminescent NMs are alternative donors in energy transfer–based luminescent sensors [78,79]. The luminescence of upconversion NMs is excited with the near-infrared sources instead of ultraviolet and visible light. Upconversion NM–based imaging allows the light penetration deep in tissues, and avoids the background interference due to auto-fluorescence from biological samples. Li et al. have used the upconversion

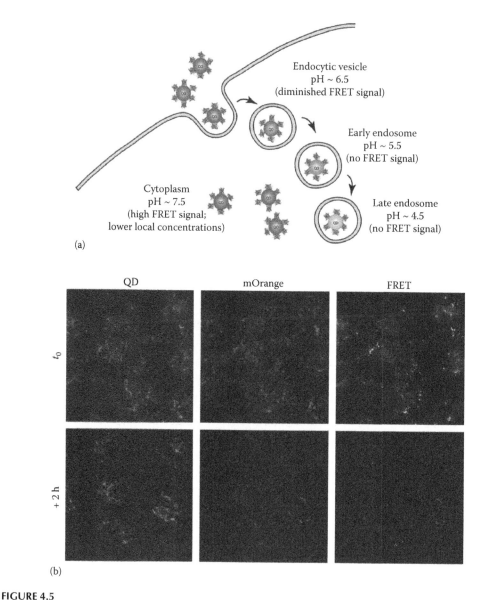

(a)

(b)

FIGURE 4.5
(See color insert.) Cellular imaging with the pH-sensitive FRET probe made of the QD-fluorescent protein (mOrange) ensemble. (a) Schematic of color change in the fluorescent probe during progression through the endocytic pathway. (b) Fluorescence images immediately after delivery of the probe and 2 h postdelivery: The QD images (left) in the endosomes over time; images of the direct excitation of mOrange (center); and the fluorescent emission of the FRET (right) with maturation of the endosome. (Reproduced from Dennis, A.M. et al., *ACS Nano*, 6, 2917, 2012.)

nanoparticles (NaYF$_4$:Yb:Er:Tm, UCNPs) as the energy donor and the Hg^{2+}-responsive ruthenium complex N719 as the energy acceptor to monitor the change in the distribution of Hg^{2+} in living cells by upconversion luminescence bioimaging [80]. In this work, the 980 nm near-infrared excitation light was used, and the emission at 540 ± 20 nm was collected as the output signal. The distribution of Hg^{2+} in the HeLa cells was successfully imaged using the upconversion luminescence technique.

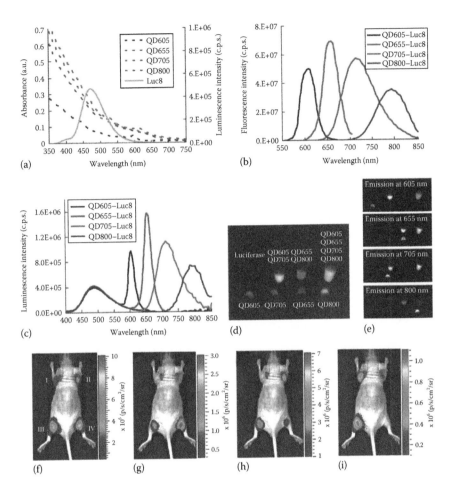

FIGURE 4.6
(See color insert.) Multiplexed imaging of QD605-Luc8, QD655-Luc8, QD705-Luc8 and QD800-Luc8 ensembles *in vitro* and in mice. (a) Bioluminescence emission of Luc8 and the absorption spectra of quantum dots. (b) Fluorescence spectra of the QD-Luc8 conjugates. (c) Bioluminescence emission spectra of the QD-Luc8 conjugates. (d) *In vitro* bioluminescence imaging of the solutions containing the QD-Luc8 conjugates shown in pseudo colors. Sample at top left contained only Luc8 in the absence of detectable long-wavelength (580–850 nm) emission. (e) *In vitro* bioluminescence imaging of the same samples in d, (f–i) *in vivo* bioluminescence imaging of the conjugates intramuscularly injected at the different sites: (I) QD800-Luc8, 15 pmol; (II) QD705-Luc8, 15 pmol; (III) a mixture of QD665-Luc8, QD705-Luc8, and QD800-Luc8; and (IV) QD655-Luc8, 5 pmol. Images were acquired with the following filters: (f) without any filter, (g) with 575–650 nm filter, (h) with x-Cy5.5 filter (680–720 nm), and (i) with ICG filter (810–875 nm). (Reproduced from So, M.K. et al., *Nat. Biotechnol.*, 24, 339, 2006.)

4.5 Applications of Charge Transfer–Based Fluorescent Sensors

Charge transfer is typically categorized into PET, Dexter interaction, and interfacial electron transfer. Interfacial electron transfer usually takes place in heterogeneous systems such as photocatalysis, photoelectrochemical cells, and solar cells, while intramolecular PET is the main type of electron transfer for the construction of fluorescent sensors. A large number of PET studies can be found in organic fluorophore–based fluorescent sensors [81].

Herein, we briefly introduce the recent results of PET fluorescent sensors based on NMs and nanostructures. Previous investigations have demonstrated that double-stranded DNA can act as the electronic transport channel [82,83]. Willner et al. have employed the electronic transport property of double-stranded DNA to develop a fluorescent sensor for the multiplexed detection of Hg^{2+} and Ag^+, as well as the logic gate [84]. In this sensor, the QDs acted as the host fluorescent material conjugated with the deliberately designed single-stranded DNA. Upon the addition of Hg^{2+} or Ag^+, the rigid hairpin structure was formed due to the formation of $T-Hg^{2+}-T$ or $C-Ag^+-C$ complexes. The hairpin structure enabled the electron transport from the QDs to the positive Hg^{2+} or Ag^+through double-stranded DNA. Consequently, the fluorescence of the QDs was quenched. Furthermore, this design can be used for the detection of multiple cations, as confirmed by Willner. The PET-based fluorescence sensing is simple, low-cost, and efficient.

The authors have developed a label-free sensor for Hg^{2+} detection with the water-soluble GO as the fluorophore (Figure 4.7b) [85]. A single-stranded aptamer was

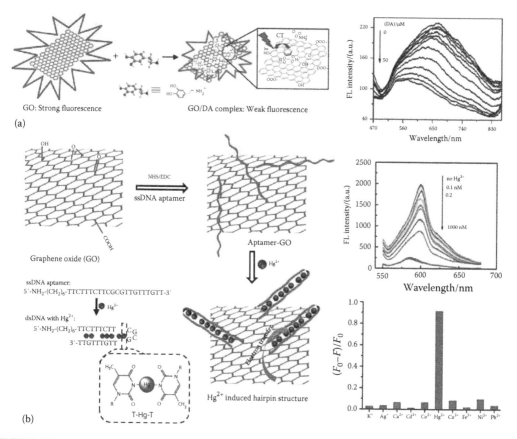

FIGURE 4.7
(a) Sketch showing the graphene (GO)-based biosensor based on the photo-induced charge transfer for detection of dopamine, and the fluorescence spectra of 25 µg/mL GO solution under excitation at 450 nm at various dopamine concentrations in a 5.0 mM Tris-HCl solution (0, 0.25, 0.5, 1.0, 2.0, 3.0, 5.0, 10, 20, 30, 40, and 50 µM). (Reproduced from Chen, J.L. et al., *Anal. Chem.*, 83, 8787, 2011.) (b) The GO-based fluorescent sensor for detection of Hg^{2+} ions, and the fluorescence spectra of the aptamer-GO conjugates in the assay solution containing various concentrations (0, 0.1, 0.2, 0.5, 1, 2, 10, 20, 50, 100, 500, and 1000 nM) of Hg^{2+} ions. (Reproduced from Li, M. et al., *Biosens. Bioelectron.*, 41, 889, 2013.)

covalently conjugated to the GO sheets. The GO–aptamer conjugate emitted the fluorescence under light excitation. When Hg^{2+} ions were present in the assay, the aptamer was subject to the conformation change due to the formation of the T-Hg^{2+}-T complex. As a result, electrons can transfer from the GO to Hg^{2+} ions *via* the double-stranded DNA, leading to the fluorescence quenching of the GO sheets. This sensor achieved a LOD of 0.92 nM in an aqueous solution. Due to the water-solubility feature and low-cost preparation of GO, the GO-based fluorescent sensors are superior in comparison with those QD-based sensors.

One appealing characteristic of GO is that some types of biomacromolecules such as DNA and aptamer can be physically adsorbed through the π–π stacking interaction [86–88]. Similarly, small aromatic molecules can be adsorbed on the GO sheets due to the π–π interaction (Figure 4.7a) [86–89]. These unique features render the possibility of label-free sensing with GO. Yan et al. have reported a GO-based PET biosensor for the detection of dopamine. The multiple noncovalent interactions between GO and dopamine resulted in the effective self-assembly of dopamine molecules on the surface of GO. And the fluorescence of the GO underwent ultrafast decay at the picoseconds range. The dopamine concentration was determined *via* the direct readout of the near-IR fluorescence of GO. This sensor reached a LOD of 94 nM toward dopamine.

4.6 Future Direction and Perspectives

Significant progress has been made on the fluorescent sensors based on energy transfer and charge transfer processes. In particular, the incorporation of NMs into fluorescent sensors has brought great benefits to the performance of fluorescent sensors including sensitivity, photostability, and multiplexed capability. In addition, the use of aptamers as the molecular recognition probes provides great flexibility for the design of fluorescent sensors. However, there are still many challenges to be resolved. A lot of sensor research is at the proof-of-concept stage. There is still a long way to go before commercialization.

When NMs are used as the fluorophores in the complex sample matrix, their fluorescence could be quenched by the nonspecific molecules and ions.

Although NMs-based fluorescent sensors have been demonstrated in both *in vitro* and *in vivo* sensing and bioimaging, the *in vivo* application is less common. To extend their applications in *in vivo* bioimaging, near-infrared fluorophores need to be developed to make the fluorescence emission penetrate in deep tissues. It is desirable to reduce or even avoid the use of external excitation sources, which will reduce the noise background and simplify the design of sensing systems.

In vitro and *in vivo* bioimaging have been demonstrated with QDs. However, the potential toxicity of QDs still needs to be evaluated. It is essential to develop biocompatible and benign QDs.

Fluorescent sensors have great potential in the rapid, high-throughput monitoring of environmental toxins and biomarkers. However, many fluorescent sensors reported previously can be operated only in the buffer solution, and their performance becomes deleterious in the real-world samples. Tedious sample preparation and preconcentration are necessary prior to the use of sensors. An efficient solution to this problem is to integrate the fluorescent sensors with the microfluidic channels and the controllers in a single chip to form a highly automated lab-on-chip.

Acknowledgments

This work was financially supported by a NSF grant (CBET-1336205). The resource and facilities used were partially supported by NSF (EPS 1003907) and a Research Challenge Grant, from the State of West Virginia (EPS08-01), the West Virginia University Research Corporation, and the West Virginia EPSCoR Office. N.W. is also grateful to the partial support of the George D. Hott Memorial and John Mathew Gay Brown Family Foundation. The use of the WVU Shared Research Facilities was acknowledged.

References

1. Vendrell, M., Zhai, D., Er, J. C., and Chang, Y.-T. Combinatorial strategies in fluorescent probe development. *Chem. Rev.* 2012, 112, 4391–4420.
2. Roy, R., Hohng, S., and Ha, T. A practical guide to single-molecule FRET. *Nat. Methods* 2008, 5, 507–515.
3. Gao, Y. Q., Georgievskii, Y., and Marcus, R. A. On the theory of electron transfer reactions at semiconductor electrode/liquid interfaces. *J. Chem. Phys.* 2000, 112, 3358–3369.
4. Dexter, D. L. A theory of sensitized luminescence in solids. *J. Chem. Phys.* 1953, 21, 836–850.
5. Lakowicz, J. R. *Principles of Fluorescence Spectroscopy*, 3rd edn. Springer Academic, New York, 2006.
6. Chen, H., Ratner, M. A., and Schatz, G. C. Time-dependent theory of the rate of photo-induced electron transfer. *J. Phys. Chem. C* 2011, 115, 18810–18821.
7. Barbara, P. F., Meyer, T. J., and Ratner, M. A. Contemporary issues in electron transfer research. *J. Phys. Chem.* 1996, 100, 13148–13168.
8. Franzen, S., Lao, K., and Boxer, S. G. Electric field effects on kinetics of electron transfer reactions: Connection between experiment and theory. *Chem. Phys. Lett.* 1992, 197, 380–388.
9. Subotnik, J. E., Vura-Weis, J., Sodt, A. J., and Ratner, M. A. Predicting accurate electronic excitation transfer rates via Marcus theory with boys or Edmiston-Ruedenberg localized diabatizatio. *J. Phys. Chem. A* 2010, 114, 8665–8675.
10. Marcus, R. A. On the theory of oxidation-reduction reactions involving electron transfer. I. *J. Chem. Phys.* 1956, 24, 966–978.
11. Tvrdy, K., Frantsuzov, P. A., and Kamat, P. V. Photoinduced electron transfer from semiconductor quantum dots to metal oxide nanoparticles. *PNAS* 2011, 108, 29–34.
12. Weller, A. Photoinduced electron-transfer in solution-exciplex and radical ion pair formation three enthalpies and their solvent dependence. *Z. Phys. Chem. Neue Folge* 1982, 133, 93–98.
13. Gill, R., Willner, I., Shweky, I., and Banin, U. Fluorescence resonance energy transfer in CdSe/ZnS-DNA conjugates: Probing hybridization and DNA cleavage. *J. Phys. Chem. B* 2005, 109, 23715–23719.
14. Rantanen, T., Järvenpää, M.-L., Vuojola, J., Kuningas, K., and Soukka, T. Fluorescence-quenching-based enzyme-activity assay by using photon upconversion. *Angew. Chem. Int. Ed.* 2008, 47, 3811–3813.
15. Makhal, A., Sarkar, S., Bora, T., Baruah, S., Dutta, J., Raychaudhuri A. K., and Pal, S. K. Role of resonance energy transfer in light harvesting of zinc oxide-based dye-sensitized solar cells. *J. Phys. Chem. C* 2010, 114, 10390–10395.
16. Clapp, A. R., Medintz, I. L., Mauro, J. M., Fisher, B.R., Bawendi, M. G., and Mattoussi, H. Fluorescence resonance energy transfer between quantum dot donors and dye-labeled protein acceptors. *J. Am. Chem. Soc.* 2004, 126, 301–310.

17. Li, M., Cushing, S. K., Wang, Q., Shi, X., Hornak, L. A., Hong, Z., and Wu, N. Size-dependent energy transfer between CdSe/ZnS quantum dots and gold nanoparticles. *J. Phys. Chem. Lett.* 2011, 2, 2125–2129.
18. Pons, T., Medintz, I. L., Sapsford, K. E., Higashiya, S., Grimes, A. F., English, D. S., and Mattoussi, H. On the quenching of semiconductor quantum dot photoluminescence by proximal gold nanoparticles. *Nano Lett.* 2007, 7, 3157–3164.
19. Mayilo, S., Kloster, M. A., Wunderlich, M., Lutich, A., Klar, T. A., Nichtl, A., Kürzinger, K., Stefani, F. D., and Feldmann, J. Long-range fluorescence quenching by gold nanoparticles in a sandwich immunoassay for cardiac troponin T. *Nano Lett.* 2009, 9, 4558–4563.
20. Huang, C.-C. and Chang, H.-T. Selective gold-nanoparticle-based "turn-on" fluorescent sensors for detection of mercury(II) in aqueous solution. *Anal. Chem.* 2006, 78, 8332–8338.
21. Zhang, C., Yuan, Y., Zhang, S., Wang, Y., and Liu, Z. Biosensing platform based on fluorescence resonance energy transfer from upconverting nanocrystals to graphene oxide. *Angew. Chem. Int. Ed.* 2011, 50, 6851–6854.
22. Dong, H., Gao, W., Yan, F., Ji, H., and Ju, H. Fluorescence resonance energy transfer between quantum dots and graphene oxide for sensing biomolecules. *Anal. Chem.* 2010, 82, 5511–5517.
23. Jennings, T. L., Singh, M. P., and Strouse, G. F. Fluorescent lifetime quenching near d = 1.5 nm gold nanoparticles: Probing NSET validity. *J. Am. Chem. Soc.* 2006, 128, 5462–5467.
24. Gueroui, Z. and Libchabe, A. Single-molecule measurements of gold-quenched quantum dots. *Phys. Rev. Lett.* 2004, 93, 166108.
25. Yun, C. S., Javier, A., Jennings, T., Fisher, M., Hira, S., Peterson, S., Hopkins, B., Reich, N. O., and Strouse, G. F. Nanometal surface energy transfer in optical rulers, breaking the FRET barrier. *J. Am. Chem. Soc.* 2005, 127, 3115–3119.
26. Swathi, R. S. and Sebastian, K. L. Resonance energy transfer from a dye molecule to graphene. *J. Chem. Phys.* 2008, 129, 054703.
27. Swathi, R. S. and Sebastian, K. L. Long range resonance energy transfer from a dye molecule to graphene has (distance)$^{-4}$ dependence. *J. Chem. Phys.* 2009, 130, 086101.
28. Huang, P. J. J. and Liu, J. DNA-length-dependent fluorescence signaling on graphene oxide surface. *Small* 2012, 8, 977–983.
29. Zhao, S., Huang, Y., Shi, M., Liu, R., and Liu, Y. M. Chemiluminescence resonance energy transfer-based detection for microchip electrophoresis. *Anal. Chem.* 2010, 82, 2036–2041.
30. Qin, G., Zhao, S., Huang, Y., Jiang, J., and Ye, F. Magnetic bead-sensing-platform-based chemiluminescence resonance energy transfer and its immunoassay application. *Anal. Chem.* 2012, 84, 2708–2712.
31. Sapsford, K. E., Berti, L., and Medintz, I. L. Materials for fluorescence resonance energy transfer analysis: Beyond traditional donor–acceptor combinations. *Angew. Chem. Int. Ed.* 2006, 45, 4562–4588.
32. Ling, J. and Huang, C. Z. Energy transfer with gold nanoparticles for analytical applications in the fields of biochemical and pharmaceutical sciences. *Anal. Methods* 2010, 2, 1439–1447.
33. Ai, K., Zhang, B., and Lu, L. Europium-based fluorescence nanoparticle sensor for rapid and ultrasensitive detection of an anthrax biomarker. *Angew. Chem. Int. Ed.* 2008, 47, 1–6.
34. Zhang, F., Haushalter, R. C., Haushalter, R. W., Shi, Y., Zhang, Y., Ding, K., Zhao, D., and Stucky, G. D. Rare-earth upconverting nanobarcodes for multiplexed biological detection. *Small* 2011, 7, 1972–1976.
35. Chan, W. C. W. and Nie, S. Quantum dot bioconjugates for ultrasensitive nonisotopic detection. *Science* 1998, 281, 2016–2018.
36. Shang, L. and Dong, S. Sensitive detection of cysteine based on fluorescent silver clusters. *Biosens. Bioelectron.* 2009, 24, 1569–1573.
37. Gaponik, N., Hickey, S. G., Dorfs, D., Rogach, A. L., and Eychmüller, A. Progress in the light emission of colloidal semiconductor nanocrystals. *Small* 2010, 6, 1364–1378.
38. Kagan, C. R., Murray, C. B., Nirmal, M., and Bawendi, M. G. Electronic energy transfer in CdSe quantum dot solids. *Phys. Rev. Lett.* 1996, 76, 1517.

39. Mandal, P. K. and Chikan, V. Plasmon–phonon coupling in charged n-type CdSe quantum dots: A THz time-domain spectroscopic study. *Nano Lett.* 2007, 7, 2521–2528.

40. Goldman, E. R., Medintz, I. L., Whitley, J. L., Hayhurst, A., Clapp, A. R., Uyeda, H. T., Deschamps, J. R., Lassman, M. E., and Mattoussi, H. A hybrid quantum dot-antibody fragment fluorescence resonance energy transfer-based TNT sensor. *J. Am. Chem. Soc.* 2005, 127, 6744–6751.

41. Medintz, I. L., Clapp, A. R., Brunel, F. M., Tiefenbrunn, T., Uyeda, H. T., Chang, E. L., Deschamps, J. R., Dawson, P. E., and Mattoussi, H. Proteolytic activity monitored by fluorescence resonance energy transfer through quantum-dot–peptide conjugates. *Nat. Mater.* 2006, 5, 581–589.

42. Han, M., Gao, X., Su, J. Z., and Nie, S. Quantum-dot-tagged microbeads for multiplexed optical coding of biomolecules. *Nat. Biotechnol.* 2001, 19, 631–635.

43. Geißer, D., Charbonnière, L. J., Ziessel, R. F., Butlin, N. G., Löhmannsröben, H., and Hildebrandt, N. Quantum dot biosensors for ultrasensitive multiplexed diagnostics. *Angew. Chem. Int. Ed.* 2010, 49, 1396–1401.

44. Goldman, E. R., Clapp, A. R., Anderson, G. P., Uyeda, H. T., Mauro, J. M., Medintz, I. L., and Mattoussi, H. Multiplexed toxin analysis using four colors of quantum dot fluororeagents. *Anal. Chem.* 2004, 76, 684–688.

45. Clapp, A. R., Medintz, I. L., Uyeda, H. T., Fisher, B. R., Goldman, E. R., Bawendi, M. G., and Mattoussi, H. Quantum dot-based multiplexed fluorescence resonance energy transfer. *J. Am. Chem. Soc.* 2005, 127, 18212–18221.

46. Algar, W. R., Massey, M., and Krull, U. J. The application of quantum dots, gold nanoparticles and molecular switches to optical nucleic-acid diagnostics. *Trends Anal. Chem.* 2009, 28, 292–306.

47. Jun, B. H., Kim, J. E., Rho, C., Byun, J. W., Kim, Y. H., Kang, H., Kim, J. H., Kang, T., Cho, M. H., and Lee, Y. S. Immobilization of aptamer-based molecular beacons onto optically encoded micro-sized beads. *J. Nanosci. Nanotechnol.* 2011, 11, 6249–6252.

48. Hwang, E., Smolyaninov, I. I., and Davis, C. C. Surface plasmon polariton enhanced fluorescence from quantum dots on nanostructured metal surfaces. *Nano Lett.* 2010, 10, 813–820.

49. Pfeiffer, M., Lindfors, K., Wolpert, C., Atkinson, P., Benyoucef, M., Rastelli, A., Schmidt, O. G., Giessen, H., and Lippitz, M. Enhancing the optical excitation efficiency of a single self-assembled quantum dot with a plasmonic nanoantenna. *Nano Lett.* 2010, 10, 4555–4558.

50. Pustovit, V. N. and Shahbazyan, T. V. Resonance energy transfer near metal nanostructures mediated by surface plasmons. *Phys. Rev. B* 2011, 83, 085427.

51. Chan, Y.-H., Chen, J., Wark, S. E., Skiles, S. L., Son, D. H., and Batteas, J. D. Using patterned arrays of metal nanoparticles to probe plasmon enhanced luminescence of CdSe quantum dots. *ACS Nano* 2009, 3, 1735–1744.

52. Lu, G., Li, W., Zhang, T., Yue, S., Liu, J., Hou, L., Li, Z., and Gong, Q. Plasmonic-enhanced molecular fluorescence within isolated bowtie nano-apertures. *ACS Nano* 2012, 6, 1438–1448.

53. Zhou, L., Ding, F., Chen, H., Ding, W., Zhang, W., and Chou, S. Y. Enhancement of immunoassay's fluorescence and detection sensitivity using three-dimensional plasmonic nano-antenna-dots array. *Anal. Chem.* 2012, 84, 4489–4495.

54. Reil, F., Hohenester, U., Krenn, J. R., and Leitner, A. Förster-type resonant energy transfer influenced by metal nanoparticles. *Nano Lett.* 2008, 8, 4128–4133.

55. Zhao, L., Ming, T., Shao, L., Chen, H., and Wang, J. Plasmon-controlled Förster resonance energy transfer. *J. Phys. Chem. C* 2012, 116, 8287–8296.

56. Zhang, J., Fu, Y., Chowdhury, M. H., and Lakowicz, J. R. Enhanced Förster resonance energy transfer on single metal particle. 2. Dependence on donor-acceptor separation distance, particle size, and distance from metal surface. *J. Phys. Chem. C* 2007, 111, 11784–11792.

57. Sekiguchi, S., Niikura, K., Iyo, N., Matsuo, Y., Eguchi, A., Nakabayashi, T., Ohta, N., and Ijiro, K. pH-Dependent network formation of quantum dots and fluorescent quenching by Au nanoparticle embedding. *ACS Appl. Mater. Interfaces* 2011, 3, 4169–4173.

58. Mandal, G., Bardhan, M., and Ganguly, T. Occurrence of Förster resonance energy transfer between quantum dots and gold nanoparticles in the presence of a biomolecule. *J. Phys. Chem. C* 2011, 115, 20840–20848.

59. Kondon, M., Kim, J., Udawatte, N., and Lee, D. Origin of size-dependent energy transfer from photoexcited CdSe quantum dots to gold nanoparticles. *J. Phys. Chem. C* 2008, 112, 6695–6699.
60. Li, M., Wang, Q., Shi, X., Hornak, L. A., and Wu, N. Detection of mercury(II) by quantum dot/DNA/gold nanoparticle ensemble based nanosensor via nanometal surface energy transfer. *Anal. Chem.* 2011, 83, 7061–7065.
61. Darbha, G. K., Ray, A., and Ray, P. C. Gold nanoparticle-based miniaturized nanomaterial surface energy transfer probe for rapid and ultrasensitive detection of mercury in soil, water, and fish. *ACS Nano* 2007, 1, 208–214.
62. Griffin, J., Singh, A. K., Senapati, D., Rhodes, P., Mitchell, K., Robinson, B., Yu, E., and Ray, P. C. Size- and distance-dependent nanoparticle surface-energy transfer (NSET) method for selective sensing of hepatitis C virus RNA. *Chem. Eur. J.* 2009, 15, 342–351.
63. Jander, S., Kornowski, A., and Weller, H. Energy transfer from CdSe/CdS nanorods to amorphous carbon. *Nano Lett.* 2011, 11, 5179–5183.
64. Guo, S. and Dong, S. Graphene and its derivative-based sensing materials for analytical devices. *J. Mater. Chem.* 2011, 21, 18503–18516.
65. Li, J. L., Bao, H. C., Hou, X. L., Sun, L., Wang, X. G., and Gu, M. Graphene oxide nanoparticles as a nonbleaching optical probe for two-photon luminescence imaging and cell therapy. *Angew. Chem. Int. Ed.* 2012, 51, 1830–1834.
66. Freeman, R., Liu, X., and Willner, I. Chemiluminescent and chemiluminescence resonance energy transfer (CRET) detection of DNA, metal ions, and aptamer–substrate complexes using hemin/G-quadruplexes and CdSe/ZnS quantum dots. *J. Am. Chem. Soc.* 2011, 133, 11597–11604.
67. Liu, X., Freeman, R., Golub, E., and Willner, I. Chemiluminescence and chemiluminescence resonance energy transfer (CRET) aptamer sensors using catalytic hemin/G-quadruplexes. *ACS Nano* 2011, 5, 7648–7655.
68. Freeman, R., Willner, B., and Willner, I. Integrated biomolecule–quantum dot hybrid systems for bioanalytical applications. *J. Phys. Chem. Lett.* 2011, 2, 2667–2677.
69. Lee, J. S., Joung, H. A., Kim, M. G., and Park, C. B. Graphene-based chemiluminescence resonance energy transfer for homogeneous immunoassay. *ACS Nano* 2012, 24, 2978–2983.
70. Rasnik, I., Mckinney, S. A., and Ha, T. Surfaces and orientations: Much to FRET about? *Acc. Chem. Res.* 2005, 38, 542–548.
71. Morgner, F., Geißer, D., Stufler, S., Butlin, N. G, Löhmannsröben, H. G., and Hildebrandt, N. A quantum-dot-based molecular ruler for multiplexed optical analysis. *Angew. Chem. Int. Ed.* 2010, 49, 7570–7574.
72. Singh, A. K., Lu, W., Senapati, D., Khan, S. A., Fan, Z., Senapati, T., Demeritte, T., Beqa, L., and Ray, P. C. Long-range nanoparticle surface-energy-transfer ruler for monitoring photothermal therapy response. *Small* 2011, 7, 2517–2525.
73. Talaga, D. S., Lau, W. L., Roder, H., Tang, J., Jia, Y., DeGrado, W. F., and Hochstrasser, R. M. Dynamics and folding of single two-stranded coiled-coil peptides studied by fluorescent energy transfer confocal microscopy. *Proc. Natl. Acad. Sci. U.S.A.* 2000, 97, 13021–13026.
74. Kim, H. D., Nienhaus, G. U., Ha, T., Orr, J. W., Williamson, J. R., and Chu, S. Mg2+-dependent conformational change of RNA studied by fluorescence correlation and FRET on immobilized single molecules. *Proc. Natl. Acad. Sci. U.S.A.* 2002, 99, 4284–4289.
75. Nyk, M., Kumar, R., Ohulchanskyy, T. Y., Bergey, E. J., and Prasad, P. N. High contrast in vitro and in vivo photoluminescence bioimaging using near infrared to near infrared Up-conversion in Tm^{3+} and Yb^{3+} doped fluoride nanophosphors. *Nano Lett.* 2008, 8, 3834–3838.
76. Dennis, A. M., Rhee, W. J., Sotto, D., Dublin, S. N., and Bao, G. Quantum dot–fluorescent protein FRET probes for sensing intracellular pH. *ACS Nano* 2012, 6, 2917–2924.
77. So, M. K., Xu, C., Loening, A. M., Gambhir, S. S., and Rao, J. Self-illuminating quantum dot conjugates for in vivo imaging. *Nat. Biotechnol.* 2006, 24, 339–343.
78. Haase, M. and Schäfer, H. Upconverting nanoparticles. *Angew. Chem. Int. Ed.* 2011, 50, 5808–5829.
79. Yang, Y., Shao, Q., Deng, R., Wang, C., Teng, X., Cheng, K., Cheng, Z., Huang, L., Liu, Z., Liu, X., and Xing, B. In vitro and in vivo uncaging and bioluminescence imaging by using photocaged upconversion nanoparticles. *Angew. Chem. Int. Ed.* 2012, 51, 3125–3129.

80. Liu, Q., Peng, J., Sun, L., and Li, F. High-efficiency upconversion luminescent sensing and bio-imaging of Hg(II) by chromophoric ruthenium complex-assembled nanophosphors. *ACS Nano* 2011, 5, 8040–8048.

81. Englich, F. V., Foo, T. C., Richardson, A. C., Ebendorff-Heidepriem, H., Sumby, C. J., and Monro, T. M. Photoinduced electron transfer based ion sensing within an optical fiber. *Sensors* 2011, 11, 9560–9572.

82. Haas, C., Kräling, K., Cichon, M., Rahe, N., and Carell, T. Excess electron transfer driven DNA does not depend on the transfer direction. *Angew. Chem.* 2004, 116, 1878–1880.

83. Boon, E. M., Ceres, D. M., Drummond, T. G., Hill, M. G., and Barton, J. K. Mutation detection by electrocatalysis at DNA-modified electrodes. *Nat. Biotechnol.* 2000, 18, 1096–1100.

84. Freeman, R., Finder, T., and Willner, I. Multiplexed analysis of Hg^{2+} and Ag^+ ions by nucleic acid functionalized CdSe/ZnS quantum dots and their use for logic gate operations. *Angew. Chem. Int. Ed.* 2009, 48, 7958–7961.

85. Li, M., Zhou, X., Ding, W., Guo, S., and Wu, N. Q. Fluorescent aptamer-functionalized graphene oxide biosensor for label-free detection of mercury(II). *Biosens. Bioelectron.* 2013, 41, 889–893.

86. Patil, A. J., Vickery, J. L., Scott, T. B., and Mann, S. Aqueous stabilization and self-assembly of graphene sheets into layered bio-nanocomposites using DNA. *Adv. Mater.* 2009, 21, 3159–3164.

87. Wang, Y., Li, Z., Wang, J., Li, J., and Lin, Y. Graphene and graphene oxide: Biofunctionalization and applications in biotechnology. *Trends Biotechnol.* 2011, 29, 205–212.

88. Wang, Y., Li, Z., Hu, D., Lin, C.-T., Li, J., and Lin, Y. Aptamer/graphene oxide nanocomplex for in situ molecular probing in living cells. *J. Am. Chem. Soc.* 2010, 132, 9274–9276.

89. Chen, J. L., Yan, X. P., Meng, K., and Wang, S. F. Graphene oxide based photoinduced charge transfer label-free near-infrared fluorescent biosensor for dopamine. *Anal. Chem.* 2011, 83, 8787–8793.

5

Graphene-Based Optical Biosensors and Imaging

Zhiwen Tang, Shijiang He, Hao Pei, Dan Du, Chunhai Fan, and Yuehe Lin

CONTENTS

5.1 Introduction

Graphene is the fundamental building element of many carbon allotropes including graphite, charcoals, carbon nanotubes, buckminsterfullerene, and other buckyballs, etc. Graphene comprises a single layer of six-atom rings in a honeycombed network and can be conceptually considered as a true planar aromatic macromolecule.[1] Interestingly the theory of graphene was explored in 1947 and scientists believed that graphene could not exist by itself due to thermodynamic instability at the nanometer scale. Though scientists investigated the reduced graphene oxide in 1962, the key advance in graphene synthesis and study was explored in 2004 by scientists at Manchester University peeling a single layer of graphene using adhesive tape and a pencil, which is often referred to as a scotch–tape or drawing method.[2] In 2005, they collaborated with another group from Columbia University and found that the quasiparticles in graphene were massless Dirac fermions. Later more important unusual properties of graphene have been unveiled such as the quantum Hall effect, the bipolar-transistor effect, the ballistic transport of charges, large quantum oscillations, etc., which led to the immediate boost of further researches and applications based on graphene. Today graphene is attracting increasing attention from the physical, chemical, and biomedical fields as a novel nanomaterial with many exceptional features including unparalleled thermal conductivity (5000 W/m/K), excellent electrical conductivity (1738 S/m), high surface-to-volume ratio (2630 m^2/g), remarkable mechanical strength (about 1100 GPa), and biocompatibility. Recently, graphene and functionalized graphene have been successfully used in many biomedical and bioassay applications and show promising potentials in these fields. These applications utilized the advantages of graphene in electrical and optical properties to construct a variety of graphene-based biosensors including electrochemical biosensors, field-effect transistor (FET) biosensors, optical biosensors, etc. Compared to carbon nanotubes, graphene lacks some bandgap-induced optical properties, but its chemical versatility and tunability nature, fluorescence, effective quencher, Raman, and NIR activity make it favorable, for fabricating optical bio-sensors. Recently, graphene-based optical nanobiosensors have been constructed to detect DNA/RNA, proteins, small molecules, and ions using different signal platforms, including fluorescence, colorimetry, SPR, SERS, etc.[3] This chapter focuses on the recent progress in graphene-based optical biosensors and discusses the design, fabrication, and application of these optical nanobiosensors. In the end, we will discuss the future opportunities and challenges in this field. Since the basics of graphene, including its synthesis and properties, has been described in Chapter 13, this chapter will not deal with it.

5.2 Graphene Oxide–Based DNA Biosensors

Graphene oxide (GO) exhibits interesting optical properties.[4] Because the disordered oxygenated functional groups on GO confine π electrons within the sp^2-carbon nanodomains, GO can fluoresce in a wide range of wavelengths (from near-infrared to ultra-violet).[4,5] Interestingly, although GO is itself fluorescent, it is also capable of quenching fluorescence.[6–8] The quenching efficiency of GO is superior to the conventional organic quenchers. It has been estimated that the quenching efficiency of pristine graphene is as large as 10^3, and the quenching even at a distance of 30 nm is attainable by GO.[9,10] On the basis of such fluorescence quenching effects, GO can serve as a good energy acceptor in fluorescence resonance energy transfer (FRET) biosensors. GO has been reported to interact strongly with nucleic acids (NAs) through π–π stacking interactions between the ring structures in the NA bases and the hexagonal cells of graphene and GO.[11] Consequently, the dye-labeled single-stranded-DNA (ssDNA) probes are attached firmly onto GO, which leads to fluorescence quenching. However, the dye-labeled ssDNA probes form a duplex with the target DNA so that it becomes rigid, and conformation changes, which, in turn, lead to the release of the duplex from the GO surface. And the subsequent termination of FRET restores the fluorescence of the initially quenched fluorophore. The mechanism is schematically shown in Figure 5.1a.

For example, He et al.[11] and Lu et al.[12] have demonstrated that the GO-based FRET DNA biosensor includes a fluorescein amidite (FAM)–labeled ssDNA, adsorbed onto the GO surface (Figure 5.1a). When the target complementary DNA (cDNA) is added, the fluorescence of FAM is recovered. The detection of target cDNA is therefore realized. In addition, because of the large planar surface of GO which allows the simultaneous quenching of multiple ssDNA probes labeled with different dyes, He et al.[11] developed a multicolor DNA analysis strategy (Figure 5.1b). In this case, a GO-based FRET biosensor is able to detect three different DNA targets using ssDNA probes with different sequences (Figure 5.1c through e). To enhance the specificity of this kind of biosensor, Tang et al.[13] have revealed that the ssDNA constrained on functionalized graphene, can be effectively protected from DNAase cleavage, which can improve the specificity of its response to target DNA (Figure 5.2a). In order to improve the sensitivity, a molecular beacon (MB) has been employed to fabricate the GO-based FRET DNA biosensor (Figure 5.2b).[14]

MB is a single-stranded oligonucleotide hybridization probe with a stem-and-loop structure in which the loop contains a probe sequence that is complementary to a target

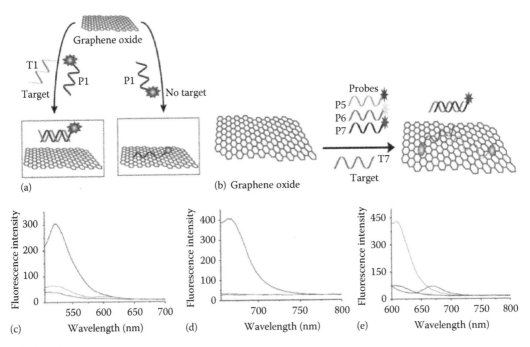

FIGURE 5.1

(a) Scheme for the fluorescent DNA detection based on the ssDNA/dsDNA discrimination ability of GO. (b) Scheme for the target hybridization-induced probe liberation from GO. (c–e) Fluorescence spectra for multicolor detection. Probe mixture in the presence of different targets T5, T6, and T7, with the excitation/emission wavelengths of (c) 494/526, (d) 643/666, and (e) 587/609 nm/nm.

sequence and the annealing of self-complementary 5′ and 3′ ends forms a stem.[15] Typically, the two ends of an MB are labeled with a fluorophore and a quencher. The target DNA molecule opens the stem–loop structure that separates the fluorophore–quencher pair, thereby restoring the fluorescence of the fluorophore.[16] Compared with linear probes, MBs provide new opportunities to detect DNA targets with high sensitivity and selectivity due to their unique thermodynamics and inherent structural constraint.[17,18] It has been reported that GO can serve as a quencher for fluorophore as well as a scaffold for MB (Figure 5.2b). The incorporation of GO with MB greatly enhances the signal-to-noise ratio of the FRET biosensor, resulting in a detection limit for the target DNA of 0.1 nM. Moreover, this method can be used for the detection of single-base mismatched target DNA. And it can be operated at high temperature (75°C) because of the high thermal stability of the MB–GO complex. It is worth noting that the quantum dots (QDs) have been introduced to the GO-based FRET biosensor to form a GO/MB-QDs sensing platform, which has displayed good selectivity and high sensitivity.[19]

5.3 Graphene-Based Optical Biosensors for Protein Assays

The chemical versatility and tunable function groups on the graphene oxide (GO) surface make GO an ideal platform to immobilize a variety of biomolecules including nucleic acids, peptides, proteins, etc. Here, we discuss the fabrications and the sensing mechanisms of

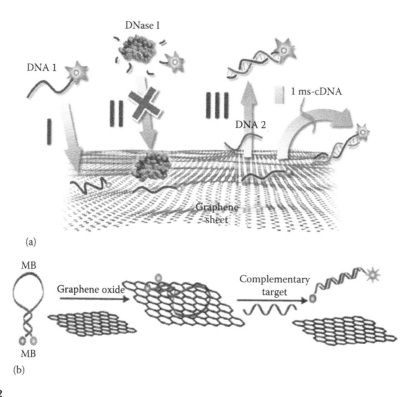

(a)

(b)

FIGURE 5.2
(a) Schematic illustration of the constraint of DNA molecules on functionalized graphene and its effects. (I) The single-stranded DNA can be effectively constrained on the surface of graphene via adsorption. (II) DNase I can digest free DNA but not graphene-bound DNA. (III) The constrained DNA show improved specificity response toward target sequences that can distinguish the complementary and single-mismatch targets. (b) Schematic presentation of nano-MBs with GO-enhanced quenching efficiency. The hairpin-structured DNA has stronger infinity with GO than dsDNA.

GO-based optical biosensors. In some protein biosensors, GO is used as the fluorescence emitter to construct the sensing transducer based on FRET or fluorescence intensity change. In other biosensors, graphene is utilized as the effective quencher. In some studies, graphene is employed as the biocompatible and convenient platform to immobilize biomolecules for sensing purpose.

Since GO has intrinsic fluorescence, GO-based biosensors have been designed by altering its intrinsic fluorescence in the presence of target biomolecules including protein, peptide, DNA/RNA, and virus.

Jung et al. have developed a GO-based biosensor to detect the virus particles by quenching the GO's intrinsic photoluminescence with gold nanoparticles.[20] The rotavirus-specific antibody is conjugated onto the GO surface via the amino and carboxyl reaction. After the capture of the rotavirus by the chemically anchored antibody, a secondary antibody conjugated with gold nanoparticles is introduced. The binding of the secondary antibody to rotavirus brings the gold nanoparticle close to the GO surface. The gold nanoparticles then efficiently quench the fluorescence of the GO. This biosensor can specifically and sensitively detect rotavirus. The authors have also successfully fabricated a microarray using this approach. This highly sensitive, specific, and rapid pathogen detection is a promising alternative to conventional time-consuming pathogen assays, which can be used for disease diagnostics, food safety inspection, and environmental pollution evaluation.

Mei and colleagues have fabricated a GO sensor on microporous membranes for the visual detection of a variety of biomolecules including peptides, proteins, and DNA.[21] The authors used a new approach different from the previous studies. In this method, silver nanoparticles (Ag NPs) modified with peptides, antibodies, and DNA are adsorbed onto the GO surface and quench the fluorescence of GO. Upon the addition of target molecules, the Ag NPs are disassociated from the GO nanosheets, resulting in the immediate restoration of fluorescence, which provides an ultrasensitive assay. In addition, the biomolecule–Ag NPs–GO complex can be easily used as the ink to print a test paper for sensitive and visual detection (Figure 5.3). This GO-based portable biosensor can be used for the convenient visual detections of peptide, protein, and DNA, which can serve as a point-of-care device.

Park and colleagues have constructed a GO-based immunosensor via the quenching of the innate fluorescence of GO in the presence of the peroxidase-catalyzed polymerization product.[22] In this study, the interleukin-5 (IL-5), a key cytokine associated with asthma pathology and eosinophilia, is used as the analyte model. After depositing the GO onto the amino-modified glass surface, one IL-5 antibody is immobilized as the capture antibody. The captured IL-5 is recognized and bound with another peroxidase-linked IL-5 antibody. In the presence of peroxide, the 3,3′-diaminobenzidine (DAB) is catalyzed to form the polymerization product, which is adsorbed on the GO surface, and effectively quenches the fluorescence of GO. The GO-based immunoassay

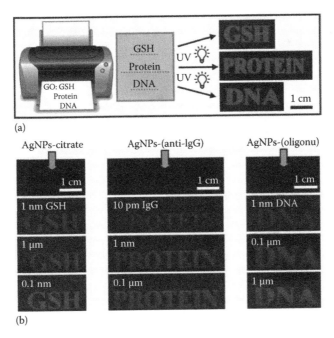

FIGURE 5.3

Visual biosensors: (a) The inkjet printing of GO-based sensing material into "words" on microporous polyvinylidene fluoride membrane. (b) Visual detections of GSH, IgG, and DNA under a UV lamp.

has demonstrated high specificity for IL-5 among other cytokines and is not affected by human serum proteins. The detection limit of IL-5 is about 5 pg/mL. This GO-based immunoassay platform can be readily adapted for the detection of other protein targets, by changing antibodies.

GO not only acts as a fluorophore but also serves as an effective fluorescence quencher. Recently, Pei et al. have developed a graphene-based sensor array for target identification with a new concept of adaptive "ensemble aptamers" (ENSaptamer), which exploits the collective recognition abilities of a small set of rationally designed, nonspecific DNA sequences to discriminatively identify molecular or cellular targets.[23] Interestingly, this graphene-based biosensor relies on the pattern recognition that mimics natural olfactory or gustatory systems, which is distinctly different from traditional, specific, "lock-and-key" recognition process. In brief, they have constructed the ENSaptamer elements by selecting a set of fluorescent dye-labeled single-stranded oligonucleotides with variation of the length, sequence, and secondary structure. Each of ENSaptamer elements is mixed with nano–graphene oxide (NGO), respectively. The flat, relatively homogeneous surface and superquenching ability of NGO ensures high reproducibility and detection sensitivity. While the target (such as proteins) is detected at the NGO–ENSaptamer sensing platform, the presence of each protein leads to differential fluorescent responses due to their interactions with NGO and ssDNA elements (Figure 5.4a and b). The fluorescent

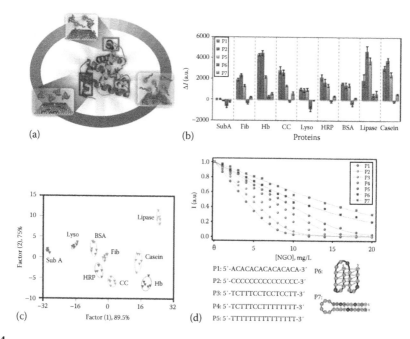

FIGURE 5.4

(a) Scheme for the ENSaptamer/NGO-based sensing platform. A set of fluorescently labeled ssDNA probes (ENSaptamers) are efficiently quenched in the presence of NGO, which are differentially displaced with the addition of molecular or cellular targets, resulting in distinctive fluorescence fingerprints for individual targets. (b) Fluorescence response patterns of ENSaptamer against various proteins, subtilisin A (SubA), fibrinogen (Fib), hemoglobin (Hb), cytochrome c (CC), lysozyme (Lyso), horseradish peroxidase (HRP), and bovine serum albumin (BSA). Error bars represent the standard deviation of six parallel measurements. (c) Canonical score plot for the NGO-ENSaptamer sensor array. All nine proteins were well separated and properly identified. (d) Fluorescence titration of fluorescently labeled ENSaptamers (P1–P7) with NGO.

response patterns are quantitatively analyzed by using a statistical technique, linear discriminant analysis (LDA). By using seven ENSaptamer elements, they could easily identify nine kinds of proteins with high precision (100%). There is no overlap between the 95% confidence ellipses on the two-dimensional canonical score plot (Figure 5.4c). The graphene-based sensor array also provides a versatile platform for the detection of cells and microorganisms. In addition, the authors have interrogated the interactions of DNA and NGO systematically (Figure 5.4d). The binding affinity of DNA to NGO is high depending on the structural information (sequence, length, and second structure) of DNA, which provides a guideline for ENSaptamer elements selection. This NGO–ENSaptamer sensing platform holds great promise for biomedical diagnostics. The concept of ENSaptamers might be extended to other affinity receptor–based applications including bioimaging and therapeutics.

Lu et al. have successfully employed GO and the pyrene-labeled peptide to construct a fluorescence nanobiosensor to study the interactions between peptide and protein,[24] which play critical roles in many biological processes. In this study, the researchers have used human immunodeficiency virus type 1 (HIV-1) glycoprotein gp120, an important protein that is involved in the receptor binding and membrane fusion as the model. The authors have assembled the pyrene-labeled V3 region peptide in the gp120 protein on the GO surface by strong adsorption via π–π stacking and hydrophobic interactions. The fluorescence of the pyrene conjugated with peptide is effectively quenched as the result of the proximity of the GO to the pyrene moiety. In the presence of anti-HIV1-gp120 antibody, the competitive binding of the antibody with GO for peptide alters the conformation of the pyrene–peptide conjugate. As a result, the pyrene moiety is moved away from the GO surface. As a result, its fluorescence signal is consequently restored. This biosensor can specifically detect the interaction between the V3 region peptide and the anti-HIV1-gp120 antibody with a detection limit of 200 pM. This design presents a universal GO-based platform to specifically and sensitively monitor the peptide–protein interactions in a homogeneous real-time manner, which is important for investigating biomolecular recognition, drug development, and biosensor fabrications.

Chen et al. have developed a concanavalin A (ConA) biosensor by using pyrene-conjugated maltose-assembled graphene based on fluorescence resonance energy transfer (FRET).[25] The authors have synthesized the maltose-grafted-aminopyrene (Mal-Apy), and immobilized the Mal-Apy on the surface of graphene by π–π stacking interaction. The fluorescence of Mal-Apy is efficiently quenched due to FRET between the pyrene moiety and graphene. The presence of ConA results in the competitive binding of ConA with glucose and disturbs the π-stacking interaction between the pyrene and graphene, which leads to the fluorescence recovery. This graphene-based biosensor can detect ConA fast and selectively in a homogenous solution in a linear range of 20 nM to 1.0 μM with a detection limit of 0.8 nM. The assay could be accomplished within 5 min. This work has demonstrated that the graphene-based FRET b platform has promising potential for protein–carbohydrate interaction studies. It could be widely used in drug screening, biomolecule recognition, and disease diagnosis.

Chang et al. have used aptamer as the sensing element to develop a highly sensitive and selective FRET aptasensor for thrombin assay.[26] In this design, the dye-labeled DNA human thrombin aptamer is self-assembled on the graphene surface due to the π-stacking and hydrophobic interactions between aptamer and graphene. The noncovalent assembly induces the effective fluorescence quenching as a result of FRET. With the introduction of thrombin, the form of DNA quadruplex–thrombin complexes alters the conformation of aptamer, leaving the dyes away from the graphene surface and leading to the fluorescence recovery. This graphene aptasensor has demonstrated high sensitivity and excellent specificity in both buffer and blood serum with a detection limit of 31.3 pM. Lu et al. have also demonstrated that GO can be used to fabricate DNA and protein nanobiosensors, based on the unique structure and the electrical properties of GO.[12] The combination of nanomaterials and biomolecule recognition units is a promising route to develop novel optical biosensors for biomedical applications.

5.4 Graphene-Based Biosensors for Ions, Small Molecule Detection

GO-based FRET biosensors can also be used for the detection of ions. Aptamers have been integrated with GO in the FRET biosensors. Aptamers are single-stranded nucleic acids isolated from random-sequence DNA or RNA libraries by an *in vitro* selection process termed the systematic evolution of ligands by exponential enrichment (SELEX).[32] Aptamers are specific to proteins, small molecules, or ions.[33] Using a T-rich mercury-specific oligonucleotide (MSO), He et al.[11] have demonstrated a GO-based FRET biosensor for mercuric ion (Hg^{2+}) detection. The presence of Hg^{2+} leads to the formation of the stem–loop structure of the FAM-labeled MSO probe, resulting in an increase in the distance between the GO and the fluorophore, which is no longer quenched by GO. The fluorescence intensity of MSO provides a quantitative readout for the Hg^{2+} concentration. This sensor exhibits excellent specificity against various interferencing metal ions, and shows a detection limit of 30 nM. With a similar detection scheme, Wen et al.[27] have reported an Ag^+ sensor using a silver (Ag^+)-specific oligonucleotide (SSO) probe that contains cytosine (C)-rich nucleic acids coupled with GO (Figure 5.5a). This sensor has a detection limit of 5 nM, which meets the requirement of US Environmental Protection Agency (EPA) for drinking water. Furthermore, the Ag^+ can be easily differentiated when other metal ions are present with a 10-fold higher concentration. Besides aptamer, DNAzyme is an interesting molecular recognition probe for metal ions. DNAzymes are typically *in vitro* selected DNA molecules with the enzyme-like catalytic activities.[28] Metal ion–dependent 8–17 DNAzymes are a class of well-characterized DNAzymes that cleave an oligonucleotide substrate containing one ribonucleotide at the cleavage site.[29,30] Wen et al.[31] have designed a fluorescent sensor for Pb^{2+} detection since Pb^{2+} could specifically modulate the interaction between GO and a Pb^{2+} dependent 8–17 DNAzyme (Figure 5.5b).

The 8–17 Pb^{2+}-dependent DNAzyme employed in this work is composed of an enzyme strand (17E) and a dye-labeled substrate strand (17S). In the presence of Pb^{2+}, the substrate strand is specifically and irreversibly cleaved at this cleavage site, resulting in the disassembly of the duplex DNAzyme into three ssDNA fragments: the 3'-and 5'-fragments of substrate strand and the enzyme strand. These ssDNA adsorb onto the GO surface via the π–π interaction between ssDNA and GO. Hence, the dye-labeled DNA probe is quenched. This is a "turn-off" strategy and this sensor has a detection limit of 0.5 nM for Pb^{2+}.

GO-based FRET biosensors have also been exploited for the detection of small molecules.[32,33] He et al.[11] have designed a GO-based FRET biosensor for adenosine triphosphate (ATP) detection. When a dye-labeled antiadenosine aptamer probe was incubated with GO, the fluorescence was largely quenched because of dye-labeled aptamers adsorbed onto the GO surface. Whereas, in the presence of adenosine, the aptamer probe was converted

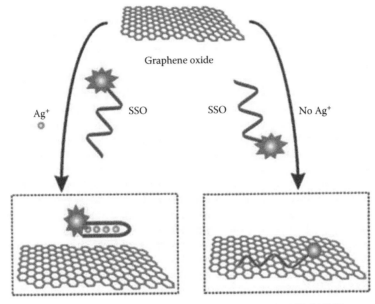

(a)   SSO: 5'-FAM-CTCTCTTCTCTCTTCATTTTTCAACACAACACAC-3'

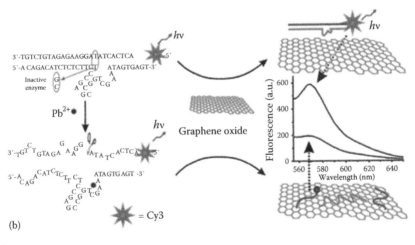

(b)

FIGURE 5.5
(a) Schematic illustration of the fluorescence sensor for Ag(I) ions based on the target-induced conformational change of a silver-specific cytosine-rich oligonucleotide (SSO) and the interactions between the fluorogenic SSO probe and graphene oxide. SSO: a FAM-labeled silver-specific oligonucleotide probe. (b) Schematic for the Pb^{2+}-modulated interactions between DNAzyme and GO. Inset is the fluorescence spectra of a mixture of DNAzyme and GO upon interaction with 0 M (top curve) and 2 mM (bottom curve) of Pb^{2+} in a Tris-HCl buffer (50 mM, pH 7.4) solution containing 50 mM of NaCl.

to a rigid tertiary structure, thereby restoring the fluorescence of the probe. This method shows high selectivity and has a detection limit of 10 μM for ATP. To increase the sensitivity of the GO-based FRET biosensor for ATP detection, Lu et al.[34] have developed an amplification strategy by exploiting the DNA-protection properties of GO.[13] This amplified aptamer-based assay has a detection limit for ATP of 40 nM.

5.5 Graphene Biosensors as Bioimaging Agents

GO has been explored for biological optical imaging due to the excellent biocompatibility, readily cellular uptake, flexible chemistry modifications, and intrinsic and tunable fluorescence of GO.[4,35-37] Recent studies have found that the intrinsic fluorescence of small GO (10 nm or less), which is referred to as graphene quantum dots (GQDs), is affected by the size, the preparation method, and the surface modifications.[38-44] Pan et al. have prepared GQDs through the hydrothermal cutting of GO, which are blue fluorescent with quantum yield less than 10%. To improve the quantum yield, Eda et al. have chemically produced GQDs with exposure to hydrazine vapor, which has significantly enhanced fluorescence.[39] Mei et al. have functionalized the GQD surface with alkylamine and observed the dramatically increased fluorescence.[43] GQDs have unique properties, including pH-dependent and upconversion fluorescence behaviors, which allow GQDs to be excited at the NIR region, to provide efficient, safe, and low-background imaging for *in vitro* and *in vivo* studies.[45] The applications of GQDs in cellular imaging have been explored.[46,47]

These studies have revealed that GO can be successfully used for *in vitro* and *in vivo* imaging in both cellular and whole-animal studies.

Sun et al. have for the first time explored the cellular uptake and imaging of the nanosized pegylated GO loaded with doxorubicin, a commonly used cancer drug, and rituxan, an antibody specifically recognize B cell surface receptor CD20.[35] The authors have functionalized the GO with pegylation to improve its solubility and compatibility in biological environments. The pegylated GO sheets are soluble in buffers and serum without aggregations. Furthermore, the GO sheets are fluorescent in the visible and near-infrared (NIR) regions. The intrinsic photoluminescence (PL) of GO facilitates the cellular imaging in the near-infrared (NIR) with low background. The same research group has also demonstrated that the pegylated GO can be used as bifunctional carrier to achieve drug delivery and biological imaging.[48] In this work, Lu et al. have successfully loaded SN38, a water-insoluble drug with pegylated GO and used it for intracellular imaging and efficient drug delivery. The authors have found that the potency of the loaded drug is not affected by the physical absorbance on the GO surface, and shows superior cytotoxicity against colon cancer cells HCT-116 over the CPT-11, the FDA-approved prodrug of SN38 for colon cancer treatment. By using the similar modification strategy, Peng et al. have constructed a PEG- and fluorescein-functionalized GO.[36] The PEG bridge has been introduced to minimize the GO-induced quenching of linked fluorescein. Interestingly, the fluorescein–PEG–GO nanocomposite exhibits excellent pH-tunable fluorescent properties. The results have demonstrated that the fluorescein–PEG–GO can be efficiently taken up by cells for intracellular imaging.

Liu et al. have developed a green and facile approach to prepare the functionalized GO based on gelatin.[49] In this study, the gelatin served not only as a reducing reagent but also as a functionalized reagent to improve the stability of the graphene nanosheets. The obtained biocompatible gelatin–GNS shows excellent solubility and stability in various physiological fluids, including cell culture media and serum. In addition, the gelatin–GNS also has good biocompatibility and is nontoxic to MCF-7 cells even at a high concentration of 200 mg mL. Furthermore, the authors have successfully loaded doxorubicin, an anticancer drug, onto the gelatin–GNS for cellular imaging and drug delivery. The study has revealed that the doxorubicin/gelatin–GNS composite does not diminish the potency of doxorubicin and exhibits a high cytotoxicity toward MCF-7 cells. Coincidentally, other researchers have also successfully employed a similar strategy for reducing and functionalizing GO as the drug delivery carrier and the imaging agent. Guo et al. have used herceptin, an antibody against the Her2 receptor, as the reducing and functionalizing reagent to prepare a new functional reduced GO in one step.[50] The obtained herceptin-rGO has low cytotoxicity and excellent solubility in buffer and cell culture media. In addition, the herceptin-functionalized rGO has a unique two-photo excitation photoluminescence property and can be readily uptaken by cells for two-photo excitation imaging. In another study, the mechanism of the cellular uptake of the protein-functionalized GO has been investigated.[51] The small GO nanosheets enter cells mainly through clathrin-mediated endocytosis, while increasing the graphene size enhances the phagocytotic internalization of the GO nanosheets. These findings have provided a fundamental understanding of interactions between the protein-functionalized GO and the biological systems, which will facilitate biomedical and toxicologic studies of GO.

Wang et al. have fabricated an aptamer–carboxyfluorescein (FAM)/graphene oxide nanosheet (GO-nS) nanocomplex for the imaging of ATP molecules in living cells.[37] The aptamer is protected from enzymatic digestion, and the fluorescence of FAM is quenched by absorbing on the GO surface. After uptake by JB6 cells, the recognition between the aptamer and the intracellular ATP induced the conformation change of the aptamer, leading to the restoration of the fluorescence of FAM (Figure 5.6). This study has provided a novel, facile, and robust approach for the intracellular tracking of biomolecules.

The QDs have been explored to conjugate with the reduced GO (rGO) for cellular imaging.[52] It is challenging to make the rGO–QDs conjugate without scarifying the fluorescence due to the quenching effect of rGO. Chen et al. have overcome this issue via linking rGO with QDs through a bridge of bovine serum albumin (BSA). The rGO–QDs conjugate could be readily uptaken by Hela cells for *in vitro* imaging.

Besides *in vitro* cellular imaging, the graphene-based bioimaging agents have been used for *in vivo* imaging. In these studies, multiple signaling technologies, including NIR, PET, NMR, etc., have been incorporated to extend the versatility and reliability of the graphene-based bioimaging platform.

Hong et al. have synthesized the PEG–GO and functionalized it with the CD105 antibody and 1,4,7-triazacyclononane-1,4,7-triacetic acid (NOTA) to facilitate the *in vivo* targeting and PET scan.[53] The CD105 (endoglin) is a vascular marker for tumor angiogenesis, and NOTA is one of the best chelators of ^{62}Cu for PET agent. The functionalized GO shows excellent stability and target specificity in cellular assay. Furthermore, the authors have demonstrated that the functionalized GO could be specifically accumulated to the tumor neovasculature *in vivo* via the targeting of CD105, which has suggested that the functionalized nanographene could be utilized for cancer-targeted drug delivery and/or photothermal therapy to further improve the therapeutic efficacy and to enable cancer theranostics.

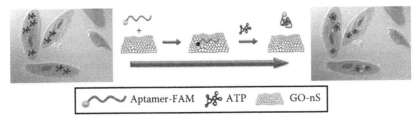

FIGURE 5.6
In situ molecular probing in living cells using the aptamer/GO-nS nanocomplex.

Ganesh et al. have developed a novel ecofriendly synthesis approach to make multi-functional graphene (MFG) and explored its biomedical application for *in vitro* and *in vivo* imaging.[54] The authors have utilized a microwave-assisted reduction and magnetization process to convert the GO into magnetic graphene in a one-min treatment, which is further covalently linked with fluorescein o-methacrylate (FMA) to generate MFG. The synthesized MFG presents excellent stability in aqueous solution (~2.5 g/L), strong magnetization, bright fluorescence and good biocompatibility. The MFG has been microinjected into zebrafish 2-cells and fully developed embryos to study the *in vivo* toxicity and imaging. MFG does not induce any significant abnormalities nor affects the survival rate. The whole animal-imaging study presents excellent colocalization and biodistribution from head to tail in the zebrafish (Figure 5.7). Hence, MFG holds a promising potential as a multifunctional probe in biomedical research and applications.

Yang et al. have fabricated a multifunctional rGO for *in vivo* imaging and minimal-invasion photothermal therapy.[55] In this design, a nanoscale rGO has been produced with the cogeneration of the iron oxide nanoparticle (rGO–IONP). The complex has then been non-covalently functionalized with PEG and fluorescence dye. The obtained rGO–IONP–PEG nanocomposite possesses excellent physiological stability, strong NIR optical absorbance, and superparamagnetic properties. The authors have used this rGO-based nanoprobe to perform the fluorescence, photoacoustic, and magnetic resonance imaging study in mice. The *in vivo* fluorescence and MR image has confirmed that the nanocomposite is accumulated in tumor site due to the EPR effect (Figure 5.8). Furthermore, the MR imaging–guided PTT treatment achieved highly efficient tumor ablation with low laser power density at 0.5 W/cm². This study highlights the great potential of graphene for cancer diagnosis applications.

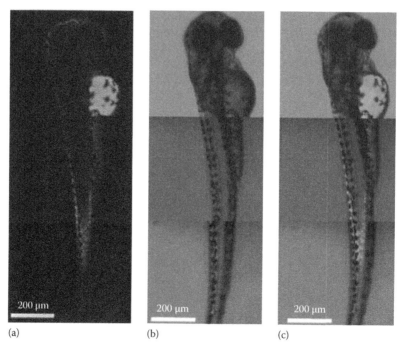

(a)   (b)   (c)

FIGURE 5.7
(See color insert.) Distribution of MFG inside a fully developed (72 hpf) zebrafish using CLSM (a) fluorescence image of MFG with a FITC filter, (b) DIC image, and (c) overlay image.

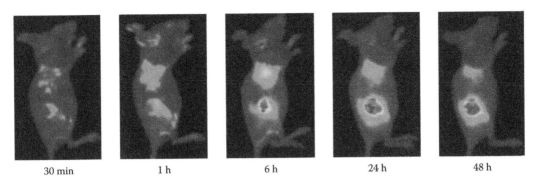

| 30 min | 1 h | 6 h | 24 h | 48 h |

FIGURE 5.8
(See color insert.) *In vivo* fluorescence imaging using Cy5 labeled RGO–IONP–PEG. The Cy5 fluorescence signals from tumor sites increase after intravenous injection and became quite strong at 48 h, suggesting high passive accumulation of RGO–IONP–PEG at tumor site.

5.6 Graphene-Related SPR and SERS Biosensor

Graphene-related materials may enhance the performance of the surface plasmon resonance (SPR)-based biosensor. The SPR biosensor utilizes surface plasmon polariton waves to probe the interactions between biomolecules and the sensor surface.[56] Wu et al.[57] have proposed a novel SPR biosensor, which consists of a graphene sheet over a gold thin film,[58] and is substantially more sensitive than the conventional SPR biosensor. The improved sensitivity comes from two properties of graphene: (1) the coated graphene can enhance the adsorption of biomolecules onto the metal/dielectric interface; (2) the optical property of graphene modifies the SPR curves and increases the sensitivity of the SPR response. Choi et al.[59] have numerically proposed that the graphene-on-silver substrate can enhance the SPR sensitivity toward DNA hybridization by three times in comparison with the conventional gold film–based SPR biosensor. In addition, graphene-on-silver can prevent the oxidation of silver due to the high impermeability property of graphene. SPR is sensitive to the refractive index and to the thickness of the test medium in the vicinity of the Au surface,[60,61] especially for the molecules with higher molecular weight such as DNA. Wang et al.[62] have demonstrated a label-free, regenerative and sensitive SPR biosensor for the detection of α-thrombin. Firstly, rGO is assembled on a positively charged Au film via electrostatic interaction. Secondly, the thrombin-specific aptamer (TBA) is noncovalently adsorbed onto the rGO layer. The target molecule (α-thrombin) binds with TBA, which will detach the aptamers from the SPR sensing surface, leading to an obvious SPR angle decrease. This graphene-based SPR biosensor exhibits excellent selectivity and a detection limit of 0.05 nM for α-thrombin.

Interestingly, graphene can effectively enhance Raman signals of absorbed organic molecules that makes it a type of useful surface-enhanced Raman scattering (SERS) substrate.[63] Due to the charge transfer between graphene and the adsorbed molecules, it was reported that graphene leads to an enhancement factor (EF) of 2–17. To increase the sensitivity of graphene-based SERS sensors, Lu et al. have decorated an rGO film with silver nanoparticles (Ag NPs) to serve as the substrate for SERS-based sensor to detect aromatic molecules.[64] This Ag NP–modified rGO substrate is more sensitive than the graphene substrate and has a detection limit in the nM range. In order to detect folic acid molecules in water and human serum, Ren et al.[65] have prepared a SERS substrate that consists of GO and poly(diallyldimethyl-ammonium chloride) (PDDA)-functionalized Ag NPs (GO/PDDA/AgNPs) using the self-assembly

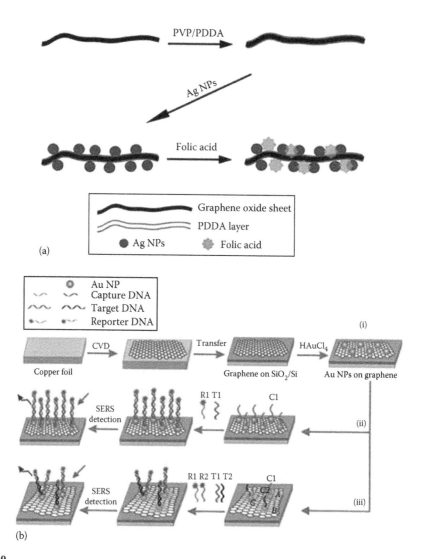

(a)

(b)

FIGURE 5.9

(a) Fabrication of the sensing interface and the detection of folic acid. (b) Schematic illustration of the preparation of SERS-active substrate and its application for DNA detection. (i) Fabrication of Au NP modified CVD-growth graphene film. (ii) Immobilize Capture DNA 1 (C1) for SERS detection of Target DNA 1 (T1) with Reporter DNA 1 (R1). (iii) Immobilize multiple capture DNAs (C1, C2) for multiplexing detection of DNA.

method (Figure 5.9a). This SERS sensor has a detection limit of 9 nM. He et al.[66] have developed a SERS-active substrate based on gold nanoparticle (Au NP)-decorated CVD-growth graphene and used it for the multiplexing detection of DNA (Figure 5.9b).

It has been reported that graphene can directly reduce metal ions, leading to the spontaneous growth of Au NPs on the graphene film. For example, an Au NP–modified CVD-growth graphene film has been prepared as the SERS substrate. The Au NPs *in situ* grown on the graphene film not only serve as the anchor spots for the assembly of the dye-labeled DNA probes, but also enhance the Raman signals of the probes. This SERS platform exhibits excellent selectivity and sensitivity with a detection limit of 10 pM. Moreover, two different DNA targets could be detected simultaneously on the same substrate using only one light source.

5.7 Summary and Perspective

Graphene and GO are finding extensive applications in bioassays, drug delivery, bioimaging, etc. Graphene-based optical biosensors have demonstrated numerous advantages over other materials due to their unique planar structure, intrinsic tunable optical properties, large surface area, facile chemistry modification, and excellent biocompatibility. In addition, the low cost, convenience, and ecofriendly production of graphene materials will promote the development of nanobiosensors as the point-of-care testing, which requires rapid, sensitive, efficient, robust, and inexpensive bioassays. Furthermore, graphene as drug carrier and imaging agent have presented promising findings. All of these successful applications paved a new avenue, to build a promising nanoplatform for biomedical studies.

Nevertheless, there remain challenges in applying graphene in biomedical applications. To overcome these challenges, we need to focus on three issues. First, the graphene synthesis should be systematically investigated to precisely control the size, morphology, surface chemistry, and composition. By doing this, the optical properties of graphene can be accurately tailored to improve the quantum yield, the fluorescence peak width, and the emission wavelength. Second, the surface modification and functionalization strategies have to be developed to provide the facile and versatile platform for the immobilization of various biomolecules, chemicals, and other nanoparticles. Third, more attention should be paid to the biocompatibility and the safety of graphene materials by studying the interactions between graphene/derivatives and biological systems, which is critical for the applications of *in vivo* imaging, drug delivery, and therapy. To achieve these goals, the collaborations among multiple disciplines, including chemistry, physics, biology, and medicine, are crucial and inevitable.

Acknowledgments

This work was supported by Grant U54 ES16015 from the National Institute of Environmental Health Sciences, the National Institute of Health (NIH), and by a DOE LDRD program at Pacific Northwest National Laboratory (PNNL). Its contents are solely the responsibility of the authors and do not necessarily represent the official views of the federal government. PNNL is operated for DOE by Battelle under Contract DE-AC05-76RL01830. YL acknowledges a fellowship from the Chinese Academy of Sciences for supporting the visit to Shanghai Institute of Applied Physics.

References

1. Geim, A. K.; Novoselov, K. S. The rise of graphene. *Nat Mater* 2007, *6*(3), 183–191.
2. Novoselov, K. S.; Geim, A. K.; Morozov, S. V.; Jiang, D.; Zhang, Y.; Dubonos, S. V.; Grigorieva, I. V.; Firsov, A. A. Electric field effect in atomically thin carbon films. *Science* 2004, *306*(5696), 666–669.
3. Wang, Y.; Li, Z.; Wang, J.; Li, J.; Lin, Y. Graphene and graphene oxide: Biofunctionalization and applications in biotechnology. *Trends Biotechnol* 2011, *29*(5), 205–212.

4. Loh, K. P.; Bao, Q. L.; Eda, G.; Chhowalla, M. Graphene oxide as a chemically tunable platform for optical applications. *Nat Chem* 2010, *2*(12), 1015–1024.

5. Luo, Z. T.; Vora, P. M.; Mele, E. J.; Johnson, A. T. C.; Kikkawa, J. M. Photoluminescence and band gap modulation in graphene oxide. *Appl Phys Lett* 2009, *94*(11).

6. Liu, Z. F.; Liu, Q.; Huang, Y.; Ma, Y. F.; Yin, S. G.; Zhang, X. Y.; Sun, W.; Chen, Y. S. Organic photovoltaic devices based on a novel acceptor material: Graphene. *Adv Mater* 2008, *20*(20), 3924–3930.

7. Swathi, R. S.; Sebastian, K. L. Resonance energy transfer from a dye molecule to graphene. *J Chem Phys* 2008, *129*(5).

8. Swathi, R. S.; Sebastian, K. L. Long range resonance energy transfer from a dye molecule to graphene has (distance)(-4) dependence. *J Chem Phys* 2009, *130*(8), 086101.

9. Xie, L. M.; Ling, X.; Fang, Y.; Zhang, J.; Liu, Z. F. Graphene as a substrate to suppress fluorescence in resonance Raman spectroscopy. *J Am Chem Soc* 2009, *131*(29), 9890–9891.

10. Kim, J.; Cote, L. J.; Kim, F.; Huang, J. X. Visualizing graphene based sheets by fluorescence quenching microscopy. *J Am Chem Soc* 2010, *132*(1), 260–267.

11. He, S. J.; Song, B.; Li, D.; Zhu, C. F.; Qi, W. P.; Wen, Y. Q.; Wang, L. H.; Song, S. P.; Fang, H. P.; Fan, C. H. A graphene nanoprobe for rapid, sensitive, and multicolor fluorescent DNA analysis. *Adv Funct Mater* 2010, *20*(3), 453–459.

12. Lu, C. H.; Yang, H. H.; Zhu, C. L.; Chen, X.; Chen, G. N. A graphene platform for sensing biomolecules. *Angew Chem Int Ed Engl* 2009, *48*(26), 4785–4787.

13. Tang, Z. W.; Wu, H.; Cort, J. R.; Buchko, G. W.; Zhang, Y. Y.; Shao, Y. Y.; Aksay, I. A.; Liu, J.; Lin, Y. H. Constraint of DNA on functionalized graphene improves its biostability and specificity. *Small* 2010, *6*(11), 1205–1209.

14. Li, F.; Huang, Y.; Yang, Q.; Zhong, Z. T.; Li, D.; Wang, L. H.; Song, S. P.; Fan, C. H. A Graphene-enhanced molecular beacon for homogeneous DNA detection. *Nanoscale* 2010, *2*(6), 1021–1026.

15. Tyagi, S.; Kramer, F. R. Molecular beacons: Probes that fluoresce upon hybridization. *Nat Biotechnol* 1996, *14* (3), 303–308.

16. Yang, R. H.; Jin, J. Y.; Chen, Y.; Shao, N.; Kang, H. Z.; Xiao, Z.; Tang, Z. W.; Wu, Y. R.; Zhu, Z.; Tan, W. H. Carbon nanotube-quenched fluorescent oligonucleotides: Probes that fluoresce upon hybridization. *J Am Chem Soc* 2008, *130*(26), 8351–8358.

17. Bonnet, G.; Tyagi, S.; Libchaber, A.; Kramer, F. R. Thermodynamic basis of the enhanced specificity of structured DNA probes. *Proc Natl Acad Sci USA* 1999, *96*(11), 6171–6176.

18. Bonnet, G.; Krichevsky, O.; Libchaber, A. Kinetics of conformational fluctuations in DNA hairpin-loops. *Proc Natl Acad Sci USA* 1998, *95*(15), 8602–8606.

19. Dong, H. F.; Gao, W. C.; Yan, F.; Ji, H. X.; Ju, H. X. Fluorescence resonance energy transfer between quantum dots and graphene oxide for sensing biomolecules. *Anal Chem* 2010, *82*(13), 5511–5517.

20. Jung, J. H.; Cheon, D. S.; Liu, F.; Lee, K. B.; Seo, T. S. A graphene oxide based immuno-biosensor for pathogen detection. *Angew Chem Int Ed* 2010, *49* (33), 5708–5711.

21. Mei, Q.; Zhang, Z. Photoluminescent graphene oxide ink to print sensors onto microporous membranes for versatile visualization bioassays. *Angew Chem Int Ed Engl* 2012, *51*(23), 5602–5606.

22. Lim, S. Y.; Ahn, J.; Lee, J. S.; Kim, M.-G.; Park, C. B. Graphene-oxide-based immunosensing through fluorescence quenching by peroxidase-catalyzed polymerization. *Small* 2012, n/a-n/a.

23. Pei, H.; Li, J.; Lv, M.; Wang, J.; Gao, J.; Lu, J.; Li, Y.; Huang, Q.; Hu, J.; Fan, C. A Graphene-based sensor array for high-precision and adaptive target identification with ensemble aptamers. *J Am Chem Soc* 2012.

24. Lu, C.-H.; Li, J.; Zhang, X.-L.; Zheng, A.-X.; Yang, H.-H.; Chen, X.; Chen, G.-N. General approach for monitoring peptide-protein interactions based on graphene-peptide complex. *Anal Chem* 2011, *83*(19), 7276–7282.

25. Chen, Q.; Wei, W.; Lin, J.-M. Homogeneous detection of concanavalin a using pyrene-conjugated maltose assembled graphene based on fluorescence resonance energy transfer. *Biosens Bioelectron* 2011, *26*(11), 4497–4502.
26. Chang, H.; Tang, L.; Wang, Y.; Jiang, J.; Li, J. Graphene fluorescence resonance energy transfer aptasensor for the thrombin detection. *Anal Chem* 2010, *82*(6), 2341–2346.
27. Wen, Y. Q.; Xing, F. F.; He, S. J.; Song, S. P.; Wang, L. H.; Long, Y. T.; Li, D.; Fan, C. H. A graphene-based fluorescent nanoprobe for silver(I) ions detection by using graphene oxide and a silver-specific oligonucleotide. *Chem Commun* 2010, *46*(15), 2596–2598.
28. Famulok, M.; Hartig, J. S.; Mayer, G. Functional aptamers and aptazymes in biotechnology, diagnostics, and therapy. *Chem Rev* 2007, *107*(9), 3715–3743.
29. Schlosser, K.; Li, Y. F. A versatile endoribonuclease mimic made of DNA: Characteristics and applications of the 8–17 RNA-cleaving DNAzyme. *Chembiochem* 2010, *11*(7), 866–879.
30. Xiao, Y.; Rowe, A. A.; Plaxco, K. W. Electrochemical detection of parts-per-billion lead via an electrode-bound DNAzyme assembly. *J Am Chem Soc* 2007, *129*(2), 262–263.
31. Wen, Y. Q.; Peng, C.; Li, D.; Zhuo, L.; He, S. J.; Wang, L. H.; Huang, Q.; Xu, Q. H.; Fan, C. H. Metal ion-modulated graphene-DNAzyme interactions: Design of a nanoprobe for fluorescent detection of lead(II) ions with high sensitivity, selectivity and tunable dynamic range. *Chem Commun* 2011, *47*(22), 6278–6280.
32. Tuerk, C.; Gold, L. Systematic evolution of ligands by exponential enrichment–RNA ligands to bacteriophage-T4 DNA-polymerase. *Science* 1990, *249*(4968), 505–510.
33. Hermann, T.; Patel, D. J. Adaptive recognition by nucleic acid aptamers. *Science* 2000, *287*(5454), 820–825.
34. Lu, C. H.; Li, J. A.; Lin, M. H.; Wang, Y. W.; Yang, H. H.; Chen, X.; Chen, G. N. Amplified aptamer-based assay through catalytic recycling of the analyte. *Angew Chem Int Edit* 2010, *49*(45), 8454–8457.
35. Sun, X.; Liu, Z.; Welsher, K.; Robinson, J. T.; Goodwin, A.; Zaric, S.; Dai, H. Nano-graphene oxide for cellular imaging and drug delivery. *Nano Res* 2008, *1*(3), 203–212.
36. Peng, C.; Hu, W.; Zhou, Y.; Fan, C.; Huang, Q. Intracellular imaging with a graphene-based fluorescent probe. *Small* 2010, *6*(15), 1686–1692.
37. Wang, Y.; Li, Z.; Hu, D.; Lin, C.-T.; Li, J.; Lin, Y. Aptamer/graphene oxide nanocomplex for in situ molecular probing in living cells. *J Am Chem Soc* 2010, *132*(27), 9274–9276.
38. Pan, D. Y.; Zhang, J. C.; Li, Z.; Wu, M. H. Hydrothermal route for cutting graphene sheets into blue-luminescent graphene quantum dots. *Adv Mater* 2010, *22*(6), 734–738.
39. Eda, G.; Lin, Y.-Y.; Mattevi, C.; Yamaguchi, H.; Chen, H.-A.; Chen, I. S.; Chen, C.-W.; Chhowalla, M. Blue photoluminescence from chemically derived graphene oxide. *Adv Mater* 2010, *22*(4), 505–509.
40. Chen, S.; Liu, J.-W.; Chen, M.-L.; Chen, X.-W.; Wang, J.-H. Unusual emission transformation of graphene quantum dots induced by self-assembled aggregation. *Chem Commun (Cambridge, England)* 2012, *48*(61), 7637–7639.
41. Morales-Narvaez, E.; Merkoci, A. Graphene oxide as an optical biosensing platform. *Adv Mater* 2012, *24*(25), 3298–3308.
42. Tang, L.; Ji, R.; Cao, X.; Lin, J.; Jiang, H.; Li, X.; Teng, K. S. et al. Deep ultraviolet photoluminescence of water-soluble self-passivated graphene quantum dots. *ACS Nano* 2012, *6*(6), 5102–5110.
43. Mei, Q.; Zhang, K.; Guan, G.; Liu, B.; Wang, S.; Zhang, Z. Highly efficient photoluminescent graphene oxide with tunable surface properties. *Chem Commun* 2010, *46*(39), 7319–7321.
44. Yan, X.; Cui, X.; Li, L.-S. Synthesis of large, stable colloidal graphene quantum dots with tunable size. *J Am Chem Soc* 2010, *132*(17), 5944–5945.
45. Shen, J.; Zhu, Y.; Chen, C.; Yang, X.; Li, C. Facile preparation and upconversion luminescence of graphene quantum dots. *Chem Commun* 2011, *47*(9), 2580–2582.
46. Zhu, S.; Zhang, J.; Qiao, C.; Tang, S.; Li, Y.; Yuan, W.; Li, B. et al. Strongly green-photoluminescent graphene quantum dots for bioimaging applications. *Chem Commun* 2011, *47*(24), 6858–6860.

47. Shen, J.; Zhu, Y.; Yang, X.; Li, C. Graphene quantum dots: Emergent nanolights for bioimaging, sensors, catalysis and photovoltaic devices. *Chem Commun* 2012, *48*(31), 3686–3699.
48. Liu, Z.; Robinson, J. T.; Sun, X.; Dai, H. Pegylated nanographene oxide for delivery of water-insoluble cancer drugs. *J Am Chem Soc* 2008, *130*(33), 10876–10877.
49. Liu, K.; Zhang, J.-J.; Cheng, F.-F.; Zheng, T.-T.; Wang, C.; Zhu, J.-J. Green and facile synthesis of highly biocompatible graphene nanosheets and its application for cellular imaging and drug delivery. *J Mater Chem* 2011, *21*(32), 12034–12040.
50. Guo, C.; Book-Newell, B.; Irudayaraj, J. Protein-directed reduction of graphene oxide and intra-cellular imaging. *Chem Commun* 2011, *47*(47), 12658–12660.
51. Mu, Q.; Su, G.; Li, L.; Gilbertson, B. O.; Yu, L. H.; Zhang, Q.; Sun, Y.-P.; Yan, B. Size-dependent cell uptake of protein-coated graphene oxide nanosheets. *ACS Appl Mater Interfaces* 2012, *4*(4), 2259–2266.
52. Chen, M.-L.; Liu, J.-W.; Hu, B.; Chen, M.-L.; Wang, J.-H. Conjugation of quantum dots with graphene for fluorescence imaging of live cells. *Analyst* 2011, *136*(20), 4277–4283.
53. Hong, H.; Yang, K.; Zhang, Y.; Engle, J. W.; Feng, L.; Yang, Y.; Nayak, T. R. et al. In vivo targeting and imaging of tumor vasculature with radiolabeled, antibody-conjugated nanographene. *ACS Nano* 2012, *6*(3), 2361–2370.
54. Gollavelli, G.; Ling, Y. C. Multi-functional graphene as an in vitro and in vivo imaging probe. *Biomaterials* 2012, *33*(8), 2532–2545.
55. Yang, K.; Hu, L.; Ma, X.; Ye, S.; Cheng, L.; Shi, X.; Li, C.; Li, Y.; Liu, Z. Multimodal imaging guided photothermal therapy using functionalized graphene nanosheets anchored with magnetic nanoparticles. *Adv Mater* 2012, *24*(14), 1868–1872.
56. Homola, J. Present and future of surface plasmon resonance biosensors. *Anal Bioanal Chem* 2003, *377*(3), 528–539.
57. Wu, L.; Chu, H. S.; Koh, W. S.; Li, E. P. Highly sensitive graphene biosensors based on surface plasmon resonance. *Opt Express* 2010, *18*(14), 14395–14400.
58. Song, B.; Li, D.; Qi, W.; Elstner, M.; Fan, C.; Fang, H. Graphene on Au(111): A highly conductive material with excellent adsorption properties for high-resolution bio/nanodetection and identification. *Chemphyschem* 2010, *11*(3), 585–589.
59. Choi, S. H.; Kim, Y. L.; Byun, K. M. Graphene-on-silver substrates for sensitive surface plasmon resonance imaging biosensors. *Opt Express* 2011, *19*(2), 458–466.
60. Li, Y.; Lee, H. J.; Corn, R. M. Detection of protein biomarkers using RNA aptamer microarrays and enzymatically amplified surface plasmon resonance imaging. *Anal Chem* 2007, *79*(3), 1082–1088.
61. Shan, X.; Patel, U.; Wang, S.; Iglesias, R.; Tao, N. Imaging local electrochemical current via surface plasmon resonance. *Science* 2010, *327*(5971), 1363–1366.
62. Wang, L.; Zhu, C. Z.; Han, L.; Jin, L. H.; Zhou, M.; Dong, S. J. Label-free, regenerative and sensitive surface plasmon resonance and electrochemical aptasensors based on graphene. *Chem Commun* 2011, *47*(27), 7794–7796.
63. Ling, X.; Xie, L. M.; Fang, Y.; Xu, H.; Zhang, H. L.; Kong, J.; Dresselhaus, M. S.; Zhang, J.; Liu, Z. F. Can graphene be used as a substrate for Raman enhancement? *Nano Lett* 2010, *10*(2), 553–561.
64. Lu, G.; Li, H.; Liusman, C.; Yin, Z. Y.; Wu, S. X.; Zhang, H. Surface enhanced Raman scattering of Ag or Au nanoparticle-decorated reduced graphene oxide for detection of aromatic molecules. *Chem Sci* 2011, *2*(9), 1817–1821.
65. Ren, W.; Fang, Y. X.; Wang, E. K. A binary functional substrate for enrichment and ultrasensitive sers spectroscopic detection of folic acid using graphene oxide/Ag nanoparticle hybrids. *ACS Nano* 2011, *5*(8), 6425–6433.
66. He, S.; Liu, K. K.; Su, S.; Yan, J.; Mao, X.; Wang, D.; He, Y.; Li, L. J.; Song, S.; Fan, C. Graphene-based high-efficiency surface-enhanced Raman scattering-active platform for sensitive and multiplex DNA detection. *Anal Chem* 2012, *84*(10), 4622–4627.

6

Biosensing Based on Surface-Enhanced Raman Spectroscopy

Gang Logan Liu, Wenwei Zheng, Pingping Zhang, and Fanqing (Frank) Chen

CONTENTS

6.1 Introduction

In view of basic science, to understand biological systems increasingly depends on our ability to dynamically and quantitatively measure the molecular processes with high sensitivity, speed, flexibility, multiplexity, throughput, and reproducibility, usually within the context of a complex biological and chemical mixture of a tiny amount. A living cell responds to its changing environment both inside and outside itself in such a dynamic way that hundreds and thousands of signaling proteins, enzymes, siRNA, DNA, mRNA, and transcription and translation factors are constantly modified or synthesized, transferred from one organelle to another, and perform appropriate cell functions in macromolecule complexes, behaving like an army of molecular machines working in perfect synchronicity and harmony. These biomolecular complexes are not only heterogeneously distributed, recombined, modified, and reassembled continuously, but perpetually changed over time with the change of surrounding microenvironments [1]. To quantitatively follow the biochemical reactions within multimolecule complexes, it is vital for the general goal of intimately following the molecular machines in cell signaling, growth, differentiation, apoptosis, cell developmental processes, and relevant diseases. In the biotechnology industry, combinatorial methods are increasingly applied to synthesize new biocatalysts or drugs, demanding the simultaneous analysis of thousands of pathogens, mutants, drug target enzymes, or therapeutic drugs themselves. Furthermore, in personalized medicine, as dictated by economic reasons, the mass application of screening and diagnostic tools have to be fast, convenient, and low cost, requiring the miniaturization, parallelization, integration, as well as automation of biosensing devices.

To address these major challenges, the best hope lies in cutting-edge biosensing research. Amongst all the biosensors, plasmon-resonant nanostructure biomolecule hybrids (nanobio hybrids), the so-called plasmonic nanobiosensors [2,3], are being developed and viewed as one key breakthrough area for real-time and parallelized biomedical analysis with high sensitivity and selectivity. Hereby, we present a solution of integrated plasmonic system by synergizing three core techniques: (1) plasmonics that manipulates EM radiation (light) at dielectric–metal interfaces by tuning the properties of nanomaterials, (2) nanofabrication and the controlled synthesis of nanomaterials containing metals (e.g., Au, Ag, Pt, and Cu), and (3) bioconjugate techniques that modify the surface of nanomaterials with various bioprobes (e.g., antibodies, enzymes, aptamers [4,5], and molecular imprint polymers [6]). Biomaterials such as proteins, DNA, or RNA have dimensions of 2–20 nm, similar to those of plasmonic nanostructures, thus, the two classes of materials are structurally compatible. Plasmonic nanomaterials exhibit unique electronic, photonic, and catalytic properties, providing the electronic or optical transduction of biological phenomena, while biomaterials have unique recognition and catalytic properties. Their integration yields plasmonic nanobiosensors with multiple synergetic advantages over the traditional molecular imaging techniques: sensitivity, stability, biocompatibility, selectivity, and spectroscopic imaging capability. Furthermore, recently, significant advancements in controlled synthesis and nanofabrication [7–9], theory and the electrodynamic modeling of optical properties [10–12], and the surface functionalization [13–15] of plasmonic nanomaterials greatly enhance the ability to control and tune the unique optical and electronic properties of plasmonic nanostructures through their sizes, structures, composition, and shapes, enabling the utilization of huge libraries of probes for different analytes, in formats such as microarray, microfluidics, MEMS, etc. Thus, plasmonic nanobiosensors promise a great potential in the development of high-throughput techniques for the parallel analysis of multiple components in samples.

These recent advancements in nanotechnology and nanoplasmonics also enable hybrid plasmonic nanostructures as powerful subnanometer and nanometer tools to directly interface with intracellular processes. The plasmonic nanobiosensors focus EM fields to significantly enhance spectral information for localized surface plasmon spectroscopy (LSPR) [16,17], surface-enhanced Raman spectroscopy (SERS) [18,19], plasmon resonance energy transfer (PRET) [20–22], and integrated photoacoustic–photothermal contrast agents [23]. In this way, we can obtain the quantitative spectral snapshots of the complex biochemical reaction over time as a result of local biochemistry-induced plasmonic changes.

Since the first observation of an enhanced Raman signal of pyridine adsorbed on a roughened silver electrode by Fleischmann et al. in 1974 [24], this effect—surface-enhanced Raman scattering (SERS)—has been a field of great scientific interest for ultrasensitive and selective biomolecular detection in biology, chemistry, and materials science [25]. An even higher enhancement is observed when the SERS technique is coupled with chemical resonance. Moreover, Raman-scattered light shows the chemical signature of chemical and biological molecules because all molecules with unique chemical compositions have unique Raman scattering spectra. Therefore, Raman scattering spectroscopy is a powerful technique to detect chemical and biological molecules without labeling and has potential applications in the ultrasensitive detection of explosives, pathogens, and contaminants in the field. In this review, we will discuss the SERS theory, summarize major nanosynthesis and nanofabrication techniques, and describe many kinds of surface biofunctionalization for SERS-based nanobiosensors. We will then give examples of the applications and summarize the synergetic relationships among these three core techniques contained in nanobiosensing to address the major aforementioned challenges in biosensing research.

6.2 Theoretical Modeling of SERS

6.2.1 Theoretical Background of SERS

Raman scattering, first demonstrated by C.V. Raman in 1928, occurs because of the inelastic scattering of light from molecules or atoms [26,27]. Then, in the mid-1970s, the explosion of activity in the field of surface-enhanced Raman scattering (SERS) started. The first measurement of a surface Raman spectrum from pyridine adsorbed on an electrochemically roughened silver electrode was reported by Fleischmann, Hendra, and McQuillan in 1974 [24], which stemmed from their pioneering work on applying Raman spectroscopy to the *in situ* study of electrode surfaces [28,29]. Till now, SERS has been developed to be a useful technique in a wide variety of research fields due to its significantly increased Raman signals from molecules, which have been attached to nanometer-sized plasmonic structures. To better understand and use SERS, the mechanism and theoretical modeling of SERS are first discussed. Before discussing the mechanism of SERS, we briefly recall the "surface plasmon resonance," which is one of the main physics behind SERS.

Plasmonics is one of the major subfields of nanophotonics. A plasmon is defined as a quantum quasiparticle representing the elementary excitations, or modes, of the charge density oscillations in a free-electron plasma. In plasmonics, the manipulation of light is based on the interaction processes between the EM radiation and the free-electron plasma (or conduction electrons) at dielectric–metal planar interfaces, or nanocurved interfaces, resulting in the surface plasmonic resonance. The surface plasmonic resonance plays an important role in the SERS mechanism and has been an area garnering major attention in recent years [17,30–37].

To understand the physics of plasmonics is important to SERS. First, the surface plasmon resonances (in fact, a certain type of plasmon resonance) are "what makes SERS possible," and are mentioned and debated as the major origin of the enhancement. Secondly, plasmonics is currently an expanding and highly active area, from which SERS can gain further insight and where SERS can play an important role in understanding plasmonic phenomena. Significant interest in understanding propagating and localized surface plasmons has been largely stimulated by investigating SERS [38,39].

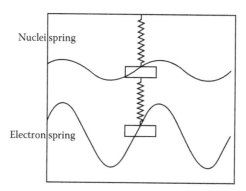

FIGURE 6.1
Coupled spring model for electron scattering and nuclei vibrations.

Researchers proposed mechanisms of both chemical and plasmon resonance–induced EM-field enhancements to explain the observed Raman enhancement on roughened metallic substrates [17,31–45].

Before the further discussion on SERS, let us first review the mechanism of Raman scattering. When light strikes molecules, the bound electrons move in the same frequency as the excitation wave. The nuclei are also subject to the dislocation due to the interaction with the bound electrons and adjacent nuclei as illustrated in the coupled spring model (Figure 6.1). Due to the coupled movement of the nuclei, the frequency of electron scattering shifts, resulting in the scattering light with the frequency different from that of the incident wave, which is called the Raman scattering light. It is clearly shown that the scattering light can be decomposed into three frequency components in the following equation:

$$P = E_0\alpha_0\cos(2\pi v_i t) + E_0\left(\frac{\partial\alpha}{\partial Q}\right)_0 A\cos(2\pi v_i t)\cos(2\pi v t)$$

$$= E_0\alpha_0\cos(2\pi v_i t) + \frac{1}{2}E_0 A\left(\frac{\partial\alpha}{\partial Q}\right)_0\cos 2\pi(v_i - v)t$$

$$+ \frac{1}{2}E_0 A\left(\frac{\partial\alpha}{\partial Q}\right)_0\cos 2\pi(v_i + v)t$$

where
  P is the molecular dipole moment
  α is the polarizability of the molecular vibration
  Q is the normal coordinate of the vibration

In this equation, $E_0\alpha_0\cos 2\pi v_i t$ represents the original molecular dipole moment with the same frequency v_i as the frequency of the incident light, which corresponds to the Rayleigh scattering light. "$1/2E_0 A(\partial\alpha/\partial Q)_0\cos 2\pi(v_i - v)t$" represents the coupled dipole moment with the frequency lower than the frequency of the incident light, which corresponds to the Stokes Raman scattering. "$1/2E_0 A(\partial\alpha/\partial Q)_0\cos 2\pi(v_i + v)t$" is the coupled dipole moment with the frequency higher than the frequency of the incident light, which corresponds to the anti-Stokes Raman scattering. The Raman scattering intensity is proportional to the intensity of excitation EM field and the coupled efficiency between the nucleic vibrations and electronic oscillations.

As mentioned earlier, Raman scattering is the inelastic scattering of a photon from a molecule in which the frequency change precisely matches the difference in vibrational energy levels. Raman spectroscopy is a highly specific Raman scattering–based technique that detects and identifies molecules by their unique vibrational fingerprints. However, as a scattering process, Raman scattering is extremely weak: Typical Raman scattering cross sections per molecule are in the range of 10^{-30} and 10^{-25} cm^2. Thus, Raman spectroscopy usually needs a relatively large volume of molecules to produce detectable scattering signal intensities. This disadvantage has prevented Raman spectroscopy from many important sensing applications such as surface and *in vivo* sensing where the number of molecules that produce Raman scattering is small. SERS is about the Raman scattering of a single molecule or an ensemble of molecules of interest appearing (e.g., by binding and absorbing) in the close proximity (within a few nanometers to the nanoparticle [NP] surface) of a plasmonic NP that will produce an enhancement of the Raman signal. It was discovered in 1974 and correctly explained in 1977. Two primary mechanisms are generally thought to be responsible for large SERS signals. First, chemical enhancement (CE) corresponds to any modification of the Raman polarizability tensors (α_R) upon the adsorption of the molecule onto the metal surface. It can result from changes in the molecular electronic state or resonant enhancements from either existing molecular excitations or newly formed charge transfer states. Second, both optical excitation and Raman scattering resonate with the LSP modes in the metal NPs simultaneously, resulting in local-field electromagnetic (EM) enhancement and radiation EM, respectively. The EM contribution is, in any case, believed to be much larger (>10^2) than the CE effect. More specifically, if we assume that g is the local field enhancement averaged over the surface of the NP, the average magnitude of the local field (E_s) around the surface will be: $E_s = g \times E_0$, where E_0 is the magnitude of the incident field. The average molecule on the surface will then be excited by the enhanced local field, E_s, resulting in the Raman-scattered light near the surface with a field strength $E_R \propto \alpha_R \times E_s \propto \alpha_R \times g \times E_0$. The Raman-scattered (or radiated) fields (E_R) at the Raman-shifted wavelength will be further enhanced by the metal NP, with the radiation enhancement factor g', in the same way as the optical excitation was, giving the magnitude of the SERS-scattered field $E_{SERS} = \alpha_R \times g' \times E_s \propto \alpha_R \times g' \times g \times E$. As the average light intensity is proportional to the square of its EM field, we will theoretically have the SERS enhancement factor (assuming that the difference in α_R between SERS and non-SERS ($E_{non-SERS} = \alpha_R \times E_0$) fields can be ignored compared to EM).

$$EF = \frac{I_{SERS}}{I_{non-SERS}} = \left(\frac{E_{SERS}}{E_{non-SERS}} \right)^2 = g^2 \cdot g'^2.$$

Assuming that $g \approx g'$, we will have *EF the fourth-power dependence on g*, the key to the extraordinary enhancements SERS provides. This approximation takes advantage of the fact that the plasmon width is generally large compared to the Stokes shift, especially the low-frequency one. However, for SERS on isolated homogeneous particles where the plasmon width is small, this assumption leads to an overestimate of the EF by factors of 3 or more.

6.2.2 Technical Rationale and Approach of SERS

As discussed in the previous section, the Raman scattering intensity is proportional to the excitation field intensity. To obtain higher Raman scattering signals, apparently, one can think of using extremely high-power light sources such as kilowatt or megawatt lasers to excite the target molecules; however, this approach is not practical because such a powerful light source is not commonly available and the corresponding optics are expensive. Alternatively, one can think of artificially creating a hotspot by concentrating the excitation energy over a million-fold while still using commonly available laser sources, such as milliwatt lasers. Therefore, we introduce nanoplasmonic devices for creating the hotspot of the electric field. A plasmon is the collective free-electron oscillation in metallic nanostructures upon the excitation of an external EM field. The free electrons in metals can be driven by optical excitations. At the plasmon resonance frequency the free-electron oscillation can maintain the highest kinetic energy level. If we carefully design a nanoplasmonic device to drive most of the free electrons to an extremely small area and bring two such areas very close to each other, we can artificially make a plasmon nanocapacitor structure as illustrated in Figure 6.2. Since the nanocapacitor dimension is more than one order of magnitude smaller than the optical wavelength, electrostatic approximations may be applied here. The electric field potential (*V*) can be described as

$$V = \frac{Q}{C} = \left(\frac{Q}{A}\right) \cdot \left(\frac{d}{\varepsilon}\right)$$

where
Q/A is the electron density
d/ε is the effective gap distance between two electrodes

Obviously the higher the electron density, the higher *V* will be. By concentrating the free electrons in an area thousand times smaller, the electron density and local electric field potential can be easily increased by 10^3 times. The actual electric field potential across a single molecule is

$$V_m = V \cdot \frac{\varepsilon_m^d}{\varepsilon_m^d}$$

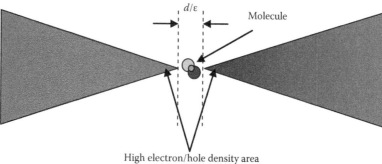

FIGURE 6.2
Hot spot in the localized electric field of a plasmon nanocapacitor or bowtie.

Here d_m and ε_m are the equivalent length and dielectric constant of the molecule. Obviously the electric field potential applied on the molecule becomes maximal, when the molecule size is close to the gap distance. The aforementioned qualitative analysis tells us from the perspective of EM enhancement that the ideal hotspot is a plasmonic nanogap structure with a small surface area, high electron or hole density and a gap distance of the same scale as the molecular size.

Considering the mechanism of chemical enhancement, when the chemical or biological molecule is in a very high electrical field in the subnanometer proximity, the effective bandgap in the target molecule becomes narrower and the molecular electrons could transfer from the highest occupied molecular orbital (HOMO) to the lowest unoccupied molecular orbital (LUMO) electronic energy level with higher coupling efficiency to the vibrational states. Hypothetically, the plasmon here serves as the mediator to facilitate the transition as shown in Figure 6.3. Therefore, matching the plasmon resonance energy with the electronic transition energy of the molecule is another key condition to assist the aforementioned chemical enhancement process [46].

We take designs of a nanoforest antenna array for theoretical modeling to explain the numerical methods. We first review the concept of a nanoforest antenna array. The design is inspired by the concept of lightning striking a tree and forest as created by mother nature (shown in Figure 6.4a). During a thunderstorm, trees can act like antennas collecting the lightning and passing superpower electric current to the ground. Here by mimicking the structure of a tree and forest, we will create nanotree and nanoforest devices to act like optical antennas that collect far-field optical excitation, generate both localized and propagating surface plasmons, and create SERS spots.

The illustration of an individual nanotree device is depicted in Figure 6.4b. The top part of the nanotree is a spherical or hemispherical gold or silver NP, and the "trunk" part of the nanotree is a short silicon nanopillar. The nanotrees are arranged side by side with sub-10 nm gap distance from each other to form a high-density nanoforest. The ground substrate underneath the nanoforest is covered with a gold or silver thin film. Due to the silicon nanopillar array, the ground metallic film is filled with ordered "nanoholes."

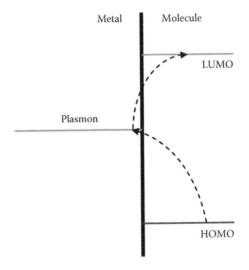

FIGURE 6.3
Energy and charge transfer between metallic SERS substrate and adsorbed molecule.

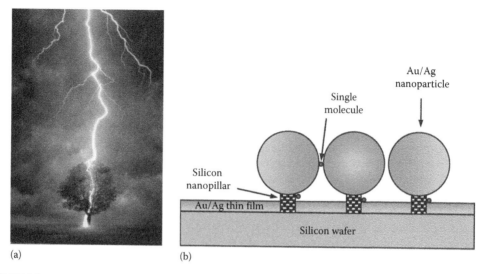

(a)   (b)

FIGURE 6.4
Biomimetic SERS substrate design. (a) Lightning striking a tree. (b) Nanotree and nanoforest array SERS substrate.

6.2.2.1 Electromagnetic Enhancement Modeling and Simulation

Due to the unconventional geometry of the 3D nanoantenna device, we will use finite-element frequency domain and finite-difference time domain methods to simulate the electrical field distribution with subnanometer spatial resolution. The general forms of Maxwell's equations are as follows:

$$\nabla \cdot D = \rho, \quad \nabla \cdot B = 0$$

$$\nabla \times H = J + \frac{\partial}{\partial t} D, \quad \nabla \times E = -\frac{\partial}{\partial t} B$$

$$D = \varepsilon_0 E + P, \quad H = \mu_0^{-1} B - M$$

$$J = \sigma E, \quad B = \mu \mu_0 H, \quad P = \varepsilon_0 \chi E$$

where
  D is the electric displacement
  E is the electric field
  B is the magnetic field
  H is the magnetic induction
  ρ is the charge density
  J is the current density
  P is the electric polarization
  M is the magnetization
  σ, μ, and χ are the conductivity, permittivity, and electric susceptibility, respectively

Analytical solutions usually only exist for simple and conformal geometries when using Maxwell equations. For nanoplasmonic devices with arbitrary geometries, numerical simulation methods are applied. The finite element method (FEM) is a method for solving partial differential equations (PDE) for arbitrary geometrical systems. This method requires the discretion of the complex geometrical domains into smaller subregions or cells in conformal geometries, such as rectangles or triangles. On each cell the function is approximated by a standard characteristic form. This method can be applied to a wide range of physical and engineering problems as long as it can be expressed as a PDE. The details related to EM simulation using FEM method can be found elsewhere [47]; only the general formulations are discussed here. For an EM wave in a time-harmonic form,

$$E(x,y,z,t) = E(x,y,z)\exp(j\omega t)$$

$$H(x,y,z,t) = H(x,y,z)\exp(j\omega t)$$

The Maxwell equation can be turned into

$$\nabla \times \left(\mu^{-1}\nabla \times E\right) - \omega^2 \varepsilon_c E = 0$$

$$\nabla \times \left(\varepsilon^{-1}\nabla \times H\right) - \omega^2 \mu H = 0$$

In this form, the time term is eliminated, and thus the equation can be directly applied to the discrete FEM cells. There are many boundary conditions in the EM FEM simulations. For nanoplasmonic structures, the low-reflecting and matched boundary conditions are used. They are defined as

$$\sqrt{\frac{\mu_0\mu_r}{\varepsilon_c}}n \times H + E - (n \cdot E)n = 2E_0 - 2(n \cdot E_0)n + 2\sqrt{\frac{\mu_0\mu_r}{\varepsilon_c}}n \times H_0$$

and

$$n \times (\nabla \times E) - j\beta\left(E - (n \cdot E)n\right) = -2j\beta\left(E_0 - (n \cdot E_0)n\right) - 2j\beta\sqrt{\frac{\mu_0\mu_r}{\varepsilon_c}}n \times H_0$$

respectively, where β is the propagation constant and E_0 and H_0 are the sources of electric and magnetic field, respectively. These formulas are applicable for three-dimensional simulations. For two-dimensional or in plane wave simulation, the wave equation and boundary conditions can be simplified as

$$\nabla \cdot \nabla E_z - \varepsilon k_0^2 E_z = 0 \text{ for transverse electric}(TE)\text{ wave}$$

$$-\nabla \cdot (\varepsilon \nabla H_z) - k_0^2 H_z = 0 \text{ for transverse magnetic}(TM)\text{ wave}$$

The low-reflecting boundary condition becomes

$$n \times \sqrt{\mu}H + \sqrt{\varepsilon}E_z = 2\sqrt{\varepsilon}E_{0z} \text{ (TE waves)}$$

$$n \times \sqrt{\varepsilon}E + \sqrt{\mu}H_z = -2\sqrt{\mu}H_{0z} \text{ (TM waves)}$$

and the matched boundary condition becomes

$$n \times (\nabla \times E_z) - j\beta E_z = -2j\beta E_{0z} \,(\text{TE waves})$$

$$n \times (\nabla \times H_z) - j\beta H_z = -2j\beta H_{0z} \,(\text{TM waves})$$

The commercial FEM simulation software COMSOL Multiphysics can be used to solve these equations. All of the simulation processes including geometry definition, FEM cell mesh generation, and equation solvers are integrated into the COMSOL software and the results can be exported into MATLAB, for further analysis.

Here, we will present the FEM simulation results for our exemplary devices. For the design of the self-organized nanohole on the nanocavity array, we show the theoretical study of SERS substrates such as periodically ordered AAO, with the deposition of the thin gold layer shown and their interactions with metallic NPs. Figure 6.5 shows the simulation results of electric amplitude enhancement under 785 nm TM-polarized-light excitation.

Furthermore, we show another exemplary model that begins to elucidate the design of an optimal nanocrescent device. In this model, the material modeled is gold, the outer radius of the nanocrescent is 200 nm, and an EM plane wave is normally incident at a free-space wavelength of 785 nm with TM polarization. Figure 6.6 shows the local field enhancement results for a typical model. By varying the tip sharpness (edge in 3D), the maximum field enhancement can vary significantly. The enhancement is also affected by varying the inner radius and the offset (center to center distance between the two spheres).

For the general time-domain EM simulation, finite-element time-domain (FDTD) simulation is generally applied. In FDTD, the time-dependent Maxwell's equations are discretized using central-difference approximations to the space and time partial derivatives. The resulting finite-difference equations are solved in a leapfrog manner: the electric field vector components in a volume of space are solved at a given instant in time; then the

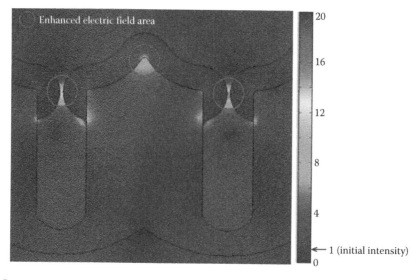

FIGURE 6.5
(See color insert.) FEM simulation results of electric field enhancement of AAO after thin gold layer deposition (cross-sectional view). The nano-hole size is 10 nm. The unit of enhancement is dB.

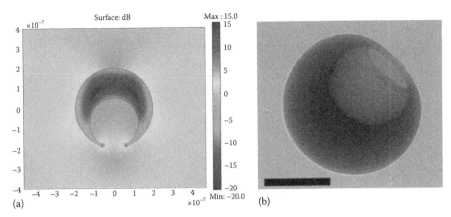

FIGURE 6.6
(See color insert.) The local field enhancement for a typical nano-crescent device. Note the high field enhancement at the sharp tips. (a) Electrical field distribution on the nano-crescent. The amplitude is normalized with respect to the incident field and shown in the unit of dB. (b) Transmission electron microscopy image of the nano-crescent. The scale bar represents 100 nm.

magnetic field vector components in the same spatial volume are solved at the next instant in time; and the process is repeated over and over again until the steady-state EM field is fully evolved. The Maxwell curl equations in Cartesian coordinates can be rewritten as

$$\frac{\partial H_x}{\partial t} = \frac{1}{\mu}\left(\frac{\partial E_y}{\partial z} - \frac{\partial E_z}{\partial y}\right), \quad \frac{\partial E_x}{\partial t} = \frac{1}{\varepsilon}\left(\frac{\partial H_z}{\partial y} - \frac{\partial H_y}{\partial z} - \sigma E_x\right)$$

$$\frac{\partial H_y}{\partial t} = \frac{1}{\mu}\left(\frac{\partial E_z}{\partial x} - \frac{\partial E_z}{\partial z}\right), \quad \frac{\partial E_y}{\partial t} = \frac{1}{\varepsilon}\left(\frac{\partial H_x}{\partial z} - \frac{\partial H_z}{\partial x} - \sigma E_y\right),$$

$$\frac{\partial H_z}{\partial t} = \frac{1}{\mu}\left(\frac{\partial E_x}{\partial y} - \frac{\partial E_y}{\partial x}\right), \quad \frac{\partial E_z}{\partial t} = \frac{1}{\varepsilon}\left(\frac{\partial H_y}{\partial x} - \frac{\partial H_x}{\partial y} - \sigma E_z\right)$$

If we define the discrete mesh grid (i, j, k) in Cartesian coordinates, these partial differential equations can be transformed to the following finite difference equations. Here, we only list the first two sets of equations and the others can be deduced in a similar fashion.

$$E_x^{n+1}\left(\frac{i+1}{2}, j, k\right) = \left[\frac{1 - \sigma(i+1/2, j, k)}{\varepsilon(i+1/2, j, k)}\right] E_x^n\left(\frac{i+1}{2}, j, k\right)$$

$$+ \frac{\Delta t}{\varepsilon}\left(\frac{i+1}{2}, j, k\right)\delta \left[\begin{array}{c} H_z^{n+1/2}\left(\frac{i+1}{2}, \frac{j+1}{2}, k\right) - H_z^{n+1/2}\left(\frac{i+1}{2}, \frac{j-1}{2}, k\right) \\[6pt] + H_y^{n+1/2}\left(\frac{i+1}{2}, j, \frac{k-1}{2}\right) + H_y^{n+1/2}\left(\frac{i+1}{2}, j, \frac{k-1}{2}\right) \\[6pt] - H_y^{n+1/2}\left(\frac{i+1}{2}, j, \frac{k+1}{2}\right) \end{array}\right]$$

$$H_x^{n+1/2}\left(i,\frac{j+1}{2},\frac{k+1}{2}\right) = H_x^{n-1/2}\left(i,\frac{j+1}{2},\frac{k+1}{2}\right) + \frac{\Delta t}{\mu\delta}\left[\begin{array}{l} E_y^n\left(i,\frac{j+1}{2},k+1\right) - E_y^n\left(i,\frac{j+1}{2},k\right) \\[2mm] +E_z^n\left(i,j,\frac{k+1}{2}\right) - E_z^n\left(i,j+1,\frac{k+1}{2}\right) \end{array}\right]$$

where
   n is the time index
   Δt is the time increment
   δ is the space increment

One can use FDTD simulation software to numerically solve these coupled equations in three dimensions, and we can also repeat the simulation for different meshing grids, Cartesian grids, or triangle grids. Using state-of-the-art, world-class supercomputing facilities, we are able to set the time increment to subfemtosecond scales and space increment to subnanometer scales.

As an example showing FDTD simulation, Figure 6.7 shows the enhancement in a silver nanocavity. The nanocavity in Figure 6.7b, adopted from the literature [48], has a width of 4 nm and a depth of 18 nm. The excitation wavelength is 582 nm and the electric field enhancement is 50 times, which agrees with the simulation results from the literature.

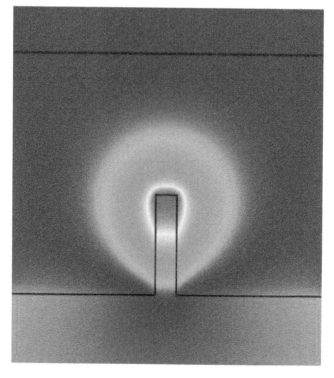

FIGURE 6.7
FDTD simulation results of a silver nanocavity.

6.2.2.2 Chemical Enhancement Modeling and Simulation

As discussed in the previous sections, chemical enhancement is another major mechanism for SERS enhancement [46]. In the quantum mechanical system, the Hamiltonian for a molecule is comprised of the terms for kinetic energies of the electrons and of the nuclei and the mutual coulombic interactions as described by the equation

$$H = \sum_{a=1,M} \left(\frac{-\hbar^2}{2m_a} \right) \nabla_a^2 + \sum_j \left[\left(\frac{-\hbar^2}{2m_e} \right) \nabla_j^2 - \frac{\sum_a z_a e^2}{r_{j,a}} \right] + \sum_{j<k} \frac{e^2}{r_{j,k}} + \sum_{a<b} \frac{z_a z_b e^2}{R_{a,b}}$$

where

m_a and m_e are the masses of the nuclei and electrons respectively

$r_{j,a}$ and $R_{a,b}$ are the distance between an electron and a nucleus and the distance between two nuclei, respectively

Clearly, in this equation, the first term is the kinetic energy of the nuclei; the second term is the kinetic and potential energy of the electrons; the third term is the coulombic interactions between electrons, and the fourth term is the coulombic interactions between nuclei.

When an EM field is present, the original Hamiltonian has to be corrected, with the addition of the interaction-time-dependent perturbation Hamiltonian shown as

$$H_{\text{int}} = \sum_j \left\{ \left(\frac{ie\hbar}{m_e c} \right) A(r_j, t) \cdot \nabla_j + \left(\frac{e^2}{2m_e c^2} \right) |A(r_j, t)|^2 \right\}$$

$$+ \sum_a \left\{ \left(\frac{iZ_a e\hbar}{m_a c} \right) A(R_a, t) \cdot \nabla_a + \left(\frac{Z_a^2 e^2}{2m_a c^2} \right) |A(R_a, t)|^2 \right\}$$

Here, $A(r, t) = 2A_0 \cos(\omega t - k \cdot r)$ is the vector potential of the excitation EM wave. The relations of the vector potential to the EM field amplitudes are $E(r, t) = \omega/c \cdot 2A_0 \sin(\omega t - k \cdot r)$, $H(r, t) = k \times A_0 2 \sin(\omega t - k \cdot r)$. As this Hamiltonian includes the term for transitions among the various electronic, vibrational, and rotational states of a molecule, it will be the major subject of our theoretical study. The first-order solution of the equation can be obtained using the Fermi "Golden Rule" to separate the time-dependent and time-independent parts. Furthermore, we will apply the "long wavelength" approximation in solving the Hamiltonian since the wavelength regime we are interested in is from ultraviolet to near-infrared wavelengths. After the approximation, for the electric dipole transition the coupling matrix between the initial states and the final states can be simplified as

$$\alpha_{f,i}(E) = \left(\frac{\omega_{f,i}}{\hbar c} \right) A_0 \cdot \left\langle \Phi_f \left| \sum_j e r_j + \sum_a Z_a e R_a \right| \Phi_i \right\rangle,$$

and the overall transition rate from the initial states to the final states after EM excitation is

$$R_{i,f} = 2\pi g(\omega_{f,i})\left|\alpha_{f,i}\right|^2 = \left(\frac{2\pi}{\hbar^2}\right)g(\omega_{f,i})\left|E_0 \cdot \left\langle \Phi_f \left| \sum_j er_j + \sum_a Z_a eR_a \right| \Phi_i \right\rangle\right|^2.$$

Here, the Φs are the eigenfunctions for all the states of the molecule. Since the transition rate is proportional to the electric field intensity, the enormous enhancement of the electric field by the SERS substrate may result in a much faster transition rate from the electronic states to the vibrational and rotational states, effectively expanding the optical cross section of Raman scattering.

The aforementioned transition dipole matrix also relates the initial and final electronic wavefunctions. The elements in the transition dipole matrix are functions of the internal vibrational coordinates of the molecule. Molecular point-group symmetry will be used to determine whether a particular transition's dipole matrix element will vanish or proceed when the applied electric field has a nonzero component along the molecule's z-axis. If we plug the eigenfunctions of the vibrational Hamiltonians associated to the initial and final electronic states and their nuclear overlap integral (known as "Frank-Condon factors") into the aforementioned rate equation, the transition rate between the electronic, vibrational states, and the vibrational coupling intensity can be calculated.

Eventually we will couple the electric field distribution at the hotspot acquired from the subnanometer resolution EM simulation with the three-dimensional quantum mechanical calculations for some model molecules. As the electric field distribution and intensity play direct roles in the vibrational state transition and coupling, we envision that the electric field enhancement and concentration would result in the enhancement of the vibrational-state transition rate and coupling intensity.

Another factor that will also be taken into account in the quantum mechanical simulation is the coupling and energy transfer between the plasmon dipole and molecular dipole. Applying the Frank–Condon principle, the rate of donor–acceptor energy transfer between the molecule and the plasmon is defined by

$$k_{pm} = \frac{2\pi}{\hbar}\left|\left\langle \psi^p_{M_D}; \psi^m_{N_A} \left| H'_{int} \right| \psi^p_{N_D}; \psi^m_{N_A} \right\rangle\right|^2 \sum_{M_D,N_D}\sum_{M_A,N_A} f\left(E^m_{N_D}\right)f\left(E^p_{M_A}\right)$$

$$\times \left|\left\langle \chi^{D^p}; \chi^{A^m} \left| \chi^{D^m}; \chi^{A^p} \right\rangle\right|^2, \cdot \delta\left(E^m_{N_D} - E^p_{M_D} + E^p_{M_A} - E^m_{N_A}\right)$$

where

H_{int} is the interaction Hamiltonian between the molecule and the plasmon
$\left\langle \chi^{D^p}; \chi^{A^m} \left| \chi^{D^m}; \chi^{A^p} \right\rangle$ is the nuclear overlap matrix
ψ is the electronic wavefunction

The interaction Hamiltonian is dependent on the size and electron density distribution of both nanoplasmonic device and molecule and the distance between them, which is

$$H_{int} = \frac{1}{4\pi\varepsilon_0}\int dr_m \int d^3_{r_p} \frac{\rho(r_m)\rho(r_p)}{\left|R - r_p + r_m\right|}.$$

For the dipole–dipole interaction, this Hamiltonian can be simplified into

$$H_{int} = \frac{1}{4\pi\varepsilon_0}\left[\frac{\mu_m \cdot \mu_p - 3(\mu_m \cdot \hat{d})(\mu_p \cdot \hat{d})}{d^3}\right],$$

Here, μ is the dipole moment operator, which is the spatial integral of charge density distribution in spherical coordinates.

The computed energy and charge transfer Hamiltonian will be coupled into the transition Hamiltonian between the electronic, vibrational, and rotational states, and a thorough quantum mechanical simulation will be carried out.

6.3 Synthesis Methods of SERS-Active Substrates

6.3.1 Controlled Synthesis and Nanofabrication of SERS Substrates

The underlying phenomena exploited for SERS-sensing applications are based on the interaction of light and matter at nanoscale surfaces. When the incoming EM radiation is coupled to the localized excitation of conductor electrons at the dielectric–metal interface of a metal NP, quantitative spectral data as a function of local environmental changes over time can be gathered [49]. Utilizing the plasmon coupling between neighboring geometrical features, the scattering cross sections of nanostructures should dominate over absorption cross sections, resulting in the enhanced scattering spectra of nearby molecular complexes for the generation of intense scattered radiation [49]. If the resulting plasmon resonance frequency matches the incoming EM radiation, the collective oscillations of the conduction electrons at the dielectric–metal interface occur in-phase, and a highly sensitive, label-free, spectral snapshot of the local biochemical environment is obtained. The strong, localized plasmon resonance exhibited by metal NPs is dependent on the surrounding environment as well as the composition, size, and shape of the NP [50]. Sharp features, such as those exhibited by nanostars, can be exploited for "lightning rod effects," where molecules adsorbed to high-curvature surfaces show enhanced Raman scattering due to the polarization of the metal in those regions resulting from the external EM field [44,49].

The ability to control the morphology of these "sensing" elements is essential for biosensing applications based on surface enhanced Raman scattering (SERS). Recent advances in the control over NPs' size and shape allow the transfer of plasmon energy as well as EM energy to be concentrated and transported [50]. Combined with nanostructured surfaces, both *in vitro* and *in vivo* static and dynamic molecular interactions of chemical and biological molecules can be detected [50].

Current SERS fabrication methods typically rely on *bottom-up* nanostructure synthesis, *top-down* nanostructure fabrication, or combinations of both processes. With *bottom-up* methods, nanocrystals are synthesized using solution-based chemical or physical processes. The composition, size, and shape of the NPs depend heavily upon the control of chemical reactions, and conditions during synthesis [16]. *Top-down* nanostructure fabrication involves lithographic techniques utilizing well-established micro-and nanofabrication tools. Modified, or hybrid, assembly fabrication may involve combinations of *bottom-up* and *top-down* processes, such as nanosphere lithography (NSL), where NPs are used as the masking template for conventional metal deposition techniques and provide another way to obtain submicron pattern spacing.

6.3.1.1 Bottom-Up Chemical Synthesis

Bottom-up nanostructure synthesis methods include sol-gel, pyrolysis, hydrothermal, micelles, and chemical precipitation from supersaturated conditions [51]. The addition of organic ligands or capping materials can achieve the size and shape control of NPs by inhibiting further crystal growth or changing the growth environment to an inert one [51]. The chemical reduction of metal salts with a stabilizer is often used to synthesize metal NPs. The stabilizer functions as a growth inhibitor in particular directions, thus controlling the shape as well as providing colloidal stability [16]. A two-step process of metal NP-seeded growth can produce diverse shapes such as rods, plates, and pyramids with high reproducibility [16]. Solution-based synthesis routes typically consist of three stages: first, nucleation; second, transformation of nuclei to seeds; finally, seed evolution into nanocrystals [52]. NP morphology is also controlled by reaction time, temperature, and the concentration of solvents, reagents, and surfactants [51]. For seeded growth, the final shape of the metal nanocrystal is determined by the structure of the seed and the capping-material binding affinity [52].

Designing NPs using wet chemical processes produces a large variety of shapes and sizes. The simplest form of NP is the nanosphere, which can be formed from seed-mediated growth, as described earlier [53,54]. The geometrical shape influences the plasmon resonance response. For solid gold colloidal nanospheres, plasmon resonance typically occurs around 520 nm and can only be tuned around that mode by approximately 50 nm [55]. The shape anisotropy of nanorods can provide additional functionality from two plasmonic resonance modes depending on the radial and longitudinal axes of the nanorod [50] and tunable by changing the aspect ratio [8]. Other synthesized shapes include cubes, tetrahedrons, octahedrons, triangular plates, bipyramids, and triangular plates [56–58]. Mixed metallic-alloy and shell-core structures have also been demonstrated [55,59]. Nanoshells, which consist of a spherical dielectric core encased in a metal shell, have tunable plasmonic properties highly sensitive to the inner and outer shell diameters [60], and have the advantage of extending into the near-infrared spectrum, a region of relative transparency for living tissues [61]. Combining the advantages of nanorod shape anisotropy and nanoshells with tunable plasmon resonances results in nanorice, a hybrid nanostructure where plasmon resonance tuning occurs by changing the nanorice length as well as varying the relative size of the inner and outer metallic shells [62]. Branched NPs, such as nanostars, are of interest due to their sharp edges and can exhibit higher SERS intensity at the tips [63,64]. Since the LSPR frequency is dependent on both the shape and the size of the nanostructures, the wide variety of NPs mentioned earlier can have their LSPR frequency varied from the entire visible to the mid-infrared part of the EM spectrum as shown in Figure 6.8, demonstrating the high tunability of plasmonic nanobiosensors, which enables a wide variety of applications in biomedical detection.

When using NPs for biosensing assay-based applications, the metal or metal–dielectric NP surfaces are functionalized with biological recognition elements that interact directly with the analytes in the aqueous solution. Some difficulties associated with functionalizing NPs in aqueous solutions include the dependency on pH, temperature, or concentration conditions [16]. The direct placement of NPs on substrates by condensation, deposition, or electrostatic interaction can be applied to avoid the unintentional aggregation of NPs in solution [16]. *Top-down* fabrication processes and tools, where the nanoscale features are produced directly on the substrate with high repeatability, may provide an alternative to the multistep process of synthesizing NPs by wet chemical means then depositing

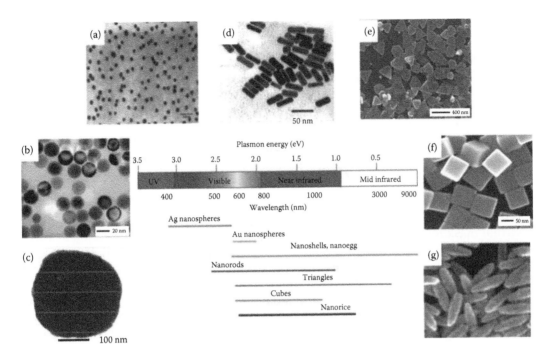

FIGURE 6.8
NP resonance range of plasmon resonances for a variety of particle morphologies [3]. TEM images of Au spheres (a), Ag spheres (b), SiO₂/Ag (core/shell) nanoshells (c), and nanorods (d); SEM images of cubes (f), nanorices (g) and (c) 2006 (triangular plates (e)). (a: From Grabar, K.C., Freeman, R.G., Hommer, M.B., and Natan, M.J.: Preparation and characterization of Au colloid monolayers. *Anal. Chem.* 1995. 67(4). 735–743; b: Wiley, B., Herricks, T., Sun, Y.G., and Xia, Y.N.: Polyol synthesis of silver NPs: Use of chloride and oxygen to promote the formation of single-crystal, truncated cubes and tetrahedrons. *Nano Lett.* 2004. 4(9). 1733–1739; c and d: Nikoobakht, B., and El-Sayed, M.A.: Preparation and growth mechanism of gold nanorods (NRs) using seed-mediated growth method. *Chem. Mater.* 2003. 15(10). 1957–1962; e: Washio, I., Xiong, Y.J., Yin, Y.D., and Xia, Y.N.: Reduction by the end groups of poly(vinyl pyrrolidone): A new and versatile route to the kinetically controlled synthesis of Ag triangular nanoplates. *Adv. Mater.* 2006. 18(13). 1745–1749; f: Wiley, B.J., Im, S.H., Li, Z.Y., Mclellan, J., Siekkinen, A., and Xia, Y.A.: Maneuvering the surface plasmon resonance of silver nanostructures through shape-controlled synthesis. *J. Phys. Chem. B.* 2006. 110(32). 15666–15675; g: Wang, H., Brandl, D.W., Le, F., Nordlander, P., and Halas, N.J.: Nanorice: A hybrid plasmonic nanostructure. *Nano Lett.* 2006. 6(4). 827–832. Copyright Wiley-VCH Verlag GmbH & Co. KGaA. Reproduced with permission.)

mono- or bilayers onto substrates. Additionally, integration with well-established micro- and nanofabrication processes and tools readily provides potential for the large-scale manufacturing of LSPR and SERS substrates. Modified, or hybrid, processes often involve a *top-down* fabrication technique either for pattern transfer or metal deposition and are also discussed in the following section.

6.3.1.2 Top-Down Nanofabrication

In addition to utilizing existing and well-established nanofabrication tools, the *top-down* fabrication of LSPR and SERS substrates can also provide reproducible control over feature size, shape, and gap distance between nanostructures. The typical process involves two steps. First, the nanoscale pattern transfer to a substrate must occur with one of the major lithographic techniques, which include electron-beam (EBL), nanoimprint (NIL), template (such as anodic aluminum oxide [AAO]), and nanosphere (NSL). The second process can involve metal deposition onto the substrate using vapor deposition via chemical (CVD), physical (PVD), oblique-angle (OAD), or glancing-angle (GLAD) methods, or an etching process. Focused-ion-beam (FIB) milling is another technique to create nanoscale features, although an unintended doping of substrates with gallium ions can modify optical properties, especially in the visible-light region [66,67]. Additional techniques to form metal nanostructures include the laser ablation of metal targets in aqueous solution, and electrodeposition, although the latter process is limited to metallic substrates [68]. Table 6.1 compares the current top-down fabrication techniques, using SERS substrates as examples for nanoplasmonic biosensors. Typically, the molecule used for SERS experiments exhibit a large Raman-scattering cross section.

6.3.1.2.1 Electron-Beam Lithography

Electron-beam lithography (EBL) is a direct-write nanopattern transfer method using a virtual mask for sequential feature exposure on a substrate. High-resolution features on the order of low 10's nm are obtainable [83]. Advantages of EBL include nanoscale feature resolution, control over beam energy and dose, elimination of physical masks, high accuracy over small regions on a wafer, reduction in defect densities, and ability for large depth of focus on changing topographies [83]. Although EBL provides an effective method for fabricating reproducible nanoscale features including nanodots [63], nanowells [84], and nanoring antennas [85], the longer writing times and higher costs are the main disadvantages of using EBL for high throughput, low cost LSPR and SERS applications.

6.3.1.2.2 Nanoimprint Lithography

A potential low-cost, large-scale method for SERS substrate fabrication is nanoimprint lithography (NIL). The process is twofold: a hard mask, typically made of metal, dielectrics, or a semiconductor material, is pressed into a thin layer of polymer heated above its glass transition temperature [86]. When pressed together, the viscous polymer conforms to the mold topography, creating thickness variations in the substrate upon the removal of the mold [87]. A reactive ion etch (RIE) of the substrate completes the pattern transfer. NIL processes have been used to create gold rectangular, cylindrical, and diamond-shaped nanoblocks based on grating mold orientation [88], flat, grated, and pillared silver nanostructures for SERS [89], and gold nanodisks [90]. A potential disadvantage of the NIL process is the embedded cost of fabricating the original mold, which requires access to high-resolution lithographic tools, such as EBL. The mold-making process involves placing resist on the mold substrate, nanopattern exposure, hard mask (metal) deposition on the template, followed by liftoff and RIE for the selective etching of the mold [91]. Once the NIL mold is fabricated, multiple transfers provide a high level of repeatability for nanoscale features.

6.3.1.2.3 Template-Based Methods

Template-based methods typically utilize the regular array of nanometer-scale holes in a hard material such as anodic aluminum oxide (AAO) for the electrochemical deposition of metals, semiconductors, or polymers [76,92]. For AAO templates, the pore diameter is controlled by changes in oxidation conditions and feature sizes can range from 5 to 500 nm [93]. Following the material deposition, which can include electrochemical or thermal vacuum evaporation, or RF sputtering, the AAO template is removed by chemical dissolution [93,94]. The advantages of AAO templates include large working areas (>1 cm^2), compatibility with different materials, and tunable size properties [93]. AAO-templated

TABLE 6.1

Comparison of Various Top-Down Nanofabrication Techniques for SERS Substrates

	EF[a]	Typical Substrate Area (cm²)	Uniformity	Reproducibility	Material/Shape[b]/Size (nm)[c]	Molecule/Laser Wavelength (nm)	Cost
EBL	10^5 for BSA, 10^7 RNase-A [69]	$<0.001 \times 0.001$ [70]	—	<20% [71]	Ag or Au/film on pillars/25 nm [71]	Rhodamine 6G (R6G) and 1,10-phenanthroline [71]/632.8 nm bovine serum albumin (BSA) and ribonuclease-A (RNase-A) [69]/632.8 nm	Expensive
NSL	10^8 [30,72,73]	1.5×1.5 [74]	—	—	5–40 nm [75]	Benzenethiol (BT) [30]	Inexpensive
Template	10^6 [76]	1×0.5 [77]	<20% [77]	<15% [77]	Au/Nanopillar /110 [77]	Thionine [77]	Inexpensive
Hybrid [78]	10^5	1×1	—	—	50 nm thick Ag	BT	Inexpensive
OAD	10^6–10^8 [79] $>10^8$ [80]	2.5×7.5 [79]	<10% [79]	<15% [79]	Ag/NR/ ~88–99 [79]/80–90 [80]	Trans-1,2-bix(4-pyridyl)ethane (BPE)/785 [80]	Moderate
GLAD	—	—	—	—	Ag/NR/20–30 [81]	R6G	Moderate
AAO/ GLAD [82]	10^5	—	—	—	Pt, Au, ITO/NT/20–200 nm	Benzenethiolate	Moderate

a Enhancement factor.
b Minimum dimension of nanostructure.
c NP, nanopillar; NR, nanorod; NT, nanotube.

nanostructures for plasmonic applications include nanorods [94,95], nanopores [96], nano-pillars [77], nanowires [76], and nanocrescents [97]. Depending on the composition of the electrochemical solution, surface roughness and different lengths of resulting nanostructures may result [95]. The branching of nanostructures at the base is also another issue with the process and pore diameters of less than 20 nm can exhibit irregular patterns [93,94]. As shown in Table 6.1, SERS-enhancement factors up to 10^5 have been demonstrated with a hybrid AAO template and glancing-angle deposition technique [82]. Block copolymers (BCP) are another technique to fabricate template-based nanostructures for LSPR applications. Nanostructure shapes such as spheres, cylinders, and lamellae are all dependent on the composition and chain structure of the polymers [98], with feature sizes ranging from 5 to 50 nm as a function of the BCP molecular weights and final self-assembled NP pattern dependent upon the BCP domain symmetry. While micrometer-scale areas are achievable, defects can exist at grain boundary edges [99]. Using a combination of *top-down* and *bottom-up* processes, examples of defect-free, large-area BCP domains on templated and lithographically defined surfaces have been demonstrated [99,100]. The high cost of extreme ultraviolet interferometric lithography limits the wide-scale application of the latter process [99], while EBL grooves combined with plasma etching are required for the former [100].

6.3.1.2.4 Nanosphere Lithography

Nanosphere lithography (NSL) is based on templating monolayer or double layer colloidal NPs for submicron- and nanometer-scale patterns. Methods for preparing NSL include electrostatic deposition, self-assembly, drop casting, spin coating, and evaporation [93,101] forming a hexagonal, close-packed monolayer on the substrate with controllable size, shape, and interparticle spacing [102]. Metal is deposited onto the NP array by thermal, e-beam, or pulsed laser deposition, then the NSL templates are removed from the substrate at high temperatures or with chemical dissolution using organic solvents [93]. NSL advantages include low cost, high throughput, compatibility with many materials, and the capability of producing well-ordered arrays on different substrates [103]. Nanostructures such as nanopillars [104], nanohole arrays [105], nanowire arrays [106], nanobowls [107], nanotriangles [102], nanorings [108], and nanocrescents [49] have been fabricated successfully for LSPR and SERS applications. However, NSL suffers from several disadvantages. First, the formation of colloidal particles into a mask has limited geometries due to the hexagonal close-packed formation [109]. Modified NSL with varying gaps can be fabricated, involving multiple processes such as etching, ion beam techniques, or spin coating prior to pattern transfer [109,110]. Since gap sizes affect the tunability of substrate plasmonic resonances [111], it is important to have flexibility while adjusting the gap between particles. Since the size of NPs and the gap distance between holes or features are interdependent, control over substrate features has additional constraints [109]. Finally, structural defects such as nanosphere polydispersity, dislocations, vacancies, polycrystalline domains, or local polystyrene (PS) or latex bead disorder are often transferred to the new substrates leaving limited defect-free areas ranging from 10 to 100 μm^2 [75,112]. The NSL method has been modified in multiple ways, including transferring monolayers via submersion in millipore water, [113] liquid/gas interface self-assembly [75], angle-resolved NSL [74], shadow NSL with annealed PS, and fabricating dimmers [16]. For SERS applications, Ag film over nanosphere substrates (AgFON) has shown a 10–100× increase in the enhancement factor [105].

6.3.1.2.5 Oblique-Angle Deposition and Glancing-Angle Deposition

Oblique-angle deposition (OAD) combines physical vapor deposition, such as electron beam deposition, with steep substrate angles >75°, relative to the vapor source. Thin films produced by PVD tend to have columnar or porous microstructures and tilting the substrate at steep angles (>75°) relative to the substrate normal leads to geometrical shadowing effects and the preferential growth of nanostructures [114]. As shown in Figure 6.9a, atoms condense and diffuse on the substrate surface then form nuclei. The region behind the nuclei does not receive additional vapor due to line-of-sight self-shadowing so that the incoming atoms deposit on the exposed face of the nuclei [115]. Columns then grow from the nuclei at an angle dependent on the incoming vapor flux direction (Figure 6.9a). Figure 6.9c shows the OAD shadowing effect on a lithographically patterned seed layer. Materials used for OAD include metals, metal oxides, silicon, silicon oxides, as well as combinations [116], and SERS enhancement factors have been demonstrated as high as 10^8 (see Table 6.1).

When combined with precise motor control, OAD becomes glancing-angle deposition technique (GLAD), a method for sculpting thin films. Figure 6.9b shows a typical GLAD apparatus [117]. The design of nanostructures depends on both substrate angle relative to the vapor source and control over the substrate, often accomplished with stepper motors controlling α and φ rotational speeds. As shown in Figure 6.10a, fabricated morphologies

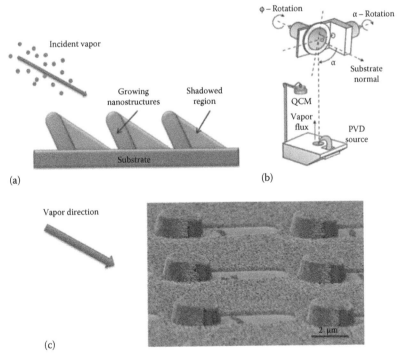

(a)

(b)

(c)

FIGURE 6.9
Schematic of oblique angle deposition (OAD) or glancing angle deposition (GLAD). (a) Conceptual illustration of column growth. (b) A typical GLAD apparatus that consists of a rotation stage with substrate angle adjustment. (c) Example of shadowing effect with lithographically patterned substrate. (b: From Steele, J.J. et al., *J. Mater. Sci. Mater. El.*, 18(4), 367, 2007.)

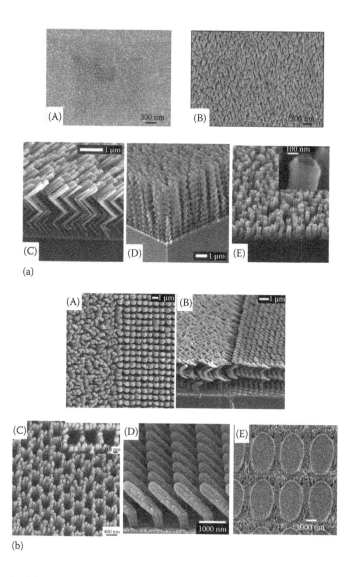

FIGURE 6.10
Various morphologies fabricated by GLAD. (a) Various non-patterned morphologies: Ag spheres (A) and tilt nanowires (B), Si chevrons (C) and helical posts (D), and nanotubes (E). (b) Various patterned nanostructures fabricated by combining GLAD with e-beam lithography (A, B), nanosphere lithography (C), and photolithography (D), and (E). (a: From Steele, J.J. and Brett, M.J., *J. Mater. Sci. Mater. El.*, 18(4), 367, 2007; Huang, Z.F. et al., *Adv. Mater.*, 21(29), 2983, 2009; b: Steele, J.J. and Brett, M.J., *J. Mater. Sci. Mater. El.*, 18(4), 367, 2007; Fu, J., Zhao, Y., Optical properties of silver/gold nanostructures fabricated by shadowing growth and their sensing applications. *Proc. SPIE* 7766(Nanostructured Thin Films III), San Diego, CA, 77660B/77661–77660B/77612, 2010; Zhou, C.M. and Gall, D., *Thin Solid Films*, 516(2–4), 433, 2007; Ye, D.X. and Lu, T.M., *Phys. Rev. B*, 76(23), 235402-235401-235408, 2007.)

range from close-packed nanospheres and tilted nanowires to chevrons, helical posts [116], and nanotubes [118]. Silicon nanowires can be used as templates for high-aspect-ratio hollow nanostructures [118]. In this case, the tube wall thickness is dependent on the reaction rate and the duration of LPCVD coating and crystallinity is a function of the temperature or a post-process anneal [118]. More complicated structures such as helical columns and zigzag nanotube arrays, and square spiral structures have also been demonstrated [118–120]. As shown in Table 6.1, Ag nanorods were fabricated and tested using R6G, although the enhancement factor was not calculated because 10^{-14} mol L^{-1} was the detection limit for the particular substrate. Although GLAD techniques show promise for the further morphology control of substrates, further optimization is required to better control the spacing, size, and shape of nanostructures [81].

Although traditional GLAD and OAD processes yield randomized nanostructure formation, which in turn produces rods of varying lengths [80], periodic arrays of lithographically patterned seed areas can restrict growth to specific regions by taking advantage of the self-shadowing effect [120]. Conventional micro- or nanofabrication tools can be used to pattern the desired seed topography. These seeds then define the initial stages of film growth by removing the randomness of nucleation sites [116]. Successful seed patterning depends on several parameters: first, the seed diameter should be of similar diameter to an individual column to avoid multiple columns growing per seed; second, column broadening can be avoided by designing the relative density of the GLAD film close to the portion of the substrate area covered by patterned seeds; finally, column formation between seeds can be prevented by careful placement of the seed shadow [117]. Seed dimensions are typically several hundred nanometers for inorganic materials with intervals of 100 nm to 1 μm and require large patterned areas (~several mm²) [116]. Figure 6.10b shows examples of patterned seed layers and the resulting GLAD nanostructure formation. GLAD techniques can also be used to fabricate heteronanostructures including gold-coated silicon "matchsticks" for biosensing applications [121] and gold–titanium dioxide–gold sandwich structures for LSPR substrates [122]. For OAD seed-patterned silver nanorods, SERS intensities were also shown to increase as both diameter and rod spacing decreased [123], indicating that morphology control may help improve SERS detection.

6.3.2 Instrumentation and Experimental Conditions for Optimization

6.3.2.1 Far-Field Optical Characterization

6.3.2.1.1 Darkfield Scattering Imaging and Spectroscopy

The scattering spectrum of a single and arrayed plasmonic NPNP is usually measured in the microscopy system shown in Figure 6.11. The device is mounted on a white light darkfield microscopy system with a true-color camera and a spectrometer to characterize the scattering image and spectrum of individual NPNPs. The excitation light only illuminates on the device sample from very oblique angles and the collection objective lens has a smaller numerical aperture, therefore not the direct excitation light but the scattering light is picked up by the microspectroscopy system.

As the scattering spectra of the nanoplasmonic devices directly reflect their plasmon resonance modes, the scattering peak wavelength is equivalent to the plasmon resonance wavelength. The darkfield scattering spectroscopy and imaging can not only experimentally characterize the plasmon resonance modes of device, but directly measure the relative local light intensity enhancement from far-field given submicron spatial resolution in microscopy. The hotspot may be imaged as super bright pixels in darkfield imaging when compared with negative control samples. However, due to the spatial resolution limit in optical microscopy, only qualitative information can be obtained with this technique; the EM field enhancement factors measured in the case are averaged results, which may not directly correspond to designed and simulated data.

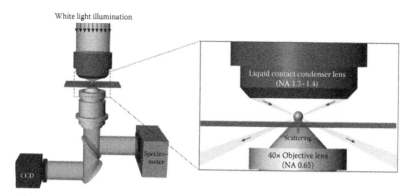

FIGURE 6.11
Darkfield microscopy system for measuring scattering spectra of nanoplasmonic devices.

6.3.2.1.2 Photoluminescence Imaging and Spectroscopy

Photoluminescence is a process in which a chemical compound absorbs photons, jumps to a higher electronic energy state and then radiates photons back out, returning to a lower energy state. Typically the absorption and emission process is extremely fast, in the order of 10 ns, but the period of this process may be significantly shortened or elongated when placing the resonance molecule in the SERS hotspot. The local electric field enhancement and charge transfer effect at the SERS hotspot will lead to the rate change of the electronic state transition and vibration state coupling.

As the photoluminescence is a fairly short event, we will use picosecond pulse laser to excite the molecule and use a high-speed microspectroscopy system to measure the time-dependent emission intensity. The measured emission decay curves will provide us the information to assess the transition rate change of the molecule, validate our quantum-mechanical simulations, and verify our modeling results.

6.3.2.1.3 Far-Field SERS Spectroscopy

Far-field SERS measurements are the most common practice. Far-field SERS spectroscopy will be able to provide a direct evaluation of the enhancement effect of SERS substrate devices. If using the comparative methods between SERS and Raman measurements for the target molecule and control molecule respectively, one can calculate the effective SERS enhancement factors, although the direct SERS enhancement factor can be only measured in nearfield.

A scanning confocal Raman microspectroscopy system can be used to acquire Raman scattering spectra from SERS substrates. As shown in Figure 6.12, a typical system consisted of a Carl Zeiss Axiovert 200 inverted microscope (Carl Zeiss, Germany) equipped with a 300 mm focal-length monochromator (Acton Research, MA) with a 1024×256-pixel cooled spectrograph CCD camera (Roper Scientific, NJ). A visible-wavelength laser can be used as the excitation source of Raman scattering, and the laser beam was focused by a 100× objective lens on the SERS substrate. The excitation power is adjustable by using different neutral-density filters. The Raman scattering light was then collected through the same optical pathway through a long-pass filter and analyzed by the spectrometer. The sample is mounted on a piezoelectric motorized stage with nanometer travel resolution, so a two-dimensional SERS spectral image may be generated using this system.

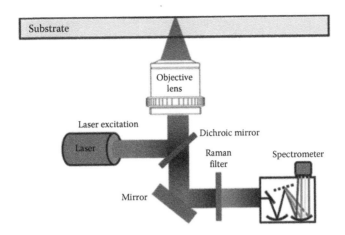

FIGURE 6.12
Raman scattering microspectroscopic system.

6.3.2.2 Near-Field Optical Characterization

6.3.2.2.1 Near-Field Scanning Optical Microscopy

Near-field Scanning Optical Microscopy (NSOM) is a microscopic technique for nanostructure investigation that breaks the far-field resolution limit by directly directing the near-field emission or scattering. This is done by placing the detector very close ($\ll$ wavelength, typically a few nanometers) to the specimen surface. This allows for the surface optical inspection with high spatial, spectral, and temporal resolving power. One can use NSOM to characterize the nearfield scattering intensity from the SERS hotspot and hope to establish the two-dimensional field distributions corresponding to our simulation results.

NSOM can be operated in both, an aperture and a nonaperture mode. As illustrated in Figure 6.13, the tips used in the apertureless mode are very sharp and do not have a metal coating.

The aperture-mode NSOM system resembles an atomic-force microscopy system. The primary components of an NSOM setup include the light source, the feedback mechanism, the scanning tip, the detector, and the piezoelectric sample stage. One can use the same laser for exciting the SERS signal as the light source in NSOM measurements. The laser light can be focused into an optical fiber through a polarizer, a beam splitter, and a coupler. The polarizer and the beam splitter serve to remove stray light from the returning reflected light. The scanning tip is an etched optical fiber coated with metal except at the tip. Avalanche photodiode (APD) can be used to pick up the scattering light. For the

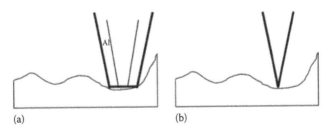

FIGURE 6.13
Configurations of the NSOM tip in (a) aperture mode and (b) non-aperture mode.

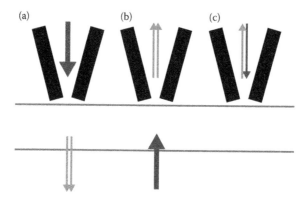

FIGURE 6.14
Illustrations of three operational methods in aperture-mode NSOM. (a) Near-field excitation far-field collection. (b) Far-field excitation near-field collection. (c) Near-field excitation near-field collection.

same system configurations, there are still many different ways of near-field excitation and detection. Figure 6.14 illustrates three possible methods usually used in characterization experiments, and they are nearfield illumination far-field collection, far-field illumination nearfield collection as well as nearfield illumination nearfield collection. The far-field illumination nearfield collection method is most close to the real situation in the common far-field SERS spectroscopy. In this case, the focused laser light will excite a sample device from far-field but the scattering light will be only picked up at the NSOM tip. By scanning the NSOM tip, the two-dimensional Rayleigh scattering light tomograph can be obtained, which can be directly compared to simulation results. The light enhancement factor can also be acquired directly.

6.3.2.2.2 Near-Field SERS Spectroscopy
Besides the nearfield Rayleigh scattering measurement, one can couple the NSOM system with our Raman spectroscopy system to measure the SERS spectra in the nearfield.

6.4 Surface Biofunctionalization of SERS Substrates

The significant advancement in controlled nanofabrication offers researchers the capability to tune the plasmonic properties of nanomaterials. However, the surface of plasmonic nanomaterials (gold and silver NPs are the most common) cannot interact with the biological analyte selectively. To overcome this limit, the surface functionalization techniques of nanomaterials by biological recognition elements (bioreceptors or bioprobes) have recently been developed to form hybrid nanomaterials that incorporate the highly selective catalytic and recognition properties of biomaterials such as enzymes and DNA, with the highly sensitive and easily tunable electronic and photonic features of plasmonic nanomaterials [13,15,127].

Often, NPs synthesized in an organic medium tend to aggregate to form clusters in an aqueous solution that is generally required by biomedical applications. Therefore, before they can be modified by any bioreceptors, water-solubilization is required, during which the colloidally unstable NPs are stabilized in an aqueous solution by conjugating with hydrophilic ligands. One way to stabilize NPs is by coulombic repulsion. It requires the ligands to be ionic. Another way to stabilize NPs is steric stabilization, during which NP aggregation is prevented by coating with a physical barrier. The barriers include polymeric ligands, such as poly (ethylene glycol) (PEG) [128], and small-molecular ligands like bis(*p*-sulfonatophenyl) phenylphosphine surfactants [32]. All these ligands for water-solubilization are then replaced by phase transfer or ligand exchange or modified by ligand addition with the desired biofunctional ligands [13]. Water-solubilization may be performed either as the final stage of the biofunctionalization process of NPs or as an intermediate stage.

Four strategies are generally used to functionalize the surface of plasmonic nanomaterials (typically Au, Ag, and Cu surfaces) with biomolecules such as bioreceptors. The first is the electrostatic adsorption of positively charged biomolecules to negatively charged NPs, or vice versa. For example, gold and silver NPs synthesized by citrate reduction are stabilized by citrate ligands at pH slightly above their isoelectric point, resulting in the anionic citrate-coated NPs that can be bound to the positively charged amino acid side chains of immunoglobulin G (IgG) molecules [129]. The second strategy is ligand-like binding to the metallic surface of plasmonic nanomaterials by the chemisorption of thiol groups. Metal nanostructures can be functionalized with L-cysteine through the Au–S bonds and then bound to target proteins through peptide bonds with the cysteine moieties [130]. They can also be directly bound to thiol-derivative analytes such as protein-containing cysteine residues (e.g., serum albumin) [131] or thiolated DNA [132,133]. The third strategy is covalent binding through biofunctional linkers, exploiting functional groups on both particles and biomolecules. The bifunctional linkers have anchor groups that can be attached to NP surfaces and functional groups that can be further covalently coupled to the target biomolecules. They are extensively used to covalently conjugate biomolecules with various NPs [134], especially when no linking moieties like thiol groups are available in biomolecules. The common anchor groups include thiols, disulfides, and phosphine ligands that are used to bind the bifunctional linkers to Au, Ag, CdS, and CdSe NPs. The fourth strategy is based on noncovalent, affinity-based receptor–ligand systems. More specifically, NPs are functionalized with bioreceptors (e.g., antibodies) that provide affinity sites for the binding of the corresponding ligand (e.g., antigens) or ligand-modified proteins and oligonucleotides. The most well-known example in the last several decades is the avidin–biotin system [135,136]. For example, biotinylated proteins (e.g., immunoglobulins and serum albumins) or biotinylated oligonucleotides (e.g., single-stranded DNA [ssDNA]) [133] have been widely used to modify streptavidin-functionalized Au NPs by affinity binding [134]. Regarding molecular recognition, the system consists of the small-molecule biotin (vitamin H) as ligand, and the globular protein avidin that is present in egg whites as a receptor. Avidin consists of four identical subunits, yielding four binding pockets that specifically recognize and bind to biotin. The dissociation constant is of the order of 1015 M and the affinity bond, though not covalent, is found to be extremely stable, resisting harsh chemical and physical (e.g., elevated temperature) conditions.

6.5 Applications of SERS Based on LSPR

Surface-enhanced Raman scattering (SERS) has a variety of applications including rapid DNA sequencing, pathogen detection, trace detection, chemical reaction, and food analysis [138]. We will provide some examples to demonstrate SERS applications in more detail.

6.5.1 Trace Detection of Biomaterials Based on SERS

In the SERS-based biosensing of biomaterials, it is important to get a biocompatible substrate [137]. Vanadates, important biocompatible materials, have wide applications in biology, and could be rapidly associated with transferrin (Tf) proteins. Mingwang Shao and coworkers [138] reported that silver vanadate nanoribbons, a biocompatible substrate, can identify human serum transferrin and human serum apotransferrin at the concentration of 10 μM by SERS.

These uniform and high-purity $AgVO_3$ nanoribbons (Figure 6.15) were synthesized via a facile hydrothermal approach. They showed an interesting SERS effect with sufficient reproducibility and stability to monitor the conversion of apoTf and Tf in turn (Figure 6.16).

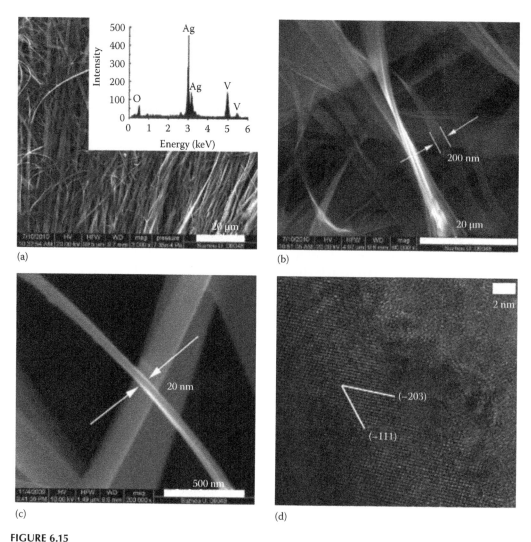

(a)

(b)

(c)

(d)

FIGURE 6.15

SEM images of $AgVO_3$ nanoribbons (a) in lower magnification, (b) and (c) in higher magnification. Inset is the EDS spectrum of $AgVO_3$; (d) HRTEM image of $AgVO_3$ nanoribbons. (From Zhou, Q. et al., *Appl. Phys. Lett.*, 98, 193110, 2011.)

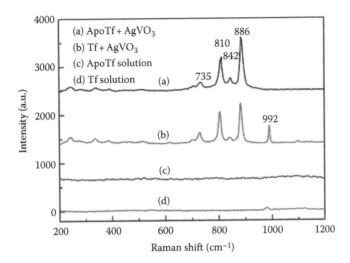

FIGURE 6.16
Raman spectra of (a) apoTf/AgVO$_3$, (b) Tf/AgVO$_3$, (c) 10 μM apoTf, and (d) 10 μM Tf. (From Zhou, Q. et al., *Appl. Phys. Lett.*, 98, 193110, 2011.)

The low-cost and low-interference monitoring might be valuable in the classification and detection of biological materials.

They also reported that a new kind of silver NPs (Figure 6.17) can be prepared by the mechanochemical reaction of copper foil and beta-silver vanadate nanoribbons. This silver NP SERS substrate was successfully employed to detect the dopamine down to 0.1 nM in a single mouse brain cell as shown in Figure 6.18. This ultrasensitive substrate might be used as an *in situ* monitor in biomedical fields.

6.5.2 Coupling LSPR with SERS

For a particular Raman band, Van Duyne and his team found that the optimal condition is achieved when the LSPR λ_{max} equals the excitation wavelength (in absolute wavenumbers) minus one-half the Stokes shift of the Raman scattering band [30]. Furthermore, the LSPR can be easily tuned by changing the size and shape of NPs. Therefore, LSPR nanobiosensors become ideal candidates for a complementary molecular identification platform to SERS [17] so that the Raman fingerprint could be used to identify unknown molecules that cannot be achieved by the biological recognition elements of LSPR nanobiosensors. The team demonstrated the complementary nature of LSPR spectral-shift assays and SERS molecular identification with the antidinitrophenyl immunoassay system [140]. The binding of the antidinitrophenyl ligand to 2,4-dinitrobenzoic acid was quantified by measuring the LSPR shift while SERS was used to verify the identity of the adsorbed molecules.

Notably, G. L. Liu and his coworker present a unique solid surface of high-aspect-ratio silver-coated silicon nanocone arrays that allows a highly uniform molecular deposition and thus subsequent uniform optical imaging and spectroscopic molecular detection without any surface chemistry modification [141] (Figure 6.19). Both dye molecules and unlabeled oligopeptides are printed on the metallic nanocone photonic substrate surface as circular spot arrays. In comparison with the printed results on ordinary glass slides

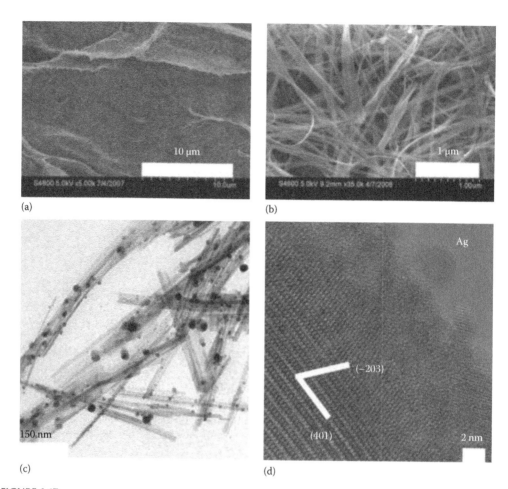

FIGURE 6.17
The SEM image of SVNs in (a) low magnification and (b) high magnification; (c) TEM and (d) HRTEM images of the resultant of silver vanadate reacted with copper foil. (From Cheng, L. et al., *Sci. Adv. Mater.*, 2(3), 386, 2010.)

and silver-coated glass slides, not only high printing density but uniform molecular distribution in every deposited spot is achieved. The high uniformity and repeatability of molecular depositions on the "coffee stain"–free nanocone surface is confirmed by laser scanning fluorescence imaging and SERS imaging experiments (Figure 6.20). The physical mechanism for the uniform molecular deposition is attributed to the superhydrophobicity and localized pinned liquid–solid–air interface on the silver-coated silicon nanocone surface. The unique surface properties of the presented nanocone surface enabled high-density, high-uniformity probe spotting beneficial for genomic and proteomic microarrays and surface molecular imaging.

6.5.3 Single-Molecule SERS Using Nanowire Functionalized by Nanoparticles of Metal or Metallic Compound

Mingwang Shao and coworkers reported simple approaches to prepare ultrasensitive, reproducible, and stable SERS substrates, such as silicon nanowires (SiNWs) modified with

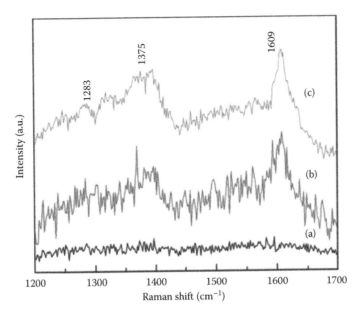

FIGURE 6.18
SERS spectra of dopamine using silver modified vanadates as substrate at different concentrations: (a) 0.01 nM; (b) 0.1 nM and (c) 1 nM. (From Cheng, L. et al., *Sci. Adv. Mater.*, 2(3), 386, 2010.)

NPs of metals [142,143], or metallic compounds [144]. The SERS enhancement is mostly due to two kinds of effects: an EM effect associated with large local fields due to resonances occurring in the nanostructure on the metal surface, and a chemical effect involving a scattering process associated with the chemical interaction between the molecule and the metal surface.

For the SERS substrates based on SiNW, they report two kinds of silicon nanowires used for the basic materials. One kind of SiNWs was prepared by oxide-assisted growth via the thermal evaporation of the SiO powder and the sequential removal of the oxide with HF (Figure 6.21). The resulting SiNWs were then used to reduce silver ions to form a highly decorated Ag-embedded surface or were directly modified with AgI NPs. Such modified SiNW substrates demonstrated ultrahigh SERS sensitivity [142] (Figure 6.22).

NPThey reported the other kind of SiNW arrays produced through the chemical etching of the n-Si(100) wafer. The resulting SiNWs were used to grow AgNPs directly through the galvanic redox reaction without any organic contamination (Figure 6.23) [143]. Their extinction spectrum revealed strong surface plasmon absorption in a broad range (from 200 to 1000 nm) indicating that the surface plasmon induced by the incident laser could resonate with incident and scattering photons in a broad wavelength region. The substrate exhibited a reproducible SERS signal down to a few percent. The observed substrate SERS enhancement factor was 10^8–10^{10}, which is several orders of magnitude higher than that of common substrates. The amounts of Sudan dye down to 10^{-17} mol of molecules on the substrate could still display molecular-specific Raman bands (Figure 6.24). Moreover, the easy fabrications of those functionalized SiNW good SERS substrates make it possible to be widely employed in nanodevices and biodetection.

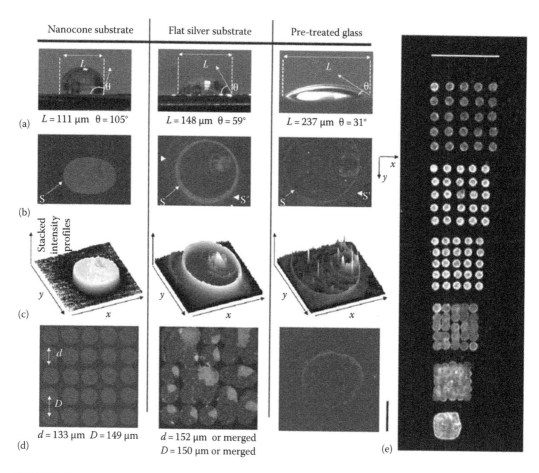

FIGURE 6.19

Liquid droplets and molecule depositions on various substrate surfaces. (a) Side view images of liquid droplets dispensed on the silver-coated nanocone substrate, flat silver surface, and pre-treated glass slide, respectively from left to right. The diameter *(D)* and contact angles (θ) of the liquid droplets are annotated. The water droplet contains 100 μM Rhodamine 6G (R6G) molecules. (b) Laser scanning fluorescence images of R6G molecules deposited on the earlier three kinds of substrate surfaces after the droplets dried. The boundaries of the main molecule deposition patterns are denoted by S and those of the peripheral deposition are denoted by S'. (c) A three-dimensional (3D) image representation to evaluate optical homogeneity of molecule deposition. Intensity profiles from two-dimensional (2D) images in (b) are converted to a 3D surface plot in which the height represents the fluorescence intensity or molecule density. (d) Fluorescence images of a 5 × 5 array of molecule deposition spots. Dimensions of deposition (spot center-to-center *(D)* and diameter *(d)*) are measured and annotated. The scale bar on the right represents 200 μm. (e) Array printing images on the silver-coated nanocone substrate with the spacing between spots of 200, 150, 100, and 50 μm from top to bottom. The scale bar on the top represents 1 mm distance. (From Coppe, J.P. et al., *Nanotechnology*, 22(24), 245710, 2011.)

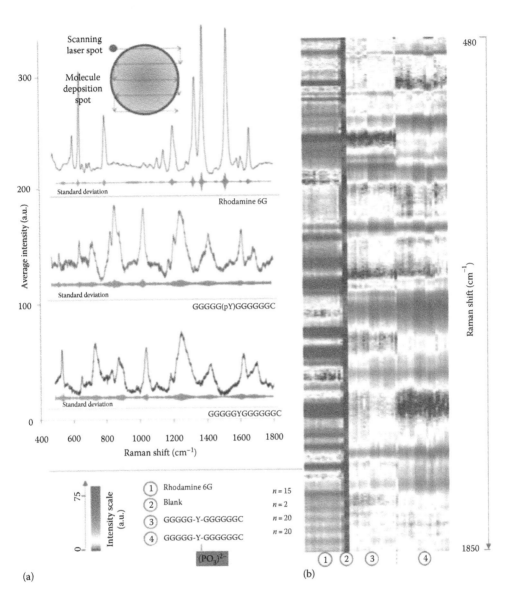

FIGURE 6.20
Uniformity testing of low concentration molecule deposition by SERS. (a) Averaged spectra and standard deviations of 2D laser scanning SERS spectroscopy measurements over the deposition spots of 100 nM R6G molecules, peptides, and phosphor-peptides. The averaged spectra are the arithmetic average of all the SERS spectra acquired from each individual deposition spot. (b) Gray scale graphical representation of multiple scanning SERS spectra from the molecule deposition spots. Raw SERS spectra obtained from either R6G (spectra number $n = 15$), peptides ($n = 20$), phosphor-peptides ($n = 20$), or blank area are shown. Normalized (intensity = 0–100) SERS spectral intensities are converted using a gray scale ranging from dark gray (intensity = 0) to white (intensity = 10) to light gray (intensity > 75), and linearly represented (from 480 to 1850 cm^{-1}). Gray-scaling of spectra allows side-by-side representation of all datasets for rapid visual assertion of similarities and/or differences to assess the molecule deposition uniformity. (From Coppe, J.P. et al., *Nanotechnology*, 22(24), 245710, 2011.)

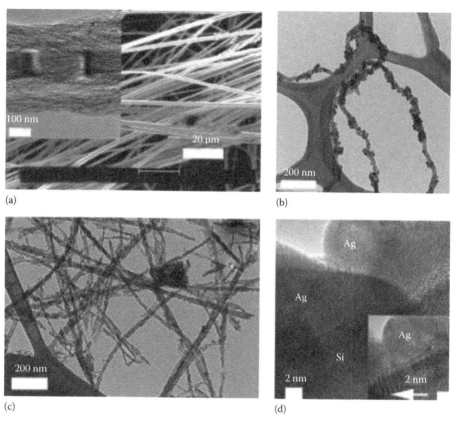

(a)

(b)

(c)

(d)

FIGURE 6.21
(a) SEM and TEM (inset) images of as-prepared SiNWs; (b) TEM image of Ag-modified SiNWs; (c) TEM image of HF-etched SiNWs showing many nanopores on the surface; and (d) HRTEM image of Ag-modified SiNW, the Moiré fringes marked with arrow, (inset) indicating that Ag NPs are embedded on the surface. (From Shao, M.W. et al., *Appl. Phys. Lett.*, 93, 233118, 2008.)

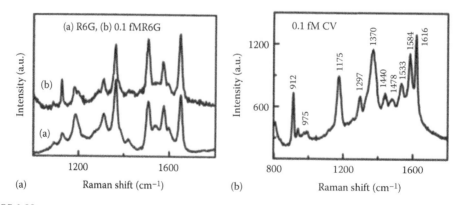

(a)

(b)

FIGURE 6.22
Raman spectra obtained from Ag-modified SiNWs coated with 25 µm of (a) 10^{-16} M R6G solution, (b) 10^{-16} M crystal violet solution, (From Shao, M.W. et al., *Appl. Phys. Lett.*, 93, 233118, 2008.)

(continued)

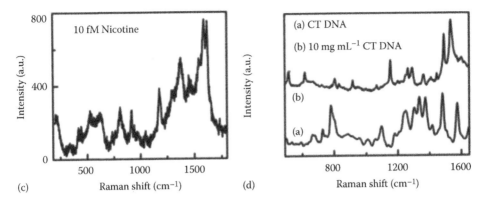

FIGURE 6.22 (continued)
Raman spectra obtained from Ag-modified SiNWs coated with 25 μm of (c) 10^{-14} M nicotine solution, and (d) 10^{-8} mg mL^{-1} CT DNA solution in water. (Note: In d), (a) and (b) are the Raman spectra collected from R6G powder and solid CT DNA, respectively. (From Shao, M.W. et al., *Appl. Phys. Lett.*, 93, 233118, 2008.)

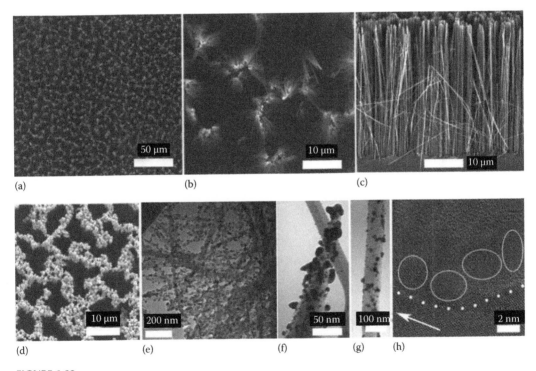

FIGURE 6.23
Characterization of SERS substrate. Top view and cross section view SEM images of SiNWs array are shown in (a–c). SEM image of SiNWs coated with AgNPs are shown in (d). TEM image of large amount of AgNPs-SiNWs is shown in (e). The tip part of a AgNPs-SiNW is shown in (f); the representative body part of a AgNPs-SiNW is shown in (g). HRTEM image of a AgNPs-SiNW is shown in (h). The dot curve indicates the interface between SiNW and AgNPs, and the loops emphasize the adjoining AgNPs. (From Zhang, M.L. et al., *J. Phys. Chem. C*, 114(5), 1969, 2010.)

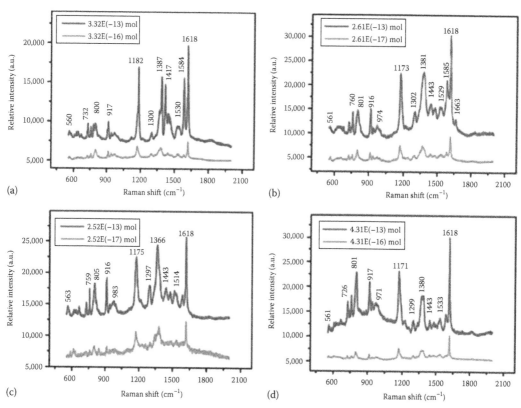

FIGURE 6.24

Raman spectra of Sudan dyes with different amounts on the SERS substrate. The darker curves show Raman spectra from about 10^{-13} mol Sudan dye molecules, and the lighter curves show Raman spectra from about 10^{-16} or 10^{-17} mol Sudan dye molecules. (a) SDII, (b) SDIII, (c) SDIV, (d) SDG. (From Zhang, M.L. et al., *J. Phys. Chem. C*, 114(5), 1969, 2010.)

They also grew AgI NPs on the surface of the SiNWs. First, SiNWs were prepared and then modified with Ag NPs; the AgI NPs were then synthesized through the reaction between Ag NPs and I_2 (Figure 6.25). The SERS of the AgI-modified SiNW substrate was also observed due to the surface plasmon resonance of AgX (X = Cl, Br, and I) (Figure 6.26). Though the SERS of the AgI-modified SiNWs was not as sensitive as that of Ag NP-modified SiNWs as reported previously, the temperature-dependent ionic conductivity, combined with the SERS, will find wide application in nanodevices and biological detection.

6.6 Executive Summary and Future Perspective

In the last decades, the Raman methods and instrumentation have been developed rapidly, which offer sophisticated tools well-suited for particular needs (e.g., high selectivity) in biospectroscopy. Typical problems in Raman biospectroscopy are low scattering cross-section and fluorescent interference. To overcome these drawbacks, the new techniques

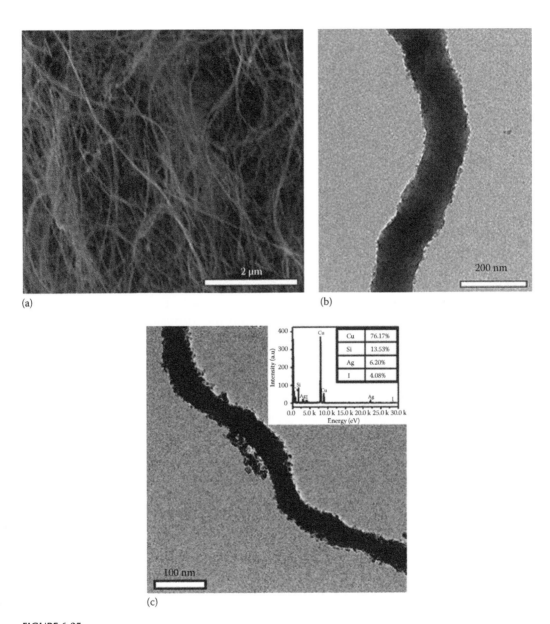

FIGURE 6.25

(a) SEM image of the as-prepared SiNWs; and (b) TEM image of the Ag/SiNW nanostructure. (c) TEM image of the AgI/SiNW nanostructure, showing that the AgI NPs were attached on the surface of the SiNWs. The inset is the EDS of the AgI/SiNW nanostructure, revealing that the products are composed of Ag, I, and Si elements. (From Cheng, L. et al., *CrystEngComm*, 14, 601, 2012.)

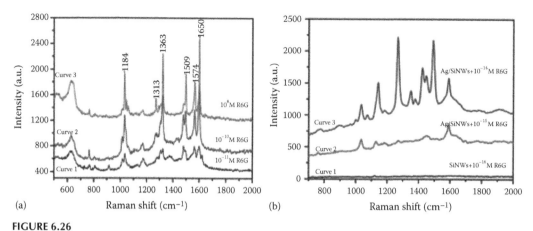

FIGURE 6.26
(a) SERS spectra of R6G CH_3OH solution using AgI/SiNW nanostructure as substrate at different concentrations: (curve 1) 10^{-11} M, (curve 2) 10^{-10} M, and (curve 3) 10^{-9} M. (b) SERS spectra of 10^{-11} M R6G CH_3OH solution using different substrates: (curve 1) SiNWs, (curve 2) AgI/SiNWs, and (curve 3) Ag NPs/SiNWs. (From Cheng, L. et al., *CrystEngComm*, 14, 601, 2012.)

in Raman spectroscopy were developed, for example, plasmonic signal enhancement and fluorescence quenching techniques. Furthermore, each biological system requires a careful selection of the most appropriate experimental setup, the adequate excitation source, and particular sample preparation to obtain structural information from biological molecules at the extremely low concentration. Biosensors based on SERS devices are being developed and viewed as one key breakthrough area to address these major challenges in biosensing research and personalized medicine: real-time and parallelized biomedical analysis with high selectivity and sensitivity.

Surface plasmons include nonpropagating localized surface plasmon–polaritons (LSPs) and propagating surface plasmon–polaritons (SPPs). Both of them are essential for biosensors based on SERS devices. Current fabrication methods for SERS substrates typically rely on bottom-up nanostructure synthesis, top-down nanostructure fabrication, or combinations of both processes to achieve the control of the size, shape, composition, and configuration of plasmonic nanostructures. Surface functionalization techniques of nanomaterials by biological recognition elements have recently been developed to incorporate the highly selective catalytic and recognition properties of biomaterials into biosensors based on SERS devices. Biosensors based on SERS devices synergize three core techniques: (1) plasmonics that manipulates light at nanoscale dielectric–metal interfaces for high sensitivity due to the resulting surface-enhanced light; (2) nanofabrication and controlled synthesis of nanomaterials containing metals (e.g., Ag and Au) for high tunability, and (3) bioconjugate techniques for high selectivity.

In conclusion, from a speculative viewpoint, the field will evolve in 5–10 years' time mainly in the following directions: (1) Biosensors based on SERS with much higher sensitivity than conventional biosensors; (2) biosensors based on the SERS device made by advanced nanomanufacturing methods to improve stability and reproducibility; (3) beyond the molecular level, advances in complex systems and detection background, such as intracellular and tissue-level detection with sensor devices based on SERS; (4) functional genomic and proteomic sensing by SERS devices; (5) the combination of current SERS nanomaterials with other nanomaterials such as quantum dots and metamaterials to improve tunability and sensitivity and enable new synergized advantages; (6) the combination of different sensing techniques such as SERS and LSPR; (7) overcome the challenges in using SERS sensing as a laboratory tool for molecular biology; and (8) overcome the challenges in using SERS sensing as a medical diagnostic and imaging tool.

Acknowledgments

The work was funded by a generous gift from Agilent Foundation, NIEHS grant 1RC2ES018812-01, National Natural Science Foundation of China Grant NSFC-30828010, DOD grant W81XWH-07-1-0663_BC061995, U.S. DOE contract DE-AC03-76SF00098, DARPA, and MEMS fundamental science program.

References

1. Spiller DG, Wood CD, Rand DA, and White MRH: Measurement of single-cell dynamics. *Nature* 465(7299), 736–745 (2010).
2. Anker JN, Hall WP, Lyandres O, Shah NC, Zhao J, and Van Duyne RP: Biosensing with plasmonic nanosensors. *Nat. Mater.* 7(6), 442–453 (2008).
3. Lal S, Link S, and Halas NJ: Nano-optics from sensing to waveguiding. *Nat. Photonics* 1(11), 641–648 (2007).
4. Nguyen T, Hilton JP, and Lin Q: Emerging applications of aptamers to micro-and nanoscale biosensing. *Microfluid. Nanofluid.* 6(3), 347–362 (2009).
5. O'sullivan CK: Aptasensors—The future of biosensing. *Anal. Bioanal. Chem.* 372(1), 44–48 (2002).
6. Ge Y and Turner APF: Too large to fit? Recent developments in macromolecular imprinting. *Trends Biotechnol.* 26(4), 218–224 (2008).
7. Lu XM, Rycenga M, Skrabalak SE, Wiley B, and Xia YN: Chemical synthesis of novel plasmonic NPs. *Annu. Rev. Phys. Chem.* 60, 167–192 (2009).
8. Stewart ME, Anderton CR, Thompson LB et al.: Nanostructured plasmonic sensors. *Chem. Rev.* 108(2), 494–521 (2008).
9. Xia YN and Halas NJ: Shape-controlled synthesis and surface plasmonic properties of metallic nanostructures. *MRS Bull.* 30(5), 338–344 (2005).
10. Zhao J, Pinchuk AO, Mcmahon JM et al.: Methods for describing the electromagnetic properties of silver and gold NPs. *Acc. Chem. Res.* 41(12), 1710–1720 (2008).
11. Pitarke JM, Silkin VM, Chulkov EV, and Echenique PM: Theory of surface plasmons and surface-plasmon polaritons. *Rep. Prog. Phys.* 70(1), 1–87 (2007).
12. Prodan E, Radloff C, Halas NJ, and Nordlander P: A hybridization model for the plasmon response of complex nanostructures. *Science* 302(5644), 419–422 (2003).
13. Thanh NTK and Green LW: Functionalisation of NPs for biomedical applications. *Nano Today* 5(3), 213–230 (2010).
14. Genevieve M, Vieu C, Carles R et al.: Biofunctionalization of gold NPs and their spectral properties. *Microelectron. Eng.* 84(5–8), 1710–1713 (2007).
15. Wang CG, Ma ZF, Wang TT, and Su ZM: Synthesis, assembly, and biofunctionalization of silica-coated gold nanorods for colorimetric biosensing. *Adv. Funct. Mater.* 16(13), 1673–1678 (2006).

16. Sepulveda B, Angelome PC, Lechuga LM, and Liz-Marzan LM: LSPR-based nanobiosensors. *Nano Today* 4(3), 244–251 (2009).
17. Willets KA and Van Duyne RP: Localized surface plasmon resonance spectroscopy and sensing. *Annu. Rev. Phys. Chem.* 58, 267–297 (2007).
18. Wachsmann-Hogiu S, Weeks T, and Huser T: Chemical analysis in vivo and in vitro by Raman spectroscopy-from single cells to humans. *Curr. Opin. Biotechnol.* 20(1), 63–73 (2009).
19. Stiles PL, Dieringer JA, Shah NC, and Van Duyne RR: Surface-enhanced Raman spectroscopy. *Annu. Rev. Anal. Chem.* 1, 601–626 (2008).
20. Choi YH, Kang T, and Lee LP: Plasmon resonance energy transfer (PRET)-based molecular imaging of cytochrome c in living cells. *Nano Lett.* 9(1), 85–90 (2009).
21. Choi Y, Park Y, Kang T, and Lee LP: Selective and sensitive detection of metal ions by plasmonic resonance energy transfer-based nanospectroscopy. *Nat. Nanotechnol.* 4(11), 742–746 (2009).
22. Liu GL, Long YT, Choi Y, Kang T, and Lee LP: Quantized plasmon quenching dips nanospectroscopy via plasmon resonance energy transfer. *Nat. Methods* 4(12), 1015–1017 (2007).
23. Kim JW, Galanzha EI, Shashkov EV, Moon HM, and Zharov VP: Golden carbon nanotubes as multimodal photoacoustic and photothermal high-contrast molecular agents. *Nat. Nanotechnol.* 4(10), 688–694 (2009).
24. Fleischmann M, Hendra PJ, and Mcquilla AJ: Raman spectra of pyridine adsorbed at a silver electrode. *Chem. Phys. Lett.* 26, 163–166 (1974).
25. Hering K, Cialla D, Ackermann K, Dörfer T, Möller R, Rösch P, and Popp J: SERS: A versatile tool in chemical and biochemical diagnostics. *Anal. Bioanal. Chem.* 390, 113–124 (2008).
26. Ra man CVKKS: A new type of secondary radiation, *Nature* 121, 501 (1928).
27. Schrader B and Bougeard D: *Infrared and Raman Spectroscopy: Methods and Applications.* Wiley-VCH: Weinheim, Germany (1995).
28. Fleischmann M, Hendra PJ, and Mcquillan AJ: Raman spectra from electrode surfaces. *J. Chem. Soc. Chem. Commun.* 3, 80–81 (1973).
29. Fleischmann M and Hill IR: Raman spectroscopy. In *Comprehensive Treatise of Electrochemistry*; White RE, Bockris JO'M., Conway BE, Yeager E, Eds. Plenum Press: New York, Vol. 8, p. 373 (1984).
30. McFarland AD, Young MA, Dieringer JA, and Van Duyne RP: Wavelength-scanned surface-enhanced Raman excitation spectroscopy. *J. Phys. Chem. B* 109, 11279–11285 (2005).
31. Zou S and Schatz GC: Silver NP array structures that produce giant enhancements in electromagnetic fields. *Chem. Phys. Lett.* 403, 62–67 (2005).
32. Zeman EJ and Schatz GC: An accurate electromagnetic theory study of surface enhancement factors for silver, gold, copper, lithium, sodium, aluminum, gallium, indium, zinc, and cadmium. *J. Phys. Chem.* 91, 634–643 (1987).
33. Moskovits M: Surface roughness and the enhanced intensity of Raman scattering by molecules adsorbed on metals. *J. Chem. Phys.* 69, 4159–4161 (1978).
34. Haynes CL and Van Duyne RP: Nanosphere lithography: A versatile nanofabrication tool for studies of size-dependent NP optics. *J. Phys. Chem. B* 105, 5599–5611 (2001).
35. Sherry LJ, Chang SH, Schatz GC, Van Duyne RP, Wiley BJ, and Xia Y: Localized surface plasmon resonance spectroscopy of single silver nanocubes. *Nano Lett.* 5, 2034–2038 (2005).
36. Sylvia JM, Janni JA, Klein JD, and Spencer KM: Surface-enhanced Raman detection of 1,4-dinitrotoluene impurity vapor as a marker to locate landmines. *Anal. Chem.* 72(23), 5834 (2000).
37. Kneipp K, Moskovits M, and Kneipp H: *Surface-Enhanced Raman Scattering: Physics and Applications.* Springer: Berlin/Germany (2006).
38. Jeanmarie DL and Van Duyne RP: Surface Raman spectroelectrochemistry, part 1: heterocyclic, aromatic, and aliphatic amines adsorbed on the anodized silver electrode. *J. Electroanal. Chem.* 84, 1–201 (1977).
39. Albrecht MG and Creighton JA: Anomalously intense Raman spectra of pyridine at a silver electrode. *J. Am. Chem. Soc.* 99, 5215–5217 (1977).

40. Otto A, Mrozek I, Grabhorn H, and Akemann W: Surface-enhanced Raman scattering. *J. Phys. Condens. Matter.* 4, 1143–1212 (1992).

41. Gersten J and Nitzan A: Electromagnetic theory of enhanced Raman scattering by molecules adsorbed on rough surfaces. *J. Chem. Phys.* 73(7), 3023–3037 (1980).

42. Metiu H and Das P: The electromagnetic theory of surface enhanced spectroscopy. *Annu. Rev. Phys. Chem.* 35, 507–536 (1984).

43. Schatz GC: Theoretical studies of surface enhanced Raman scattering. *Acc. Chem. Res.* 17, 370–376 (1984).

44. Wokaun A: Surface enhancement of optical fields: Mechanism and applications. *Mol. Phys.* 56, 1–33 (1985).

45. Wokaun A: Surface-enhanced electromagnetic processes. *Solid State Phys.* 38, 223–294 (1984).

46. Gartia MR, Bond TC, and Liu GL: Metal-molecule Schottky junction effects in surface enhanced Raman scattering. *J. Phys. Chem. A.* 115(3), 318–328 (2011).

47. Jin J: The Finite Element Method in Electromagnetics. Wiley: New York (2002).

48. Webb KJ and Li J: Waveguide cavity surface-enhanced Raman scattering. *Phys. Rev. B* 73(7), 073404 (2006).

49. Lee SE and Lee LP: Biomolecular plasmonics for quantitative biology and nanomedicine. *Curr. Opin. Biotechnol.* 21(4), 489–497 (2010).

50. Liu GL: Nanoplasmonic-particle-enhanced optical molecular sensing. *IEEE J. Sel. Top. Quant.* 16(3), 662–671 (2010).

51. Burda C, Chen X, Narayanan R, and El-Sayed MA: Chemistry and properties of nanocrystals of different shapes. *Chem. Rev.* 105(4), 1025 (2005).

52. Xia Y, Xiong Y, Lim B, and Skrabalak SE: Shape-controlled synthesis of metal nanocrystals: Simple chemistry meets complex physics. *Angew. Chem. Int. Ed.* 48(1), 60–103 (2009).

53. Grabar KC, Freeman RG, Hommer MB, and Natan MJ: Preparation and characterization of Au colloid monolayers. *Anal. Chem.* 67(4), 735–743 (1995).

54. Wiley B, Herricks T, Sun YG, and Xia YN: Polyol synthesis of silver NPs: Use of chloride and oxygen to promote the formation of single-crystal, truncated cubes and tetrahedrons. *Nano Lett.* 4(9), 1733–1739 (2004).

55. Sun Y, Mayers B, and Xia Y: Metal nanostructures with hollow interiors. *Adv. Mater.* 15(7–8), 641–646 (2003).

56. Tao AR, Habas S, and Yang P: Shape control of colloidal metal nanocrystals. *Small* 4(3), 310–325 (2008).

57. Wiley BJ, Im SH, Li ZY, Mclellan J, Siekkinen A, and Xia YA: Maneuvering the surface plasmon resonance of silver nanostructures through shape-controlled synthesis. *J. Phys. Chem. B* 110(32), 15666–15675 (2006).

58. Washio I, Xiong YJ, Yin YD, and Xia YN: Reduction by the end groups of poly(vinyl pyrrolidone): A new and versatile route to the kinetically controlled synthesis of Ag triangular nanoplates. *Adv. Mater.* 18(13), 1745–1749 (2006).

59. Jackson JB and Halas NJ: Silver nanoshells: Variations in morphologies and optical properties. *J. Phys. Chem. B* 105(14), 2743–2746 (2001).

60. Halas N: Playing with plasmons: Tuning the optical resonant properties of metallic nanoshells. *MRS Bull.* 30, 362–367 (2005).

61. Svoboda K and Block SM: Biological applications of optical forces. *Annu. Rev. Biophys. Biomol. Struct.* 23(1), 247–285 (1994).

62. Wang H, Brandl DW, Le F, Nordlander P, and Halas NJ: Nanorice: A hybrid plasmonic nanostructure. *Nano Lett.* 6(4), 827–832 (2006).

63. Grzelczak M, Perez-Juste J, Mulvaney P, and Liz-Marzan LM: Shape control in gold NP synthesis. *Chem. Soc. Rev.* 37(9), 1783–1791 (2008).

64. Barbosa S, Agrawal A, Rodriguez-Lorenzo L et al.: Tuning size and sensing properties in colloidal gold nanostars. *Langmuir* 26(18), 14943–14950 (2010).

65. Nikoobakht B and El-Sayed MA: Preparation and growth mechanism of gold nanorods (NRs) using seed-mediated growth method. *Chem. Mater.* 15(10), 1957–1962 (2003).

66. Lin Y, Zou Y, Mo Y, Guo J, and Lindquist RG: E-Beam patterned gold nanodot arrays on optical fiber tips for localized surface plasmon resonance biochemical sensing. *Sensors-Basel* 10(10), 9397–9406 (2010).

67. Fu Y and Bryan N: Investigation of physical properties of quartz after focused ion beam bombardment. *Appl. Phys. B* 80(4), 581–585 (2005).

68. Hutter E and Fendler JH: Exploitation of localized surface plasmon resonance. *Adv. Mater.* 16(19), 1685–1706 (2004).

69. David C, Guillot N, Shen H, Toury T, and De La Chapelle ML: SERS detection of biomolecules using lithographed NPs towards a reproducible SERS biosensor. *Nanotechnology* 21(47), 475501 (2010).

70. Tripp RA, Dluhy RA, and Zhao YP: Novel nanostructures for SERS biosensing. *Nano Today* 3(3–4), 31–37 (2008).

71. De Jesus MA, Giesfeldt KS, Oran JM, Abu-Hatab NA, Lavrik NV, and Sepaniak MJ: Nanofabrication of densely packed metal-polymer arrays for surface-enhanced Raman spectrometry. *Appl. Spectrosc.* 59(12), 1501–1508 (2005).

72. Camden JP, Dieringer JA, Zhao J, and Van Duyne RP: Controlled plasmonic nanostructures for surface-enhanced spectroscopy and sensing. *Acc. Chem. Res.* 41(12), 1653–1661 (2008).

73. Haynes CL and Van Duyne RP: Plasmon-sampled surface-enhanced Raman excitation spectroscopy, Ä⁺. *J. Phys. Chem. B* 107(30), 7426–7433 (2003).

74. Haynes CL, Mcfarland AD, Smith MT, Hulteen JC, and Van Duyne RP: Angle-resolved nanosphere lithography: Manipulation of NP size, shape, and interparticle spacing. *J. Phys. Chem. B* 106(8), 1898–1902 (2002).

75. Rybczynski J, Ebels U, and Giersig M: Large-scale, 2D arrays of magnetic NPs. *Colloids Surf. Physicochem. Eng. Asp.* 219(1–3), 1–6 (2003).

76. Du Y, Shi L, He T, Sun X, and Mo Y: SERS enhancement dependence on the diameter and aspect ratio of silver-nanowire array fabricated by anodic aluminium oxide template. *Appl. Surf. Sci.* 255(5), 1901–1905 (2008).

77. Ruan C, Eres G, Wang W, Zhang Z, and Gu B: Controlled fabrication of nanopillar arrays as active substrates for surface-enhanced Raman spectroscopy. *Langmuir* 23(10), 5757–5760 (2007).

78. Jung D, Lee YM, Lee Y, Kim NH, Kim K, and Lee J-K: Facile fabrication of large area nanostructures for efficient surface-enhanced Raman scattering. *J. Mater. Chem.* 16(30), 3145–3149 (2006).

79. Driskell JD, Shanmukh S, Liu Y et al.: The use of aligned silver nanorod arrays prepared by oblique angle deposition as surface enhanced Raman scattering substrates. *J. Phys. Chem. C* 112(4), 895–901 (2008).

80. Chaney SB, Shanmukh S, Dluhy RA, and Zhao YP: Aligned silver nanorod arrays produce high sensitivity surface-enhanced Raman spectroscopy substrates. *Appl. Phys. Lett.* 87(3), 031908-031903 (2005).

81. Zhou Q, Li Z, Yang Y, and Zhang Z: Arrays of aligned, single crystalline silver nanorods for trace amount detection. *J. Phys. D: Appl. Phys.* 41(15), 152007 (2008).

82. Dickey MD, Weiss EA, Smythe EJ, Chiechi RC, Capasso F, and Whitesides GM: Fabrication of arrays of metal and metal oxide nanotubes by shadow evaporation. *ACS Nano* 2(4), 800–808 (2008).

83. Madou MJ: *Fundamentals of microfabrication: The science of miniaturization.* (2nd edn.). CRC Press: Boca Raton, FL. (2002).

84. Li K, Clime L, Tay L, Cui B, Geissler M, and Veres T: Multiple surface plasmon resonances and near-infrared field enhancement of gold nanowells. *Anal. Chem.* 80(13), 4945–4950 (2008).

85. Clark AW and Cooper JM: Nanogap ring antennae as plasmonically coupled SERRS substrates. *Small* 7(1), 119–125 (2011).

86. Chou SY, Krauss PR, and Renstrom PJ: Imprint of sub-25 nm vias and trenches in polymers. *Appl. Phys. Lett.* 67(21), 3114–3116 (1995).

87. Chou SY, Krauss PR, and Renstrom PJ: Nanoimprint lithography. *J. Vac. Sci. Technol. B* 14(6), 4129–4133 (1996).

88. Lucas BD, Kim J-S, Chin C, and Guo LJ: Nanoimprint lithography based approach for the fabrication of large-area, uniformly oriented plasmonic arrays. *Adv. Mater.* 20(6), 1129–1134 (2008).

89. Alvarez-Puebla R, Cui B, Bravo-Vasquez J-P, Veres T, and Fenniri H: Nanoimprinted SERS-active substrates with tunable surface plasmon resonances. *J. Phys. Chem. C* 111(18), 6720–6723 (2007).

90. Lee S-W, Lee K-S, Ahn J, Lee J-J, Kim M-G, and Shin Y-B: Highly sensitive biosensing using arrays of plasmonic Au nanodisks realized by nanoimprint lithography. *ACS Nano* 5(2), 897–904 (2011).

91. Guo LJ: Nanoimprint lithography: Methods and material requirements. *Adv. Mater.* 19(4), 495–513 (2007).

92. Masuda H and Fukuda K: Ordered metal nanohole arrays made by a two-step replication of honeycomb structures of anodic alumina. *Science* 268(5216), 1466–1468 (1995).

93. Lei Y, Yang S, Wu M, and Wilde G: Surface patterning using templates: Concept, properties and device applications. *Chem. Soc. Rev.* 40(3), 1247–1258 (2011).

94. Broglin BL, Andreu A, Dhussa N et al.: Investigation of the effects of the local environment on the surface-enhanced Raman spectra of striped gold/silver nanorod arrays. *Langmuir* 23(8), 4563–4568 (2007).

95. Bok H-M, Shuford KL, Kim S, Kim SK, and Park S: Multiple surface plasmon modes for a colloidal solution of nanoporous gold nanorods and their comparison to smooth gold nanorods. *Nano Lett.* 8(8), 2265–2270 (2008).

96. Choi D, Choi Y, Hong S, Kang T, and Lee LP: Self-organized hexagonal-nanopore SERS array. *Small* 6(16), 1741–1744 (2010).

97. Qin Y, Pan A, Liu L, Moutanabbir O, Yang RB, and Knez M: Atomic layer deposition assisted template approach for electrochemical synthesis of Au crescent-shaped half-nanotubes. *ACS Nano* 5(2), 788–794 (2011).

98. Bang J, Jeong U, Ryu DY, Russell TP, and Hawker CJ: Block copolymer nanolithography: Translation of molecular level control to nanoscale patterns. *Adv. Mater.* 21(47), 4769–4792 (2009).

99. Kim SO, Solak HH, Stoykovich MP, Ferrier NJ, De Pablo JJ, and Nealey PF: Epitaxial self-assembly of block copolymers on lithographically defined nanopatterned substrates. *Nature* 424(6947), 411–414 (2003).

100. Cheng JY, Mayes AM, and Ross CA: Nanostructure engineering by templated self-assembly of block copolymers. *Nat. Mater.* 3(11), 823–828 (2004).

101. Deckman HW and Dunsmuir JH: Natural lithography. *Appl. Phys. Lett.* 41(4), 377–379 (1982).

102. Malinsky MD, Kelly KL, Schatz GC, and Van Duyne RP: Nanosphere lithography: Effect of substrate on the localized surface plasmon resonance spectrum of silver NPs. *J. Phys. Chem. B* 105(12), 2343–2350 (2001).

103. Hulteen JC, Treichel DA, Smith MT, Duval ML, Jensen TR, and Van Duyne RP: Nanosphere lithography: Size-tunable silver NP and surface cluster arrays. *J. Phys. Chem. B* 103(19), 3854–3863 (1999).

104. Kuo C-W, Shiu J-Y, Chien F-C, Tsai S-M, Chueh D-Y, and Chen P: Polymeric nanopillar arrays for cell traction force measurements. *Electrophoresis* 31, 3152–3158 (2010).

105. Masson J-F, Murray-Methot M-P, and Live LS: Nanohole arrays in chemical analysis: Manufacturing methods and applications. *Analyst* 135, 1483–1489 (2010).

106. Peng K, Zhang M, Lu A, Wong N-B, Zhang R, and Lee S-T: Ordered silicon nanowire arrays via nanosphere lithography and metal-induced etching. *Appl. Phys. Lett.* 90, 163123 (2007).

107. Xu M, Lu N, Xu H, Qi D, Wang Y, and Chi L: Fabrication of functional silver nanobowl arrays via sphere lithography. *Langmuir* 25(19), 11216–11220 (2009).

108. Aizpurua J, Hanarp P, Sutherland DS, Kall M, Bryant GW, and Garcia De Abajo FJ: Optical properties of gold nanorings. *Phys. Rev. Lett.* 90(5), 057401 (2003).

109. Vossen DLJ, Fific D, Penninkhof J, Van Dillen T, Polman A, and Van Blaaderen A: Combined optical tweezers/ion beam technique to tune colloidal masks for nanolithography. *Nano Lett.* 5(6), 1175–1179 (2005).

110. Jiang P and Mcfarland MJ: Wafer-scale periodic nanohole arrays templated from two-dimensional nonclose-packed colloidal crystals. *J. Am. Chem. Soc.* 127, 3710–3711 (2005).

111. Masson J-F, Gibson KF, and Provencher-Girard A: Surface-enhanced Raman spectroscopy amplification with film over etched nanospheres. *J. Phys. Chem. C* 114(51), 22406–22412 (2010).

112. Haynes CL and Van Duyne RP: Nanosphere lithography: A versatile nanofabrication tool for studies of size-dependent NP optics. *J. Phys. Chem. B* 105(24), 5599–5611 (2001).

113. Burmeister F, Schafle C, Matthes T, Bohmisch M, Boneberg J, and Leiderer P: Colloid monolayers as versatile lithographic masks. *Langmuir* 13(11), 2983–2987 (1997).

114. Hawkeye MM, and Brett MJ: Glancing angle deposition: Fabrication, properties, and applications of micro-and nanostructured thin films. *J. Vac. Sci. Technol. A* 25(5), 1317–1335 (2007).

115. Brett MJ and Hawkeye MM: New materials at a glance. *Science* 319(5867), 1192–1193 (2008).

116. Steele JJ and Brett MJ: Nanostructure engineering in porous columnar thin films: Recent advances. *J. Mater. Sci-Mater. El.* 18(4), 367–379 (2007).

117. Jensen MO and Brett MJ: Periodically structured glancing angle deposition thin films. *IEEE Trans. Nanotechnol.* 4(2), 269–277 (2005).

118. Huang Z, Harris KD, and Brett MJ: Morphology control of nanotube arrays. *Adv. Mater.* 21(29), 2983–2987 (2009).

119. Robbie K, Brett MJ, and Lakhtakia A: Chiral sculptured thin films. *Nature* 384(6610), 616–616 (1996).

120. Kennedy SR, Brett MJ, Toader O, and John S: Fabrication of tetragonal square spiral photonic crystals. *Nano Lett.* 2(1), 59–62 (2002).

121. Fu J, Park B, Siragusa G et al.: An Au/Si hetero-nanorod-based biosensor for Salmonella detection. *Nanotechnology* 19(15), 155502-155501-155507 (2008).

122. Fu J and Zhao Y: Optical properties of silver/gold nanostructures fabricated by shadowing growth and their sensing applications. *Proceedings of the SPIE* 7766 (Nanostructured Thin Films III), San Diego, CA, 77660B/77661–77660B/77612 (2010).

123. Liu YJ, Zhang ZY, Dluhy RA, and Zhao YP: The SERS response of semiordered Ag nanorod arrays fabricated by template oblique angle deposition. *J. Raman Spectrosc.* 41(10), 1112–1118 (2010).

124. Huang ZF, Harris KD, and Brett MJ: Morphology control of nanotube arrays. *Adv. Mater.* 21(29), 2983–2987 (2009).

125. Zhou CM and Gall D: Surface patterning by nanosphere lithography for layer growth with ordered pores. *Thin Solid Films* 516(2–4), 433–437 (2007).

126. Ye DX and Lu TM: Ballistic aggregation on two-dimensional arrays of seeds with oblique incident flux: Growth model for amorphous Si on Si. *Phys. Rev. B* 76(23), 235402-235401-235408 (2007).

127. Wang X, Liu LH, Ramstrom O, and Yan MD: Engineering nanomaterial surfaces for biomedical applications. *Exp. Biol. Med.* 234(10), 1128–1139 (2009).

128. Cobley CM, Chen JY, Cho EC, Wang LV, and Xia YN: Gold nanostructures: A class of multifunctional materials for biomedical applications. *Chem. Soc. Rev.* 40(1), 44–56 (2011).

129. Shenton W, Davis SA, and Mann S: Directed self-assembly of NPs into macroscopic materials using antibody-antigen recognition. *Adv. Mater.* 11(6), 449–452 (1999).

130. Naka K, Itoh H, Tampo Y, and Chujo Y: Effect of gold NPs as a support for the oligomerization of L-cysteine in an aqueous solution. *Langmuir* 19(13), 5546–5549 (2003).

131. Hayat MA: *Colloidal Gold: Principles, Methods, and Applications.* Academic Press: San Diego, CA (1989).

132. Mirkin CA, Letsinger RL, Mucic RC, and Storhoff JJ: A DNA-based method for rationally assembling NPs into macroscopic materials. *Nature* 382(6592), 607–609 (1996).

133. Sonnichsen C, Reinhard BM, Liphardt J, and Alivisatos AP: A molecular ruler based on plasmon coupling of single gold and silver NPs. *Nat. Biotechnol.* 23(6), 741–745 (2005).

134. Niemeyer CM: NPs, proteins, and nucleic acids: Biotechnology meets materials science. *Angew. Chem. Int. Ed.* 40(22), 4128–4158 (2001).

135. Green NM: Avidin. *Adv. Protein Chem.* 29, 85–133 (1975).

136. Wilchek M and Bayer EA: The avidin biotin complex in bioanalytical applications. *Anal. Biochem.* 171(1), 1–32 (1988).

137. Ling X, Xie LM, Fang Y, Xu H, Zhang HL, Kong J, Dresselhaus MS, Zhang J, and Liu ZF: Can graphene be. Used as a substrate for Raman enhancement. *Nano Lett.* 10, 553–561 (2010).
138. Zhou Q, Shao MW, Que RH, Cheng L, Zhuo SJ, Tong YH, and Lee ST: Silver vanadate nanoribbons: A label-free bioindicator in the conversion between human serum transferrin and apotransferrin via surface-enhanced Raman scattering. *Appl. Phys. Lett.* 98, 193110 (2011).
139. Cheng L, Shao MW, Zhang ML, and Ma DDD: An ultrasensitive method to detect dopamine from single mouse brain cell: Surface-enhanced Raman scattering on Ag NPs from beta-silver vanadate and copper. *Sci. Adv. Mater.* 2(3), 386–389 (2010).
140. Yonzon CR, Zhang XY, and Van Duyne RP: Localized surface plasmon resonance immunoassay and verification using surface-enhanced Raman spectroscopy. *Proc. SPIE* 5224, 78 (2003).
141. Coppe JP, Xu ZD, Chen Y, and Liu GL: Metallic nanocone array photonic substrate for high-uniformity surface deposition and optical detection of small molecules. *Nanotechnology* 22(24), 245710 (2011).
142. Shao MW, Zhang ML, Wong NB, Ma DDD, Wang H, Chen WW, and Lee ST: Ag-modified silicon nanowires substrate for ultrasensitive surface-enhanced Raman spectroscopy. *Appl. Phys. Lett.* 93, 233118 (2008).
143. Zhang ML, Fan X, Zhou HW, Shao MW, Zapien JA, Wong NB, and Lee ST: A high-efficiency surface-enhanced Raman scattering substrate based on silicon nanowires array decorated with silver NPs. *J. Phys. Chem. C* 114(5), 1969–1975 (2010).
144. Cheng L, Shao MW, Yin K, and Liu Z: AgI modified silicon nanowires: Synthesis, characterization and properties of ionic conductivity and surface-enhanced Raman scattering. *CrystEngComm* 14, 601–604 (2012).

7

In Vivo Biodetection Using Surface-Enhanced
Raman Spectroscopy

Seunghyun Lee, Ulhas S. Kadam, Ana Paula Craig, and Joseph Irudayaraj

CONTENTS

7.1 Introduction

Nanophotonics engages with light–material interaction behaviors that occur on wavelength or subwavelength scales, where the electromagnetic field is confined to the surface of designed nanostructures with unique and tunable optical properties. In particular, "plasmonics" using surface plasmon polaritons (SPPs), simply called surface plasmon, is diverse and a rapidly growing field in nanophotonics. Over the recent decades, the emergence of novel nanomaterials and fabrication of diverse nanostructures on surfaces allow the manipulation of their optical properties as well as develop a methodology to increase inherent sensitivity that lead to new insights at this highly interdisciplinary field for many applications. The confinement of the SPPs is empowered to enhance the electromagnetic field at the interfacial surface that gives rise to remarkable sensitivity to surface conditions and environment surrounding the media refractive index, which is widely employed for biological and chemical sensing. In addition, the enhancement contributes to surface optical properties such as Raman scattering.

When a surface plasmon is confined to a metal nanoparticle with a size equal to the subwavelength of light, nonpropagating excitation of the free electrons on the surface of the nanoparticle in the oscillating electromagnetic fields gives rise to localized surface plasmon resonance (LSPR) (Hutter and Fendler 2004). LSPR results in strong optical extinction, which can be tuned throughout the visible and near-infrared (NIR) wavelengths by adjusting the particle's size and shape (Oldenburg et al. 1998; Link et al. 1999; Lu et al. 2009).

Vibrational spectroscopy has played a significant role in identifying molecular structure, bonding, and verification of the interfacial correlation between the adsorbates at surfaces and the surface performance properties. Vibrational transitions of the elements occur intrinsically through interaction with electromagnetic radiation. Among vibrational techniques, Surface-enhanced Raman scattering (SERS) was first demonstrated by Feischman et al. (1974). In this study, unusually enhanced Raman scattering was observed from pyridine adsorbed on the highly roughened surface of a silver electrode. Later, Jeanmaire and Van Duyne (1977) and separately Albrecht and Creighton (1977) proposed that the enhancement of Raman scattering could be increased by a factor of 10^6 and the remarkable enhancement of the Raman signal originated from the increased large number of adsorption sites of the roughened surface. In 1997, Kneipp et al. and Nie et al. independently achieved single molecule detection using silver colloidal nanoparticles by the Raman scattering with estimated enhancements by factors up to 10^{15} (Kneipp et al. 1997; Nie and Emery 1997). The tremendous enhancement of Raman scattering is called surface-enhanced Raman scattering (SERS). SERS originates from the highly enhanced electromagnetic field at the adjacent surface of the metal nanoparticles or nanostructures with the localized surface plasmon resonance (LSPR). Also, the SERS signals enhanced by electromagnetic fields are highly confined to the "hotspot," which is the very small gap when two or more nanoparticles are assembled closely within about a couple of nanometers.

The complex of molecule–metal absorbs the excited energy from the incident light via this charge transfer process, leading to an increase in the Raman scattering cross section by resonance. It is called the chemical enhancement. This enhancement provides an additional boost to the overall SERS enhancement. The chemical enhancement factor ranges typically from 10 to 10^3. Second, the electromagnetic theory attributes the enhancement to the large local electromagnetic fields caused by surface plasmon resonance that can be optically excited at certain wavelengths for metal nanoparticles with different sizes and shapes or closely packed nanoparticles with very small interstices much smaller than the wavelength. Usually, the local enhancement in the hotspots can reach several orders of magnitude 10^{10} or even 10^{12} for optimal conditions. Generally, the electromagnetic enhancement due to excitations of LSPR is considered as a more dominant factor in the total enhancement.

SERS can provide molecular information and extraordinary sensitivity of the surface structure and behavior of molecules for chemical or biological analysis. In addition, SERS has several advantages over noninvasive measurement, simple sample preparation, compatibility with aqueous solution, and observation at low frequency. Thus, a number of geometries of the nanoparticles/nanostructures or their ensembles have been extensively investigated to generate larger enhancement for reproducible and controllable SERS-active platforms because the field enhancement due to LSPR from "hot spots" in morphological features, such as sharp tips and edges, can create strong spatially confined field enhancement, which makes a major contribution to the total enhancement of Raman scattering (Kneipp et al. 2006e; Schlücker 2011).

Recently, SERS is being applied increasingly to living systems. The complexity of the environmental conditions of living system's environment may cause unexpected nonspecific binding to the SERS-active substrate and can disturb the SERS signals of interest. Nevertheless, SERS applications have been demonstrated due to the remarkable molecular and chemical specificity, sensitivity, and multiplex sensing over the past decade (Zhang et al. 2011; Dougan and Faulds 2012; Tu and Chang 2012). Investigations in SERS span the building blocks of life (DNA, RNA) to functional complex structures (peptides, proteins) to whole cells and tissues. Since *in vitro* SERS detection was reported by Kneipp et al. (2002) using colloidal AuNPs in single living cells, many research groups have demonstrated the use of SERS for, not only *in vitro*, but also *in vivo* applications. In the next few sections we provide a brief account of nanomaterials and then discuss *in vitro* and *in vivo* applications.

7.2 Nanomaterials for SERS

7.2.1 Nanomaterial Basics: Types and Basic Properties

The optical properties of materials are described by their complex dielectric function, which are composed of real and imaginary parts at a given wavelength of incident light. Simply, this function can characterize the polarization of materials interacting with electromagnetic waves because most materials behave differently to incident electromagnetic waves with different wavelength. The quantity of the real part expresses how much a material is polarized due to the electric dipoles in the material by an applied electric field. And the quantity of the imaginary part represents the losses occurring in polarizing the materials and it is connected with absorption in the materials. A transparent material has zero value, but the imaginary part is going to be nonzero value when absorption (energy loss) happens. And the dielectric functions of metals among attenuating materials are complex numbers. Therefore, materials with small value of imaginary part are preferred for lower energy loss (West et al. 2010; Schlücker 2011).

Gold and silver are well-known plasmonic materials and the most widely used metals for SERS-active substrate as both metals have high ratios of real and imaginary parts of the dielectric function and relatively lower loss from near-UV (~300 nm) to near-IR region (~900 nm) (Le Ru and Etchegoin 2009). These characteristics contribute to enhancement of local electromagnetic fields, which is one of the important properties of plasmonic materials. In fact, dielectric functions of gold and silver show similar plasmonic properties except over 600 nm wavelength, where gold generates more dissipation of surface plasmon resonance. Especially, in terms of technological applications, gold as a substrate is chemically inert and not prone to surface oxidation, hence chemical modification of gold can be compatible and readily prepared under ambient conditions.

Apart from gold and silver, various types of materials such as copper (Allen and Vanduyne 1981; Xue et al. 1991; Kim and Lee 2005; Wu et al. 2008; Chen et al. 2009) aluminum (Joo and Suh 1995; Du et al. 2008; Gutes et al. 2010; Yang et al. 2011), titanium oxide (Musumeci et al. 2009; Teguh et al. 2012), and quantum dots (Quagliano 2004; Wang et al. 2008; Livingstone et al. 2010; Fan et al. 2012) have been used as SERS substrates. Very recently, graphene (Jung et al. 2010; Ling and Zhang 2010; Ling et al. 2010; Qiu et al. 2011) and mixed metals (Olivares-Amaya et al. 2012) have been explored for their contribution to enhancement of Raman scattering. However, the enhancements of quantum dots, graphene, and mixed metal as a SERS-active substrate were ascribed to the charge transfer and chemical enhancement. Hence, their enhancements were much smaller than normal electromagnetic enhancement (Sharma et al. 2012).

7.2.2 Fabrication of SERS Nanostructures

SERS requires a substrate that has structure and can enhance the Raman scattering to detect an analyte of interest effectively. To fulfill its demands, a SERS-active substrate can be configured as follows: (1) high sensitivity due to a very large enhancement factor, (2) high reproducibility of detected analytes through homogeneous distribution of hot spots, (3) reusability after a simple cleaning step, (4) feasibility of ease of sample preparation to detect the analyte of interest.

The developments of SERS substrate have been extensively performed using nanoparticles or nanostructures to create a uniform and higher number of "hot spots" as much as possible for large local field enhancement. In early studies, roughened surface by electrochemical treatment (Tuschel et al. 1986) was used for SERS and later controlled nanoparticles' assembly and well-defined nanostructures through lithographical methods have been produced. SERS efforts on nanoparticles have been exploited by drop-and-dry (Wang and Halas 2008; Xie et al. 2008; Esenturk and Walker 2009), controllable self-assembly (Kuncicky et al. 2006; Alvarez-Puebla et al. 2011; Adams et al. 2012; Watanabe et al. 2012; Yap et al. 2012), physical deposition, or lithographic (Shanmukh et al. 2006; Zhang et al. 2006; Yan et al. 2009; Casadio et al. 2010; Barcelo et al. 2012) arrays constructed on a template (Wang et al. 2006; Li et al. 2010; Yang et al. 2010; Lee et al. 2012). Furthermore, the evolution of novel nanoparticles with complicated geometries or multiple sharp protrusions has offered intriguing possibilities and boosted the fabrication of SERS substrate with good performance.

First, in the drop-and-dry method for SERS substrate, the nanoparticles' shapes are emphasized as their geometrical patterns are unique, which allows to generate plentiful "hot spots" by local field enhancement at the protrusions on the surface of nanoparticle. Figure 7.1 shows closed-packed layer of the gold meatball and nanoflowers as examples of protruded or multibranched nanoparticles. Second, the controllable self-assembly method enables the individual nanoparticle to form relatively uniform cluster arrays, patterns, and three-dimensional (3D) colloidal crystal with periodic structure shown in Figure 7.2. To achieve these goals, various factors such as electrostatic force, the temperature for convective flow, and chemical functionality on the different polymer surfaces are tuned. The local field enhancement on these structures was attributed to a repetitive formation with contiguous or closed-packed nanoparticles. This feature can also provide reliable SERS signal. Third, the lithographical tools including physical deposition methods are widely employed as SERS substrates. One of the widely known substrates is metal film over nanospheres (MFON), in which drop-coated polymer spheres' single layer of closed-packed structure was prepared on a glass slide and silver film was deposited, then alumina film was fabricated via a go through atomic layer deposition. This produced periodically uniform metal structure and a stable surface against oxidation and high temperature as shown in Figure 7.3a and b. Another example in Figure 7.3c is the silver nanorod array substrate fabricated by oblique angle deposition (OAD) method. This angle-dependent metal deposition is utilized for various SERS substrates (Baumberg et al. 2005; Lu et al. 2005). Nanoimprint and e-beam lithographic techniques fabricated patterned array/cluster of nanoparticles with nanometer scale spacing. In addition, prepatterned surface as a template by the lithographic

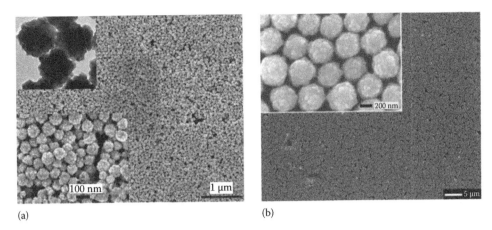

(a)   (b)

FIGURE 7.1
(a) FESEM and TEM images of Au nanoflowers with a variety of shapes and sizes. (Adapted with permission from Xie, J. P., Zhang, Q.B., Lee, J.Y., and Wang, D.I.C., The synthesis of SERS-active gold nanoflower tags for *in vivo* applications, *ACS Nano*, 2(12), 2473–2480. Copyright 2008 American Chemical Society.) (b) SEM image of a monolayer of a close-packed submicrometer Au sphere arrays formed on a glass slide. (From Wang, H. and Halas, N.J.: Mesoscopic Au "Meatball" particles. *Adv. Mater.* 2008. 20(4). 820–825. Copyright Wiley-VCH Verlag GmbH & Co. KGaA. Adapted with permission.)

method has been used for nanoparticle cluster array via self-assembly. Figure 7.3d illustrates the SERS substrate with well-defined and homogeneously clustered nanostructures by a nanoimprinting technique, which showed highly reproducible signals of targeting analyte and greater enhancement factor rather than randomly aggregated nanoparticle and conventional nanopatterned array. Fourth, SERS substrates based on template are capable of creating nanostructures conveniently over a large area with controlled size and shape in accordance with their template' structural parameters. One of the widely used templates is anodized aluminum oxide (AAO). Fabrication of silver nanoparticles based on AAO template can control the distance between adjacent nanoparticles, which is a significant aspect to produce stronger electromagnetic coupling. In case of using AAO template, an etching process is crucial to the regulation of narrow interparticle gaps within 10 nm presented in Figure 7.4a. The substrate represented uniform and highly reproducible SERS-active properties. Another material as a template is titanium dioxide (TiO$_2$), which has high photocatalytic activity to degrade organic pollutants and nontoxicity. Also, TiO$_2$ has self-cleaning function when it is exposed to UV irradiation, which makes it reusable. Figure 7.4b presents the schematic diagram of its working process with scanning and transmission electron microscope (SEM and TEM) images of the SERS substrate structures. Thus, a composite of TiO$_2$ and plasmonic materials such as gold could enhance the detection of organic pollutants and recycling. SERS-based polymer mesoparticles have also been used. Here, the spin-coated polymer particle's single layer was processed through the thermal treatment and plasma etching in order. Subsequently, silver thin film was deposited onto the polymer particle layer via electrophoretic deposition, which can modulate the diameter, the surface roughness, and the interparticle gaps. An alternative choice as a template material is carbon nanotube. In fact, SERS substrate using noble metals decorated on carbon nanotubes have been studied (Corio et al. 2000; Chu et al. 2009; Sun et al. 2010). Recently, gold nanoparticles decorated along vertically aligned carbon nanotubes with 3D SERS-active volumes were achieved, where highly dense vertically aligned carbon nanotubes with millimeter length were utilized as a template in Figure 7.4c. When the carbon nanotubes were exposed to the

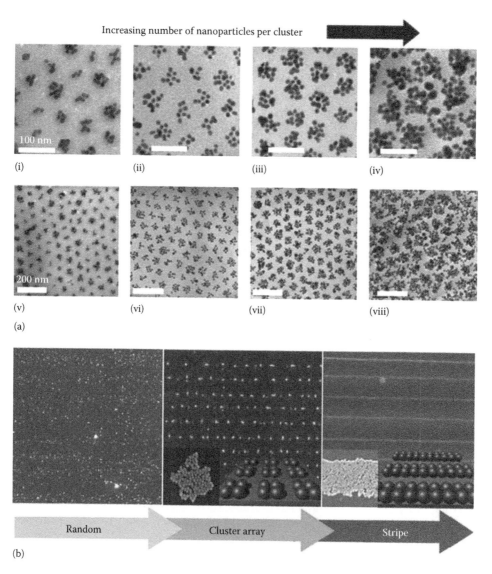

FIGURE 7.2

(a) Fabrication of gold nanoparticle cluster arrays using block copolymer thin film on a silicon or glass surface. Representative plan-view TEM images showing gold nanoparticle clusters with systematically increasing number of particles per cluster. (Adapted with permission from Yap, F.L., Thoniyot, P., Krishnan, S., and Krishnamoorthy, S., Nanoparticle Cluster arrays for high-performance SERS through directed self-assembly on flat substrates and on optical fibers, *ACS Nano*, 6(3), 2056–2070. Copyright 2012 American Chemical Society.) (b) Optical micrograph and SEM image of 60 nm gold particles with different patterns. Each formation can be controlled by temperatures and nanoparticle concentration regime. (Adapted with permission from Watanabe, S., Mino, Y., Ichikawa, Y., and Miyahara, M.T., Spontaneous formation of Cluster array of gold particles by corrective Self-assembly, *Langmuir*, 28(36), 12982–12988. Copyright 2012 American Chemical Society.)

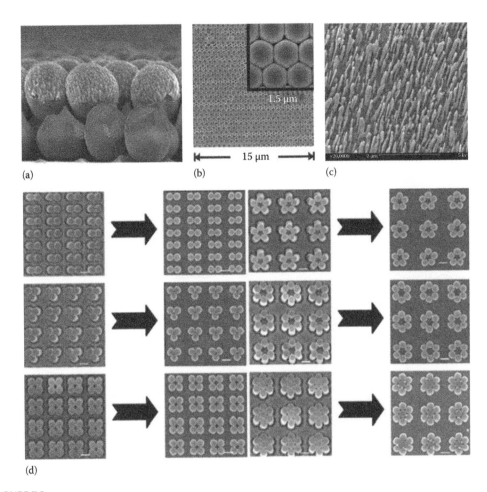

(a) (b) (c)

(d)

FIGURE 7.3
(a) SEM image of AgFON (silver film over the nanospheres). (Adapted with permission from Casadio, F., Leona, M., Lombardi, J.R., and Van Duyne, R., Identification of organic colorants in fibers, paints, and glazes by surface enhanced Raman Spectroscopy, *Acc. Chem. Res.*, 43(6), 782–791. Copyright 2010 American Chemical Society.) (b) SEM image of alumina-modified AgFON substrates. (Adapted with permission from Zhang, X.Y., Zhao, J., Whitney, A.V., Elam, J.W., and Van Duyne, R.P., Ultrastable substrates for surface-enhanced Raman Spectroscopy: Al$_2$O$_3$ overlayers fabricated by atomic layer deposition yield improved anthrax biomarker detection, *J. Am. Chem. Soc.*, 128(31), 10304–10309. Copyright 2006 American Chemical Society.) (c) SEM image of silver nanorod array with 868 nm of height fabricated by oblique angle deposition. (Adapted with permission from Shanmukh, S., Jones, L., Driskell, J., Zhao, Y.P., Dluhy, R., and Tripp, R.A., Rapid and Sensitive detection of respiratory virus molecular signatures using a silver nanorod array SERS Substrate, *Nano Lett.*, 6(11), 2630–2636. Copyright 2006 American Chemical Society.) (d) SEM images showing the versatility and deterministic control of nanoparticle assemblies by using a nanoimprint transfer process. All scale bars are 200 nm. (Adapted with permission from Barcelo, S.J., Kim, A., Wu, W., and Li, Z.Y., Fabrication of deterministic nanostructure assemblies with sub-nanometer spacing using a nanoimprinting transfer technique, *ACS Nano*, 6(7), 6446–6452. Copyright 2012 American Chemical Society.)

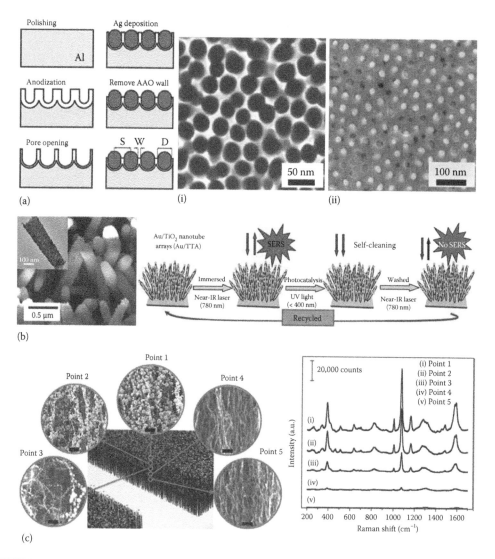

FIGURE 7.4

(a) Schematic showing the process for fabricating silver-filled porous anodic alumina substrates. (i) Top-view SEM image of an AAO substrate with D=25 nm and W=5 nm before growth of Ag nanoparticles, (ii) SEM image of silver nanoparticles array substrates. (From Wang, H.H., Liu, C.Y., Wu, S.B., Liu, N.W., Peng, C.Y., Chan, T.H., Hsu, C.F., Wang, J.K., and Wang, Y.L. Highly Raman-enhancing substrates based on silver nanoparticle arrays with tunable sub-10 nm gaps. *Adv. Mater.* 2006. 18(4). 491–495. Copyright Wiley-VCH Verlag GmbH & Co. KGaA. Adapted with permission.) (b) SEM/TEM image of gold-coated TiO$_2$ nanotube arrays substrate and scheme of the reversible SERS behavior of the SERS substrate. (From Li, X.H., Chen, G.Y., Yang, L.B., Jin, Z., and Liu, J.H.: Multifunctional Au-coated TiO$_2$ nanotube arrays as recyclable SERS substrates for multifold organic pollutants detection. *Adv. Funct. Mater.* 2010. 20(17). 2815–2824. Copyright Wiley-VCH Verlag GmbH & Co. KGaA. Adapted with permission.) (c) Scheme and SEM images of Au NPs formed on vertically aligned CNTs along the perpendicular axis. Populations of the Au NPs are decreased from the top to the bottom of the CNTs. The distance between the points is 30 μm. All of the scale bars are 100 nm. SERS spectra measured from the side view of the CNTs sample on different points and they display higher intensities along the perpendicular axis to the top surface of the CNTs sample. (From Lee, S., Hahm, M.G., Vajtai, R., Hashim, D.P., Thurakitseree, T., Chipara, A.C., Ajayan, P.M., and Hafner, J.H.: Utilizing 3D SERS active volumes in aligned carbon nanotube scaffold substrates. *Adv. Mat.* 2012. 24(38). 5261–5266. Copyright Wiley-VCH Verlag GmbH & Co. KGaA. Adapted with permission.)

solution including target molecules and subsequently the solution was evaporated, the 3D volume of carbon nanotubes was dramatically decreased due to their strong van der Waals interactions. At this time, the spacing between gold nanoparticles decorated on carbon nanotubes also decreased and simultaneously generated abundant "hot spots" for better SERS performance. Its detection sensitivity was at 10 fM.

7.3 SERS-Based Applications

7.3.1 SERS-Based Devices and Construction

SERS detections based on microfluidic devices have been developed to boost the advantages of both SERS and microfluidics technology. However, there are a few studies focused on the SERS-active substrate in the device due to the complexity of fabrication of nanostructures (Liu and Lee 2005; Connatser et al. 2008). Thus, optofluidic device for SERS detection has attracted attention. Herein, interaction between the plasmonic nanoparticles and target analytes inside fluidic channel is very important for reproducible SERS detection. On the other hand, design of plasmonic nanoparticle with large Raman enhancement is also important, as well as the formation of their aggregation in live cell for biological application (Kneipp et al. 2006b,c,d).

7.3.2 SERS for *In Vitro* Systems

7.3.2.1 *DNA Sequence Detection*

Detection of specific DNA sequences is central to modern molecular biology and molecular diagnostics where identification of a particular disease is based on nucleic acid identification. Although fluorescence spectroscopy, with different assay formats, dominates the detection technologies employed, there are many drawbacks. As this technique arises due to the nature of the fluorescence emission spectrum, which is broad, it gives limited characteristic information about the target analyte. The large spectral overlap that occurs from more than one fluorophore makes the detection of multiple analytes in a mixture difficult (MacAskill et al. 2009). Recently, significant progress has been made in the development of nonfluorescence DNA assays. Among them, SERS must be highlighted, with relevant studies published on cancer gene expression. Detection schemes utilizing SERS have the advantage in that the peaks are more distinct than in fluorescence, and in theory, a clinically significant number of markers can be multiplexed in a single sample using different SERS reporters (Lowe et al. 2010).

Highly sensitive SERS technique has been applied for the detection of nucleotides in aqueous solution at submicromolar concentrations (Bell and Sirimuthu 2006, 2008). In sequence, silver-nanorod SERS-based approach was used for the detection of microRNAs. The single-stranded nucleic acids and RNA/DNA hybrid complexes showed variable binding affinities depending on target RNA transcripts (Driskell and Tripp 2010; Driskell et al. 2010). In another study, AgNPs in conjunction with AuNP as nanotips were found to be a highly sensitive SERS substrate used to probe microRNA gene expression. The use of silicon (Si) nanotips with AuNPs and AgNPs improved substantially the signal (Lo et al. 2011a,b). A dramatic increase in the reproducibility of the SERS spectra of ssDNA was achieved in a

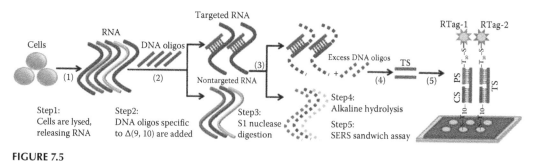

FIGURE 7.5

(See color insert.) Detection schematic integrating S1 nuclease digestion and an SERS sandwich assay to quantify splice variants from targets obtained directly from cancer cells. (Adapted with permission from Sun, L. and Irudayaraj, J., *Biophys. J.*, 96(11), 4709. Copyright 2009 Biophysical Society.)

novel approach using Au nanoshells. An improved detection reproducibility was obtained because the cycling pretreatment resulted in a relaxation of the DNA molecules into what was believed to be an extended linear conformation (Barhoumi et al. 2008a,b).

Moreover, quantitative detection of gene expression in breast cancer cells has been reported (Sun et al. 2007, 2008; Sun and Irudayaraj 2009a,b). Sun and Irudayaraj (2009b) developed a sandwich assay to quantify gene expression from cancer cells without the need for any amplification steps (Figure 7.5). Recently, Lee et al. (2011) demonstrated the feasibility of using DNA–gold nanoparticle probes to achieve dual marker detection of three breast cancer cells in an efficient multiplexed approach. In their work, gold nanoparticle network was grown using DNA hybridization on the cell surface marker sites, providing an efficient platform for detection with SERS. As this network structure is reversible, the signal enhancement during formation and dissipation could be dynamically monitored on cell surfaces. Further, our group has shown the application of SERS to detect different alternatively spliced patterns of BRC1 gene, which is involved in development of breast cancer in humans, and to detect gene expression in plants (unpublished data, Irudayaraj).

7.3.2.2 Other Methodologies for Disease Diagnostics

Folic acid (FA), known as a widely distributed water-soluble vitamin, is reported to be a very significant component for human health, which relates to a series of diseases and has also drawn attention as a possible targeting agent of cancer cells because folate receptors (FRs) are often overexpressed on the membranes of various human cancer cells (Ren et al. 2011; Zong et al. 2012). Therefore, Ren and collaborators (2011) fabricated a graphene oxide/ Ag nanoparticle hybrid (GO/PDDA/AgNPs), where the modified GO with positive potential could concentrate the negatively charged FA molecules due to electrostatic interaction. This label-free SERS method was able to detect FA in human serum with a linear response ranging from 9 to 180 nM.

7.3.2.3 Interactions between Nucleic Acids and Small Molecules

Investigation of the nature of interactions between small molecules and nucleic acids not only sheds light on understanding the chemical basis for the antitumor mechanism of drugs and the carcinogenicity of pollutants, but also gives chemists and pharmacologists opportunities to discover or design new drug candidates (Wang and Yang 2009). Wang and Yang (2009) employed SERS and other techniques to explore the interaction of toluidine blue (TB), a potential antitumor drug for photodynamic therapy of tumor, with calf thymus DNA (ctDNA). The SERS experiment was based on the Raman spectroscopy analysis of solutions prepared with TB, ctDNA, and silver colloid. Based on the intensity of specific peaks of the spectra, it was proposed that TB could partially intercalate into DNA with ring C_1NC_1 buried into DNA base pairs, while the steric hindrance resulting from the substituents blocked the insertion from the C_6NC_6 side of TB.

7.3.2.4 Monitoring of Conformational Changes Induced by Target Molecules

Aptamers are single-stranded DNA/RNA oligomers that fold into 3D conformations in the presence of specific molecular targets. Although many aptamer-based detection methods have been reported, these techniques typically require complex labeling and sample preparation. The direct optical detection of aptamer–target binding still remains a key analytical challenge (Neumann et al. 2009). A direct, label-free, optical method based on SERS for monitoring the binding of an aptamer to its target and the conformational changes induced was proposed by Neumann and others (2009). These changes in the conformation of the aptamer molecules were quantified by obtaining several SERS spectra and calculating the pairwise spectral correlation function, Γ, before and after exposure to the target analyte. Nanoshell substrates were treated with thiolated aptamer SAMs specific to a protein platelet-derived growth factor (PDGF-BB) and a small molecule, cocaine, allowing the examination of two distinct detection regimes, high and low specificity, respectively. In both situations, the exposure of anti-PDGF and anticocaine aptamer SAMs to PDGF-BB and cocaine, respectively, provided a dramatic reduction in reproducibility of the SERS spectra. The specificity of the methodology was evaluated using control molecules. This type of measurement may provide a method for assessing the degree of specificity of an aptamer for its target. Conversely, since the values for each target analyte are distinct and reproducible, this limited degree of specificity may lead to new optics-based strategies for the identification of multiple targets by a single aptamer where aptamer-target specificity is inherently limited.

7.3.2.5 Pathogen Detection

SERS was successfully applied as a diagnostic method for bacterial infectious disease medicine, without the need for extrinsic labeling (Patel et al. 2008). Spectra of *cereus* group of *Bacillus* bacteria were obtained using the *in situ* grown, aggregated Au-nanoparticle-covered SiO_2 substrates, combining attributes of the chemically produced colloids with the ease of use and reproducibility of the solid state. PCA plots and HCA dendograms illustrated the high specificity and sensitivity obtained from the SERS approach, which allowed for sample discrimination in specie- and strain-level. The ability to rapidly distinguish between avirulent and virulent *B. anthracis* strains demonstrates the potential of SERS to be used as a bacterial diagnostic testing for causative agent of anthrax disease.

SERS has also been extensively studied and considered a valuable alternative to current foodborne pathogen diagnostic tools for onsite food inspection. Silver NPs were used as substrates for the detection and discrimination between gram types, species, strains, and viability of generic *Escherichia coli*, *E. coli* O157:H7, *E. coli* DH 5α, *Staphylococcus aureus*, *Staphylococcus epidermidis*, *Salmonella typhimurium*, *Listeria monocytogenes*, and *Enterococcus faecelis*. Depending on the methodology applied, LODs varied from 10 UFC/mL to single cells (Chu et al. 2008; Wang et al. 2010; Fan et al. 2011). He et al. (2008) successfully employed the commercial Klarite substrate made of silicon wafers coated with gold to detect single

Bacillus spores and discriminate five *Bacillus* strains (*B. cereus* ATCC 13061, *B. cereus* ATCC 10876, *B. cereus* sp., *B. subtilis* sp., and *B. stearothermophilus* sp.). AuNPs and magnetic NPs were applied via sandwich immunoassays for detection and enumeration of *E. coli* achieving correlation coefficients and limits of detection close to and comparable to the classical counting methods in real water samples, respectively. In addition, the authors described that the total analysis time was less than 70 min, quite short when compared with other novel immunoassays as ELISA (1 day) and PCR (5 h) (Temur et al. 2010; Guven et al. 2011).

While there has been significant progress in biosensor design, simultaneous detection of multiple pathogens is often accompanied by compromises in either precision or sensitivity (Ravindranath et al. 2011). Thus, a novel immunomagnetic SERS biosensor based on a sandwich assay for the separation and detection of multiple pathogens was proposed by Wang and collaborators (2011). First, the pathogens of a food matrix were captured and separated using a silica-coated magnetic probe functionalized with specific pathogen antibodies. In a second step, AuNPs integrated with a Raman reporter and functionalized with corresponding antibodies were allowed to form a sandwich assay. Using the developed tool, *S. enterica* serovar Typhimurium and *S. aureus* were separately detected in spinach wash and peanut butter at a limit of 10^3 CFU/mL. A similar methodology was proposed by Ravindranath et al. (2011), but rather than magnetic separation, a millipore nanoporous membrane (pore size ~450 nm) was used to retain the pathogens bounded with the nanoprobes functionalized with antiligands. This membrane with the probes tethered to the captured bacteria can be directly analyzed by the Raman spectrometer without any additional sample processing steps. Using the aforementioned platform the authors could simultaneously detect *S. typhimurium*, *S. aureus*, and *E. coli* O157:H7 with a LOD ranging between 10^2 and 10^3 CFU/mL.

7.3.3 SERS for *In Vivo* Systems

7.3.3.1 Detection of Biomolecules at a Single Cell Level

Gold nanoparticles with high plasmonic capabilities are the most common substrates for SERS-based intracellular detection, as they have small sizes and high surface areas and low toxicity (Kneipp and Kneipp 2006; Kneipp et al. 2006d). Kneipp and coworkers have pioneered the SERS-based live cells monitoring, where gold nanoparticles with sizes ranging from 30 to 50 nm were introduced into immortalized rat renal proximal tubule (IRPT) cells and mouse microphage cell line (J774), via endocytosis (Kneipp et al. 2006a,b,d). To minimize background autofluorescence, 786 nm was used as the excitation source for the measurement of SERS spectra at different time points. The pattern of SERS intensity changed over time with the spectra after particles' internalization showing the largest number of bands and highest intensity. Thus, SERS is a sensitive tool for label-free biomolecule identification inside an individual living cell. But, because any chemical species near the nanoparticle surface could result in a Raman signal, this problem still exists (Kneipp et al. 2006b,c,d; Jarvis et al. 2008). For selective detection of a particular biomolecule in samples of complex biological origin, nanoparticles conjugated with chemical receptors are pursued as SERS-based sensors. Recently, gold nanoparticles functionalized with redox-active chemicals were shown to respond to redox potential changes in NIH/3T3 fibroblast cells (Kneipp et al. 2010a; Auchinvole et al. 2012).

One example is the pH monitoring in endosomal compartments over time (Bishnoi et al. 2006; Ochsenkuhn et al. 2009), which is of basic interest for a better understanding of a broad range of physiological and metabolic processes, including pathologies such as certain cancers and cystic fibrosis (Kokkonen et al. 2004). Considering this, Kneipp et al. (2010b) applied a pH-dependent nanosensor to explore the dynamics of pH in the endosomal compartment of NIH/3T3 (mouse fibroblast cells) live cells. The mobile nanosensor used was produced from gold nanoaggregates with 4-mercaptobenzoic acid (pMBA) attached as a reporter that reversibly follows changes of pH in the environment in the time scale of a few seconds. The pH value in the environment of the sensor was inferred from the signal ratio of two specific Raman lines at 1423 and 1076 cm^{-1} in comparison with a calibration curve generated from the nanosensor dispersed in aqueous solution of known pH. Exploiting signals of pairs of Raman lines in the same spectrum enables quantitative measurements without any correction regarding optical cellular background signals that can be pointed as an advantage of SERS over pH sensors based on fluorescence.

More recently, Zong et al. (2012) developed a SERS and fluorescence dual mode cancer cell targeting probe based on CdTe quantum dots (QDs) conjugated with silica coated Au-Ag core–shell nanorods (Au-Ag NRs). FA was used as targeting ligand for the detection of folate receptor (FR) overexpressed cancer cells. HeLa cells were used as target cells and MRC-5 cells with low FR expression level as the negative control, and the SERS and fluorescence results proved that the proposed probe can recognize FR overexpressed cancer cells with high selectivity.

7.3.3.2 Raman Imaging for In Vivo Analysis

In addition to intracellular detection, SERS imaging has been applied for extracellular analysis of cells, tissues, and bacteria. Such imaging can provide location=specific chemical information, for example, size, concentration, and distribution of the macromolecules present. Such studies improve our understanding of trafficking of macromolecules and their association at specific sites. For this SERS should be coupled with high-spatial resolution capabilities. The tip-enhanced Raman spectroscopy (TERS) is one of the most common methods to improve spatial resolution for SERS imaging. In this approach, an accurately positioned nanotip (SERS-active substrate) was used to confine enhancement to reach subdiffraction limited spatial resolution. For TERS, the improved tips of scanning probe microscopy (SPM) are used with SERS-active metals. For example, SERS coupled with near-field scanning optical microscopy (NSOM) was able to resolve and detect chemical images of multitrace ions (Betzig et al. 1986; Deckert et al. 1998; Zeisel et al. 1998). SPMs, such as atomic force microscopy (AFM) and scanning tunneling microscopy (STM) coupled to SERS can resolve sub diffraction-limited chemical imaging (Pettinger et al. 2004; Ren et al. 2004; Neugebauer et al. 2006a,b). Particularly, AFM tip with silver coating is able to provide both surface features and SERS spectral evidence membranes of bacteria. SERS was able to show the different protein and carbohydrate components of the cell surface (Neugebauer et al. 2006b).

However, TERS has limited applications to study static/fixed sample analysis, because it needs longer duration to acquire the images. This limitation of TERS could be addressed by employing nanoprobes with coherent fiber-optic imaging bundles coupled to SERS for real-time subdiffraction-limited chemical imaging (Hankus et al. 2006; Aksu et al. 2011; Holthoff et al. 2011). Such SERS nanoimaging probes can resolve spatiotemporal chemical species in the sample, allowing the dynamics and trafficking of molecules across membranes. The proof-of-concept studies using such probes show ability to characterize samples with spatial resolution below <100 nm (Hankus et al. 2006). Furthermore, images at different time points allowed monitoring diffusion of chemicals to the millisecond resolution (Hankus et al. 2006; Aksu et al. 2011). The dynamic visualization of biomolecules associated with cell membranes validates the prospects of such probes to explore the physiological role of cellular membranes in maintaining homeostasis (Hankus et al. 2006).

7.3.3.3 Applications of Raman Imaging

In vivo applications of SERS for analysis of biological samples represent a relevant development (Schlücker 2009). This has particular implications in the field of medical diagnostics where SERS functionalized nanotags have been used as pathophysiological markers for disease detection (El-Said et al. 2010; Wang et al. 2011). Antibodies tagged with SERS-active molecules have been used for protein identification and localization in tissues (Jehn et al. 2009). Additionally, the possibility of localizing label-free biomarkers in living cells using gold nanoarrays (Almond et al. 2011; Horsnell et al. 2012) was also demonstrated.

For rapid *in vivo* analysis a number of SERS-based approaches were pursued to enhance Raman signals in mammals, including human dermal tissue targeting. The composition of pigments, proteins, and other biomolecules in skin is well known. For Raman spectroscopy–based approaches using optical probes the diagnosis of skin cancers was reported (Nijssen et al. 2007; Lieber et al. 2008a,b). This procedure is noninvasive, inexpensive, and requires less time, which makes Raman-based methods an attractive analytical tool. Raman analysis of skin samples is highly consistent, sensitive, and specific. The feasibility of these methods was demonstrated in biomedical diagnosis (Nijssen et al. 2007).

Typical Raman applications require the NIR laser power source to avoid nonspecific background due to autofluorescence from biological samples. With advancement of technology in high-throughput and optical speedy data acquisition methods, it is possible to perform real-time dermal tissue analysis. *In vivo* applications to diagnose tumors in different body parts have been reported in the last 5 years, using narrow-diameter fiber-optic Raman probes (Motz et al. 2006; Sćepanović et al. 2006). Further, *in vivo* Raman analysis permits to probe stages in breast cancer development mastectomy and is also able to classify malignant and benign tissues in 3D cell cultures (Irudayaraj, unpublished data). Approaches to detect SERS probes in animal models have also been developed (Figure 7.6). An enhanced sensitivity by a factor of 10^2 compared to fluorescence-based approaches (Qian et al. 2008) was noted. Moreover, developments on the use of CARS microscopy for *in vivo* imaging have been used to probe changes in structure of lipids in adipose tissue of mouse ears (Evans et al. 2005) and other targets (Légaré et al. 2006). Thus a variety of detection modalities exist using Raman.

7.4 Future Trends

Raman spectroscopy has evolved as an attractive bioanalytical tool with a range of sensing modalities. Advances in lasers, optics, and detector coupled with the availability of Raman active probes have significantly improved Raman adaptability to a wide range of biological samples for both label-free chemical fingerprinting and highly sensitive detection. However, continuous improvements in Raman-based approaches both from SERS substrate fabrication, technology development, and miniaturization have made it possible to expand its applicability in a range of areas. While routine applications in quality control are already in place for pharmaceutical quality control, SERS-integrated devices for high-throughput analysis might be more relevant for routine molecular biology. Further, the increased

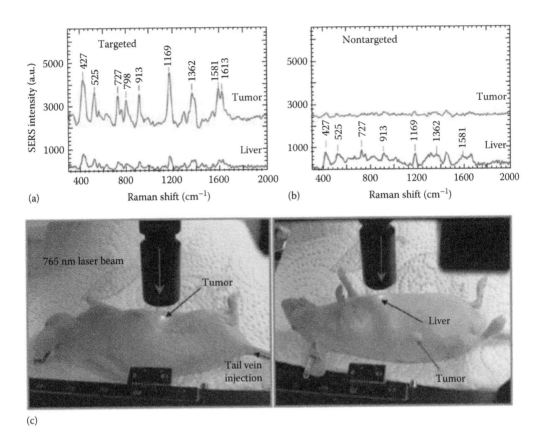

FIGURE 7.6

(See color insert.) *In vivo* cancer targeting and surface-enhanced Raman detection by using ScFv antibody conjugated gold nanoparticles that recognize the tumor biomarker EGFR. (a, b) SERS spectra obtained from the tumor and the liver locations by using targeted (a) and nontargeted (b) nanoparticles. Two nude mice bearing human head-and-neck squamous cell carcinoma (Tu686) xenograft tumor (3-mm diameter) received 90 mL of ScFv EGFR-conjugated SERS tags or PEGylated SERS tags (460 pM). The particles were administered via tail vein single injection. SERS spectra were taken 5 h after injection. (c) Photographs showing a laser beam focusing on the tumor site or on the anatomical location of liver. *In vivo* SERS spectra were obtained from the tumor site (red) and the liver site (blue) with 2-s signal integration and at 785 nm excitation. The spectra were background subtracted and shifted for better visualization. The Raman reporter molecule is malachite green, with distinct spectral signatures as labeled in A and B. Laser power, 20 mW. (Adapted with permission from Macmillan Publishers Ltd. *Nat. Biotechnol.*, Qian, X., Peng, X.H., Ansari, D.O., Yin-Goen, Q., Chen, G.Z., Shin, D.M., Yang, L.A., Young, N., Wang, M.D., and Nie, S., 26(1), 83–90. Copyright 2008.)

sensitivity of SERS will make it an ideal candidate to detect trace level of analytes relating to biomedicine or environment. Significant strides in applications can be expected because of the contribution of the multidisciplinary efforts and expertise in this exciting field.

Acknowledgments

The authors gratefully acknowledge financial support from the Center for Food Safety Engineering (CFSE) at Purdue University and the Brazilian Government Agency CNPq.

References

Adams, S. M., S. Campione, J. D. Caldwell, F. J. Bezares, J. C. Culbertson, F. Capolino, and R. Ragan. 2012. Non-lithographic SERS substrates: Tailoring surface chemistry for Au nanoparticle cluster assembly. *Small* 8(14):2239–2249.

Aksu, S., M. Huang, A. Artar, A. A. Yanik, S. Selvarasah, M. R. Dokmeci, and H. Altug. 2011. Flexible plasmonics on unconventional and nonplanar substrates. *Advanced Materials* 23(38):4422–4430.

Albrecht, M. G. and J. A. Creighton. 1977. Anomalously intense Raman-spectra of pyridine at a silver electrode. *Journal of the American Chemical Society* 99(15):5215–5217.

Allen, C. S. and R. P. Vanduyne. 1981. Molecular generality of surface-enhanced Raman-spectroscopy (SERS)—A detailed investigation of the hexacyanoruthenate ion adsorbed on silver and copper electrodes. *Journal of the American Chemical Society* 103(25):7497–7501.

Almond, L. M., J. Hutchings, N. Shepherd, H. Barr, N. Stone, and C. Kendall. 2011. Raman spectroscopy: A potential tool for early objective diagnosis of neoplasia in the oesophagus. *Journal of Biophotonics* 4(10):685–695.

Alvarez-Puebla, R. A., A. Agarwal, P. Manna, B. P. Khanal, P. Aldeanueva-Potel, E. Carbo-Argibay, N. Pazos-Perez et al. 2011. Gold nanorods 3D-supercrystals as surface enhanced Raman scattering spectroscopy substrates for the rapid detection of scrambled prions. *Proceedings of the National Academy of Sciences of the United States of America* 108(20):8157–8161.

Auchinvole, C. A., P. Richardson, C. McGuinnes, V. Mallikarjun, K. Donaldson, H. McNab, and C. J. Campbell. 2012. Monitoring intracellular redox potential changes using SERS nanosensors. *ACS Nano* 6(1):888–896.

Barcelo, S. J., A. Kim, W. Wu, and Z. Y. Li. 2012. Fabrication of deterministic nanostructure assemblies with sub-nanometer spacing using a nanoimprinting transfer technique. *ACS Nano* 6(7):6446–6452.

Barhoumi, A., D. Zhang, and N. J. Halas. 2008a. Correlation of molecular orientation and packing density in a dsDNA self-assembled monolayer observable with surface-enhanced Raman spectroscopy. *Journal of the American Chemical Society* 130(43):14040–14041.

Barhoumi, A., D. Zhang, F. Tam, and N. J. Halas. 2008b. Surface-enhanced Raman spectroscopy of DNA. *Journal of the American Chemical Society* 130(16):5523–5529.

Baumberg, J. J., T. A. Kelf, Y. Sugawara, S. Cintra, M. E. Abdelsalam, P. N. Bartlett, and A. E. Russell. 2005. Angle-resolved surface-enhanced Raman scattering on metallic nanostructured plasmonic crystals. *Nano Letters* 5(11):2262–2267.

Bell, S. E. and N. M. Sirimuthu. 2006. Surface-enhanced Raman spectroscopy (SERS) for submicromolar detection of DNA/RNA mononucleotides. *Journal of American Chemical Society* 128(49):15580–15581.

Bell, S. E. and N. M. Sirimuthu. 2008. Quantitative surface-enhanced Raman spectroscopy. *Chemical Society Reviews* 37(5):1012–1024.

Betzig, E., A. Lewis, A. Harootunian, M. Isaacson, and E. Kratschmer. 1986. Near-field scanning optical microscopy (NSOM)—Development and biophysical applications. *Biophysical Journal* 49(1):269–279.

Bishnoi, S. W., C. J. Rozell, C. S. Levin, M. K. Gheith, B. R. Johnson, D. H. Johnson, and N. J. Halas. 2006. All-optical nanoscale pH meter. *Nano Letters* 6(8):1687–1692.

Casadio, F., M. Leona, J. R. Lombardi, and R. Van Duyne. 2010. Identification of organic colorants in fibers, paints, and glazes by surface enhanced Raman spectroscopy. *Accounts of Chemical Research* 43(6):782–791.

Chen, L. Y., J. S. Yu, T. Fujita, and M. W. Chen. 2009. Nanoporous copper with tunable nanoporosity for SERS applications. *Advanced Functional Materials* 19(8):1221–1226.

Chu, H., Y. Huang, and Y. Zhao. 2008. Silver nanorod arrays as a surface-enhanced Raman scattering substrate for foodborne pathogenic bacteria detection. *Applied Spectroscopy* 62(8):922–931.

Chu, H. B., J. Y. Wang, L. Ding, D. N. Yuan, Y. Zhang, J. Liu, and Y. Li. 2009. Decoration of gold nanoparticles on surface-grown single-walled carbon nanotubes for detection of every nanotube by surface-enhanced Raman spectroscopy. *Journal of the American Chemical Society* 131(40):14310–14316.

Connatser, R. M., M. Cochran, R. J. Harrison, and M. J. Sepaniak. 2008. Analytical optimization of nanocomposite surface-enhanced Raman spectroscopy/scattering detection in microfluidic separation devices. *Electrophoresis* 29(7):1441–1450.

Corio, P., S. D. M. Brown, A. Marucci, M. A. Pimenta, K. Kneipp, G. Dresselhaus, and M. S. Dresselhaus. 2000. Surface-enhanced resonant Raman spectroscopy of single-wall carbon nanotubes adsorbed on silver and gold surfaces. *Physical Review B* 61(19):13202–13211.

Deckert, V., D. Zeisel, R. Zenobi, and T. Vo-Dinh. 1998. Near-field surface enhanced Raman imaging of dye-labeled DNA with 100-nm resolution. *Analytical Chemistry* 70(13):2646–2650.

Dougan, J. A. and K. Faulds. 2012. Surface enhanced Raman scattering for multiplexed detection. *Analyst* 137(3):545–554.

Driskell, J. D. and R. A. Tripp. 2010. Label-free SERS detection of microRNA based on affinity for an unmodified silver nanorod array substrate. *Chemical Communications* 46(19):3298–3300.

Driskell, J. D., Y. Zhu, C. D. Kirkwood, Y. Zhao, R. A. Dluhy, and R. A. Tripp. 2010. Rapid and sensitive detection of rotavirus molecular signatures using surface enhanced Raman spectroscopy. *PLoS One* 5(4):e10222.

Du, Y. B., L. F. Shi, T. C. He, X. W. Sun, and Y. J. Mo. 2008. SERS enhancement dependence on the diameter and aspect ratio of silver-nanowire array fabricated by anodic aluminium oxide template. *Applied Surface Science* 255(5):1901–1905.

El-Said, W. A., T. H. Kim, H. Kim, and J. W. Choi. 2010. Detection of effect of chemotherapeutic agents to cancer cells on gold nanoflower patterned substrate using surface-enhanced Raman scattering and cyclic voltammetry. *Biosensors and Bioelectronics* 26(4):1486–1492.

Esenturk, E. N. and A. R. H. Walker. 2009. Surface-enhanced Raman scattering spectroscopy via gold nanostars. *Journal of Raman Spectroscopy* 40(1):86–91.

Evans, C. L., E. O. Potma, M. Puoris'haag, D. Côté, C. P. Lin, and X. S. Xie. 2005. Chemical imaging of tissue in vivo with video-rate coherent anti-Stokes Raman scattering microscopy. *Proceedings of the National Academy of Sciences of the United States of America* 102(46):16807–16812.

Fan, C., Z. Hu, A. Mustapha, and M. Lin. 2011. Rapid detection of food-and waterborne bacteria using surface-enhanced Raman spectroscopy coupled with silver nanosubstrates. *Applied Microbiology and Biotechnology* 92(5):1053–1061.

Fan, Y. Q., H. H. Cheng, C. Zhou, X. J. Xie, Y. Liu, L. M. Dai, J. Zhang, and L. T. Qu. 2012. Honeycomb architecture of carbon quantum dots: A new efficient substrate to support gold for stronger SERS. *Nanoscale* 4(5):1776–1781.

Fleischm.M, P. J. Hendra, and A. J. Mcquilla. 1974. Raman-spectra of pyridine adsorbed at a silver electrode. *Chemical Physics Letters* 26(2):163–166.

Gutes, A., C. Carraro, and R. Maboudian. 2010. Silver dendrites from galvanic displacement on commercial aluminum foil as an effective SERS substrate. *Journal of the American Chemical Society* 132(5):1476–1477.

Guven, B., N. Basaran-Akgul, E. Temur, U. Tamer, and I. H. Boyaci. 2011. SERS-based sandwich immunoassay using antibody coated magnetic nanoparticles for *Escherichia coli* enumeration. *Analyst* 136(4):740–748.

Hankus, M. E., H. Li, G. J. Gibson, and B. M. Cullum. 2006. Surface-enhanced Raman scattering-based nanoprobe for high-resolution, non-scanning chemical imaging. *Analytical Chemistry* 78(21):7535–7546.

He, L., Y. Liu, M. Lin, A. Mustapha, and Y. Wang. 2008. Detecting single *Bacillus* spores by surface enhanced Raman spectroscopy. *Sensing and Instrumentation for Food Quality and Safety* 2(4):247–253.

Holthoff, E. L., D. N. Stratis-Cullum, and M. E. Hankus. 2011. A nanosensor for TNT detection based on molecularly imprinted polymers and surface enhanced Raman scattering. *Sensors* 11(3):2700–2714.

Horsnell, J. D., J. A. Smith, M. Sattlecker, A. Sammon, J. Christie-Brown, C. Kendall, and N. Stone. 2012. Raman spectroscopy—A potential new method for the intra-operative assessment of axillary lymph nodes. *Surgeon* 10(3):123–127.

Hutter, E. and J. H. Fendler. 2004. Exploitation of localized surface plasmon resonance. *Advanced Materials* 16(19):1685–1706.

Jarvis, R. M., N. Law, I. T. Shadi, P. O'Brien, J. R. Lloyd, and R. Goodacre. 2008. Surface-enhanced Raman scattering from intracellular and extracellular bacterial locations. *Analytical Chemistry* 80(17):6741–6746.

Jeanmaire, D. L. and R. P. Vanduyne. 1977. Surface Raman spectroelectrochemistry. 1. Heterocyclic, aromatic, and aliphatic-amines adsorbed on anodized silver electrode. *Journal of Electroanalytical Chemistry* 84(1):1–20.

Jehn, C., B. Küstner, P. Adam, A. Marx, P. Ströbel, C. Schmuck, and S. Schlücker. 2009. Water soluble SERS labels comprising a SAM with dual spacers for controlled bioconjugation. *Physical Chemistry Chemical Physics* 11(34):7499–7504.

Joo, Y. and J. S. Suh. 1995. SERS on silver formed in anodic aluminum-oxide nanotemplates. *Bulletin of the Korean Chemical Society* 16(9):808–810.

Jung, N., A. C. Crowther, N. Kim, P. Kim, and L. Brus. 2010. Raman enhancement on graphene: Adsorbed and intercalated molecular species. *ACS Nano* 4(11):7005–7013.

Kim, K. and H. S. Lee. 2005. Effect of Ag and Au nanoparticles on the SERS of 4-aminobenzenethiol assembled on powdered copper. *Journal of Physical Chemistry B* 109(40):18929–18934.

Kneipp, J., G. Balakrishnan, R. Chen, T. J. Shen, S. C. Sahu, N. T. Ho, J. L. Giovannelli, V. Simplaceanu, C. Ho, and T. G. Spiro. 2006a. Dynamics of allostery in hemoglobin: Roles of the penultimate tyrosine H bonds. *Journal of Molecular Biology* 356(2):335–353.

Kneipp, J., H. Kneipp, and K. Kneipp. 2006b. Two-photon vibrational spectroscopy for biosciences based on surface-enhanced hyper-Raman scattering. *Proceedings of the National Academy of Sciences of the United States of America* 103(46):17149–17153.

Kneipp, J., H. Kneipp, M. McLaughlin, D. Brown, and K. Kneipp. 2006d. In vivo molecular probing of cellular compartments with gold nanoparticles and nanoaggregates. *Nano Letters* 6(10):2225–2231.

Kneipp, J., H. Kneipp, B. Wittig, and K. Kneipp. 2010a. Novel optical nanosensors for probing and imaging live cells. *Nanomedicine* 6(2):214–226.

Kneipp, J., H. Kneipp, B. Wittig, and K. Kneipp. 2010b. Following the dynamics of pH in endosomes of live cells with SERS nanosensors. *Journal of Physical Chemistry C* 114(16):7421–7426.

Kneipp, K., A. S. Haka, H. Kneipp, K. Badizadegan, N. Yoshizawa, C. Boone, K. E. Shafer-Peltier, J. T. Motz, R. R. Dasari, and M. S. Feld. 2002. Surface-enhanced Raman spectroscopy in single living cells using gold nanoparticles. *Applied Spectroscopy* 56(2):150–154.

Kneipp, K. and H. Kneipp. 2006. Single molecule Raman scattering. *Applied Spectroscopy* 60(12):322A–334A.

Kneipp, K., H. Kneipp, and J. Kneipp. 2006c. Surface-enhanced Raman scattering in local optical fields of silver and gold nanoaggregates—From single-molecule Raman spectroscopy to ultra-sensitive probing in live cells. *Accounts of Chemical Research* 39(7):443–450.

Kneipp, K., M. Moskovits, and H. Kneipp. 2006e. *Surface-Enhanced Raman Scattering: Physics and Applications, Topics in Applied Physics*. Berlin, Germany: Springer.

Kneipp, K., Y. Wang, H. Kneipp, L. T. Perelman, I. Itzkan, R. Dasari, and M. S. Feld. 1997. Single molecule detection using surface-enhanced Raman scattering (SERS). *Physical Review Letters* 78(9):1667–1670.

Kokkonen, N., A. Rivinoja, A. Kauppila, M. Suokas, I. Kellokumpu, and S. Kellokumpu. 2004. Defective acidification of intracellular organelles results in aberrant secretion of cathepsin D in cancer cells. *Journal of Biological Chemistry* 279(38):39982–39988.

Kuncicky, D. M., B. G. Prevo, and O. D. Velev. 2006. Controlled assembly of SERS substrates templated by colloidal crystal films. *Journal of Materials Chemistry* 16(13):1207–1211.

Le Ru, E. C. and P. G. Etchegoin. 2009. *Principles of Surface-Enhanced Raman Spectroscopy: And Related Plasmonic Effects*. Amsterdam, the Netherlands: Elsevier Science.

Lee, K., V. P. Drachev, and J. Irudayaraj. 2011. DNA-gold nanoparticle reversible networks grown on cell surface marker sites: Application in diagnostics. *ACS Nano* 5(3):2109–2117.

Lee, S., M. G. Hahm, R. Vajtai, D. P. Hashim, T. Thurakitseree, A. C. Chipara, P. M. Ajayan, and J. H. Hafner. 2012. Utilizing 3D SERS active volumes in aligned carbon nanotube scaffold substrates. *Advanced Materials* 24(38):5261–5266.

Légaré, F., C. L. Evans, F. Ganikhanov, and X. S. Xie. 2006. Towards CARS endoscopy. *Optics Express* 14(10):4427–4432.

Li, X. H., G. Y. Chen, L. B. Yang, Z. Jin, and J. H. Liu. 2010. Multifunctional Au-coated TiO_2 nanotube arrays as recyclable SERS substrates for multifold organic pollutants detection. *Advanced Functional Materials* 20(17):2815–2824.

Lieber, C. A., E. M. Kanter, and A. Mahadevan-Jansen. 2008a. Comparison of Raman spectrograph throughput using two commercial systems: Transmissive versus reflective. *Applied Spectroscopy* 62(5):575–582.

Lieber, C. A., S. K. Majumder, D. Billheimer, D. L. Ellis, and A. Mahadevan-Jansen. 2008b. Raman microspectroscopy for skin cancer detection in vitro. *Journal of Biomedical Optics* 13(2):024013.

Ling, X., L. M. Xie, Y. Fang, H. Xu, H. L. Zhang, J. Kong, M. S. Dresselhaus, J. Zhang, and Z. F. Liu. 2010. Can graphene be used as a substrate for Raman enhancement? *Nano Letters* 10(2):553–561.

Ling, X. and J. Zhang. 2010. First-layer effect in graphene-enhanced Raman scattering. *Small* 6(18):2020–2025.

Link, S., M. B. Mohamed, and M. A. El-Sayed. 1999. Simulation of the optical absorption spectra of gold nanorods as a function of their aspect ratio and the effect of the medium dielectric constant. *Journal of Physical Chemistry B* 103(16):3073–3077.

Liu, G. L. and L. P. Lee. 2005. Nanowell surface enhanced Raman scattering arrays fabricated by soft-lithography for label-free biomolecular detections in integrated microfluidics. *Applied Physics Letters* 87(7): 074101.

Livingstone, R., X. C. Zhou, M. C. Tamargo, J. R. Lombardi, L. C. Quagliano, and F. Jean-Mary. 2010. Surface enhanced Raman spectroscopy of pyridine on CdSe/ZnBeSe quantum dots crown by molecular beam epitaxy. *Journal of Physical Chemistry C* 114(41):17460–17464.

Lo, H. C., H. I. Hsiung, S. Chattopadhyay, H. C. Han, C. F. Chen, J. P. Leu, K. H. Chen, and L. C. Chen. 2011b. Label free sub-picomole level DNA detection with Ag nanoparticle decorated Au nanotip arrays as surface enhanced Raman spectroscopy platform. *Biosensors and Bioelectronics* 26(5):2413–2418.

Lo, Y. L., C. F. Hsiao, Y. S. Jou, G. C. Chang, Y. H. Tsai, W. C. Su, K. Y. Chen et al. 2011a. Polymorphisms of MLH1 and MSH2 genes and the risk of lung cancer among never smokers. *Lung Cancer* 72(3):280–286.

Lowe, A. J., Y. S. Huh, A. D. Strickland, D. Erickson, and C. A. Batt. 2010. Multiplex single nucleotide polymorphism genotyping utilizing ligase detection reaction coupled surface enhanced Raman spectroscopy. *Analytical Chemistry* 82(13):5810–5814.

Lu, X. M., M. Rycenga, S. E. Skrabalak, B. Wiley, and Y. N. Xia. 2009. Chemical synthesis of novel plasmonic nanoparticles. *Annual Review of Physical Chemistry* 60:167–192.

Lu, Y., G. L. Liu, J. Kim, Y. X. Mejia, and L. P. Lee. 2005. Nanophotonic crescent moon structures with sharp edge for ultrasensitive biomolecular detection by local electromagnetic field enhancement effect. *Nano Letters* 5(1):119–124.

MacAskill, A., D. Crawford, D. Graham, and K. Faulds. 2009. DNA sequence detection using surface-enhanced resonance Raman spectroscopy in a homogeneous multiplexed assay. *Analytical Chemistry* 81(19):8134–8140.

Motz, J. T., M. Fitzmaurice, A. Miller, S. J. Gandhi, A. S. Haka, L. H. Galindo, R. R. Dasari, J. R. Kramer, and M. S. Feld. 2006. In vivo Raman spectral pathology of human atherosclerosis and vulnerable plaque. *Journal of Biomedical Optics* 11(2):021003.

Musumeci, A., D. Gosztola, T. Schiller, N. M. Dimitrijevic, V. Mujica, D. Martin, and T. Rajh. 2009. SERS of semiconducting nanoparticles (TiO_2 hybrid composites). *Journal of the American Chemical Society* 131(17):6040.

Neugebauer, U., P. Rosch, M. Schmitt, J. Popp, C. Julien, A. Rasmussen, C. Budich, and V. Deckert. 2006a. On the way to nanometer-sized information of the bacterial surface by tip-enhanced Raman spectroscopy. *ChemPhysChem* 7(7):1428–1430.

Neugebauer, U., U. Schmid, K. Baumann, U. Holzgrabe, W. Ziebuhr, S. Kozitskaya, W. Kiefer, M. Schmitt, and J. Popp. 2006b. Characterization of bacterial growth and the influence of antibiotics by means of UV resonance Raman spectroscopy. *Biopolymers* 82(4):306–311.

Neumann, O., D. Zhang, F. Tam, S. Lal, P. Wittung-Stafshede, and N. J. Halas. 2009. Direct optical detection of aptamer conformational changes induced by target molecules. *Analytical Chemistry* 81(24):10002–10006.

Nie, S. M. and S. R. Emery. 1997. Probing single molecules and single nanoparticles by surface-enhanced Raman scattering. *Science* 275(5303):1102–1106.

Nijssen, A., K. Maquelin, L. F. Santos, P. J. Caspers, T. C. Bakker Schut, J. C. den Hollander, M. H. Neumann, and G. J. Puppels. 2007. Discriminating basal cell carcinoma from perilesional skin using high wave-number Raman spectroscopy. *Journal of Biomedical Optics* 12(3):034004.

Ochsenkuhn, M. A., P. R. Jess, H. Stoquert, K. Dholakia, and C. J. Campbell. 2009. Nanoshells for surface-enhanced Raman spectroscopy in eukaryotic cells: Cellular response and sensor development. *ACS Nano* 3(11):3613–3621.

Oldenburg, S. J., R. D. Averitt, S. L. Westcott, and N. J. Halas. 1998. Nanoengineering of optical resonances. *Chemical Physics Letters* 288(2–4):243–247.

Olivares-Amaya, R., D. Rappoport, P. A. Munoz, P. Peng, E. Mazur, and A. Aspuru-Guzik. 2012. Can mixed-metal surfaces provide an additional enhancement to SERS? *Journal of Physical Chemistry C* 116(29):15568–15575.

Patel, I. S., W. R. Premasiri, D. T. Moir, and L. D. Ziegler. 2008. Barcoding bacterial cells: A SERS-based methodology for pathogen identification. *Journal of Raman Spectroscopy* 39(11):1660–1672.

Pettinger, B., B. Ren, G. Picardi, R. Schuster, and G. Ertl. 2004. Nanoscale probing of adsorbed species by tip-enhanced Raman spectroscopy. *Physical Review Letters* 92(9):096101.

Qian, X., X. H. Peng, D. O. Ansari, Q. Yin-Goen, G. Z. Chen, D. M. Shin, L. Yang, A. N. Young, M. D. Wang, and S. Nie. 2008. In vivo tumor targeting and spectroscopic detection with surface-enhanced Raman nanoparticle tags. *Nature Biotechnology* 26(1):83–90.

Qiu, C. Y., H. Q. Zhou, H. C. Yang, M. J. Chen, Y. J. Guo, and L. F. Sun. 2011. Investigation of n-layer graphenes as substrates for Raman enhancement of crystal violet. *Journal of Physical Chemistry C* 115(20):10019–10025.

Quagliano, L. G. 2004. Observation of molecules adsorbed on III-V semiconductor quantum dots by surface-enhanced Raman scattering. *Journal of the American Chemical Society* 126(23):7393–7398.

Ravindranath, S. P., Y. Wang, and J. Irudayaraj. 2011. SERS driven cross-platform based multiplex pathogen detection. *Sensors and Actuators B-Chemical* 152(2):183–190.

Ren, B., G. Picardi, B. Pettinger, R. Schuster, and G. Ertl. 2004. Tip-enhanced Raman spectroscopy of benzenethiol adsorbed on Au and Pt single-crystal surfaces. *Angewandte Chemie International Edition in English* 44(1):139–142.

Ren, W., Y. Fang, and E. Wang. 2011. A binary functional substrate for enrichment and ultrasensitive SERS spectroscopic detection of folic acid using graphene oxide/Ag nanoparticle hybrids. *ACS Nano* 5(8):6425–6433.

Sćepanović, O. R., M. Fitzmaurice, J. A. Gardecki, G. O. Angheloiu, S. Awasthi, J. T. Motz, J. R. Kramer, R. R. Dasari, and M. S. Feld. 2006. Detection of morphological markers of vulnerable atherosclerotic plaque using multimodal spectroscopy. *Journal of Biomedical Optics* 11(2):021007.

Schlücker, S. 2009. SERS microscopy: Nanoparticle probes and biomedical applications. *ChemPhysChem* 10(9–10):1344–1354.

Schlücker, S. 2011. *Surface Enhanced Raman Spectroscopy: Analytical, Biophysical and Life Science Applications*. Weinheim, Germany: Wiley-VCH.

Shanmukh, S., L. Jones, J. Driskell, Y. P. Zhao, R. Dluhy, and R. A. Tripp. 2006. Rapid and sensitive detection of respiratory virus molecular signatures using a silver nanorod array SERS substrate. *Nano Letters* 6(11):2630–2636.

Sharma, B., R. R. Frontiera, A. I. Henry, E. Ringe, and R. P. Van Duyne. 2012. SERS: Materials, applications, and the future. *Materials Today* 15(1–2):16–25.

Sun, L. and J. Irudayaraj. 2009a. PCR-free quantification of multiple splice variants in a cancer gene by surface-enhanced Raman spectroscopy. *The Journal of Physical Chemistry B* 113 (42):14021–14025.

Sun, L. and J. Irudayaraj. 2009b. Quantitative surface-enhanced Raman for gene expression estimation. *Biophysical Journal* 96(11):4709–4716.

Sun, L., C. Yu, and J. Irudayaraj. 2007. Surface-enhanced Raman scattering based nonfluorescent probe for multiplex DNA detection. *Analytical Chemistry* 79(11):3981–3988.

Sun, L., C. Yu, and J. Irudayaraj. 2008. Raman multiplexers for alternative gene splicing. *Analytical Chemistry* 80(9):3342–3349.

Sun, Y. H., K. Liu, J. Miao, Z. Y. Wang, B. Z. Tian, L. N. Zhang, Q. Q. Li, S. S. Fan, and K. L. Jiang. 2010. Highly sensitive surface-enhanced Raman scattering substrate made from superaligned carbon nanotubes. *Nano Letters* 10(5):1747–1753.

Teguh, J. S., F. Liu, B. G. Xing, and E. K. L. Yeow. 2012. Surface-enhanced Raman scattering (SERS) of nitrothiophenol isomers chemisorbed on TiO$_2$. *Chemistry: An Asian Journal* 7(5):975–981.

Temur, E., I. H. Boyaci, U. Tamer, H. Unsal, and N. Aydogan. 2010. A highly sensitive detection platform based on surface-enhanced Raman scattering for *Escherichia coli* enumeration. *Analytical and Bioanalytical Chemistry* 397(4):1595–1604.

Tu, Q. and C. Chang. 2012. Diagnostic applications of Raman spectroscopy. *Nanomedicine-Nanotechnology Biology and Medicine* 8(5):545–558.

Tuschel, D. D., J. E. Pemberton, and J. E. Cook. 1986. SERS and SEM of roughened silver electrode surfaces formed by controlled oxidation reduction in aqueous chloride media. *Langmuir* 2(4):380–388.

Wang, G., R. J. Lipert, M. Jain, S. Kaur, S. Chakraboty, M. P. Torres, S. K. Batra, R. E. Brand, and M. D. Porter. 2011. Detection of the potential pancreatic cancer marker MUC4 in serum using surface-enhanced Raman scattering. *Analytical Chemistry* 83(7):2554–2561.

Wang, H. and N. J. Halas. 2008. Mesoscopic Au "Meatball" particles. *Advanced Materials* 20(4):820–825.

Wang, H. H., C. Y. Liu, S. B. Wu, N. W. Liu, C. Y. Peng, T. H. Chan, C. F. Hsu, J. K. Wang, and Y. L. Wang. 2006. Highly Raman-enhancing substrates based on silver nanoparticle arrays with tunable sub-10 nm gaps. *Advanced Materials* 18(4):491–495.

Wang, J. and X. Yang. 2009. Multiplex binding modes of toluidine blue with calf thymus DNA and conformational transition of DNA revealed by spectroscopic studies. *Spectrochimica Acta Part A: Molecular and Biomolecular Spectroscopy* 74(2):421–426.

Wang, Y., K. Lee, and J. Irudayaraj. 2010. Silver nanosphere SERS probes for sensitive identification of pathogens. *Journal of Physical Chemistry C* 114(39):16122–16128.

Wang, Y., S. Ravindranath, and J. Irudayaraj. 2011. Separation and detection of multiple pathogens in a food matrix by magnetic SERS nanoprobes. *Analytical and Bioanalytical Chemistry* 399(3):1271–1278.

Wang, Y. F., J. H. Zhang, H. Y. Jia, M. J. Li, J. B. Zeng, B. Yang, B. Zhao, W. Q. Xu, and J. R. Lombardi. 2008. Mercaptopyridine surface-functionalized CdTe quantum dots with enhanced Raman scattering properties. *Journal of Physical Chemistry C* 112(4):996–1000.

Watanabe, S., Y. Mino, Y. Ichikawa, and M. T. Miyahara. 2012. Spontaneous formation of cluster array of gold particles by convective self-assembly. *Langmuir* 28(36):12982–12988.

West, P. R., S. Ishii, G. V. Naik, N. K. Emani, V. M. Shalaev, and A. Boltasseva. 2010. Searching for better plasmonic materials. *Laser & Photonics Reviews* 4(6):795–808.

Wu, D. Y., X. M. Liu, S. Duan, X. Xu, B. Ren, S. H. Lin, and Z. Q. Tian. 2008. Chemical enhancement effects in SERS spectra: A quantum chemical study of pyridine interacting with copper, silver, gold and platinum metals. *Journal of Physical Chemistry C* 112(11):4195–4204.

Xie, J. P., Q. B. Zhang, J. Y. Lee, and D. I. C. Wang. 2008. The synthesis of SERS-active gold nanoflower tags for in vivo applications. *ACS Nano* 2(12):2473–2480.

Xue, G., J. F. Ding, P. Lu, and J. Dong. 1991. SERS, XPS, and electroanalytical studies of the chemisorption of benzotriazole on a freshly etched surface and an oxidized surface of copper. *Journal of Physical Chemistry* 95(19):7380–7384.

Yan, B., A. Thubagere, W. R. Premasiri, L. D. Ziegler, L. Dal Negro, and B. M. Reinhard. 2009. Engineered SERS substrates with multiscale signal enhancement: Nanoplarticle cluster arrays. *ACS Nano* 3(5):1190–1202.

Yang, S. K., W. P. Cai, L. C. Kong, and Y. Lei. 2010. Surface nanometer-scale patterning in realizing large-scale ordered arrays of metallic nanoshells with well-defined structures and controllable properties. *Advanced Functional Materials* 20(15):2527–2533.

Yang, Z. L., Q. H. Li, B. Ren, and Z. Q. Tian. 2011. Tunable SERS from aluminium nanohole arrays in the ultraviolet region. *Chemical Communications* 47(13):3909–3911.

Yap, F. L., P. Thoniyot, S. Krishnan, and S. Krishnamoorthy. 2012. Nanoparticle cluster arrays for high-performance SERS through directed self-assembly on flat substrates and on optical fibers. *ACS Nano* 6(3):2056–2070.

Zeisel, D., V. Deckert, R. Zenobi, and T. Vo-Dinh. 1998. Near-field surface-enhanced Raman spectroscopy of dye molecules adsorbed on silver island films. *Chemical Physics Letters* 283(5–6):381–385.

Zhang, X. Y., J. Zhao, A. V. Whitney, J. W. Elam, and R. P. Van Duyne. 2006. Ultrastable substrates for surface-enhanced Raman spectroscopy: Al_2O_3 overlayers fabricated by atomic layer deposition yield improved anthrax biomarker detection. *Journal of the American Chemical Society* 128(31):10304–10309.

Zhang, Y., H. Hong, D. V. Myklejord, and W. B. Cai. 2011. Molecular imaging with SERS-active nanoparticles. *Small* 7(23):3261–3269.

Zong, S., Z. Wang, J. Yang, C. Wang, S. Xu, and Y. Cui. 2012. A SERS and fluorescence dual mode cancer cell targeting probe based on silica coated Au@Ag core-shell nanorods. *Talanta* 97:368–375.

8

Photonic Crystal Biosensors

Bashar Hamza, Maurya Srungarapu, Anand Kadiyala,
Jeremy Dawson, and Lawrence Hornak

CONTENTS

8.1 Photonic Crystal Basics

The use of engineered nanoscale lattice structures, or photonic crystals, to control light energy propagation was pioneered by Yablonoivitch (1987) and John (1987). Their objective was to inhibit spontaneous emission and study light localization in periodic dielectric structures. They realized that the periodicity of the engineered lattice and the materials it comprises define energy propagation regimes in the crystal-like structure. While this was the first rigorous examination of engineered lattices, such structures existed in nature well before they were replicated by the scientific community (see, e.g., Vukusic and Sambles 2003, Welch et al. 2007). Any periodic dielectric structure made up of two materials with sufficient difference in refractive index, and features that are on the order of the wavelength of the interacting electromagnetic energy, will possess an optical bandgap analogous to that found in semiconductors and the unique optical properties that arise from it (Benisty et al. 2005; Saleh and Teich 2007; Joannopoulos et al. 2008; Prather et al. 2009). This optical bandgap can easily be observed in butterfly wings, insect carapaces, and certain

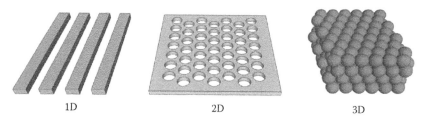

1D   2D   3D

FIGURE 8.1
(See color insert.) Three types of photonic crystals (PhCs).

minerals, which possess color not due to pigmentation, but rather due to nanoscale periodic lattice structures made up of proteins or other materials. Photonic crystal (PhC) periodicity can occur in one, two, or three directions, as shown in Figure 8.1.

A typical example of a one-dimensional (1D) photonic crystal is the well-studied distributed Bragg reflector (DBR), comprised two or more different optical materials stacked on top of each other in a periodic fashion. Although these DBRs are now considered a 1D class of PhCs, they were studied for several years before the findings of Yablonoivitch and John (Bykov 1972, 1975, 1978). Currently, these structures are employed in a wide variety of optoelectronic devices (Prather et al. 2009). Two-dimensional (2D) PhCs occur when the dielectric variation is engineered to be periodic in two directions and can be considered constant along the third direction. This is achieved by either introducing holes of a low dielectric material with specific symmetry in a higher dielectric material, or simply the opposite case in which pillars of a high dielectric material are surrounded by a low dielectric background. In three-dimensional (3D) PhCs, the refractive index is varied periodically in all three dimensions. This 3D order can be achieved using modified top-down fabrication methods used in the semiconductor industry or bottom-up approaches that take advantage of self-assembly of proteins or engineered nanoparticles. Fabrication methods will be discussed later in this chapter.

The most significant characteristic of PhCs is the ability to engineer optical bandgaps for wavelengths spanning the visible spectrum. This feature has made PhCs attractive for a wide variety of applications, such as waveguides and optical filters (Prather et al. 2009). Another attribute of the PhC lattice is the potential for creating localized regions of optical behavior through the introduction of defects in an otherwise ordered PhC lattice. High quality factor resonators, beam splitters, lasers, and light emitting diodes (LEDs) are among the most common device applications for PhCs (Prather et al. 2009).

In addition to the objective of creating integrated nanophotonic devices, PhC lattices have also been the focus of intensive research involving optical-based sensors that have the potential to exhibit single-molecule detection limits, beyond what can be achieved using conventional mechanical and electrochemical methods alone (Nair and Vijaya 2010). The design of these PhC-based sensor solutions is aimed at meeting the high demand for accurate sensors that allow untrained operators to detect trace amounts of target analyte using high-throughput, portable platforms in health, defense, and even biometric applications. Since the photonic bandgap of a PhC is determined by the indices of refraction of the lattice materials and the dimensions of the lattice features, any change in these characteristics has the potential to measurably change the optical properties. This behavior can be exploited in "active" sensor modalities in which the presence of a target analyte affects the measurable light interaction with the lattice, such as transmission and reflection properties. The photonic bandgap can also be exploited in "passive" detection methodologies, where the transmission and reflection properties of the lattice or localized defect regions are used to enhance the emission wavelength of naturally fluorescent or labeled analytes.

This chapter provides a review of the theoretical concepts necessary for PhC design and modeling, as well as a description of common fabrication methods. A literature review providing a survey of active and passive PhC biosensor devices is provided, accompanied by a discussion of future trends and applications of PhC biosensors.

8.1.1 Photonic Crystal Theory

To fully understand the behavior of electromagnetic waves in photonic bandgap materials, it is better to first discuss the similarities between the Schrodinger and Maxwell equations that govern the motion of electrons and photons, respectively. The electron behavior is described using the Schrodinger equation (Benisty et al. 2005; Saleh and Teich 2007; Joannopoulos et al. 2008; Prather et al. 2009)

$$\left[\frac{-h^2}{8\pi^2 m^*}\nabla^2 + V(r)\right]\varphi(r) = E\varphi(r) \tag{8.1}$$

where

$[(-h^2/8\pi^2 m^*)\nabla^2 + V(r)]$ is the Hamiltonian operator
h is Planck's constant
m^* is the effective mass of the electron
$V(r)$ is the potential function
E is the total energy
$\varphi(r)$ is the wave function of the electron, which is interpreted as the probability amplitude function

For a defect-free crystal lattice, the potential is periodic; $V(r) = V(r+R)$, where R is a vector that represents the displacement between plane waves that are modulated by an amplitude function relative to the periodicity of the lattice. These waves are commonly known as Bloch waves (Prather et al. 2009). On the other hand, the electromagnetic fields are governed by classic electromagnetic theory. The fields are described using four equations that relate the electric field to the magnetic field and to other present sources or charges within the medium. These are called Maxwell's equations and in the absence of magnetic media, two of the four equations can be combined, as will be explained in the following section, to yield the final *master* PhC equation

$$\left[\nabla \times \frac{1}{\varepsilon(r)}\nabla \times\right]H(r) = \left(\frac{\omega}{c}\right)^2 H(r) \tag{8.2}$$

where
$\left[\nabla \times \left(1/\varepsilon(r)\right)\nabla \times\right]$ is Maxwell's operator

$H(r)$ is the magnetic field
ω is the angular frequency
c is the speed of light in vacuum
$\varepsilon(r)$ is the dielectric permittivity

Similar to the atomic crystalline lattice, photonic crystals have a periodic dielectric structure, $\varepsilon(r) = \varepsilon$ $(r + R)$, and solutions are also Bloch waves. It is obvious that both Equations 8.1 and 8.2, are of the eigenvalue/eigenfunction type. They both describe a wave-like function in space, $\varphi(r)$ in (8.1) and $H(r)$ in (8.2), and each wave exists in a periodic medium characterized by a periodic potential V (for electrons) and a periodic permittivity ε (for photons).

Photonic crystals have discrete translational symmetry that is not invariant under translations of any distance, but rather, only distances that are a multiple of some fixed step length commonly known as the lattice constant. The simplest example of such a system is the 1D PhC (Figure 8.2). For this system, a continuous translational symmetry can be observed in the x and z directions and a discrete translational symmetry in the y direction with a basic step length, which is called the lattice constant, a. In other words, the dielectric constant is only varying along the y direction. The discrete symmetry will allow us to write the dielectric function in terms of the lattice constant as follows (Benisty et al. 2005; Saleh and Teich 2007; Joannopoulos et al. 2008; Prather et al. 2009):

$$\varepsilon(r) = \varepsilon(r \pm a) \tag{8.3}$$

By repeating this translation, we see that $\varepsilon(r) = \varepsilon(r \pm R)$ for any R that is an integral multiple of a; $R = la$ where l is an integer. The discrete periodicity in the y direction leads to a y-dependency for H that is simply the product of a plane wave with a y-periodic function. The plane wave is similar to that in free space but modulated by a periodic function because of the periodic lattice as shown in the following (Joannopoulos et al. 2008):

$$H(\ldots, y, \ldots) \, \alpha \, e^{ik_y y} \cdot u_{k_y}(y, \ldots) \tag{8.4}$$

The modes can then be written as follows:

$$H_{k_y}(r) = e^{ik_y y} \cdot u_{k_y}(r) = e^{ik_y y} \cdot u_{k_y}(r + R) \tag{8.5}$$

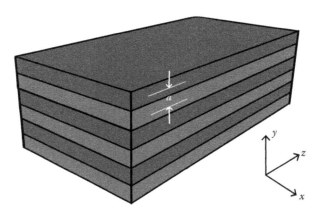

FIGURE 8.2
A 1D photonic crystal with varying dielectric constant in the y direction. Dark layers can represent high refractive index regions while light colored layers can represent low refractive index regions.

This result is commonly known as Bloch's theorem. In solid state physics, the form of Equation 8.4 is known as a Bloch state (Benisty et al. 2005; Saleh and Teich 2007; Joannopoulos et al. 2008; Prather et al. 2009). Bloch states with a wave vector k_y and that of a wave vector $k_y + mb$ where m is an integer, are identical. In fact, all the k_ys that differ by an integral multiple of $b = 2\pi/a$ are not different from a physical point of view. This allows us to consider only k_ys that exist in the range $(-\pi/a) < k_y \leq (\pi/a)$, which is the region of nonredundant values of k_y. This region is commonly known as the Brillouin zone, which is explained later in this section. In this region, the dielectric is invariant under translations through a multitude of lattice vectors and $R = la_1 + ma_2 + na_3$ for some integers l, m, and n (Joannopoulos et al. 2008). The real space vectors, a_1, a_2, and a_3, give rise to three primitive reciprocal lattice vectors, b_1, b_2, and b_3, defined in such a way that $a_i.b_j = 2\pi\delta_{ij}$. These reciprocal vectors, which will also be explained later in this section, span a reciprocal lattice of their own, which is inherited by wave vectors (Benisty et al. 2005; Saleh and Teich 2007; Joannopoulos et al. 2008; Prather et al. 2009).

The modes of a 3D periodic system are Bloch states that can be labeled by a Bloch wave vector $k = k_1b_1 + k_2b_2 + k_3b_3$, where k lies in the Brillouin zone. Each value of the wave vector k inside the Brillouin zone identifies an eigenstate of L with frequency $\omega(k)$ and an eigenvector H_k of the following form:

$$H_k(r) = e^{ik.r}u_k(r) \tag{8.6}$$

where $u_k(r)$ is a periodic function on the lattice $u_k(r) = u_k(r + R)$ for all lattice vectors R. The wave vector k is a conserved quantity in a periodic system and hence the addition of a reciprocal lattice vector does not change an eigenstate or its propagation direction. This is different from the free-space case, in which all wave vectors represent physically distinct states (Prather et al. 2009).

Equation 8.6 demonstrates how the electromagnetic modes of a PhC with discrete periodicity can be written as Bloch states. All of the information about these modes is given by the wave vector k and the periodic function $u_k(r)$. To solve for $u_k(r)$, the Bloch state can be inserted into the master equation to get the following:

$$\hat{L}_k u_k(r) = \left(\frac{\omega(k)}{c}\right)^2 u_k(r) \tag{8.7}$$

where $\hat{L}_k$ is the new Hermitian operator defined as $\hat{L}_k = (ik + \nabla) \times (1/\varepsilon(r))(ik + \nabla) \times$. The function u and the mode profiles are determined by the eigenvalue problem that is restricted to a single unit cell of the photonic crystal lattice to create a discrete spectrum of eigenvalues. Hence, for each value of k, an infinite set of modes with discretely spaced frequencies can be found, which we can label by a band index n. And since k enters as a continuous parameter in $\hat{L}$, the frequency of each band varies continuously as k varies. Therefore, the modes of a PhC are simply a set of continuous functions $\omega_n(k)$ indexed in the order of increasing frequency by the band number. The information contained in these functions is called the band structure of the PhC. Studying the band structure of a crystal supplies us with most of the information we need to predict its optical properties.

For a given PhC with a periodic dielectric function $\varepsilon(r)$, we can use powerful computational tools that solve Equation 8.7 as a standard eigenvalue equation in an iterative

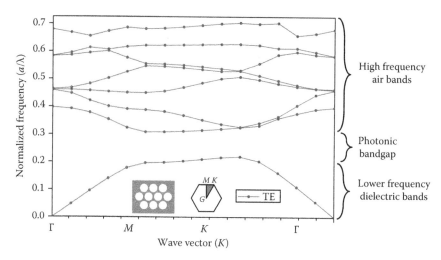

FIGURE 8.3
TE band diagram of a two-dimensional infinitely thick photonic crystal of triangular lattice of air holes in silicon.

minimization technique for each value of k. The electromagnetic variational theorem states that "the lowest frequency mode of a system is the field pattern that minimizes the electromagnetic energy functional," (Nightingale 2008) and this is accomplished by concentrating electric field energy in the high dielectric regions. Therefore, the definition of a PhC's *dielectric* and *air* bands is analogous to a semiconductor's valence and conduction bands. A band diagram of a 2D infinitely long PhC of triangular lattice of air holes in silicon is shown in Figure 8.3. In this figure, the lower frequency dielectric bands have their electric field energy mostly concentrated in higher dielectric regions, while higher frequency air bands have the electric field energy of their modes concentrated in lower dielectric regions.

The photonic bandgap is that frequency range in the middle in which there are no solutions for the master PhC equation for any k value as shown in Figure 8.3. The origin of the photonic bandgap arises due to the fact that the lower frequency band's electric field energy becomes concentrated in the higher dielectric regions, and since the electromagnetic variational theorem requires that each allowable mode be orthogonal to the modes below it in frequency, the second band modes would ideally be concentrated in the same high dielectric regions as well (Nightingale 2008). However, the orthogonality requirement causes the electric field energy of this second band of modes to be concentrated in the lower dielectric regions instead. A significant increase in the frequency of the second band compared to the first would then be sufficient to create a region of no modes that is known as the "photonic bandgap."

If $f(r)$ is a periodic function on a lattice with $f(r) = f(r + R)$ for all vectors R that connect one lattice point to the next, then the dielectric function $\varepsilon(r)$ in PhCs is considered an example of such a function (Prather et al. 2009). To analyze PhCs, which are essentially periodic lattices, it is common to take the Fourier transform and build a periodic function $f(r)$ out of plane waves with various wave vectors. This function represents light interaction with the lattice. Given a lattice with a set of lattice vectors R, all of the reciprocal lattice vectors G can be determined once the condition $G \cdot R$ is some integer

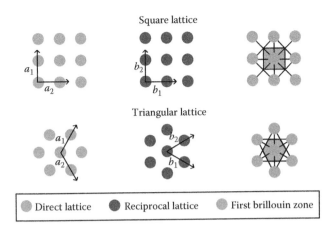

FIGURE 8.4
(See color insert.) Primitive lattice vectors, reciprocal lattice vectors, and Brillouin zones for the square (top row) and triangular lattices (bottom row). (Adapted from Joannopoulos, J.D. et al., *Photonic Crystals: Molding the Flow of Light*, Princeton University Press, Princeton, NJ, 2008.)

multiple of 2π for every R. Every lattice vector R can be written in terms of primitive lattice vectors, which are the smallest set of vectors pointing from one lattice to another. For example, on a simple cubic lattice with a lattice constant a, the vectors R are of the form: $R = la_1\hat{x} + ma_2\hat{y} + na_3\hat{z}$ where (l,m,n) are integers and a_1, a_2, and a_3 are the primitive lattice vectors (Joannopoulos et al. 2008).

An interesting feature of Bloch states is that different values of k can lead to the same mode. For example, a mode with wave vector k and a mode with a wave vector $k+G$ are considered the same mode, if G is a reciprocal lattice vector. Therefore, when k is incremented by G, the phase between cells is incremented by $G \cdot R$ which is $2\pi N$ and the result is the same physical mode. This means that there is a redundancy in the label k (Joannopoulos et al. 2008). To eliminate this redundancy, a finite zone in reciprocal space must be found in which adding increments of G will not lead to the same mode. The zone that is closest to $k=0$ is called the (first) Brillouin zone. Determination of the Brillouin zone can be accomplished geometrically by drawing perpendicular bisector line segments that connect lattice points. Each bisector divides the lattice into two half-planes, and the intersection of all the half-planes is the first Brillouin zone. Examples of square and triangular primitive lattice vectors, reciprocal vectors, and their Brillouin zones are shown in Figure 8.4.

8.1.2 Photonic Crystal Modeling and Design

In the previous section, the origin of the photonic band diagram was discussed. Due to the complexity of solving multidimensional partial differential equations, computational tools are often used to determine the photonic bandgap and other properties of PhC lattices. Only a few lattice geometries can be analyzed using exact analytical tools. The PhC behaviors and characteristics that can be modeled by currently available computational tools can be grouped into three categories (Joannopoulos et al. 2008):

- *Frequency-domain eigenproblems*: Finding the eigenvectors and eigenvalues. Band structure and the corresponding fields can also be derived from eigenvalues.

TABLE 8.1

PhC Modeling Tools

Software	Technique Used	Output	License	References
MIT photonic bands (MPB)	Frequency-domain	Eigenstates and eigenvalues	Open-source	MIT Photonic Bands–AbInitio (n.d.)
MIT electromagnetic equation propagation (MEEP)	Time-domain	Field Evolution	Open-source	Meep–AbInitio (n.d.)
Cavity modeling framework (CAMFR)	Both	Eigenstates, eigenvalues, and field evolution	Open-source	CAMFR Home Page (n.d.)
OptiWave OptiFDTD	Time-domain	Field evolution	Commercial	Optiwave Systems Inc. (n.d.)
RSoft photonic suite	Both	Eigenstates, eigenvalues, and field evolution	Commercial	RSoft Design Group (n.d.)

- *Frequency-domain responses*: Given a current source at a certain frequency, the resulting fields at a given frequency can be determined.
- *Time-domain simulations*: Given a time-dependent current source, electric and magnetic fields propagating in time can be determined.

Numerical methods that are used in solving the partial differential equations over the PhC lattice include: finite difference, finite element, spectral functions, and boundary-element methods (Joannopoulos et al. 2008). Table 8.1 provides a listing of available PhC modeling tools and the modeling techniques they use.

While these tools may use different numerical methods to model PhC characteristics, they are all based on frequency and/or time domain techniques. Generally, frequency domain techniques, such as MPB, are eigensolvers that use the plane-wave expansion method. Time-domain techniques, such as MEEP employ the finite difference time-domain (FDTD) method. Although all eigenstates that define the band structure of the PhC can be calculated from a single field (electric or magnetic) that arises due to an applied source, there are several disadvantages to this technique. First, because of the uncertainty principle of the Fourier transform, frequency resolution is inversely proportional to the length of time needed to complete the simulation. Second, if a steady-state response is required, a large time variable is required in order to eliminate transient effects in the solution. Third, the time-step size is directly proportional to the spatial resolution, hence, increasing the spatial resolution for the same frequency increases the temporal resolution resulting in longer simulation times. Fourth, to determine the eigenmodes the simulation must be repeated for each eigenstate for a time inversely proportional to spacing between each state (Joannopoulos et al. 2008). In frequency-domain methods, eigenstates and eigenvectors are calculated at the same time. Because of the iterative nature of these methods, error in frequency decreases exponentially. One disadvantage of frequency-domain methods is that all eigenstates must be calculated until the desired solution is obtained, which greatly increases simulation times. Keeping these advantages and disadvantages in mind, one has to choose between these techniques based on the complexity of the design and application.

The plane-wave expansion method, which makes use of the fact that normal modes in periodic structures can be expressed as a superposition of a set of plane waves, is the most convenient method to understand and demonstrate light interaction with periodic PhC lattices (Benisty et al. 2005; Saleh and Teich 2007; Joannopoulos et al. 2008; Prather et al. 2009). In this method, the master equation is converted to a matrix eigenvalue problem that is solved using standard numerical techniques to obtain the dispersion relations inside a PhC. The eigenfrequency solutions are plotted as functions of the in-plane wave vectors tracing the edges of the irreducible Brillouin zone. The resulting dispersion diagram becomes simply a geographical representation of the frequencies that correspond to waves propagating within a PhC lattice with various wave vectors.

Because the results of bandgap simulations are unitless for some software tools, an extra calculation step is necessary to determine real parameters based on the desired wavelength of operation. The y-axis of the band diagram shown in Figure 8.5 represents the normalized frequency, a/λ, where a is the lattice constant, and the x-axis is wave vector, k. As Maxwell's equations are *scale-invariant*, the band diagram can be used to design PhC lattices for different frequencies. The lattice constant for a certain frequency is obtained by using the following equations:

Band midgap frequency

$$= \frac{\text{Lowest frequency of higher order band} + \text{Higest frequency of lower order band}}{2}$$

$$= \frac{x+y}{2} \tag{8.8}$$

$$\text{Lattice constant } (a) = \text{Band midgap frequency} \times \text{Wavelength}(\lambda) \tag{8.9}$$

For example, the lowest frequency of higher order band and highest frequency of lower order band are x and y, then band midgap frequency is $(x+y)/2$. Then, for a PhC to have bandgap at 632 nm, the lattice constant must be calculated using $((x+y)/2) \times 632$ nm.

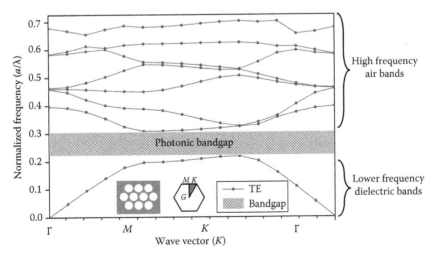

FIGURE 8.5
TE band diagram of a two-dimensional infinitely thick photonic crystal of triangular lattice of air holes in silicon. Shaded region band shows the photonic bandgap.

The bandgap for a given lattice is typically characterized by its width, which can be calculated using the following formula (Joannopoulos et al. 2008):

Bandgap width (%)

$$= \frac{\text{Lowest frequency of higher order band} - \text{Highest frequency of lower order band}}{\text{Band midgap frequency}}$$

$$= \frac{(x - y)}{((x + y)/2)} \tag{8.10}$$

The remainder of this section will focus on the design methodology for 2D PhC lattices and defect structures. The reader should consult (Ogawa et al. 2004; Yan et al. 2005a; Joannopoulos et al. 2008) for more information on the design of 1D and 3D PhC structures.

8.1.2.1 Design of Two-Dimensional Photonic Crystals (Infinitely Long)

A 2D PhC is periodic along two of its axes and homogeneous along its third axis (Figure 8.6). Any mode that propagates parallel to the plane of the PhC is invariant under reflections through that plane (Joannopoulos et al. 2008). The symmetry of the 2D PhC lattice allows for the classification of the modes into two polarizations: transverse-electric (TE) modes having H normal to the plane and E in the plane and transverse-magnetic (TM) modes having just the opposite of that (Joannopoulos et al. 2008). The band diagrams for TE and TM modes can be completely different. It is, therefore, possible to observe a wide photonic bandgap for one polarization and not for the other for a specific lattice. In this section, the band diagram of an infinitely long PhC will be discussed. The diagrams for square and triangular lattices of silicon rods surrounded by air are shown in Figures 8.7 and 8.8. It is obvious how a complete overlapping bandgap cannot be extracted from either lattice. The minima and maxima of the first and second bands, respectively, determine the bandgap frequencies and almost always occur at the

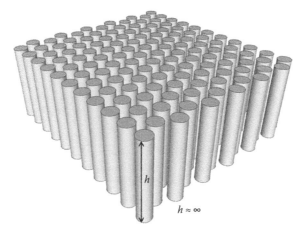

FIGURE 8.6
Infinitely long 2D PhC with a triangular lattice symmetry of dielectric rods.

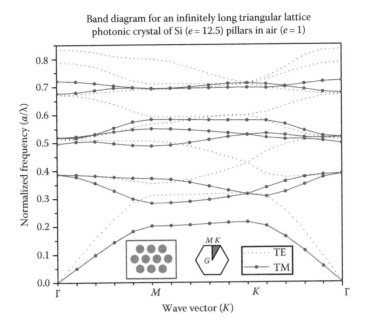

FIGURE 8.7
Band diagram of triangular lattice of silicon rods surrounded by air, solved using MIT Photonic Bands (MPB).

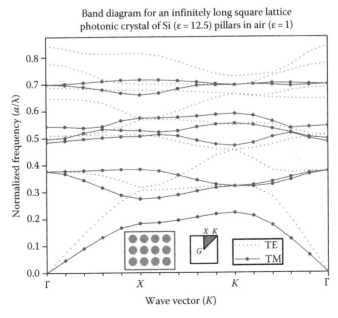

FIGURE 8.8
Band diagram of square lattice of silicon rods surrounded by air, solved using MPB.

irreducible Brillouin zone edges, and often at a corner. Therefore, the wave vector is normally plotted along the edges of this irreducible Brillouin zone.

8.1.2.2 Design of Two-Dimensional Photonic Crystal Slabs

Two-dimensional PhC slabs (Figure 8.9) are similar to infinitely long PhCs in their in-plane periodicity, but differ in that they have a finite thickness, typically chosen to allow the slab to act as a waveguide structure. This property allows the PhC lattice to be employed in sensors and devices based on guided wave operation, as will be discussed in the literature review presented in this chapter. However, 2D calculations cannot be applied directly to finite-thickness slab structures. In the previous section, the band diagram of a 2D PhC structure was shown in Figures 8.7 and 8.8. This may be applied to a 3D structure only when these periodic structures extend infinitely in that third dimension (Johnson et al. 1999). These previous diagrams demonstrated 2D bands that correspond to states with no vertical wavevector component that is perpendicular to the PhC plane. When vertical wave vectors are included in the calculations, a continuum of states is produced throughout all frequencies above the first band and this ultimately cancels the bandgap of the 2D structure (Johnson et al. 1999, 2000; Johnson, 2001). Moving from an infinitely long structure to one with a finite thickness recreates the bandgap in the guided slab modes. The system then becomes fundamentally 3D and distinct from the 2D calculations with a new set of parameters that must be considered such as slab thickness, effective refractive index contrast of the slab and its background, and mirror symmetry of the PhC slab (Johnson et al. 1999).

The band diagram of a PhC slab is calculated by first finding the states of the slab and then the light cone is overlaid as an opaque region on the band diagram (Johnson, 2001). The light cone consists of radiation "leaky" modes that extend infinitely in the region above and below the slab. This region is normally referred to as the background. Guided modes, on the other hand, are simply the localized states within the slab and exist in the regions of the band diagram that are outside the light cone. The slab guided modes are computed using preconditioned conjugate-gradient minimization of the Rayleigh quotient in a plane-wave basis (Johnson 2001). This requires a periodic cell, which is already achieved in the plane of the PhC and this periodicity is extended to the third dimension by generating a sequence of slabs separated by a background region (low-ε medium). It is important that this background is of a sufficient thickness so that the periodic vertical slabs do not affect the mode solutions of each other.

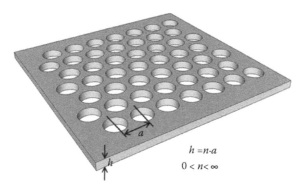

$h = n \cdot a$

$0 < n < \infty$

FIGURE 8.9
A two-dimensional photonic crystal slab.

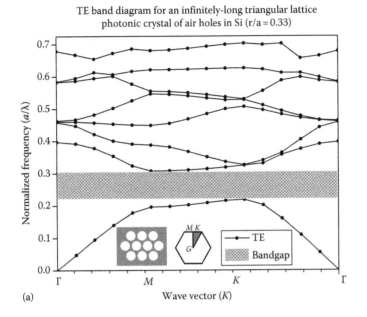

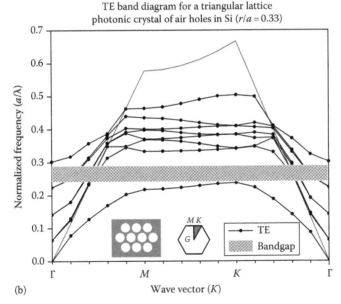

FIGURE 8.10

TE band diagram of a triangular lattice of an infinitely long photonic crystal of air holes in Si (a) and a triangular lattice of a slab photonic crystal of air holes in Si (b). The photonic bandgap is indicated by the shaded region.

The light cone is normally depicted as a uniform shaded area that does not reflect the varying density of states in this region. Figure 8.10 demonstrates the TE band diagram of a slab PhC compared to that of an infinitely long PhC of a triangular lattice of air holes in silicon. The light cone is an important feature that distinguishes slabs from infinitely long PhCs. The guided modes that lie below the light cone in the bottom band diagram of Figure 8.10 do not couple with modes in the bulk background. These guided states extend infinitely in the PhC plane and decay exponentially into the background region (Johnson et al. 1999). The resulting confinement is somewhat similar to the total internal reflection (TIR) in which the guided modes remain in the higher effective index of the silicon slab and become resonant when they reach the edge of the light cone but due to loss effects, they cannot remain resonant permanently within the slab and start to leak to the background. These structures are still referred to as "photonic crystals" due to the existence of a photonic bandgap. This bandgap, however, is different than that for an infinitely long PhC lattice. It contains the range of frequencies in which no "guided" modes exist. Therefore, it is not a real bandgap as there are radiation losses that have a major impact on the overall functionality of the PhC lattice. However, several research groups have successfully used slab PhCs with defined bandgaps to successfully develop efficient light emitting diodes (LEDs) and lasers when they managed to control the background radiation using slab PhCs with defined bandgaps (Prather et al. 2009).

The guided modes within the PhC slab are divided into two classes that are not purely TE or TM polarized. The reason is due to the lack of a discrete translational symmetry in the vertical direction. However, when considering the horizontal symmetry plane that bisects the slab, guided modes then can be classified as even or odd with respect to reflections through this plane. These even and odd states are very similar to TE and TM states for the infinitely long PhCs (Johnson et al. 2000).

As mentioned earlier, the slab thickness plays an important role in determining whether or not a photonic bandgap exists for a specific PhC slab. Thick slabs will cause the generation of higher-order modes that lie slightly above the first band and hence either canceling or severely narrowing the photonic bandgap to a point of no use. On the other hand, thin slabs will be considered a very weak perturbation of the background dielectric constant and therefore guided modes within the slab will hardly exist (Johnson et al. 1999). Johnson et al. (1999) proposed a method of calculating the optimal slab thickness. It is suggested to be on the order of half the 2D gap-bottom wavelength. The group justified this by explaining that the gap-bottom frequency was used instead of the midgap because the state at the bottom of the gap is the basis for both the state at the lower edge of the slab gap and the excited states at the upper edge. When the slab thickness is at least an order of the wavelength, then the small energy barrier will prevent the generation of higher-order states via a nodal plane. On the other hand, slabs of less than half the wavelength in thickness will not be sufficient for the existence of any guided modes (Johnson et al. 1999).

It is also very important to consider the effective refractive index of the background medium above and below the slab because in most applications this medium will not be air at all times. Therefore, if the slab is sandwiched between some background with an effective refractive index that is lower than that of the slab, index guiding will still allow the generation of guided bands. However, it must be noted that the localization of the guided modes within the slab and the creation of bandgaps means that the substrate must be sufficiently thick (several wavelengths). The increased effective refractive index surrounding the slab pulls down the frequencies of the guided modes and confines them under the narrow light cone. However, the guided modes become less localized within the slab and it has been measured that 89% of the energy of the lowest band remains within the height of the slab with a dielectric background of 2, versus 96% for that of an air background (Johnson et al. 1999).

8.1.2.3 Designing Defects in Two-Dimensional Photonic Crystals

It has been discussed previously that a photonic bandgap of a 2D PhC represents the range of wavelengths that are prohibited from propagating in the periodicity plane of the PhC.

However, by breaking the lattice symmetry at specific locations, single localized modes or a set of closely spaced modes can be generated within the bandgap. This can be accomplished by either removing a single pillar or hole (or rows of these features) from the lattice of a PhC within a specific background or replacing it with another one of different size, shape, or dielectric constant. This perturbation disrupts the discrete translational symmetry of the lattice.

The main interest in these defects is the frequencies that they support as well as the associated quality factor (Q-factor) of each mode. As its name indicates, the Q-factor is simply a measure of the quality of this cavity or how efficient it is in storing energy. It is equal to the number of oscillations the cavity can support before the trapped energy decays by $e^{-2\pi}$ ($\sim 0.2\%$) (Johnson 2001). The total quality factor for the cavity, $Q_{tot,}$ is represented as follows:

$$\frac{1}{Q_{tot}} = \frac{1}{Q_1} + \frac{1}{Q_2} \tag{8.11}$$

where
Q_1 is the quality factor of radiating modes outside of the slab
Q_2 is the quality factor of the guided modes in the plane of the PhC

The in-plane leakage occurs due to tunneling effects. This leakage can be minimized by increasing the number of unaltered PhC periods surrounding the cavity. The guided-modes' quality factor, Q_2, then becomes very large and its reciprocal in Equation 8.2, $1/Q_2$ approaches zero making the following approximation valid (Johnson 2001):

$$Q_{tot} \approx Q_1 \tag{8.12}$$

Another way of measuring a specific cavity's Q-factor is done by examining the sharpness of the cavity's resonance peak. The width of this peak is inversely proportional to the cavity Q factor,

$$Q = \frac{\lambda_0}{\Delta\lambda} \tag{8.13}$$

where
λ_0 is the center resonant frequency
$\Delta\lambda$ is the spectral full-width half-maximum (FWHM) of the resonance

A high Q-factor PhC nanocavity is the one that can maintain its trapped photons over more radiation cycles than a lower Q-factor nanocavity but can support much fewer resonant frequencies than the lower Q-factor cavities. These resonant cavities, in general, can be classified as acceptor or donor defects depending on their size and their index of refraction. Acceptor defects are formed by removal of high index material from a specific lattice location as shown in Figure 8.11a, which represents an enlarged air hole within a 2D triangular lattice of air holes in silicon. The defect frequencies normally occur near the bottom edge of the photonic bandgap. On the other hand, donor defects are formed by the addition of high index material at a lattice location as shown in Figure 8.11b. This defect is created by filling out a range of air holes with the same refractive index material as that of the slab, silicon here. Donor defect resonant frequencies normally occur near the top edge of the photonic bandgap.

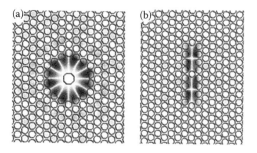

FIGURE 8.11

(a) A resonant cavity in which the defect is generated by filling in the holes with high dielectric material surrounding a central lower dielectric circular opening. (b) A resonant cavity in which six holes on top and bottom of a central hole are filled with high dielectric region. Extending this filling technique to the edge of the photonic crystal can generate a W1 waveguide.

8.2 Fabrication Methods

In the previous section, photonics crystal theory and modeling of electromagnetic wave interaction with photonic crystals were discussed. The critical dimensions obtained from modeling are used for PhC fabrication. This section will describe top-down and bottom-up fabrication techniques used to achieve periodic nanoscale lattice features.

8.2.1 Top-Down Fabrication Methods

The main techniques used to fabricate PhC structures in top-down fabrication are electron beam lithography (EBL) for pattern generation, metal etch-mask deposition using electron beam evaporation, and substrate etching using plasma (i.e., reactive ion) etching. These tools are used in a specific sequence in order to fabricate the final PhC structure. This top-down method starts by first creating a CAD file using software tools that control the beam path of an e-beam lithography system (Nabity n.d.). Negative- or positive-tone e-beam resists are spin-coated on the top surface of the sample, with desired thicknesses determined by spin speeds and material viscosity. The pattern is then transferred into the e-beam-sensitive polymer layer, which is developed to create an intermediate mask of the pattern. Resists such as ma-N-2403, XR-1541 (Hydrogen Silesquioxane [HSQ]) are used for negative pattern generation and resists like PMMA, ZEP520 are used for positive pattern generation. Some of these materials can be used directly as an etch mask after additional curing steps. Others are not robust to reactive ion etching and require the implementation of an additional masking layer such as metal. In this case, after the development of the e-beam resist layer, a metal layer is evaporated using electron beam deposition followed by liftoff creating a negative pattern of metal. E-beam deposition is desired over sputter deposition due to the larger grain size of sputtered metal, which negatively impacts the transfer of nanoscale features into the underlying substrate.

Two general methods used to create PhCs in dielectric materials are explained in detail in this section. The first is a recipe used to produce a lattice of air holes and the second is the opposite of the first, which is to create pillars surrounded by air. These processes involve the use of EBL, metal deposition, liftoff, and plasma etching to achieve the final structure as shown in Figure 8.12. The fabrication of air holes in silicon starts off with the creation

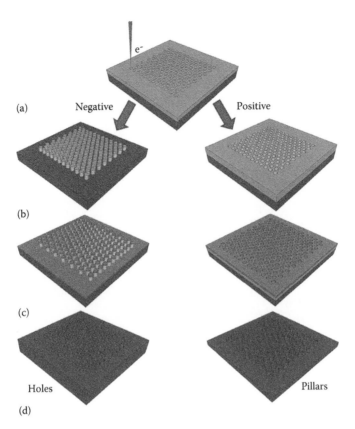

FIGURE 8.12
Top-down process flow illustrating fabrication of holes and pillars in dielectric materials. (a) EBL, (b) development, (c) metal deposition, and (d) lift off and plasma etch.

of a negative pattern of pillars with electron beam resists such as ma-N-2403 or XR-1541 (HSQ). Figure 8.13 demonstrates SEM images of structures fabricated successfully when the process is followed precisely (Hamza 2011) with some additional steps to create the suspended structure on a SOI substrate. Similarly, the fabrication of pillars in silicon starts off with creating holes in electron beam resists like PMMA or ZEP520 followed by metal deposition, liftoff and plasma etching of the pillars into silicon. Figure 8.14 shows the final fabricated structure containing pillars etched into silicon substrate. Repeating these processes several times, intricate structures like the "woodpile" structure (Joannopoulos et al. 2008) can be achieved. Techniques such as focused ion beam (FIB) lithography can eliminate intermediate steps of conventional top-down fabrication to achieve the final structure through direct milling of the pattern into the substrate (Watt et al. 2005). This method also facilitates the realization of yablonovite-like 3D PhCs (Yablonovitch et al. 1991). While able to realize more complex PhC structures, the serial nature of FIB processing is not amenable to mass production.

Top-down techniques based on e-beam lithography are generally limited to small area (~100 × 100 μm) patterns. In addition, sample preparation and processing time from start to finish lead to low-throughput fabrication for certain PhC structures. In order to improve throughput and achieve large-area PhC lattices, techniques like nanosphere lithography (NSL) and nanoimprint lithography (NIL) are used. NSL involves use of colloidal spheres

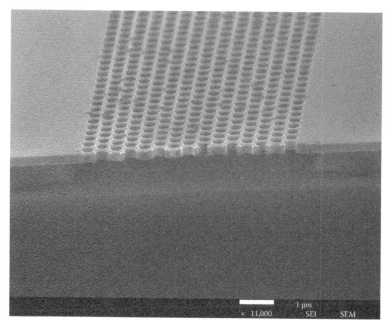

FIGURE 8.13

Cross section SEM image of the suspended PhC structures in silicon with underlying air channels. Image was captured at 85° glancing angle.

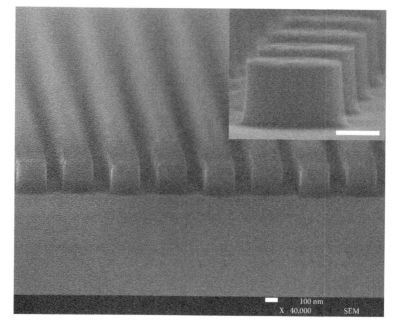

FIGURE 8.14

SEM image of the final structure of Silicon Pillars surrounded by air fabricated using HSQ. (Inset scale is equivalent to 100 nm). (From Hamza, B. et al., *Microelectron. Eng.*, 91, 70, 2012.)

TABLE 8.2

Summary of Common PhC Fabrication Processes

Name	Type	Area of Pattern	Dimensionality	Throughput
EBL	Top-down	Limited to field of view	1D and 2D	Low
FIB	Top-down	Limited to field of view	1D, 2D, and 3D	Low
NSL	Top-down	Large scale	1D and 2D	High
NIL	Top-down	Large scale	1D, 2D, and 3D	Ultrahigh
CCA	Bottom-up	Large scale	2D and 3D	Ultrahigh
Robot-aided	Bottom-up	Limited to field of view	2D and 3D	Low

spin-coated over a large area, which is used as a template for the pattern transfer onto the substrate. The patterns generated by the spheres are achieved due to either voids between close-packed colloidal arrays (Moon et al. 2005) or non-close-packed arrays (Jiang and McFarland 2005) followed by further processes to transfer the pattern to the substrate. NIL can be used to fabricate PhC using a master mold containing nanoscale features to transfer a pattern into a polymeric material controlled by pressure, temperature, or even UV light (Stephen et al. 1997; Guo 2007). This technique is widely used for mass production of PhC structures as it yields in ultrahigh resolution and throughput. The prefabricated master mold is created using top-down fabrication methods. The choice of polymer materials used to transfer the pattern to the substrate allows for a high degree of flexibility in lattice design.

8.2.2 Bottom-Up Fabrication Methods

As described earlier, bottom-up methods rely mostly on growth or self-assembly techniques. In the majority of bottom-up PhC fabrication, colloidal particles are self-assembled to generate a pattern or an entire structure. Self-assembly of colloidal particles has proven to be an inexpensive method to fabricate 3D PhCs (Likui and Zhao 2007). Colloidal crystal arrays (CCAs) are arrays of colloidal microspheres self-assembled using various techniques like gravitational sedimentation (Zhu et al. 1997; Miguez et al. 1998), vertical deposition (VD) (Jiang et al. 1999), horizontal deposition (Yan et al. 2005b), electrophoretic deposition (Holgado et al. 1999), spin-coating (Mihi et al. 2006; Jiang and McFarland 2007), confined cell method (Park et al. 1999), Langmuir–Blodgett technique (Reculusa and Ravaine 2003), and floating self-assembly (Im and Park 2002). All these methods result in a large area of 3D PhCs. In most of the cases, the 3D PhCs form a hexagonal close-packed array (Sean et al. 2003), which is by nature close to the FCC configuration. Although FCC PhC lattices do not typically contain a photonic bandgap, altering the structure of the CCAs by polymerization and creating inverse lattices, a photonic bandgap can be achieved, as explained in the literature review section of this chapter. Table 8.2 gives a brief summary of the fabrication techniques previously discussed.

8.3 Active Photonic Crystal Biosensors

8.3.1 Concept

Several critical parameters play a role in determining the optical bandgap properties of PhCs. Considering a simple 2D PhC lattice of triangular symmetry comprised of low-ε

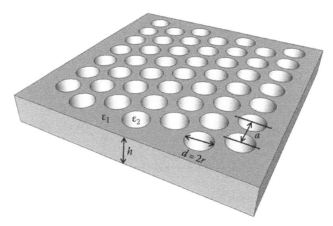

FIGURE 8.15
Critical parameters of a 2D PhC slab.

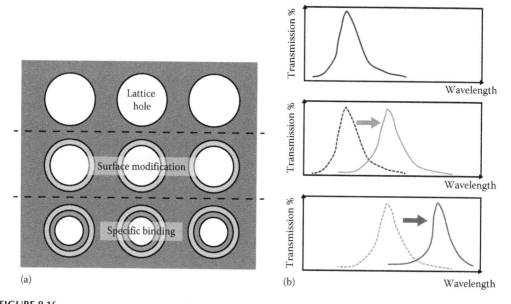

(a)   (b)

FIGURE 8.16
Active PhC sensing concept: defect (a) Probe and Target molecules modifying the surface of lattice holes.
(b) Change in Photonic Bandgap with surface modification.

holes in a high-ε slab, as shown in Figure 8.15, the critical parameters are dielectric constant of the slab (ε_1), dielectric constant of the hole (ε_2), slab thickness (h), lattice constant (a), and radius of the holes (r). In the active detection modality, one of these parameters is intentionally modified when target analytes interact with the PhC lattice. This translates into either changes of the radius and/or the lattice constant due to swelling effects, or changes of the effective refractive index as the target analytes replace the low-ε regions of the PhC lattice (see Figure 8.16). In most detection schemes utilizing this modality, a control sample is first tested to acquire initial information regarding the specific range of transmitted/reflected wavelengths. As the desired target is introduced, the change in one or more parameters translates into changes of the transmitted/reflected wavelengths, offering label-free detection. These changes are usually observed as red or blue shifts that are directly related to the local density of the adsorbed molecules, and are very sensitive to the target type and quantity. A variety of PhC-sensors have been developed based on this active detection modality.

8.3.2 Active Photonic Crystal Devices

Polymerized crystalline colloidal arrays (PCCAs) are self-assembled 3D PhC lattices that result from the electrostatic repulsion between highly charged spheres (Lee and Asher 2000). The repulsion allows the spheres to align in either a face-centered cubic (FCC) or a body-centered cubic (BCC) array and can significantly Bragg-diffract visible wavelengths. The unique characteristic of these arrays is their target-induced volume changes that cause the diffracted light to shift accordingly. For example, a PCCA has demonstrated the unique ability to sense pH changes and the ionic strength of a specific chemical solution. By relating the diffracted wavelength to the lattice constant and the hydrogel volume, precise monitoring of the changes in pH and ionic strength is possible (Lee and Asher 2000). Moreover, the same 3D photonic-crystal arrays have been used to develop a new sensing motif for the detection and quantification of creatinine, an important small molecule marker of renal dysfunction (Sharma et al. 2004).

In a similar method, 3D crystalline colloidal arrays embedded within a polyacrylamide-poly(ethylene glycol) (PEG) hydrogel have demonstrated the ability to generate a colorimetric glucose recognition sensor (Lee et al. 2004). As glucose of different concentrations is introduced to the array, it self-assembles the boronic acid and PEG functional groups into a supramolecular complex capable of introducing blue shifts to the photonic-crystal-based diffracted wavelengths. The visually evident diffraction color shifts across the visible spectral region using this method, from red to blue over physiologically important glucose concentration ranges (Alexeev et al. 2003; Lee et al. 2004; Liu et al. 2009).

The response of a 2D PhC resonator to changes of ambient gas filling lattice cavities demonstrates another example of how PhC lattices can be actively utilized in ultrasensitive sensing platforms. These architectures could be used to enable breath-analysis-based disease diagnostics that measure specific volatile organic compounds (VOCs). One such device that could accomplish this is a 2D triangular PhC lattice fabricated in GaAs (Sünner et al. 2008). When different gases were introduced into the resonant cavity, the refractive index within the holes surrounding the cavity changes, modifying the band structure of the crystal and the resonance properties of the cavity. A shift of the resonance toward higher wavelengths was observed as the refractive index of the ambient was increased from that of vacuum to nitrogen and finally to SF_6. Moreover, air-guiding photonic bandgap fibers (PBFs) have demonstrated the ability to sense both strongly (acetylene/hydrogen cyanide) and weakly (methane/ammonia) absorbing gases (Ritari et al. 2004). PBFs are very advantageous as gas sensors due to the long optical path that they introduce, which allows more interaction between the gas and light mode field and therefore only very small sample volume is needed.

A 2D PhC slab of a triangular array of air holes in silicon can also be used to analyze protein binding on the pore walls and quantitatively measure the protein diameter. In this biosensor architecture, a partial TE bandgap was realized in the triangular lattice with a r/a ratio of approximately 0.29. Since the PhC slab lacked a TM bandgap, all experiments were carried out using a TE polarized input light at ~1.58 µm (Lee and Fauchet 2007a,b; Ouyang et al. 2007). When proteins of different sizes coated the internal walls, different amounts of resonance red shift were observed, and analyte masses as low as 2.5 fg were detected. Device performance was verified by measuring the red shift corresponding to the binding of glutaraldehyde and bovine serum albumin (BSA) (Lee and Fauchet 2007a,b).

Understanding protein–DNA interactions is very important for the understanding of a variety of cellular processes. The study of such interactions has been limited to the observation of small molecule disruptors. However, there are very few methods available for the rapid identification of compounds that disrupt protein–DNA interactions (Chan et al. 2008). Adsorption of these molecules on the surface of a PhC transducer has proven to be a very effective method of allowing such an interaction to be examined with a variety of protein types. Two very different protein–DNA interactions were successfully analyzed using this method; the bacterial MazEF complex, which binds to its promoter DNA in a sequence-specific manner, and the human AIF, a protein that binds nonspecifically to chromosomal DNA [26]. The sensor system utilizing these structures was capable of identifying compounds that prevent protein–DNA binding. The group predicted that the generality and simplicity of this PhC biosensor could enable such structures to find broad utility for identification of compounds that inhibit protein–DNA binding (Chan et al. 2008).

A PhC has been used within a microscope-based detection system to measure the resonant mode shifts caused by changes in refractive index due to dissolved avidin concentrations as low as 15 nM (Scullion et al. 2011). The advantage of this sensor is its low sensing area (2.2 μm^2), enabling high density sensing elements. Hosseinibalam et al. have proposed a sensor with a PhC coupled to ring cavity resonator to increase the resonant mode shift. They have numerically demonstrated a high sensitivity of 293 nm/RIU (Hosseinibalam et al. 2012).

Porous silicon (PSi) can be used to form 1D PhCs through the control of pore size during HF etch by altering current density and dissolution rate. PhCs from PSi are functionalized to capture specific cells. Resonant mode shifts caused by the secretion of metalloprotease enzymes from living macrophage cells can be used as a diagnostic/theranostic tool with single-cell detection capability (Tang et al. 2012). This sensor modality can also be used to study the effect of therapeutics on the release of protease enzymes from cells.

8.4 Passive Photonic Crystal Biosensors

8.4.1 Concept

In the active modality explained in Section 8.3 the introduction of a specific target to the system incorporating PhC lattices causes a critical change in one or more of the PhC parameters, which then is translated into red or blue shifts of the transmitted/reflected incident light. The concept for *passive* detection utilizing PhCs is different in that all parameters are designed to remain essentially constant throughout the detection event. The PhC lattice or defect region acts as a structure that controls and guides the emission from labeled molecules in the direction of the detector, leading to an enhancement in the number of photons per unit area that reach the detector (Figure 8.17). In addition, the waveguiding properties of PhC slabs can be used to deliver excitation light along a path orthogonal to the observation direction. Therefore, it is fair to say that the PhC lattices alone are not sensors. They are simply passive elements within their sensors that effectively manipulate and guide light to propagate toward conventional detectors that read the produced signal.

The passive PhC sensing modality is mostly utilized for biosensing applications, although it is less common than the active modality due to the increased interest in

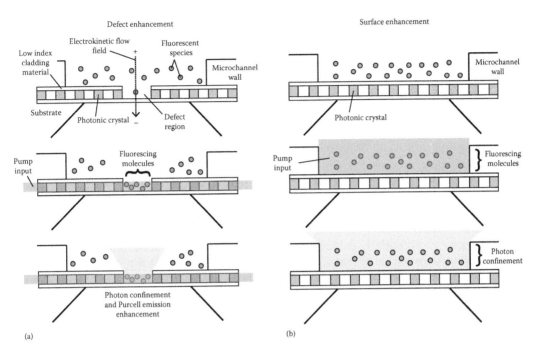

FIGURE 8.17
Passive PhC sensing concept: defect (a) and surface (b) fluorescence enhancement.

developing label-free biosensors. However, for many sensing applications, including the emerging field of rapid DNA analysis, laser induced fluorescence (LIF) is considered the most reliable method for detecting labeled or naturally fluorescing biomolecules at very low concentrations (VanEngelenburg and Palmer 2008; Aye-Han et al. 2009; Selid et al. 2009). Modern benchtop fluorescence analysis instruments are capable of generating accurate quantitative measurements of specific target analytes, leading to widespread use in biomedical and environmental applications. Fluorescence spectroscopy offers excellent sensitivity and low detection limits for a wide range of fluorescent label/molecule combinations. However, the benchtop nature of diagnostic systems that employ these methods does not lend itself well to sample analysis outside of dedicated laboratories in point-of-use or point-of-care scenarios. The following section will explain common detection methods in which PhC lattices with specific photonic bandgaps are utilized to achieve enhancement of the fluorescence signal from labeled molecules on the surface of the PhC or within high quality-factor resonant cavities.

8.4.2 Passive Sensing PhC Devices

Labeling target analytes for visualization and quantification purposes is very important to life science procedures that involve imaging of cells and their components as well as gene expression profiling. Research on the effects of metals on enhancing fluorescence and specifically that of surface plasmon resonance has demonstrated promising results (Homola et al. 1999; Hung et al. 2006; Skorobogatiy and Kabashin 2006; Aslan et al. 2007; Hoa et al. 2007; Yao et al. 2007). However, it was soon observed that such fluorescence enhancement on metal surfaces can also undergo nonuniform enhancement when colloidal nanoparticles serve as the substrate. Nanopatterned metal structures have been pursued to resolve this issue, but the challenge of large-area fabrication of such nanostructures has limited the application of these methods. Moreover, fluorophore quenching of labeled molecules that are in the vicinity of the metal substrates (~20 nm) is another factor that limits these methods from being employed in large-scale enhancement sensors (Ray et al. 2007). In addition to these approaches, PhCs are being used to enhance the laser excitation used in SERS. Using a PhC in a SERS architecture, a 21-fold enhancement was demonstrated (Cunningham 2010).

One solution to the previous limitations is the use of PhCs, which have demonstrated capabilities of fluorescence enhancement through mechanisms similar to those observed with metal nanostructures. PhCs fabricated in dielectric materials have proven to be very effective at reducing quenching effects of fluorophores close to the PhC surface (Mathias et al. 2008). After careful design, dielectric-based PhCs allow for narrow-band reflections with spectral properties determined by the lattice dimensions. Since the narrow-band reflections of the proposed 1D PhC vary with position at a fixed illumination angle, a single device can potentially exhibit reflections at a range of wavelengths including that of fluorophore's excitation wavelength. To achieve this functionality, a thin high refractive index TiO_2 layer was deposited on a dielectric-based 1D PhC. By coating the device with a monolayer of Cy5-conjugated protein and scanning it at normal incidence with a microarray scanner, a spatial map of enhanced fluorescence was generated in order to determine the reflected wavelength that corresponds to the greatest enhancement. The group reported PhC an 18-fold fluorescence enhancement when such a reflection overlaps the fluorophore excitation wavelengths (Mathias et al. 2008).

In a recent work demonstrated by the same group, a 1D PhC was used to experimentally demonstrate that the detection of fluorescent molecules on a PhC surface can be substantially enhanced through the combined effects of resonance-enhanced excitation of the fluorescent dye, resonance-enhanced extraction of the fluorescence emission, and a dielectric nanorod surface coating increasing the surface area available for fluorophore–PC interaction (Wu et al. 2010). Enhanced excitation is obtained by engineering a high-Q TM resonant mode to efficiently couple with an incident TM-polarized $\lambda = 633$ nm laser for exciting cyanine-5 (Cy5). Enhanced extraction results from a low-Q TE resonance designed to spectrally overlap the Cy5 emission spectrum for channeling TE-polarized emission toward the detection instrument. To increase the emission based on surface area, the entire surface is coated with TiO_2 nanorods that allows more fluorophores to penetrate into the region of enhanced near-electric fields. Experimental results reveal a 588-fold enhancement in fluorescence intensity relative to an unpatterned glass surface. Pokhriyal et al. have designed a biosensor comprising a PhC fabricated on a quartz substrate to reduce background autofluorescence. This arrangement has resonant modes present in the absorption and emission regions of fluorophores, resulting in a 7500-fold enhancement factor for LD-700 when compared with fluorescence on a conventional glass surface. In addition to enhancement, SNR has improved 330-fold and limit of detection has lowered 140-fold (Pokhriyal et al. 2010a,b). This sensor was further extended for multicolor fluorescence enhancement, which can be used in biological assays with multiple fluorescent dyes, such as gene expression microarrays (Pokhriyal et al. 2010a,b). In a biosensor presented by the same group, PhCs are used for detecting a panel of cancer biomarkers in microarray format (Huang et al. 2011). In this case, the PhC is designed to enhance emission from Cy-5 fluorophore labeled analyte, enabling detection of 2 pg/mL of cancer biomarker in a mixed solution with a 3.8- to −6.6-fold increase in SNR and 6%–89% decrease in detection limits depending upon antibody–antigen interaction. Chaudhery et al. (2011) presented a PhC label-free imaging biosensor imaging combined with enhanced fluorescence. A label-free image of the attached molecule regions is used to selectively maximize the enhancement factor of captured region of cells and minimize enhancement factor in the region between spots. With this approach, concentrations as low as 0.97 pg/mL of protein biomarkers in buffer were detected. In a sensor presented by Lidstone et al. (2011), photonic crystal enhanced microscopy was used to measure the cell attachment and/or attachment modulation properties of HepG2/C3 hepatic carcinoma cells, Panc-1 pancreatic cancer cells, etc. Here, PhC resonator cavities were incorporated into commercially available microplate wells, and shifts in the resonant bandgap modes were measured.

In the PhC-based transduction mechanism developed by the authors' group (Paturi et al. 2005; Dawson et al. 2008; Hamza et al. 2008, 2011a,b; Tompkins et al. 2008; Yalamanchili et al. 2009; Andagana and Henry 2010), the PhC structure is considered a passive element that can enhance emission from labeled molecules that fall within its bandgap. The enhancement results from the fact that frequencies that fall within the bandgap of a 2D PhC slab are not allowed to leak outside of the slab if the slab contained at least 14 periods of varying dielectric constant regions. Therefore, a 2D PhC slab is designed to have a bandgap surrounding the emission wavelength of the label, in this case, quantum dots (QDs) that emit around 1100 nm. Exciting the quantum dots from within the PhC forces the emitted light to be confined within the PhC region and leak only vertically where a detector is placed. Using this method, 27-fold enhancement of the emitted light has been experimentally recorded. Achieving much higher enhancement factors is possible through the incorporation of resonant cavities within the PhC lattices. The resonant cavities confine the emitted wavelengths that originally fall within the bandgap into much smaller volumes. As the volume of the cavity is reduced, Purcell's effect can cause larger enhancement factors by increasing the spontaneous emission rate of the QDs within a PhC point defect nanocavity. This can lead to more photons per unit time and area, resulting in an enhancement in fluorescence that is proportional to the quality factor (Q) of the defect.

8.5 Future Trends

An increasing number of research efforts in PhC biosensing are focused on new high-throughput fabrication methods, many of which are biologically inspired, with the intention of biomimetic device operation. Tang et al. have presented polypyrrole-containing PhC structures, which are synthesized from Morpho butterfly wing replicas. Polypyrrole replicas were used in sensing dopamine for preliminary testing and the polypyrrole replicas have shown high biological activity (Guan et al. 2011). The Blue Morpho wing nanostructure has been used as a template for the fabrication of magnetophotonic crystal (MPC) materials that can be red-shifted with an increase of the external magnetic field strength (Peng et al. 2012). This structure could be used in biosensing approaches that employ magnetic beads to "label" analytes. Beyond conventional PhC lattices, a novel class of biomimetic photonic chiral composites with three-dimensional cubic symmetry have been fabricated that exhibit strong circular dichroism (Turner et al. 2011). These devices show promise as a new class of nanophotonic devices. A 1D PhC consisting of poly(1,2-butadiene) (PB) and Os multilayers that mimic the exoskeleton of the jewel beetle Elytra have been demonstrated (Yabu et al. 2011). Control of the position of peak reflective wavelength was achieved via controlled swelling of the PB layers using a solvent, which could be exploited as a sensing modality.

Although conventional photolithography processing is high-throughput in production facilities, its use for fabricating PhCs is limited by the feature sizes that can be achieved. This disadvantage can be overcome by a novel technique called nanospherical-lens lithography (Hou et al. 2005; Chang et al. 2012). On top of a photoresist layer, a monolayer of polystyrene nanospheres is formed and when the surface is exposed to UV light, nanospheres act as lens and collimate the exposure energy. After the photoresist is developed, the process of metal deposition, liftoff, and etching are performed as discussed in a top-down approach.

A diamond lattice of spheres possesses photonic bandgap, but the fabrication of such intricate structures is not easily achieved, even with the conventional self-assembly techniques. Use of robot-aided fabrication (Morishita and Hatamura 1993; Garcia-Santamaria 2001) shows potential for enabling the fabrication of 3D diamond lattice PhC structures.

References

Alexeev, V. L. et al. High ionic strength Glucose-sensing Photonic crystal. *Anal. Chem.* 75 (2003): 2316–2323.

Andagana, J. and B. Henry. Nanofabrication of optofluidic photonic crystal resonators for biosensing. Master's thesis, West Virginia University, Morgantown, WV, 2010.

Aslan, K., M. Stuart, and G. Chris. Metal-enhanced fluorescence from gold surfaces: Angular dependent emission. *J. Fluoresc.* 17 (2007): 7–13.

Aye-Han, N-N., Q. Ni, and J. Zhang. Fluorescent biosensors for real-time tracking of post-translational modification dynamics. *Curr. Opin. Chem. Biol.* 13 (2009): 392–397.

Benisty, H., V. Berger, J-M. Gerard, D. Maystre, and A. Tchelnokov. *Photonic Crystals: Towards Nanoscale Photonic Devices.* New York: Springer, 2005.

Bykov, V. P. Spontaneous emission in a periodic structure. *Sov. J. Exp. Theor. Phys.* 35 (1972): 269–273.

Bykov, V. P. Spontaneous emission from a medium with a band spectrum. *Sov. J. Quant. Electron.* 4 (1975): 1557–1577.

Bykov, V. P. Free oscillations of elastic dipole located in periodic structure. *Zhurnal Tekhnicheskoi Fiziki* 48 (1978): 505–513.

CAMFR Home Page. August 17, 2007. http://camfr.sourceforge.net/ (accessed August 29, 2013).

Chan, L. L., M. Pineda, J. T. Heeres, P. J. Hergenrother, and B. T. Cunningham. A general method for discovering inhibitors of protein-DNA interactions using photonic crystal biosensors. *ACS Chem. Biol.* 3(7) (2008): 437–448.

Chang, Y-C., J-S. Huang, and H-C. Chung. Controlled fabrication of photonic crystals in situ using nanospherical-lens lithography. *SPIE Newsroom*, April 11, 2012.

Chaudhery, V., C-S. Huang, A. Pokhriyal, J. Polans, and B. T. Cunningham. Spatially selective photonic crystal enhanced fluorescence and application to background reduction for biomolecule detection assays. *Opt. Express* 19(23) (2011): 23327–23340.

Cunningham, B. T. Biosensing with photonic crystal surfaces. *Annual Meeting of the IEEE Photonics Society.* Denver, CO, 2010.

Dawson, J. M, J. R. Nightingale, R. P. Tompkins, T. H. Myers, L. A. Hornak, X. Cao, and D. Korakakis. GaN photonic crystal-based, enhanced fluorescence biomolecule detection system. *Proceedings of. Materials Research Society.* Boston, MA, 2008.

Garcia-Santamaria, F. et al. Opal-like photonic crystal with diamond lattice. *Appl. Phys. Lett.* 79 (2001): 2309.

Guan, B. et al. Mesoporous silicon photonic crystal microparticles: Towards single-cell optical biosensors. *Faraday Discuss.* 149 (2011): 301–317.

Guo, L. J. Nanoimprint lithography: Methods and material requirements. *Adv. Mater.* 19 (2007): 495–513.

Hamza, B. Two-dimensional polymer and thin-film semiconductor-based photonic crystals for biosensing applications. Master's thesis, West Virginia University Libraries, Morgantown, WV, 2011.

Hamza, B., A. Kadiyala, L. A. Hornal, Y. Liu, and J. M. Dawson. Direct fabrication of two-dimensional photonic crystal structures in silicon using positive and negative Hydrogen Silsesquioxane (HSQ) patterns. *Microelectron. Eng.* 91 (2012): 70–74.

Hamza, B., A. Kadiyala, C. Kilemi, Y. Liu, and J. Dawson. Fluorescence enhancement in a polymer-based photonic crystal biosensor. *Proc. SPIE 7888.* San Francisco, CA. (2011): 788804.

Hamza, B. M., H. Yalamanchili, H. Cao, X. Andagana, L. A Hornak, J. M. Dawson, and D. Korakakis. Top-down approach to the fabrication of GaN-based photonic crystal biosensor. *Proceedings of the Materials Research Society.* Boston, MA, 2008.

Hoa, X. D., A. G. Kirk, and M. Tabrizian. Towards integrated and sensitive surface plasmon resonance biosensors: A review of recent progress. *Biosens. Bioelectron.* 23 (2007): 151–160.

Holgado, M., F. Garcia-Santamaria, A. Blanco, M. Ibisate, and A. Cintas. Electrophoretic deposition to control artificial. *Langmuir* 15 (1999): 4701.

Homola, J., S. S. Yee, and G. Gauglitz. Surface plasmon resonance sensors: Review. *Sens. Actuat. B: Chem.* 54 (1999): 3–15.

Hosseinibalam, F., S. Hassanzadeh, A. Ebnali-Heidari, and C. Karnutsch. Design of an optofluidic biosensor using the slow-light effect in photonic crystal structures. *Appl. Opt.* 51(5) (2012): 568–576.

Hou, C-H. et al. Output power enhancement of light-emitting diodes via two-dimensional hole arrays generated by a monolayer of microspheres. *Appl. Phys. Lett.* 95 (2005): 133105.

Huang, C-S. et al. Application of photonic crystal enhanced fluorescence to cancer biomarker microarrays. *Anal. Chem.* 83 (2011): 1425–1430.

Hung, Y-J., I. I. Smolyaninov, C. C. Davis, and H-C. Wu. Fluorescence enhancement by surface gratings. *Opt. Express* 14 (2006): 10825–10830.

Im, S. H., and O. O. Park. Effect of evaporation temperature on the quality of colloidal crystals at the water-air interface. *Langmuir* 18 (2002): 9642–9646.

Jiang, P., J. F. Bertone, K. S. Hwang, and V. L. Colvin. Single-crystal colloidal multilayers of controlled thickness. *Chem. Mater.* 11 (1999): 2132–2140.

Jiang, P., and M. J. McFarland. Wafer-scale periodic nanohole arrays templated from two-dimensional nonclose-packed colloidal crystals. *J. Am. Chem. Soc.* 127(11) (2005): 3710–3711.

Jiang, P., and M. J. McFarland. Large-scale fabrication of wafer-size colloidal crystals, macroporous polymers, and nanocomposites by spin-coating. *J. Am. Chem. Soc.* 126 (2007): 13778–13786.

Joannopoulos, J. D., S. G. Johnson, J. N. Winn, and R. D. Meade. *Photonic Crystals: Molding the Flow of Light.* Princeton, NJ: Princeton University Press, 2008.

John, S. Strong localization of photons in certain disordered dielectric superlattices. *Phys. Rev. Lett.* 58 (1987): 2486–2489.

Johnson, S. G. Photonic crystals: From theory to practice. PhD thesis, Department of Physics, Massachusetts Institute of Technology, Cambridge, MA, 2001.

Johnson, S. G., S. Fan, P. R. Villeneuve, and J. D. Joannopoulos. Guided modes in photonic crystal slabs. *Phys. Rev. B* 60 (1999): 5751–5758.

Johnson, S. G., P. R. Villeneuve, S. Fan, and J. D. Joannopoulos. Linear waveguides in photonic-crystal slabs. *Phys. Rev. B* 62 (2000): 8212–8222.

Kadiyala, A., L. A. Hornak, and J. M. Dawson. Modeling of a 3-D tunable photonic crystal for camouflage coating. *Proc. SPIE 7781.* San Diego, CA. (2010): 77810U.

Lee, K., and S. A. Asher. Photonic crystal chemical sensors: pH and ionic strength. *J. Am. Chem. Soc.* 122 (2000): 9534–9537.

Lee, M. R., and P. M. Fauchet. Nanoscale microcavity sensor for single particle detection. *Opt. Lett.* 32 (2007a): 3284–3286.

Lee, M. R., and P. M. Fauchet. Two-dimensional silicon photonic crystal based biosensing platform for protein detection. *Opt. Express* 15 (2007b): 4530–4535.

Lee, Y.-J., S. A. Pruzinsky, and P. V. Braun. Glucose-sensitive inverse opal hydrogels: Analysis of optical diffraction response. *Langmuir* 20 (2004): 3096–3106.

Lidstone, E. A. et al. Label-free imaging of cell attachment with photonic crystal enhanced microscopy. *Analyst* 136 (2011): 3608–3615.

Likui W. and X. S. Zhao. Fabrication of crack-free colloidal crystals using a modified vertical deposition method. *J. Phys. Chem.* 111 (2007): 8538–8542.

Liu, Y., Y. Zhang, and Y. Guan. New polymerized crystalline colloidal array for glucose sensing. *Chem. Commun.* 2009: 1867–1869.

Mathias, P. C, N. Ganesh, W. Zhang, and B. T. Cunningham. Graded wavelength one-dimensional photonic crystal reveals spectral characteristics of enhanced fluorescence. *J. Appl. Phys.* 103 (2008): 094320.

Meep–AbInitio. October 3, 2012. http://ab-initio.mit.edu/meep/ (accessed August 29, 2013).

Miguez, H., F. Meseguer, C. Lopez, A. Blanco, and J. S. Moya. Control of the Photonic Crystal Properties of fcc-Packed Submicrometer SiO$_2$ Spheres by Sintering. *Adv. Mater.* 10 (1998): 480–483.

Mihi, A., M. Ocana, and H. Miguez. Oriented colloidal-crystal thin films by spin-coating microspheres dispersed in volatile media. *Adv. Mater.* 18 (2006): 2244.

MIT Photonic Bands–AbInitio. n.d. http://ab-initio.mit.edu/mpb/ (accessed July 17, 2012).

Moon, J. H., W. S. Kim, J-W. Ha, S. G. Jang, S-M. Yang, and J-K. Park. Colloidal lithography with crosslinkable particles: Fabrication of hierarchical nanopore arrays. *Chem. Commun.* 32 (2005): 4107–4109.

Morishita, H., and Y. Hatamura. Development of ultra micromanipulator system under stereo SEM observation. *IEEE/RSJ International Conference on Intelligent Robots and Systems*, Tokyo, Japan, 1993.

Nabity, J. C. *NPGS: Overview*. JC Nabity lithography systems. June 27, 2013. http://www.jcnabity.com/overview.htm (accessed June 29, 2012).

Nair, R. V., and R. Vijaya. Photonic crystal sensors: An overview. *J. Prog. Quant. Electron.* 34 (2010): 89–134.

Nightingale, J. R. Optical biosensors: Sparrow biosensor and photonic crystal-based fluorescence enhancement. Master's thesis, West Virginia University Libraries, Morgantown, WV, 2008.

Ogawa, S., M. Imada, S. Yoshimoto, M. Okano, and S. Noda. Control of light emission by 3D photonic crystals. *Science* 305 (July 9, 2004): 227–229.

Optiwave Systems Inc. *Photonic Crystal*. 2013. http://www.optiwave.com/products/fdtd_overview.html (accessed August 29, 2013).

Ouyang, H., L. A. DeLouise, B. L. Miller, and P. M. Fauchet. Label-free quantitative detection of protein using macroporous silicon photonic bandgap biosensors. *Anal. Chem.* 79 (2007): 1502–1506.

Park, S. H., B. Gates, and Y. N Xia. A three-dimensional photonic crystal operating in the visible region. *Adv. Mater.* 11 (1999): 462.

Paturi, N., C. R. Vemuri, D. Korakakis, and L. A. Hornak. Analysis of cluster defects in photonic crystals for biosensor applications. *Proc. SPIE.* (2005): pp. 146–151.

Peng, W. et al. 3D network magnetophotonic crystals fabricated on morpho butterfly wing templates. *Adv. Funct. Mat.* 22(10) (2012): 2072–2080.

Pokhriyal, A., M. Lu, V. Chaudhery, C-S. Huang, S. Schulz, and B. T. Cunningham. Photonic crystal enhanced fluorescence using a quartz substrate to reduce limits of detection. *Opt. Express* 18(24) (2010): 24193–24808.

Pokhriyal, A., M. Lu, C-S. Huang, S. Schulz, and B. T. Cunningham. Multicolor fluorescence enhancement from a photonics crystal surface. *Appl. Phys. Lett.* 97 (2010): 121108.

Prather, D. W., S. Shi, A. Sharkawy, J. Murakowski, and G. J. Schneider. *Photonic Crystals: Theory, Applications, and Fabrication*. Hoboken, NJ: John Wiley & Sons Inc., 2009.

Ray, K., H. Szmacinski, J. Enderlein, and J. R. Lakowicz. Distance dependence of surface plasmon-coupled emission observed using Langmuir-Blodgett films. *Appl. Phys. Lett.* 90 (2007): 251116.

Reculusa, S., and S. Ravaine. Synthesis of colloidal crystals of controllable thickness through the Langmuir–Blodgett technique. *Chem. Mater.* 15(2) (2003): 598–605.

Ritari, T. et al. Gas sensing using air-guiding photonic bandgap fibers. *Opt. Express* 12 (2004): 4080–4087.

Synopsys' Optical Solutions Group. *RSoft Products-Synopsys Optical Solutions.* http://optics.synopsys.com/rsoft/ (accessed August 29, 2013).

Saleh, B. E. A., and M. C. Teich. *Fundamentals of Photonics.* Hoboken, NJ: John Wiley & Sons Inc., 2007.

Scullion, M., A. D. Falco, and T. Krauss. Slotted photonic crystal cavities with integrated microfluidics for biosensing applications. *Biosens. Bioelectron.* 27 (2011): 101–105.

Sean W., V. Kitaev, and G. A. Ozin. Colloidal crystal films: Advances in universality and perfection. *J. Am. Chem. Soc.* 125(50) (2003): 15589–15598.

Selid, P. D., H. Xu, E. M. Collins, M. S. Face-Collins, and J. X. Zhao. Sensing mercury for biomedical and environmental monitoring. *Sensors* 9 (2009): 5446–5459.

Sharma, A. C. et al. A general photonic crystal sensing motif: Creatinine in bodily fluids. *J. Am. Chem. Soc.* 126 (2004): 2971–2977.

Skorobogatiy, M., and A. V. Kabashin. Photon crystal waveguide-based surface plasmon resonance biosensor. *Appl. Phys. Lett.* 89 (2006): 148518.

Stephen, Y. C. et al. Sub-10 nm imprint lithography and applications. *J. Vac. Sci. Technol. B* 15 (1997): 2897.

Sünner, T. et al. Photonic crystal cavity based gas sensor. *Appl. Phys. Lett.* 92 (2008): 261112.

Tang, J. et al. Replication of polypyrrole with photonic structures from butterfly wings as biosensor. *Mater. Chem. Phys.* 131 (2012): 706–713.

Tompkins, R. P., J. M. Dawson, L. A. Hornak, and T. H. Myers. Optofluidic photonic crystals for biomolecular fluorescence enhancement—A bottom-up approach for fabricating GaN-based biosensors. *Proc. SPIE 7056.* San Diego, CA. (2008): 70560J.

Turner, M. D., G. E. Schröder-Turk, and M. Gu. Fabrication and characterization of three-dimensional biomimetic chiral composites. *Opt. Express* 19(10) (2011): 10001–10008.

VanEngelenburg, S. B., and A. E. Palmer. Fluorescent biosensors of protein function. *Curr. Opin. Chem. Biol.* 12 (2008): 60–65.

Vukusic, P., and J. R. Sambles. Photonic structures in biology. *Nature* 24 (2003): 852–855.

Watt, F., A. A. Bettiol, J. A. Van Kan, E. J. Teo, and M. B. H. Breese. Ion beam lithography and Nanofabrication: A Review. *Int. J. Nanosci.* 4(3) (2005): 269–286.

Welch, V., V. Lousse, O. Deparis, A. Parker, and J. P. Vigneron. Orange reflection from a three-dimensional photonic crystal in the scales of the weevil Pachyrrhynchus congestus pavonius (Curculionidae). *Phys. Rev. E Stat. Nonlin. Soft. Matter. Phys.* 75(4) (2007): 041919.

Wu, H-Y., W. Zhang, P. C. Mathias, and B. T. Cunningham. Magnification of photonic crystal fluorescence enhancement via TM resonance excitation and TE resonance extraction on a dielectric nanorod surface. *Nanotechnology* 21 (2010): 125203.

Yablonovitch, E. Inhibited spontaneous emission in solid-state physics and electronics. *Phys. Rev. Lett.* 58(20) (May 1987): 2059–2062.

Yablonovitch, E., T. J. Gmitter, and K. M. Leung. Photonic band structure: The face-centered-cubic case employing nonspherical atoms. *Phys. Rev. Lett.* 67(17) (October 1991): 2295–2298.

Yabu, H., T. Naknishi, Y. Hirai, and M. Shimomura. Black thin layers generate strong structural colors: A biomimetic approach for creating one-dimensional (1D) photonic crystals. *J. Mater. Chem.* 21(39) (2011): 15154–15156.

Yalamanchili, H., L. A. Hornak, D. Korakakis, and J. M. Dawson. Bandgap tuning of Photonic crystals on III-V Nitride thin films. *Proc. SPIE 7402.* San Diego, CA. (2009): 740212.

Yan, Q., Z. Zhou, X. S. Zhao, and S. J. Chua. Line defects embedded in three-dimensional photonic crystals. *Adv. Mater.* 17(15) (2005b): 1917–1920.

Yan, Q. F., Z. C. Zhou, and X. S. Zhao. Inward-growing self-assembly of colloidal crystal films on horizontal substrates. *Langmuir* 21 (2005a): 3158.

Yao, Y., B. Yi, J. Xiao, and Z. H. Li. Surface plasmon resonance biosensors and its application. *ICBBE.* Wuhan, China, 2007, pp. 1043–1046.

Zhu, J. X., M. Li, R. Rogers, W. Meyer, R. H. Ottewill, and W. B. Russell. Crystallization of hard-sphere colloids in microgravity. *Nature* 387 (1997): 883–885.

9

Nanomaterial-Based Electrochemiluminescence Biosensors

Rongfu Huang and Liang-Hong Guo

CONTENTS

9.1 Introduction

Electrogenerated chemiluminescence (ECL), also called electrochemiluminescence, is briefly described as chemiluminescence (CL) produced directly or indirectly as a result of electrochemical reactions. When an appropriate potential is applied to an electrode, an ECL-emitting species is generated at the electrode surface and subsequently emits light (Bard 2004; Forster et al. 2009; Hu and Xu 2010; Miao 2008). In principle, ECL not only retains the advantages of sensitivity (low background resulting from no excitation light source) and selectivity inherent to conventional CL methodology, but also offers many additional advantages as follow. First of all, because light emission is initiated by electrochemical reactions on the surface of an electrode, great temporal and spatial control can be easily imposed. Secondly, the excited state ECL emitter can be generated by electrochemically oxidizing or reducing the stable ground state counterpart. Therefore, ECL reagent storage and shelf life are not a problem. Thirdly, deliberate variation of the electrochemical potential or current allows further control over the ECL reaction and can improve selectivity. Fourthly, some inactive compounds in CL reaction can be electrochemically modified on the surface of electrode and can further take part in CL reaction, extending the application range of ECL analysis. The first ECL phenomenon was described in the 1920s as light emission during electrolysis (Dufford et al. 1927; Harvey 1929), and detailed ECL study was reported by Hercules and Bard et al. in the middle of the 1960s (Hercules 1964; Santhanam and Bard 1965; Visco and Chandross 1964). Now ECL has become a very powerful analytical technique. Coupled with capillary electrophoresis, high-performance liquid chromatography (HPLC), flow injection analysis (FIA), and micro total analysis (μ-TAS) (Yin et al. 2004), ECL has been successfully used as a sensitive detection method in the area of medical diagnostics, food safety, environmental monitoring, and biowarfare agent detection (Bard 2004).

A biosensor is an analytical device that combines a biological component that interacts (binds or recognizes) with an analyte of interest with a physicochemical detector or transducer. The transducer converts the interaction of the analyte with the biological element into a signal (optical, electrochemical, piezoelectric, thermometric, magnetic, micromechanical, etc.) that can be measured and quantified. ECL biosensors provide a powerful tool for the ultrasensitive detection and quantification of a wide range of analytes, which combines the advantages offered by the selectivity of the biological recognition reactions and the high sensitivity of ECL technique.

The application of nanomaterials in biosensors is of considerable interest in the biosensor field owing to their unique physical and chemical properties, which has led to novel biosensors that exhibit significantly improved sensitivity, selectivity, and dynamic range in comparison with conventional biosensors. In this chapter, we review the design, fabrication, and applications of ECL biosensors that incorporate nanomaterials. The functions of nanomaterials in ECL biosensing systems are divided into four major categories: (1) nanomaterials as the electrode materials that can catalyze the electrochemical reaction of ECL coreactants or facilitate the electron transfer of ECL emitters, (2) nanomaterials as the solid phase for biomolecule immobilization to increase their surface coverage and biological reactivity, (3) nanomaterials as the carriers of conventional ECL emitting molecules for enhanced signal, and (4) nanomaterials as the new ECL emitters. The aim of this chapter is to provide a general review of the recent development and application of nanomaterials in ECL biosensors. Particular emphasis will be given to the application of metallic, carbon, semiconductor, and polymeric nanomaterials.

9.2 Principles of ECL

ECL can be produced by two dominant pathways, that is, annihilation and coreactant pathway. In each case, two species are generated electrochemically, and those two species undergo homogeneous redox reactions to produce an emissive species. In the annihilation process, the oxidized form and reduced form of a chemical are first produced either at a

$$DPA - e^- \longrightarrow DPA^{\bullet+} \text{ (oxidation at the electrode)}$$

$$DPA + e^- \longrightarrow DPA^{\bullet-} \text{ (reduction at the electrode)}$$

$$DPA^{\bullet-} + DPA^{\bullet+} \longrightarrow DPA + DPA^* \text{ (annihilation process)}$$

$$DPA^* \longrightarrow DPA + h\nu \ (\lambda = 425 \text{ nm})$$

SCHEME 9.1

Ion annihilation reaction of DPA. (Adapted from *Biosens. Bioelectron.*, 24, Bertoncello, P. and Forster, R.J., Nanostructured materials for electrochemiluminescence (ECL)-based detection methods: Recent advances and future perspectives, 3191–3200. Copyright 2009 with permission from Elsevier.)

single electrode by using an alternating potential, or at two separate electrodes in close proximity to each other with each electrode holding at an appropriate potential. The two species then react in solution to produce an electronically excited state, which emits light when relaxing to the ground state. The earliest ECL study originated with ion annihilation, and a typical example of ion annihilation process is the ECL of 9,10-diphenylanthracene (DPA), which is based on the following processes (Santhanam and Bard 1965; Visco and Chandross 1964; Scheme 9.1)

From the view of thermodynamics, ion annihilation process involves two routes: "S-route" and "T-route." If the enthalpy related to the ion annihilation reaction exceeds the energy required to produce the lowest excited states from the ground state, then the reaction is defined as "energy sufficient" singlet route "S-route." In contrast, if the enthalpy is lower than the energy required to produce the lowest excited state but still exceeds the triple state energy, the emitting species is formed via a triplet–triplet annihilation "T-route." The typical example of "T-route" annihilation is the ECL of rubrene and of $Ru(bpy)_3^{2+}$ (bpy = bi-pyridine) or its derivatives. In addition, when excimers (excited dimers) and exciplexes (excited complexes) are formed in ion annihilation, the system is said to follow the "E-route". The major advantage of the annihilation process is that it requires only the ECL species, solvent, and supporting electrolyte in order to generate light. However, the potential window of water is often not sufficiently wide to allow the species to be both oxidized and reduced, making it necessary to use organic solvents such as acetonitrile or N,N-dimethylformamide (DMF).

The second dominant pathway to produce ECL is defined as "coreactant ECL," on which modern ECL applications are almost exclusively based. In this process, ECL is usually generated by one-directional potential scan or step on the electrode in the presence of both the emitter and coreactant. Using anodic scan as an example, both the coreactant and ECL emitter get oxidized during the potential scan. The oxidized coreactant undergoes a chemical decomposition to form a strongly reducing intermediate, which then reacts with the oxidized emitter to generate the excited state. In this pathway, excited species can be regenerated while the coreactant is consumed via the catalytic route. A good coreactant should possess good water solubility, stability, rapid electrochemical kinetics, and low ECL background. Thus, the most commonly used coreactants for ECL are oxalate ($C_2O_4^{2-}$), tertiary amines, and peroxydisulfate ($S_2O_8^{2-}$). The major advantage of using the coreactant approach is to promote the generation of ECL in aqueous solution, which opens up a wide range of applications in biochemical analysis. Because the ECL signal is often proportional to the concentration of the coreactant or emitter, ECL method can be used in the analysis of the coreactant, the emitter, or the species tagged with the emitter.

9.2.1 ECL with Ru(bpy)$_3^{2+}$ Analogues as Emitters

According to literature reports, a wide variety of molecules exhibit ECL behaviors and can be classified into three types based on their chemical nature: transition metal complexes, organic molecules, and semiconductor nanomaterials. However, the vast majority of publications are concerned with coreactant ECL pathway employing Ru(bpy)$_3^{2+}$ or its derivatives as the emitting species and tripropylamine (TPA) or oxalate as the coreactant. These systems exhibit excellent chemical, electrochemical, and photochemical properties (as high as 4.2% luminescence quantum yield in water [Van Houten and Watts 1976]) even in aqueous media and in the presence of oxygen. In 1972, Tokel and Bard (1972) first reported the observation of Ru(bpy)$_3^{2+}$ ECL. Orange emission centered at 610 nm was observed when Ru(bpy)$_3^{3+}$ reacted with Ru(bpy)$_3^+$ and yielded excited state Ru(bpy)$_3^{2+*}$, following the "T-route" of the ion annihilation process.

In 1981, Bard's group reported the ECL of Ru(bpy)$_3^{2+}$ in the presence of oxalate (Rubinstein and Bard 1981). They found that the homogeneous reaction of oxalate with Ru(bpy)$_3^{3+}$, which was produced electrochemically at the electrode produced a highly reducing intermediate (CO$_2$$^{·-}$ [Butler and Henglein 1980]) that could reduce Ru(bpy)$_3^{3+}$ to give ECL signal. This is called "oxidative-reduction" coreactant mechanism (Bolleta et al. 1982; White and Bard 1982). In acetonitrile, however, it was shown that oxalate was oxidized directly at the electrode to produce the intermediate (Chang et al. 1977). The contribution of directly oxidized oxalate to the overall ECL generation depends on the electrode material, the hydrophobicity of electrode surface, the concentration of oxalate, and the electrode potential applied. A typical example of coreactants used for "reductive-oxidation" ECL is peroxydisulfate (S$_2$O$_8^{2-}$). Upon electrochemical reduction, S$_2$O$_8^{2-}$ is reduced to SO$_4$$^{·-}$ either directly at the electrode or by electro-generated Ru(bpy)$_3^+$. SO$_4$$^{·-}$ then reacts with Ru(bpy)$_3^+$ to give ECL signal (White and Bard 1982).

The ECL of Ru(bpy)$_3^{2+}$/amine system has been studied extensively in the past 20 years or so. It has been found that tertiary amines are more effective than secondary and primary amines and other types of amine coreactants (Leland and Powell 1990; Noffsinger and Danielson 1987). In 1990 Leland and Powell (1990) reported the first detailed study on the ECL of Ru(bpy)$_3^{2+}$ and TPA as a coreactant, and Blackburn et al. (1991) soon developed ECL immunoassays and DNA probe assays using TPA as coreactant and Ru(bpy)$_3^{2+}$ derivative as the label.

ECL reaction mechanism of Ru(bpy)$_3^{2+}$/TPA is very complicated with multiple pathways (Miao et al. 2002), as shown in Scheme 9.2. In general, the light-emitting species is the excited state of Ru(bpy)$_3^{2+}$, which is produced by the reaction of Ru(bpy)$_3^{3+}$ with a strongly reducing species. In the Ru(bpy)$_3^{2+}$/TPA system, electrochemical oxidation generates Ru(bpy)$_3^{3+}$ and TPA$^{·+}$. The latter undergoes rapid deprotonation and converts to a highly reducing radical TPA·. Alternatively, homogeneous redox reaction between Ru(bpy)$_3^{3+}$ and TPA also produces TPA$^{·+}$ and subsequently TPA·. In both routes, Ru(bpy)$_3^{3+}$ can be reduced by the highly reducing radical TPA· directly to the excited state of Ru(bpy)$_3^{2+}$. Alternatively, it can be reduced to Ru(bpy)$_3^+$, and an ion annihilation reaction takes place between Ru(bpy)$_3^+$ and Ru(bpy)$_3^{3+}$ to produce the excited state of Ru(bpy)$_3^{2+}$. The relative contribution of the two routes to the formation of excited state Ru(bpy)$_3^{2+}$ and ECL emission depends on the electrode potential, the relative concentration of Ru(bpy)$_3^{2+}$ and TPA, and the rate of TPA oxidation at the electrode (including the surface property of the electrode, halide ions, and surfactants) (Cole et al. 2003; Factor et al. 2001; Li and Zu 2004; Zu and Bard 2000, 2001). In bioanalytical systems where the concentration of Ru(bpy)$_3^{2+}$ as an ECL label is very low, the dominant route of radical generation is via direct electrochemical oxidation of TPA.

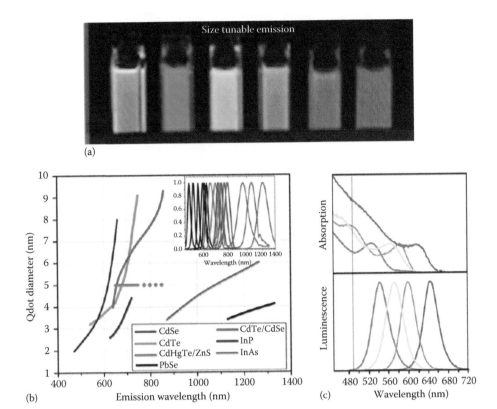

(a)

(b)

(c)

FIGURE 2.2

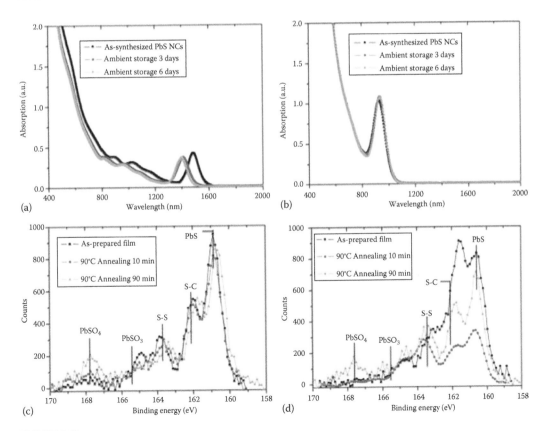

(a)

(b)

(c)

(d)

FIGURE 2.13

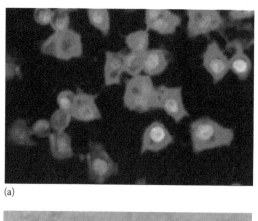

(a)

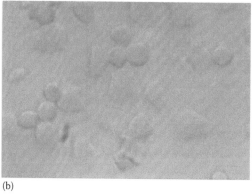

(b)

FIGURE 3.6

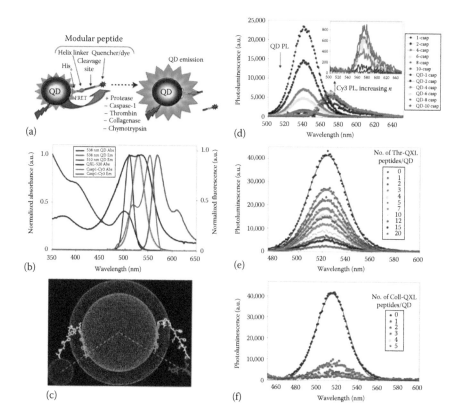

FIGURE 4.3

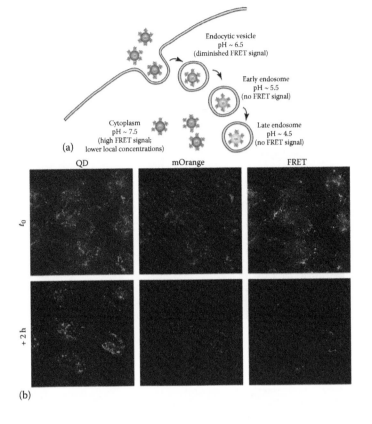

FIGURE 4.5

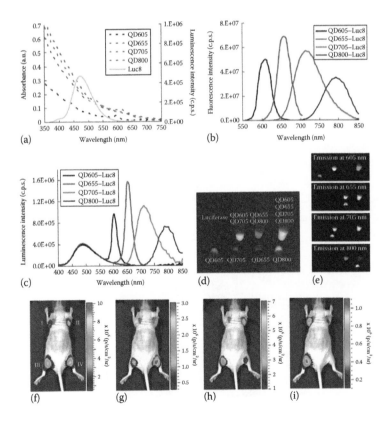

FIGURE 4.6

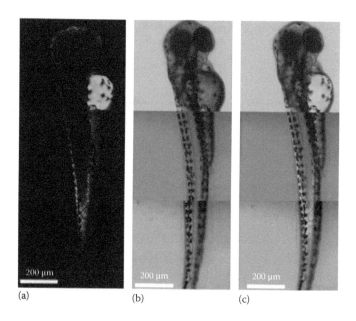

(a)　(b)　(c)

FIGURE 5.7

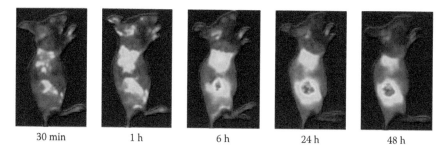

30 min　　1 h　　6 h　　24 h　　48 h

FIGURE 5.8

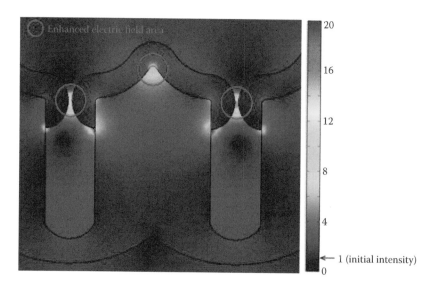

FIGURE 6.5

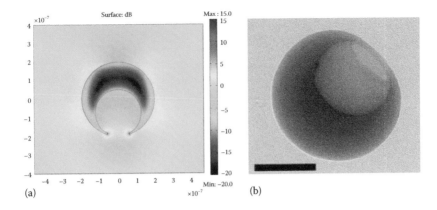

(a)

(b)

FIGURE 6.6

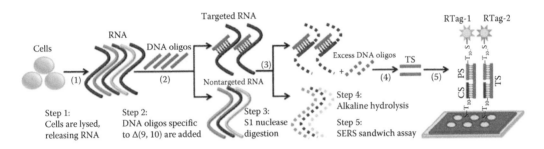

Step 1:
Cells are lysed,
releasing RNA

Step 2:
DNA oligos specific
to Δ(9, 10) are added

Step 3:
S1 nuclease
digestion

Step 4:
Alkaline hydrolysis

Step 5:
SERS sandwich assay

FIGURE 7.5

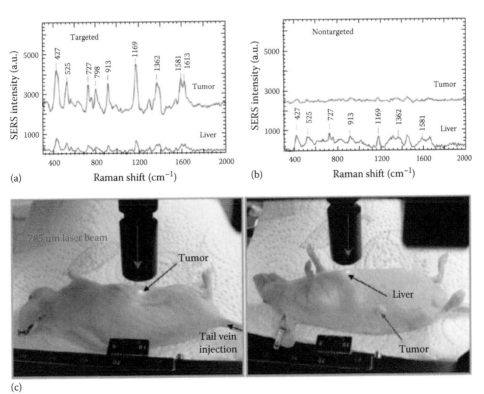

(a)

(b)

(c)

FIGURE 7.6

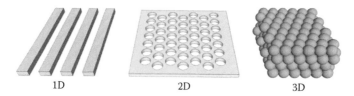

FIGURE 8.1

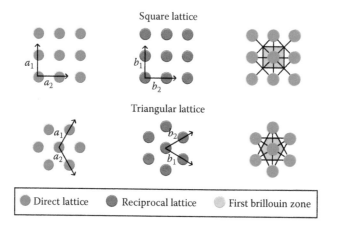

FIGURE 8.4

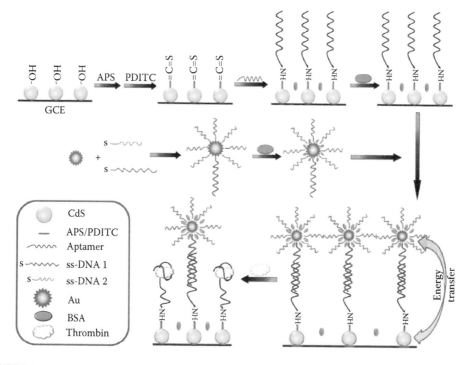

FIGURE 9.2

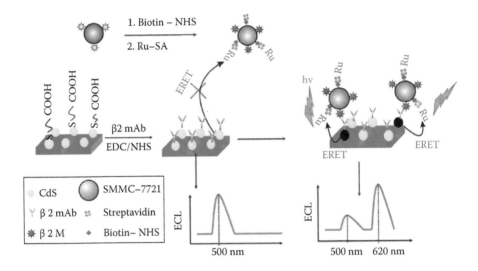

FIGURE 9.7

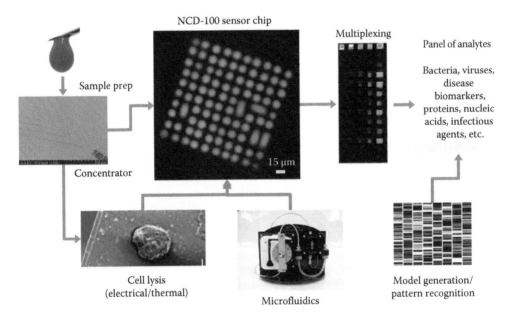

FIGURE 10.1

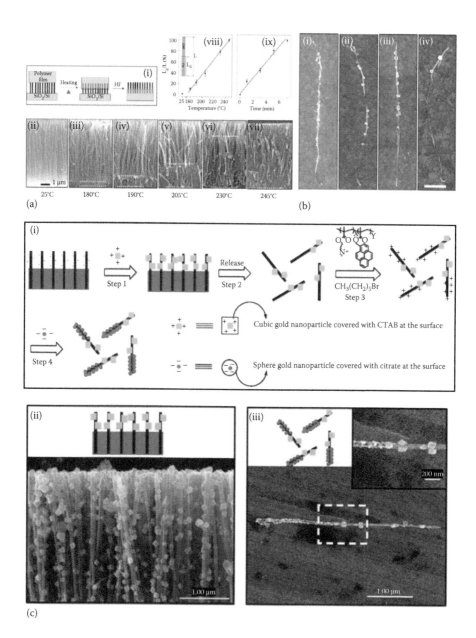

FIGURE 11.8

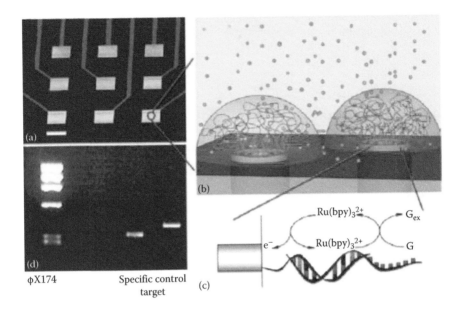

(a)

(b)

Ru(bpy)$_3^{2+}$ — G$_{ex}$

Ru(bpy)$_3^{2+}$ — G

e$^-$

(c)

(d)

φX174   Specific control
                    target

FIGURE 11.15

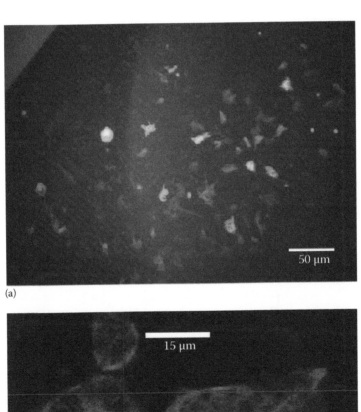

50 μm

(a)

15 μm

(b)

FIGURE 12.6

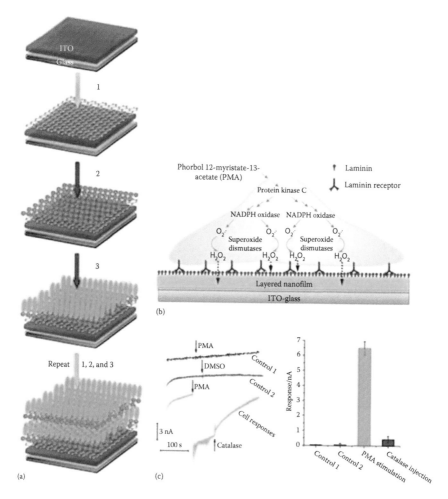

ITO
Glass

1

2

3

Repeat 1, 2, and 3

(a)

Phorbol 12-myristate-13-
acetate (PMA)   Laminin

                                                Laminin receptor
        Protein kinase C

    NADPH oxidase   NADPH oxidase

O₂·⁻   O₂·⁻   O₂·⁻   O₂·⁻
    Superoxide   Superoxide
    dismutases   dismutases
H₂O₂   H₂O₂   H₂O₂   H₂O₂

                Layered nanofilm
                ITO-glass

(b)

PMA
                                Control 1
DMSO
PMA
                                Control 2

                            Cell responses

3 nA
                        Catalase
100 s

(c)

Control 1   Control 2   PMA stimulation   Catalase injection

FIGURE 13.4

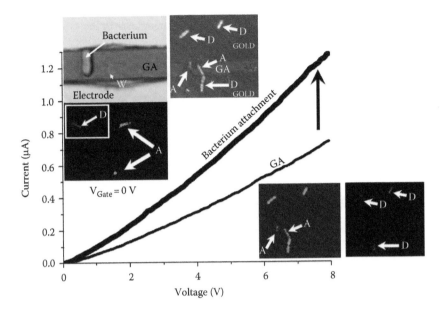

FIGURE 14.2

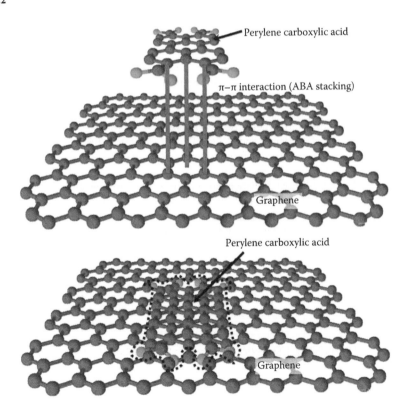

FIGURE 14.4

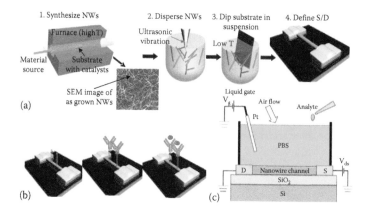

FIGURE 15.3

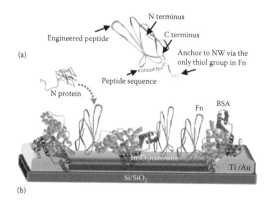

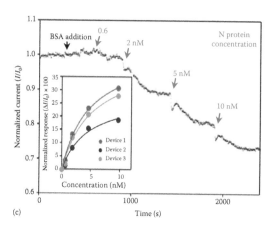

FIGURE 15.7

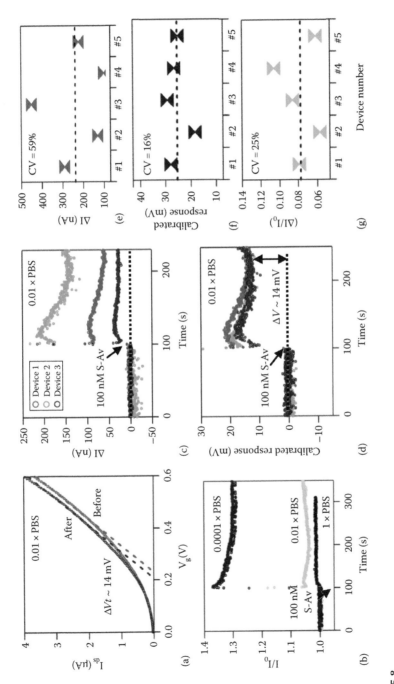

FIGURE 15.8

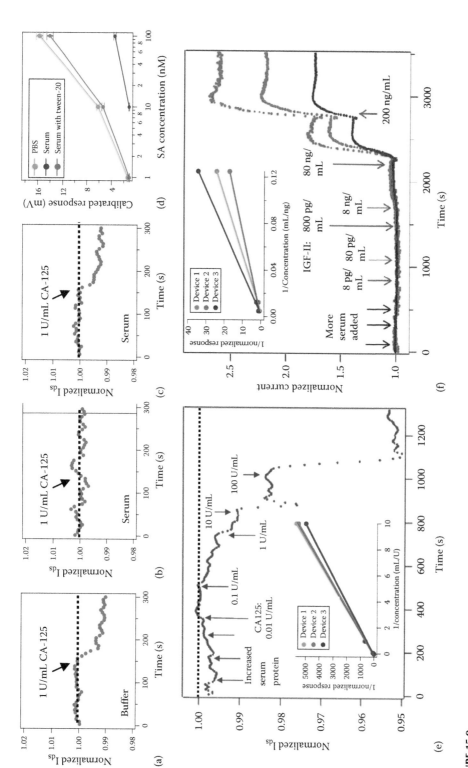

FIGURE 15.9

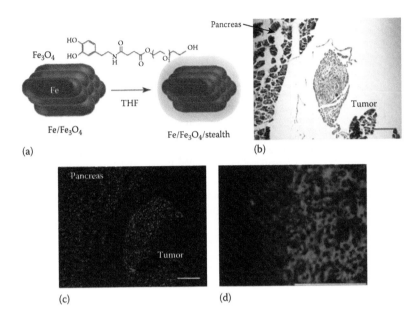

FIGURE 16.20

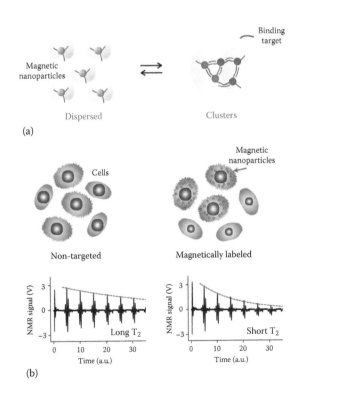

FIGURE 16.22

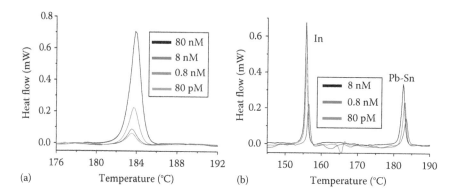

(a)   (b)

FIGURE 17.4

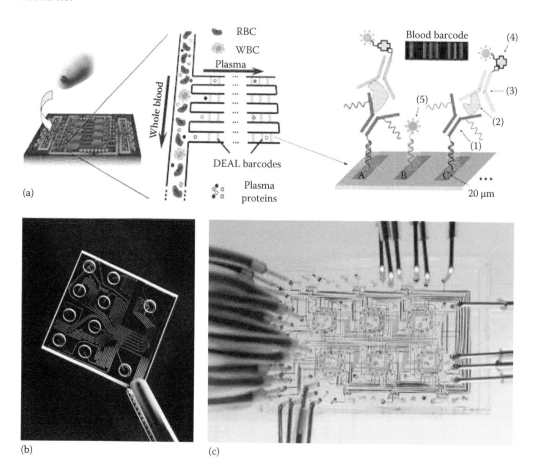

FIGURE 18.1

$Ru(bpy)_3^{2+} - e^- \longrightarrow Ru(bpy)_3^{3+}$ (oxidation on the electrode)

$Ru(bpy)_3^{3+} + (CH_3CH_2CH_2)_3N \longrightarrow Ru(bpy)_3^{2+} + (CH_3CH_2CH_2)_3N^{\cdot+}$

$(CH_3CH_2CH_2)_3N - e^- \longrightarrow (CH_3CH_2CH_2)_3N^{\cdot+}$ (oxidation on the electrode)

$(CH_3CH_2CH_2)_3N^{\cdot+} \longrightarrow (CH_3CH_2CH_2)_2NC^\cdot HCH_2CH_3 + H^+$

$Ru(bpy)_3^{3+} + (CH_3CH_2CH_2)_2NC^\cdot HCH_2CH_3 \longrightarrow Ru(bpy)_3^{2+*} + (CH_3CH_2CH_2)_2N^+ = CHCH_2CH_3$

$Ru(bpy)_3^{2+} + (CH_3CH_2CH_2)_2NC^\cdot HCH_2CH_3 \longrightarrow Ru(bpy)_3^+ + (CH_3CH_2CH_2)_2N^+ = CHCH_2CH_3$

$Ru(bpy)_3^+ + Ru(bpy)_3^{3+} \longrightarrow Ru(bpy)_3^{2+*} + Ru(bpy)_3^{2+}$

$Ru(bpy)_3^{2+*} \longrightarrow Ru(bpy)_3^{2+} + h\nu$

SCHEME 9.2
ECL reaction mechanism of $Ru(bpy)_3^{2+}$/TPA system. (Adapted with permission from Miao, W., Choi, J., and Bard, A., Electrogenerated Chemiluminescence 69: The tris (2,2′-bipyridine) ruthenium (II), ($Ru(bpy)_3^{2+}$)/tei-n-propylamine (TPrA) system revisited—A new route involving TPrA⁺⁺ cation radicals. *J. Am. Chem. Soc.*, 124, 14478–14485. Copyright 2002 American Chemical Society.)

$(CH_3CH_2CH_2)_2N - e^- \longrightarrow (CH_3CH_2CH_2)_3N^{\cdot+}$ (oxidation on the electrode, $E^{0'} \sim 0.9$ V SCE)

$(CH_3CH_2CH_2)_3N^{\cdot+} \longrightarrow (CH_3CH_2CH_2)_2NC^\cdot HCH_2CH_3 + H^+$

$Ru(bpy)_3^{2+} + (CH_3CH_2CH_2)_2NC^\cdot HCH_2CH_3 \longrightarrow Ru(bpy)_3^+ + (CH_3CH_2CH_2)_2N^+ = CHCH_2CH_3$

$Ru(bpy)_3^+ + (CH_3CH_2CH_2)_3N^{\cdot+} \longrightarrow Ru(bpy)_3^{2+*} + (CH_3CH_2CH_2)_3N$

$Ru(bpy)_3^{2+*} \longrightarrow Ru(bpy)_3^{2+} + h\nu$

SCHEME 9.3
Low-oxidation-potential ECL mechanism of $Ru(bpy)_3^{2+}$/TPA system. (Adapted with permission from Miao, W., Choi, J., and Bard, A., Electrogenerated Chemiluminescence 69: The tris (2,2′-bipyridine) ruthenium (II), ($Ru(bpy)_3^{2+}$)/tei-n-propylamine (TPrA) system revisited—A new route involving TPrA⁺⁺ cation radicals. *J. Am. Chem. Soc.*, 124, 14478–14485. Copyright 2002 American Chemical Society.)

Later on, Bard's group proposed a new ECL route of $Ru(bpy)_3^{2+}$/TPA system at low oxidation potentials (Miao et al. 2002), as shown in Scheme 9.3. TPA is first oxidized to TPA·⁺ at the electrode surface and then undergoes rapid decomposition to form TPA·. At low oxidation potentials, instead of oxidation at the electrode, $Ru(bpy)_3^{2+}$ is reduced to $Ru(bpy)_3^+$ by the radical TPA·. The excited state of $Ru(bpy)_3^{2+}$ is then generated by the reaction of $Ru(bpy)_3^+$ with TPA cation radical (TPA·⁺). Since no electrochemical oxidation of $Ru(bpy)_3^{2+}$ is required in this ECL route, the emission can be generated at a potential below 1.0 V vs SCE. Evident low-oxidation-potential ECL was observed at freshly polished glass carbon and fluorosurfactant modified electrodes (Li and Zu 2004; Zu and Bard 2000).

9.2.2 ECL with Luminol as Emitter

While the $Ru(bpy)_3^{2+}$/TPA system described earlier is probably the most commonly used system to generate ECL in sensing application, some other compounds were also found to produce ECL with different pathways, such as luminol (5-amino-2,3-dihydro-1,4-phthalazinedione), lucigenin, and acridinium ester. The first report on luminol ECL was published in 1954 at a dropping mercury electrode during the reduction of oxygen

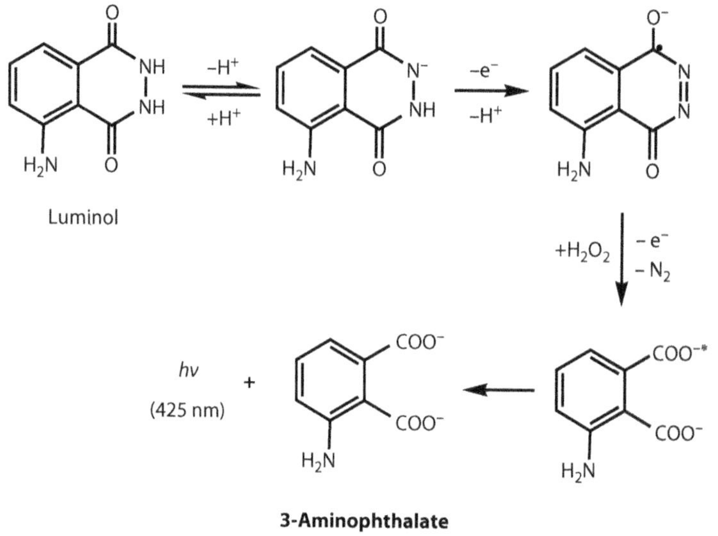

SCHEME 9.4

ECL reaction of luminol with hydrogen peroxide. (Adapted from *Talanta*, 54, Fähnrich, K.A., Pravda, M., and Guilbault, G.G., 2001, Recent applications of electrogenerated chemiluminescence in chemical analysis, 531–559. Copyright 2001 with permission from Elsevier.)

in an alkaline medium in the presence of luminol. This was followed by the studies of anodic generation of ECL in similar reaction media at a Pt electrode (Kuwana et al. 1963). Luminol ECL is often produced in alkaline solution with hydrogen peroxide upon electrochemical oxidation (Richter 2004). In alkaline medium, luminol forms an anion that is electrochemically oxidized. Further oxidation of the resulting diazo compound in the presence of hydrogen peroxide produces 3-aminophtalate in the excited state, as shown in Scheme 9.4. Different mechanistic pathways are involved in the electro-oxidation of luminol, partly depending on the applied potential. Hydrogen peroxide can participate as the peroxide anion HOO^- or as an electrochemically formed superoxide radical $O_2^{\cdot-}$ (Haapakka and Kankare 1982). Based on this reaction mechanism, luminol/H_2O_2-ECL system was allowed to detect a wide range of analytes including the species tagged with luminol, H_2O_2, enzyme reactions with the generation of H_2O_2, and some analytes acting as electrogenerated catalysts for the conventional CL-reaction. However, the relatively low quantum yield of luminol derivatives used for labeling has limited its practical application (Dodeigne et al. 2000).

9.2.3 ECL with Quantum Dots as Emitters

Quantum dots (QDs) are semiconductor nanocrystals with their size in the range of 1–10 nm. QDs are comprised of elements from the periodic groups IIB-VIA or IIIA-VA and the most typical QDs are Cd-chalcogenide nanocrystals (CdX, X = S, Se, Te). The ECL phenomenon of silicon nanocrystal QDs was first observed in 2002 by Ding and Bard (Ding et al. 2002). Since then, many QD-based ECL emitters including elemental or compound QDs have been reported. Compared with conventional organic emitters, QDs as ECL emitters show excellent advantages (e.g., high quantum yield, size or surface trap-controlled luminescence, and stability against photobleaching).

As other ECL systems, the ECL mechanism of QDs also involves general ion annihilation and coreactant ECL reaction pathways. In the annihilation pathway, both oxidized and reduced QD species are produced on the electrode surface by potential sweeping or pulsing. These species then react with each other to produce an electronically excited state, which emits light. A typical annihilation pathway is the ECL system of Si–QDs (Ding et al. 2002). When Si-NPs are oxidized or reduced by injecting holes or electrons under electrochemical conditions, electron-transfer annihilation of electrogenerated anion and cation radicals results in the production of excited state for ECL emission. Although annihilation ECL does not need additional reagent for emission, radical QDs must be chemically stable and maintain their charged states long enough to transfer charge upon colliding with oppositely charged QDs. Especially, when annihilation reaction between oxidized and reduced QDs is inefficient, the use of a coreactant may produce more intense ECL emission. In the presence of the coreactant, both QDs and coreactant are reduced at the working electrode. The coreactant is reduced to a strongly oxidizing agent, which can inject a hole into a QD species. The excited state QDs can be provided by the reaction between reduced and oxidized QDs, or by the direct injection of a hole into a reduced QD by the strongly oxidizing agent.

Thus, modern ECL applications of QDs are almost exclusively based on coreactant ECL. Oxalate and TPA are the most important "oxidative" or "oxidative–reductive" coreactants and have been widely used in analysis due to their ability to form a strongly reducing agent upon electrochemical oxidation. For example, Bard's group demonstrated strong light emission from Si–QD solution, in which CO_2^{-} injects an electron into the LUMO of an oxidized Si–QD to produce excited state that then emits light (Ding et al. 2002). Different from oxalate and TPA systems, the reduction of peroxydisulfate ($S_2O_8^{2-}$) produces a strong oxidant, SO_4^{-}, which then undergoes an electron-transfer reaction with an ECL luminophore to generate light. Bard and coworkers first demonstrated that peroxydisulfate can be used as coreactant for the ECL emission of Si–QDs (Ding et al. 2002). In addition, Zou and Ju demonstrated that the electron transfer reaction between electrochemically reduced nanocrystal species and H_2O_2 can produce ECL emission from CdSe–QDs, where H_2O_2 can be generated from the reduced dissolved oxygen and enzyme-based biological reactions (Zou and Ju 2004). In Zhu's group, they first reported the ECL property of CdS spherical nanoparticles and proposed the mechanism for ECL as annihilation mechanism (Ren et al. 2005). Next, they studied the ECL behavior of CdS nanotubes in aqueous solution and found two respective ECL peaks (Jie et al. 2007a; Miao et al. 2005). The first ECL peak at −0.9 V (vs. Ag/AgCl sat. KCl) is generated via an annihilation process between reduced and oxidized species. The second ECL peak at −1.2 V is attributed to the electron-transfer reaction between electrochemically reduced CdS nanocrystal species (CdS·$^{-}$) and coreactants ($S_2O_8^{2-}$ or H_2O_2).

9.3 Functions of Nanomaterials in ECL Sensing Systems

Nanomaterials are defined as materials having at least one dimension 100 nm or less, which constitute a bridge between molecules and infinite bulk systems. Nanomaterials encompass a broad range of materials, including nanoparticles, nanorods, nanocrystals, nanowires, and nanotubes of virtually any chemical composition. Unlike the corresponding bulk materials, nanomaterials render them with large surface area, high surface energy, spatial confinement, etc., and exhibit unique chemical, physical, and electronic properties. Due to the small dimensions, nanomaterials show extremely large surface area to volume ratio, which makes large interfacial atoms, resulting in more "surface" dependent material properties. This in turn may enhance or modify the properties of the bulk materials, such as higher chemical reactivity. Meanwhile, the nanometer feature sizes of nanomaterials also have spatial confinement effect on the materials, which bring the quantum effects. Furthermore, the energy band structure and charge carrier density in the materials can be modified quite differently from their bulk and in turn will modify the electronic and optical properties of the materials.

Bioanalysis in general and biosensor fields in particular are showing special interest in nanomaterials in the last years because of their unique optical, electrical, electrochemical, and luminescent properties, which make them an attractive material with applications in biosensing and medical diagnostics. Achieving higher sensitivities and better and more reliable analysis are the major objectives of biosensors. The incorporation of nanomaterials into sensing devices generates novel interfaces that enable sensitive optical or electrochemical detection of molecular and biomolecular analytes. Moreover, they are being used as effective labels to amplify the analysis and to design novel biomaterial architectures with predesigned and controlled functions with interest for several applications. In ECL sensing systems, the application of various types of nanomaterials including metallic nanoparticles, CNTs, semiconductor nanoparticles, and even composite nanoparticles has drastically improved ECL sensitivity and stability. Although these nanomaterials play different roles based on their unique chemical and physical properties, the basic functions in ECL sensors can be roughly classified as follows:

1. *Facilitating electrochemical reactions*: As described earlier, electrochemical reactions of an ECL emitter and coreactant are the first step in a series of reactions that eventually generate ECL. In general, these electrode reactions are rather slow in comparison with homogeneous redox reactions, and are therefore the rate-determining steps. Many nanomaterials, especially metal nanoparticles have excellent catalytic properties. The introduction of conductive nanomaterials with catalytic properties into ECL (bio)sensors as electrodes can catalyze the electrochemical oxidation/reduction of ECL emitters or coreactants. For instance, Cui's group investigated the ECL behavior of luminol on a gold nanoparticle (AuNP) modified electrode in neutral and alkaline solutions (Cui et al. 2004). The AuNP electrode exhibited excellent electrocatalytic property for luminol, showing three enhanced ECL peaks and one new ECL peak in neutral solutions. Following this study, they also investigated lucigenin ECL on AuNP modified gold disk electrode (Cui and Dong 2006). Unlike luminol, AuNPs enhanced lucigenin ECL by catalyzing the subsequent chemical reactions, exhibiting about one order of magnitude stronger ECL intensity than luminol. In the ECL system of $Ru(bpy)_3^{2+}$/TPA, it has been recognized that TPA electro-oxidation plays a critical role in ECL generation, especially in bioanalysis. Zu's group reported that gold modified indium tin oxide (ITO) electrode showed enhanced sensitivity for $Ru(bpy)_3^{2+}$ by reducing the large over-potential of TPA oxidation and the corrosive effect of ITO surface at high anodic potentials (Chen and Zu 2007). Huang et al. fabricated a highly transparent electrode for $Ru(bpy)_3^{2+}$-TPA ECL system based on ITO nanoparticle modified conductive glass (Huang et al. 2011). Due to the electrocatalysis of ITO nanoparticles, TPA oxidation potential shifted cathodically by 600 mV, leading to 24-fold increase in ECL peak intensity over the conventional ITO film electrode, and 2-fold increase in the integrated signal over the conventional gold film electrode.

2. *New solid support for biomolecule immobilization*: Nanomaterials can be employed as solid support for the immobilization of enzymes, antibodies, and DNAs in biosensors. Due to their large specific surface area and high surface free energy, nanomaterials can increase the amount of surface-immobilized biomolecules and improve their stability. In general, the adsorption of biomolecules directly onto the surface of bulk materials may result in their denaturation and loss of bioactivity. However, the adsorption of these biomolecules onto the surface of nanomaterials can retain their bioactivity due to the high biocompatibility of nanomaterials. In one such example, Dong and coworkers fabricated an alcohol dehydrogenase (ADH) biosensor by adsorbing ADH to $Ru(bpy)_3^{2+}$-containing AuNPs assembled on an ITO electrode (Zhang et al. 2007b). Because amine groups and cysteine residues of the enzyme are known to bind strongly with gold, AuNPs work as a favorable candidate for the immobilization of enzymes.

3. *Carriers of conventional ECL emitters for signal enhancement*: In ECL biosensors and bioassays, conventional (molecular) ECL emitters are attached to biomolecules as signal reporters. The number of emitters attached to a biomolecule is often limited to a few due to potential disruption of biomolecule structure and loss of activity. To improve ECL signal and biosensor sensitivity, great efforts have been made in using nanomaterials as the carriers of ECL emitters. In theory, tens or even hundreds of ECL emitters can be incorporated into one single nanoparticle, which can then be used as an ECL label with drastically enhanced luminescence intensity. The ECL emitters can be either encapsulated inside a nanoparticle, or immobilized on the surface of a nano-carrier. SiO_2 nanoparticles are widely used as the carrier of ECL emitters. Guo et al. (2004) reported a simple method of preparing $SiO_2/Ru(bpy)_3^{2+}$ multilayer films on electrodes by alternately adsorbing positively charged $Ru(bpy)_3^{2+}$ and negatively charged SiO_2 nanoparticles. Later, $Ru(bpy)_3^{2+}$ (Zhang and Dong 2006) and luminol (Zhang and Zheng 2006) were doped into nanoparticles, respectively and applied to ECL sensors. Additionally, many metallic nanoparticles and CNTs were also used as ECL emitter carriers for the fabrication of highly sensitive ECL biosensors (Sun et al. 2005; Tao et al. 2008; Wang et al. 2006).

4. *New ECL emitters*: Semiconductor nanocrystals (QDs) have been shown to possess some unique optical properties such as high luminescence intensity, wide range of excitation wavelength, narrow emission peak, and high photo-stability, and therefore have become very popular fluorescent labels and imaging agents. Similarly, some QDs also exhibit excellent ECL properties and are regarded as a new generation of ECL-emitters. The first study on ECL of elemental semiconductor, silicon nanocrystal, was reported by Bard's group in 2002 (Ding et al. 2002). They found that electron transfer reactions between positively and negatively charged nanocrystals or between charged nanocrystals and coreactants led to annihilation between electrons and holes, and subsequent emission of visible light. Following this work, the ECL emission of many other elemental or compound semiconductors in organic media or aqueous solutions was observed, including Ge (Myung et al. 2004), CdS (Jie et al. 2007b), ZnS (Shen et al. 2007), CdSe (Myung et al. 2002), and CdTe (Bae et al. 2004). The ECL mechanism of QDs also follows the general annihilation and coreactant reaction pathways as described earlier. Meanwhile, elemental semiconductors such as Si and Ge have the advantage of being relatively stable on reduction and oxidation (in the absence of water), compared to compound semiconductors (Bard et al. 2005).

9.4 Nanomaterial-Based ECL Biosensors

9.4.1 Metallic Nanoparticles

9.4.1.1 Gold Nanoparticle

In the field of ECL (bio)sensing with metal nanoparticles, AuNPs are widely used due to their excellent catalytic activity, electrical conductivity, ease of synthesis, and established surface chemistry. Wang's group employed AuNPs as solid support for the immobilization of avidin in the ECL detection of bovine serum albumin (BSA) and immunoglobulin G (IgG), as illustrated in Figure 9.1 (Yin et al. 2005). AuNPs were first covalently attached to the surface of a gold film electrode. Avidin was then covalently immobilized on the AuNP surface modified with 3-mercaptopropionic acid. Biotinylated BSA was reacted with avidin, and detected by ECL. IgG was tested via a typical sandwich-type immunoassay method. Sensitivity enhancement of 10- and 6-fold was obtained for BSA and IgG with AuNPs over direct immobilization on Au film electrodes, due to the increased electrode surface area and higher amount of immobilized avidin. Other gold nanomaterials, such as gold nanorods, have also been investigated as nanostructures for ECL (Dong et al. 2006). ECL intensity was enhanced 2- to 10-fold on the gold nanorod modified electrode in neutral solutions than a gold-nanosphere modified electrode.

AuNP modified electrodes also show catalytic effect toward the electrochemical oxidation/reduction of ECL emitters such as luminol (Cui et al. 2004) and lucigenin (Cui and Dong 2006) as well as coreactant TPA (Chen and Zu 2007). Cui's group found that AuNP electrodes enhanced the luminol–hydrogen peroxide CL signal due to the catalytic effect of AuNPs on the radical generation and electron-transfer processes during luminol CL reaction (Cui et al. 2004; Zhang et al. 2005). Liu et al. fabricated a glucose biosensor based on AuNP-catalyzed luminol ECL on a three-dimensional sol-gel network (Liu et al. 2008). The assembled AuNPs could efficiently electrocatalyze luminol ECL. Recently, Li's group reported a novel ECL biosensor using AuNPs as signal transduction

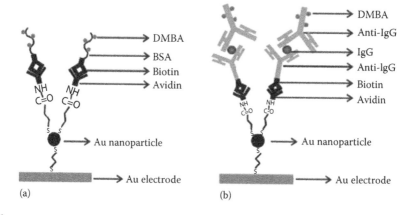

(a)   (b)

FIGURE 9.1
Schematic diagrams of immobilization of bovine serum albumin (BSA (a)) and immunoglobulin G (IgG (b)) on the gold electrode with gold nanoparticle (AuNP) amplification. (Reprinted with permission from Yin, X.B., Qi, B., Sun, X., Yang, X., and Wang, E., 4-(Dimethylamino) butyric acid labeling for electrochemiluminescence detection of biological substances by increasing sensitivity with gold nanoparticle amplification, *Anal. Chem.,* 77, 3525–3530. Copyright 2005 American Chemical Society.)

probes for the detection of kinase activity (Xu et al. 2010). The nanoparticles were conjugated specifically to the thiophosphate group after the protein phosphorylation process, amplified the ECL signal of luminol, and thus offered a highly sensitive ECL biosensor for kinase activity detection.

AuNPs were further used as ECL emitter carrier for the fabrication of highly sensitive ECL biosensors. For example, Zhang's group developed a highly sensitive ECL method for the detection of DNA hybridization event using AuNPs as a carrier for ECL label and ssDNA (Wang et al. 2006). Due to multiple signal reporters per hybridization event, a detection limit of as low as 5 pM for target ssDNA was achieved. Dong et al. (Sun et al. 2005) fabricated $Ru(bpy)_3^{2+}$-gold nanoparticle aggregates (Ru-AuNPs) via electrostatic interactions by mixing citrate-capped AuNPs and $Ru(bpy)_3^{2+}$ in aqueous medium. The aggregates were then attached to functionalized ITO electrode surface via Au–S interaction. The resulting Ru–AuNP modified ITO electrode was quite stable and exhibited excellent ECL behavior. It holds great promise for solid-state ECL detection of organic amines in capillary electrophoresis (CE) or CE microchips.

Xu's group demonstrated the interactions between electrogenerated excitons in ECL of CdS/Mn nanocrystals and ECL-induced surface plasmon resonance (SPR) of AuNPs (Shan et al. 2009b). The quenching of ECL from a CdS:Mn nanocrystal film by proximal Au nanoparticles was observed as a result of Förster energy transfer. Meanwhile, ECL enhancement took place after DNA hybridization due to energy transfer from ECL excited SPR in AuNPs to CdS:Mn at large separation. ECL intensity from CdS/Mn increased by 55% when Au NPs and CdS/Mn film were at a distance of about 10 nm. Later, they further reported greatly enhanced ECL of CdS thin films by AuNPs in the ultrasensitive detection of thrombin (Wang et al. 2011b), as illustrated in Figure 9.2. Compared to the one without AuNPs, the current system showed fivefold enhancement of ECL intensity, which is attributed to the long-distance interaction between CdS and SPR field of AuNPs.

9.4.1.2 Platinum Nanoparticle

Like AuNPs, platinum nanoparticles (PtNPs) have also been used in electrochemical sensors due to their high electrical conductivity and electroactivity. Wang and coworkers have demonstrated their use in an ECL sensor for TPA based on a novel PtNP/Eastman AQ55D cation ion-exchange polymer/$Ru(bpy)_3^{2+}$ colloidal materials (Du et al. 2006). The cation ion-exchanger was used to encapsulate $Ru(bpy)_3^{2+}$ and also as a dispersant of PtNPs. The sensor exhibited higher ECL intensity and shorter equilibration time, resulting in an extremely low detection limit of 10^{-15} M TPA.

Cui's group studied the ECL behavior of lucigenin at a glass carbon electrode in the presence of PtNPs dispersed in alkaline aqueous solutions (Guo et al. 2007). A new ECL peak appeared at −2.0 V (vs. SCE) in the presence of PtNPs. They proposed that the new ECL peak is likely due to the reductive intermediate $H_{ads}Pt^0$ formed during the hydrogen-evolution process that reduced lucigenin cation (Luc^{2+}) to monocation radial ($Luc^{.+}$). Subsequently, $Luc^{.+}$ and $H_{ads}Pt^0$ reacted with dissolved oxygen to generate $O_2^{.-}$, which interacted with $Luc^{.+}$ to produce the excited state N-methylacridone, generating light emission at 495 nm. Chen et al. (2009) also investigated the ECL behavior of luminol on PtNPs modified ITO electrode in a neutral aqueous solution. Compared with bare ITO or bulk platinum electrodes, the ECL behaviors of luminol on the PtNP modified electrode exhibited significant difference, showing two new ECL peaks at −0.44 and −1.16 V. The excellent ECL properties of luminol on the PtNP electrode in the neutral medium revealed a great potential for analytical applications of biological samples.

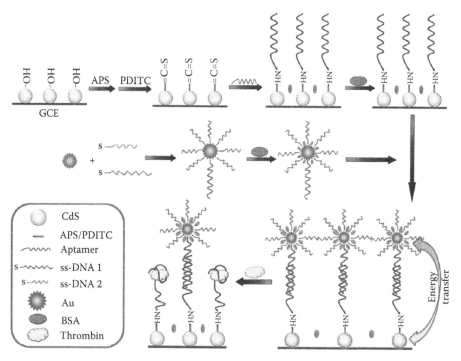

FIGURE 9.2

(See color insert.) ECL aptamer sensing platform based on energy transfer between CdS nanocrystals (NCs) and gold nanoparticles (Au NPs). (Acronym: 3-aminopropyl-triethoxysilane [APS], bovine serum albumin [BSA], 1,4-diisocyanatobenzene [PDITC]). (Reprinted with permission from Wang, J., Shan, Y., Zhao, W.W., Xu, J.J., and Chen, H.Y., Au nanoparticles enhanced electro-chemiluminescence of Cds thin film for ultrasensitive thrombin detection, *Anal. Chem.*, 83, 4004–4011. Copyright 2011b American Chemical Society.)

9.4.1.3 Silver Nanoparticles

Silver nanoparticles (AgNPs) are another type of conductive nanomaterials for ECL applications (Chang et al. 2005; Tang et al. 2005). As silver is more easily oxidized than gold, certain electrocatalytic reactions occur more rapidly with AgNPs as a catalyst than with gold. Cui and coworkers investigated the ECL behavior of luminol on AgNP modified gold electrodes in neutral and alkaline solutions (Wang and Cui 2007). The electrode exhibited excellent ECL properties for the luminol ECL system. The ECL intensity was enhanced significantly compared to bulk gold electrodes and AuNP modified electrodes. Additionally, Gao et al. (2009) proved that AgNPs could also facilitate the oxidation of $Ru(bpy)_3^{2+}$ in ECL measurements and dramatically enhance its emission intensity. Based on the synergistic catalysis of nicotinamide adenine dinucleotide hydride (NADH) and AgNPs, Wang's group later developed a signal-enhanced ECL immunosensor (Wang et al. 2011a). Recently, Pan's group fabricated a conductive, transparent electrode composed of silver nanowires and used in ECL system of $Ru(bpy)_3^{2+}$ in the presence of hydrogen peroxide (Zhu et al. 2011). Compared with bulk silver wire, glassy carbon disk, and thermally reduced transparent graphene oxide electrodes, the Ag nanowire electrode showed excellent properties for the reductive-oxidation ECL generation, which is attributed to its catalytic properties with respect to the reduction of hydrogen peroxide and its high surface area.

9.4.1.4 Metal Nanoclusters

Metal nanoclusters are composed of a very few metal atoms with a size comparable to the Fermi wavelength of electrons (0.7 nm) and therefore exhibit molecule-like properties of discrete electronic states. Due to their low toxicity compared with QDs, metal nanoclusters are promising candidates in optical systems, biosensors, and catalysis. Ras's group first illustrated the cathodic hot electron-induced ECL behavior of silver nanoclusters in the presence of $S_2O_8^{2-}$ via an "oxidation–reduction" excitation pathway (Díez et al. 2009). However, the poor stability of silver nanocluster limited its applications. Recently, gold nanoclusters (AuNCs) were synthesized with BSA as a protective coating, which displayed different ECL phenomena when using different electrodes and coreactants (Fang et al. 2011; Li et al. 2011b). Li et al. investigated the ECL mechanism on AuNCs in detail. They confirmed that the cathodic ECL originated from electron-transfer annihilation of negatively charged $Au_{25}^{\cdot-}$ and $SO_4^{\cdot-}$ radicals generated by electroreduction of $S_2O_8^{2-}$ (Li et al. 2011b). The proposed ECL mechanisms are illustrated in Figure 9.3. The ITO electrode employed in this study acted as an effective reductant for AuNCs by transferring electrons from its conduction band to the LUMO of AuNCs. Finally, the AuNC modified ITO electrode was applied to the detection of dopamine based on the enhanced ECL by formation of a charge transfer complex between dopamine and ITO.

Recently, Fang and coworkers reported the ECL generation of AuNCs with another coreactant, triethylamine (TEA), and applied the system to the determination of a heavy metal ion, Pb^{2+} (Fang et al. 2011). Unlike the previous system, the observed anodic ECL was

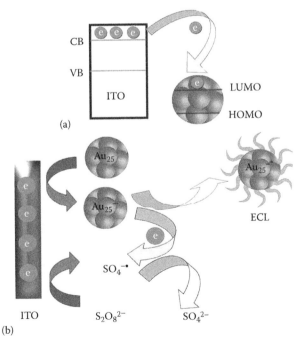

FIGURE 9.3
Schematic illustration of (a) electron transfer between indium tin oxide (ITO) and Au nanocrystals (NCs) and (b) the ECL mechanisms of gold nanocluster. (Acronym: conduction band [CB], valence band [VB], lowest unoccupied molecular orbital [LUMO], high occupied molecular orbital [HOMO]). (Reprinted with permission from Li, L., Liu, H., Shen, Y., Zhang, J., and Zhu, J.J., Electrogenerated Chemiluminescence of Au nanoclusters for the detection of dopamine, *Anal. Chem.* 83, 661–665. Copyright 2011b American Chemical Society.)

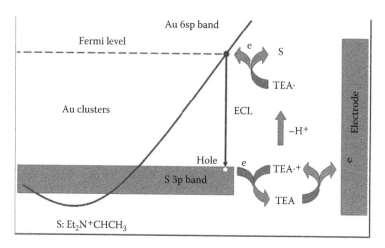

FIGURE 9.4
Schematic ECL mechanism from the Au_{25} clusters with triethylamine (TEA). (From Fang, Y.M., Song, J., Li, J. et al., Electrogenerated Chemiluminescence from Au nanoclusters, *Chem. Commun.*, 47, 2369–2371. Copyright 2011. Reprinted by permission of The Royal Society of Chemistry.)

attributed to the electrochemical oxidation of TEA rather than the nanocluster. Instead of electrochemical oxidation at the electrode, Au_{25} is oxidized to Au_{25}^{+} by the injection of holes in the 3p-band with the electrochemical oxidation product (TEA·$^{+}$). This product deprotonates to form a very reductive radical (TEA·), which injects the electrons in the 6sp-band of gold, reducing Au_{25} to Au_{25}^{-}. Light emission occurs when Au_{25}^{+} collides with Au_{25}^{-} to produce excited state (Au_{25}^{*}), as shown in Figure 9.4. Based on the quenched ECL of AuNCs by Pb^{2+}, a novel method for the selective Pb^{2+} determination was developed with *L*-cysteine as the masking agent.

9.4.2 Carbon Nanomaterials

9.4.2.1 Carbon Nanotubes

The two main types of carbon nanotubes (CNTs) are single-walled CNTs (SWCNTs) and multiwalled carbon nanotubes (MWCNTs). While they have many of the same properties as other types of carbon materials, CNTs offer unique advantages including enhanced electronic properties, large edge plane/basal plane ratio, and rapid electrode kinetics. When CNTs are incorporated into an ECL sensor, they can increase the electrode surface area and its porosity, and also act as a conducting pathway to the electrode. Therefore, CNT-based sensors generally have higher sensitivity, lower limit of detection, and faster electron transfer kinetics than conventional carbon electrodes.

Similar to metal nanoparticles, CNTs have also been employed in ECL chemo-sensors and biosensors as immobilization phase and electrode materials. ECL sensors based on CNTs/polymer/Ru(bpy)$_3^{2+}$ composite films have been developed, using polymeric materials such as Nafion (Guo and Dong 2004), Eastman-AQ55D (Du et al. 2005), SiO_2 (Tao et al. 2007), sol–gel (Choi et al. 2006), and polystyrene (PSP) (Li et al. 2007a). CNTs were first dispersed in a polymer solution before they were cast onto an electrode surface to form a film. Ru(bpy)$_3^{2+}$ was then immobilized on the electrode by encapsulation within the film. For example, Guo et al. developed a Ru(bpy)$_3^{2+}$ doped composite film of Nafion/CNTs (Guo and Dong 2004). When the film was assessed with TPA, it was found that the interfusion of CNT in Nafion resulted in high ECL intensity. This suggests that the porous composite film allows fast diffusion of $Ru(bpy)_3^{2+}$, and that the CNTs connect $Ru(bpy)_3^{2+}$ sites to the electrode surface and facilitate ECL reactions. The sensitivity for TPA detection was 2 orders of magnitude greater than when silica was used in the place of CNTs, and 3 orders of magnitude higher than pure Nafion films. Additionally, CNTs not only benefited $Ru(bpy)_3^{2+}$-ECL system, but also improved other ECL systems such as luminol. For example, Dong et al. investigated the ECL of luminol at CNTs/Nafion modified gold electrode and found that ECL was enhanced 20-fold compared with the bare gold electrode (Dong 2010). The results indicate that CNTs have a significantly catalytic effect on luminol ECL.

CNT paste electrodes were developed by Chen's group by electrically heating the mixture of MWNT powder, $Ru(bpy)_3^{2+}$, and mineral oil to form a paste and casting on an electrode (Chen et al. 2007b). Coupled with electrophoresis, this sensing system showed high sensitivity, wide dynamic range, and excellent reproducibility for the detection of organophosphate insecticides. In addition, they also developed a CNT paste electrode infused with glucose oxidase (GOx) as a glucose sensor (Chen et al. 2007a). Luminol was injected into the solution phase to react with H_2O_2, which was produced in the catalysis of glucose by GOx. Recently, room temperature ionic liquids have attracted intensive interest in electrochemistry because of their unique chemical and physical properties such as high chemical and thermal stability, a relatively wide potential window, and high ionic conductivity. Chen et al. developed a composite paste electrode consisting of MWNT and room temperature ionic liquids for the fabrication of ECL sensors (Dai et al. 2009). The sensors exhibited extraordinary stability during long-term potential cycling, and were used for the determination of methamphetamine hydrochloride.

CNTs are an ideal type of carriers for electrochemical signal reporters due to their microscale length and high electrical conductivity that ensure high loading and electrochemical accessibility to all the signaling molecules. Khairoutdinov et al. (2004) and Panhuis and coworkers (Frehill et al. 2002) reported respectively covalent attachment of ruthenium complexes to carboxylated SWCNTs and amino functionalized MWCNTs. Following these studies, Li et al. developed a sandwich DNA hybridization assay using SWCNT carried $Ru(bpy)_3^{2+}$ as an ECL label (Li et al. 2007b). Single stranded DNA probes were also loaded onto the nanotube to produce SWCNT/$Ru(bpy)_3^{2+}$ labeled DNA. After sandwich hybridization reaction between capture DNA, target DNA, and probe DNA, the composite label was brought to the electrode surface, and generated strong ECL signal (Figure 9.5). The SWCNT provided a signal enhancement platform for carrying a large number of $Ru(bpy)_3^{2+}$ and thus resulted in an ultrasensitive ECL detection of DNA hybridization, in which a detection limit of 9 fM was achieved.

9.4.2.2 Graphene

Graphene, a flat monolayer of carbon atoms tightly packed into a two-dimensional honeycomb lattice, is the basic building block for graphitic materials of all other dimensionalities. Compared with other carbon nanomaterials, graphene has some obvious advantages: no interference from metallic impurities that might exist in the synthesis of CNTs and ease of production and functionalization. As an electrode material, graphene presented excellent electron transfer ability for some enzymes (Kang et al. 2009; Wu et al. 2010) and excellent catalytic behavior toward small molecules such as dopamine, H_2O_2, O_2, NADH, and TNT (Chen et al. 2010; Shan et al. 2009a; Tang et al. 2009, 2010; Wang et al. 2009b; Zhou et al. 2009). Additionally, the large surface area of graphene and its derivatives (theoretically $2630 \ m^2 \cdot g^{-1}$ for single-layer graphene) also enables them to be an excellent carrier of signal

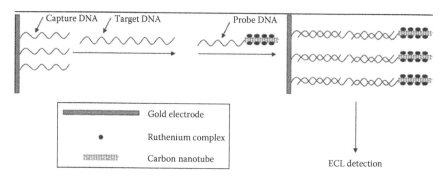

FIGURE 9.5
Schematic diagram of the ECL detection for DNA hybridization using sandwich DNA detection model and the ECL probes of carbon-nanotubes loaded with probe ss-DNA and Ruthenium complex derivative tags. (Reprinted from *Talanta*, 72, Li, Y., Qi, H., Fang, F., and Zhang, C., Ultrasensitive electrogenerated chemiluminescence detection of DNA hybridization using carbon-nanotubes loaded with tris (2,2′-bipyridyl) ruthenium derivative tags, 1704–1709. Copyright 2007, with permission from Elsevier.)

probes and active domain for biomolecule binding, offering significant enhancement of the electrochemical and ECL sensing signals (Du et al. 2010, 2011; Wan et al. 2011).

Fan et al. (2008) first reported fairly intense ECL of graphene oxide (GO) nanoparticles at a potential of 1.15 V (vs. SCE). Besides its intrinsic ECL, improved ECL performance was also achieved on graphene modified electrodes. Xu's group (Li et al. 2009) reported an ECL sensor based on Ru(bpy)$_3^{2+}$-graphene-Nafion composite film. The introduction of graphene into Nafion film not only dramatically promotes the electron transfer of Ru(bpy)$_3^{2+}$ but also significantly improves the stability of the sensor by inhibiting the migration of Ru(bpy)$_3^{2+}$ into the electrochemically inactive hydrophobic region of Nafion. This ECL sensor showed comparable detection limit to the ECL sensor based on Nafion–CNT composite, and was further used to detect oxalate in urine samples. They later fabricated a Ru(phen)$_3^{2+}$/GO modified electrode instead of Ru(bpy)$_3^{2+}$ by mixing Ru(phen)$_3^{2+}$ with GO (Yuan et al. 2012). The ECL sensor demonstrated outstanding long-term stability. Recently, Cui's group covalently grafted a Ru(II) complex onto GO by the amide reaction between the amino group of a Ru(bpy)$_3^{2+}$ analogue and carboxyl group on GO (Yu et al. 2012). The as-prepared Ru-GO showed excellent ECL activity, good solubility, and good stability.

Additionally, graphene has been applied in ECL biosensors using luminol and quantum dot (QD)-based systems. Li et al. (Wang et al. 2009d) first reported GO amplified ECL of QDs platform and its efficient selective sensing for antioxidants. They found GO facilitated the generation of CdTe QD·$^+$ and formed a high yield of CdTe QDs·, then leading to fivefold ECL amplification compared to the system without GO. Later, the same group reported cathodic ECL of luminol at ca. 0.05 V (vs. Ag/AgCl) with strong light emission on the graphene-modified glass carbon electrode, offering an excellent platform for high performance biosensing application (Xu et al. 2011). Based on the cathodic ECL, an ECL sandwich immunosensor for sensitive detection of cancer biomarkers at low potentials was developed, which employed a multiple signal amplification strategy relying on graphene composite modified electrode and gold nanorod multilabeled with glucose oxidase and secondary antibody (Figure 9.6). The introduction of functionalized graphene not only facilitated the ECL generation of luminol, but also increased the surface density of immobilized primary antibody. The as-proposed low-potential ECL immunosensor exhibited a detection range from 10 pg·mL^{-1} to 8 ng·mL^{-1} and a detection limit of as low as 8 pg·mL^{-1} for prostate antigen.

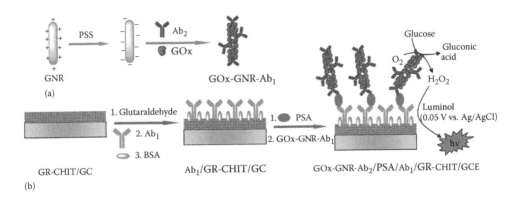

FIGURE 9.6
(a) Modification procedure of gold nanorods and (b) ECL immunoassay of PSA with multiple amplification strategy based on a graphene composite modified electrode. (Acronym: primary antibody [Ab1], secondary antibody [Ab2], bovine serum albumin [BSA], chitosan [CHIT], glass carbon electrode [GCE], gold nanorods [GNRs], glucose oxidase [GOx], graphene [GR], prostate protein antigen [PSA], poly(sodium 4-styrenesulfonate) [PSS]). (Reprinted with permission from Xu, S., Liu, Y., Wang, T., and Li, J., Positive potential operation of a cathodic electrogenerated chemiluminescence immunosensor based on luminol and graphene for cancer biomarker detection, *Anal. Chem.*, 83, 3817–3823. Copyright 2011 American Chemical Society.)

9.4.2.3 Carbon Nanocrystals

In 2004, Sun et al. reported the finding of quantum-sized carbon nanocrystals (CNCs), also called carbon dots, which upon simple surface passivation are strongly photoluminescent in both solutions and the solid state (Sun et al. 2006). They also found that these carbon dots are strongly two-photon luminescent with pulsed laser excitation in the near-infrared range, and can be used in cell imaging (Cao et al. 2007). Since then carbon dots have been prepared by a variety of methods, including laser ablation of graphite (Cao et al. 2007; Sun et al. 2006), electrochemical oxidation of graphite (Zhao et al. 2008), electrochemical treatment of MWCNTs (Zhou et al. 2007), chemical oxidation of arc-discharge SWCNTs (Bottini et al. 2006; Xu et al. 2004) and candle soot (Li et al. 2010), proton-beam irradiation of nanodiamonds (Fu et al. 2007), and thermal oxidation of suitable molecular precursors (Bourlinos et al. 2008). The generation of ECL signal of CNCs was first reported in Chi's group (Zheng et al. 2009). They used a simple and effective method for preparing water-soluble CNCs with ECL activity by applying a scanning potential to graphite rods and presented their observations on the ECL behavior during and after the preparation of CNCs. Similar to other semiconductor nanocrystals, the ECL mechanism of CNC is proposed as the formation of excited-state CNCs via electron-transfer annihilation between negatively charged and positively charged CNCs. In addition, the ECL behavior of CNC in the presence of coreactant (peroxydisulfate) was also investigated, showing the stable and greatly enhanced ECL response. This kind of CNCs provides the promising applications in the development of new types of ECL biosensors in the future based on its strong ECL emission, good water solubility, high stability, ease of production and derivation, and environmental friendliness.

9.4.3 Quantum Dots

Since the ECL of silicon QDs was reported by Bard's group in 2002, a variety of QDs with different compositions, sizes, and shapes have been synthesized as ECL emitters for bioanalysis. Especially QDs functionalized with biomolecules offer excellent ECL signal-transduction platforms for designing a new generation of biosensing devices.

Similar to conventional molecular ECL emitters, the applications of QDs in ECL sensing are mostly based on the coreactant ECL pathway, including oxalate, TPA, $S_2O_8^{2-}$, SO_3^{2-}, H_2O_2, etc. (Lei and Ju 2011). As we know, H_2O_2 is the substrate of many enzymatic reactions and also is a coreactant of QDs-based ECL systems. Therefore, a number of QDs–ECL biosensors were developed for peroxidase-related analytes by coupling with an enzymatic reaction where H_2O_2 was produced. For example, Ju et al. reported an ECL sensor for H_2O_2 detection by depositing a CdSe–QD film on a graphite electrode (Zou and Ju 2004). They found that the electron-transfer reaction between electrochemically reduced nanocrystals and oxidative coreactants such as H_2O_2 led to an ECL peak, which was dependent on the concentration of H_2O_2. This system was used to detect H_2O_2 in de-aerated solutions down to levels as low as 0.1 µM. Later, they found dissolved oxygen was a more efficient coreactant than H_2O_2, and another QDs-based ECL sensor was developed based on the consumption of dissolved oxygen during enzymatic reaction (Jiang and Ju 2007b). This strategy can be applied to detect the substrates of many oxidases.

Another sensing mechanism is based on the inhibition effect of QD ECL by the target analytes. For example, in the ECL system of thioglycolic acid–capped CdSe–QD film/peroxide, it was believed that the intermediate hydroxyl radical was the key species for producing hole-injected QDs. Thus, a highly sensitive method for the detection of both scavengers and generators of OH· was developed (Jiang and Ju 2007a). In addition, energy transfer or charge transfer involving the excited QDs also provides a strategy for biosensing. For instance, Liu et al. found that the mercaptopropionic acid–capped CdTe–QDs produced intensive anodic ECL at an ITO electrode (Liu et al. 2007). The superoxide ion generated on the ITO surface injects an electron into QDs, resulting in the formation of the excited QDs. However, in the presence of catechol derivatives (e.g., dopamine or L-adrenalin), the energy of the excited CdTe–QDs is transferred to these derivatives, leading to reduced ECL. This provides a novel way to detect catechol derivatives. Xu's group reported an ECL sensing-platform for highly sensitive and specific detection of DNA targets with CdS:Mn nanocrystal as an ECL emitter and AuNP as both ECL quencher and enhancer (Shan et al. 2009b). AuNP quenched the ECL of QDs through Förster energy transfer before hybridization, and enhanced the ECL emission due to the interactions of the excited CdS:Mn–QDs with surface-plasmon resonance of AuNP at long distance upon hybridization. Wu et al. reported a novel ECL resonance energy transfer protocol involving energy transfer from an ECL donor (CdS–QDs) to an acceptor ($Ru(bpy)_3^{2+}$) (Wu et al. 2011). The latter does not produce cathodic ECL in the potential range from 0 to −1.4 V, and therefore can serve as a sensitive energy acceptor of cathodic ECL donor (CdS–QDs). By exploiting the specific antibody–cell surface interactions, this system responded sensitively to 12.5 SMMC-7721 cells·mL^{-1} (Figure 9.7). Recently, Jin's group reported another ECL resonance energy transfer system using luminol as the donor and QD as the acceptor, which was used in the investigation of protein interactions and conformational changes (Li et al. 2011a).

Some conducting nanomaterials including graphene (oxide), metallic nanoparticles, and CNTs have been found to enhance the cathodic ECL of QDs. The enhancement was attributed to a reduced barrier for electron injection, resulting in a lower onset potential and increased ECL intensity. This enhancement is important since QDs are typically poorer ECL emitters than the more commonly used ruthenium complexes or luminol. Wang et al. developed a biosensor for acetylcholine and choline using a paraffin-impregnated graphite electrode (PIGE) incorporating MWCNT–QD conjugates (Wang et al. 2009c). The CdS QDs were synthesized on the CNTs *in situ* and the QD–CNT conjugates displayed a fivefold enhancement in ECL intensity compared to QDs alone. The enzymes, acetylcholine esterase and choline oxidase were immobilized on the QD–CNT–modified PIGE.

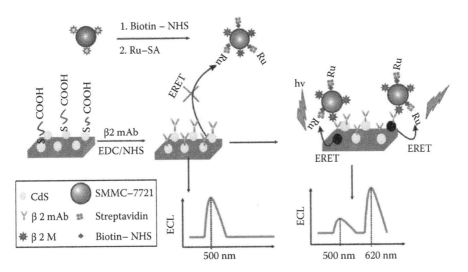

FIGURE 9.7
(See color insert.) ECL biosensor based on ECL-RET for determination of b2 M expressed cells. (Acronym: electrochemiluminescence resonance energy transfer [ERET], *N*-hydroxysuccinimide [NHS], streptavidin [SA], *N*-(3-dimethylaminopropyl)-*N*'-ethyl-carbodiimide hydrochloride [EDC]). (From Wu, M.S., Shi, H.W., Xu, J.J., and Chen, H.Y., CdS quantum dots/Ru (bpy)$_3^{2+}$ electrochemiluminescence resonance energy transfer system for sensitive cytosensing, *Chem. Commun.*, 47, 7752–7754. Copyright 2011. Reprinted by permission of The Royal Society of Chemistry.)

A byproduct of the catalytic cycles of these enzymes was hydrogen peroxide as coreactant for cathodic QD ECL. Increasing sample concentrations of acetylcholine or choline increased the observed ECL linearly, with limit of detection of 0.8 and 1.7 μM, respectively. Additionally, the incorporation of AuNPs into QD-ECL biosensor design had the effect of increasing ECL intensity. For example, Jie et al. (2008) reported a nonlabeled ECL immunosensor based on CdSe–QD by incorporating a layer of AuNPs on an electrode. The ECL intensity was enhanced ca. 17 times, which was attributed to a decreased charge transfer resistance resulting from the conductivity imparted by the AuNPs. This system was developed to detect human prealbumin (PAB, antigen) with a 10 pg·mL^{-1} LOD. Zhu's group presented an advanced ECL immunosensor for the sensitive detection of human IgG using graphene–QD composites as the ECL label (Li et al. 2011c), as shown in Figure 9.8. In the sensing system, cationic polymer PDDA-functionalized graphene was used to assemble a large number of QDs, thus enhancing the ECL performance of the QDs. After assembly on AuNPs, the graphene–CdSe composite film exhibited higher ECL intensity, better electronic conductivity, and faster response time. Then, the antibody (Ab, goat antihuman IgG) was linked to the graphene–CdSe–AuNP film. The ECL immunosensor had an extremely sensitive response to human IgG in a linear range of 0.02–2000 pg·mL^{-1} with a detection limit of 0.005 pg·mL^{-1}.

9.4.4 Magnetic Nanoparticles

Magnetic nanoparticles (MNPs) are a class of nanoparticles that consist of magnetic elements such as iron, nickel, cobalt, and their chemical compounds, and can be manipulated using magnetic fields. Currently, ferrite nanoparticles are the most explored MNPs up to date. Actually the micron-sized magnetic particles (microbeads, 0.5–500 μm) have been previously used for ECL sensing (Miao and Bard 2004a, b) and the first ECL commercial

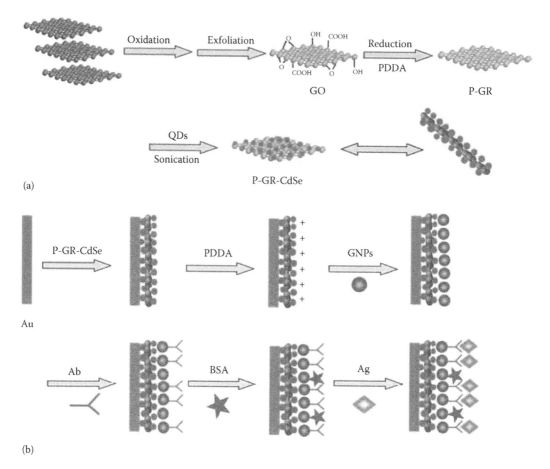

FIGURE 9.8
(a) Schematic representation of the preparation procedure of P-GR-CdSe composites: graphite (gray blocks). (b) Schematic illustration of the stepwise immunosensor fabrication process, including the formation of P-GR-CdSe composite film on the Au electrode, the linkage of PDDA to the film, the conjugation of GNPs to PDDA, the immobilization of antibody (Ab) on the electrode via GNPs, and the specific immunoreactions. (Acronym: polydiallyldimethylammonium chloride [PDDA], gold nanoparticles [GNPs], graphene [GR], quantum dots [QDs]). (From Li, L.L., Liu, K.P., Yang, G.H., Wang, C.M., Zhang, J.R., and Zhu, J.J.: Fabrication of graphene-quantum dots composites for sensitive electrogenerated chemiluminescence immunosensing. *Adv. Funct. Mater.* 2011. 21. 869–878. Copyright Wiley-VCH Verlag GmbH & Co. KGaA. Reproduced with permission.)

instrument was adapted to measure ECL labels present on the surface of magnetically responsive beads in 1994 (Yang et al. 1994). However, recent studies have mainly focused on the use of smaller-sized nanoparticles because they provide high colloidal stability, minimal nonspecific binding, and enhanced magnetic behavior. For example, Lee et al. coated magnetic nanoparticles with Nafion and used them as an immobilization matrix for $Ru(bpy)_3^{2+}$ (Kim et al. 2005). It was demonstrated that fast mass transport of $Ru(bpy)_3^{2+}$ at the Nafion-coated nanoparticles, probably due to the accessibility of the SO_3^- sites, resulted in higher sensitivity than the pure Nafion film without nanoparticles. The ECL signal decreased to 80% of the original value after 1 month storage, showing high stability. Dong's group developed a bifunctional nanoarchitecture by combing the magnetic iron oxide and the luminescent $Ru(bpy)_3^{2+}$ encapsulated in silica (Zhang et al. 2007a), in which

$Ru(bpy)_3^{2+}$ serves as a ECL marker, and Fe_3O_4 nanoparticles allow external manipulation by a magnetic field. This ECL sensor shows a wide linear range, high sensitivity, and good stability. In the work of Lee et al. (Lyu et al. 2009) monodispersed MNPs were coated with poly(3-thiopheneacetic acid) via an oxidative polymerization using $KMnO_4$ as an oxidant, and the magnetic field–driven multilayer films of the functional MNPs were formed as a matrix for immobilization of $Ru(bpy)_3^{2+}$. This ECL sensor exhibited quite a low limit of detection for TPA and also showed good reproducibility.

Recently, Jie et al. prepared a novel magnetic Fe_3O_4-CdSe composite QD and successfully applied to sensitive ECL detection of thrombin by a multiple DNA cycle amplification strategy (Jie and Yuan 2012). The composite QDs showed intense ECL, excellent magnetism and favorable biocompatibility. Xu's group reported optomagnetic interaction-induced enhancement of ECL from a CdS:Mn nanocrystal film by Fe_3O_4 nanoparticles and its application to sensitive immunosensing (Shan et al. 2010). The QD film was deposited on a glassy carbon electrode, upon which the capture antibody was immobilized. The second antibody was attached to the MNPs. In the presence of the antigen, a sandwich immuno-complex was formed, bringing the MNPs in close proximity of the QD film. ECL intensity increased greatly due to the enhancement effect, and was proportional to the antigen concentration.

9.4.5 Polymeric Nanoparticles

Bard's group investigated the electrochemical oxidation (Palacios et al. 2007) and ECL (Chang et al. 2008) of conjugated copolymer nanoparticles, poly(9,9-dioctylfluorene-co-benzothiadiazole) (F8BT), with a size of 25 ± 15 nm, as shown in Figure 9.9. ECL emission was generated when both F8BT nanoparticles and TPA were oxidized. This is the first observation of ECL from sub-25 nm single nanoparticles. And the catalytic ECL amplification by coreactant in the reaction provided a way to studying the dynamic information of single nanoparticle not seen in ensembles.

Another type of polymer nanoparticle used in ECL studies is aromatic hydrocarbon nanoparticles. Bard's group reported the preparation, characterization, and ECL characteristics of rubrene nanoparticles (diameter ~50 nm) and 9,10-diphenylanthracene (DPA) nanorods (with an average size of ~500 nm in length and ~50 nm in diameter) (Omer and Bard 2009). ECL emission from these nanoparticles was observed upon electrochemical oxidation in aqueous solutions containing different coreactants, such as TPA for rubrene and an oxalate for DPA nanorods. The ECL intensity from rubrene nanoparticles was greatly higher than that from DPA nanorods, which is attributed to the smaller size resulting in higher diffusion coefficient for rubrene as compared to DPA nanorods. Suk et al. recently reported the electrochemistry, photoluminescence, and ECL characterization of 9-naphthylanthracene (NA)-based dimer and trimer (Suk et al. 2011). Cyclic voltammetry of these two compounds showed two or three reversible, closely spaced one-electron oxidation peaks. The ECL emission resulted from the annihilation reaction in benzonitrile, and the ECL spectra showed two bands assigned to monomer and excimer emission, which was not observed in photoluminescence spectra. However, the ECL emission in the presence of coreactant, $K_2S_2O_8$, showed only monomer emission similar to PL wavelength, indicating the formation of excimer exclusively by radical ion annihilation. Furthermore, NA organic nanoparticles were synthesized by a coprecipitation method with a size of 15 ± 6 nm, which produced stable but weak ECL emission from the annihilation reaction. In the presence of the coreactant, ECL signal was strong enough to obtain an ECL spectrum.

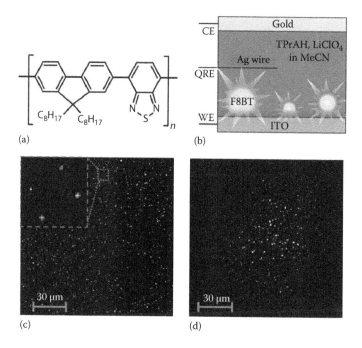

FIGURE 9.9

(a) F8BT chemical structure. (b) Schematic diagram of SMSEC cell. (c) Wide-field ECL image. (d) Wide-field photoluminescence (PL) image (same area as c) with the laser beam focused on the central area of the image (inset: expanded region showing ECL from four particles). The intensity scale (0–200 counts) and integration time (0.5 s) of images c and d are the same. (Reprinted with permission from Chang, Y.L., Palacios, R.E., Fan, F.R.F., Bard, A.J., and Barbara, P.F., Electrogenerated chemiluminescence of single conjugated polymer nanoparticles, *J. Am. Chem. Soc.*, 130, 8906–8907. Copyright 2008 American Chemical Society.)

Large-sized polymeric particles were also synthesized and applied in ECL sensing. For instance, polystyrene microspheres/beads (PSB) were synthesized by Miao et al. as the carrier of ECL emitters, tris(2,2-bipyridyl) ruthenium(II) tetrakis(pentafluorophenyl) borate (Ru(bpy)$_3$[B(C$_6$F$_5$)$_4$]$_2$), and used as labels in DNA hybridization and CRP immunoassay detection (Miao and Bard 2004a, b). PSB contained a large number of water insoluble Ru(bpy)$_3$[B(C$_6$F$_5$)$_4$]$_2$ species (7.5×10^9 molecules per bead). The detection limit of DNA and CRP was 1.0 fM and 10 ng·mL^{-1}, respectively.

9.4.6 Other Nanoparticles

1. *SiO$_2$ nanoparticles*: SiO$_2$ nanoparticles have shown some unique properties such as good biocompatibility and high optical transparency, and have been adapted to different applications in the bioanalytical field. Fang and coworkers used Ru(bpy)$_3^{2+}$-doped silica nanoparticles as ECL labels for DNA hybridization determinations (Chang et al. 2006). The doped nanoparticles were modified with complimentary target DNA, which hybridized with the capture DNA on the electrode surface. The coreactant, oxalic acid, was believed to penetrate the nanoparticles and allowed for the production of ECL proportional to the amount of target DNA. Due to the large number of Ru(bpy)$_3^{2+}$ molecules inside the nanoparticle, a detection limit at levels as low as 1.0×10^{-13} M of the target DNA was reported. Additionally, Ru(bpy)$_3^{2+}$ doped SiO$_2$ nanoparticles were conjugated with a biopolymer chitosan membrane

as a novel ECL sensor (Zhang and Dong 2006). Since a large amount of $Ru(bpy)_3^{2+}$ was immobilized three-dimensionally on the electrode, the $Ru(bpy)_3^{2+}$ ECL signal was enhanced greatly, which resulted in the increased sensitivity. This sensor showed a detection limit of 2.8 nM for TPA, which is 3 orders of magnitude lower than that observed at a Nafion-based ECL sensor. Furthermore, another important ECL emitter, luminol, was also doped into SiO_2 nanoparticles to fabricate novel ECL sensor (Zhang and Zheng 2006). The nanoparticles were then immobilized on a graphite electrode in a chitosan film through which pyrogallol diffused and was electrochemically oxidized. The resulting pyrogallol radical reduced oxygen to an anion radical, which in turn reacted with luminol to produce ECL. The emission was therefore dependent on pyrogallol concentration and a detection limit of 1.0 nM was achieved.

2. *Hybrid nanomaterials:* Recently, the application of hybrid nanomaterials consisting of two or more types of different nanomaterials in ECL sensing has received much attention. Hybrid nanomaterials based on nanosized particles and clusters have showed the possibility to tailor or integrate several different functionalities from these different nanomaterials (Guerra and Herrero 2010). For example, on graphene/metal nanocomposite modified ECL electrodes, graphene can provide large surface area for the adsorption of biomolecules, whereas the metal nanoparticle can catalyze the ECL reactions of the emitter and coreactant (Jafri et al. 2010). Zhu's group synthesized the Au nanoclusters (AuNCs) *in situ* on a bilayer graphene (Chen et al. 2011), as shown in Figure 9.10. The hybrid material was dispersible in aqueous solution and produced stable photoluminescence emission in the near-infrared range under visible light excitation. The application of this novel material for label-free detection of H_2O_2 was developed based on the ECL emission of the graphene/AuNCs hybrid in aqueous solution. Besides graphene (oxide), other types of nanomaterials such as metallic nanopartilces, CNTs, and semiconductor QDs are the most frequently used to fabricate hybrid nanomaterials in ECL sensing systems. For example, an ECL sensing technique for the detection of DNA

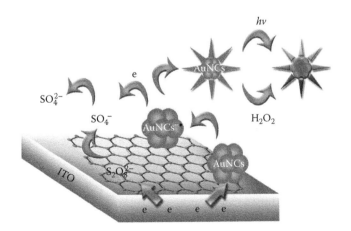

FIGURE 9.10
Schematic illustration of the ECL mechanism of the graphene/AuNCs hybrid for the detection of H_2O_2. (From Chen, Y., Shen, Y., Sun, D. et al., Fabrication of a dispersible graphene/gold nanoclusters hybrid and its potential application in electrogenerated chemiluminescence, *Chem. Commun.*, 47, 11733–11735. Copyright 2011. Reprinted by permission of The Royal Society of Chemistry.)

hybridization was developed based on a composite modified electrode prepared from AuNP and CNTs (Chu et al. 2011). Haghighi et al. fabricated a novel ECL glucose biosensor using AuNP decorated MWCNTs (Haghighi et al. 2011). This biosensor showed a remarkably improved electrocatalytic activity toward luminol oxidation and significant improvement in its ECL response. Zhu's group also presented an advanced ECL immunosensor for the sensitive detection of human IgG using graphene–QD composites as the ECL label (Li et al. 2011c).

Nanocomposites in an ordered array are expected to integrate several different functionalities required by the applications in one common structure, which are otherwise difficult to accomplish in single-component materials. In addition, the close coupling of different components on the nanoscale may significantly improve the application performance, or even create new properties. For instance, Xu's group synthesized *in situ* CdS nanocrystals on the surface of MWCNT, which reacted with hydrogen peroxide to generate strong and stable ECL emission in neutral solution (Wang et al. 2009c). Compared with pure CdS nanocrystals, the MWCNT–CdS enhanced the ECL intensity by 5.3-fold and moved the onset ECL potential more positively by about 400 mV, which reduced H_2O_2 decomposition at the electrode surface and increased detection sensitivity of H_2O_2. Later, Wang et al. prepared CdS–Ag nanocomposite array by an electrochemical approach based on CdS hierarchical nanoarrays as templates, allowing strong coupling between CdS and Ag nanoparticle (Wang et al. 2009a). Based on this nanocomposite array, a novel hydrogen peroxide ECL sensor was fabricated and showed a low detection limit of 15 nM.

9.5 Conclusions and Perspectives

In the past two decades or so, design, fabrication, and applications of nanomaterial-based ECL biosensors have advanced rapidly. Nanomaterials with various chemical compositions, sizes, and shapes have been incorporated into ECL biosensors for the exploitation of their unique electrical, optical, and chemical properties. Used as electrode or electrode modification materials, metallic and carbon nanomaterials offer drastically increased specific surface area for the immobilization of capture molecules in bio-affinity reactions. Due to the high surface to volume ratio, the active sites on the surface of some noble metal, carbon, and doped metal oxide nanomaterials possess high electrocatalytic activities, which benefit ECL detection tremendously as electrochemical reactions of ECL coreactants are often very sluggish on conventional electrodes and thus rate-limiting. Due to the internal porous structure, SiO_2 and polystyrene nanoparticles are capable of encapsulating a large number of molecular ECL emitters. Alternatively, the emitters can be covalently attached to the surface of metal and carbon nanomaterials in large quantity. These emitter-loaded nanomaterials can be visualized as Christmas trees that light up intensely upon electrochemical excitation. Some silicon, semiconductor, and conjugating polymer nanoparticles are a new generation of ECL emitters that have demonstrated improved ECL performance over the molecular emitters in terms of high luminescence intensity, good stability, and long emission wavelength. The application of the earlier nanomaterials in ECL biosensors has led to significantly improved sensor performance, particularly in detection sensitivity. These days, detection limits of ppt or fM in bio-affinity assays are routinely obtained.

However, some challenges still remain in the field of ECL nanobiosensors. On the fundamental side, although the electrocatalytic activity of some conducting nanomaterials has been demonstrated, the detailed mechanism is still unclear. In some studies, side-by-side comparison with bulk material was missing, and the increased surface area of the nanomaterial was not accounted for. Therefore, the observation of several-fold increase in ECL intensity is not conclusive evidence for the increased catalytic activity of the nanomaterials. In addition, unlike fluorescent QDs, the size effect of nanomaterials on ECL emission has not been demonstrated, and is an interesting direction for future studies. On the performance side, although sensitivity has improved tremendously, other parameters of ECL nanobiosensors such as specificity, reproducibility, and stability are not as impressive. How to take advantage of the high reactivity of nanomaterials and at the same time prevent it from compromising sensor stability and reproducibility is quite a challenge. On the application side, most of the sensor studies up to date have focused on the ECL electrodes or labels, which are understandably the core elements of ECL sensors. However, the protocols for the preparation of nanomaterial electrodes and labels, as well as ECL detection, are still too complex for the nonspecialists to follow. It is hoped that, with further studies on the ECL mechanisms of nanomaterials, further improvement on ECL nanobiosensor reproducibility and stability, integrated, automated devices or even instruments can be assembled and used by researchers of different interests and backgrounds for the detection of environmental pollutants, food contaminants, chemical and biowarfare agents, pathogens, and disease markers.

References

Bae, Y., Myung, N., and Bard, A.J. 2004. Electrochemistry and electrogenerated chemiluminescence of CdTe nanoparticles. *Nano Lett.* 4: 1153–1161.

Bard, A.J. 2004. *Electrogenerated Chemiluminescence*. New York: Marcel Dekker.

Bard, A.J., Ding, Z.F., and Myung, N. 2005. Electrochemistry and electrogenerated chemiluminescence of semiconductor nanocrystals in solutions and in films. In *Semiconductor Nanocrystals and Silicate Nanoparticles*, eds. X. Peng and D.M.P. Mingos, pp. 1–57. Berlin, Germany: Springer-Verlag.

Bertoncello, P. and Forster, R.J. 2009. Nanostructured materials for electrochemiluminescence (ECL)-based detection methods: Recent advances and future perspectives. *Biosens. Bioelectron.* 24: 3191–3200.

Blackburn, G.F., Shah, H.P., Kenten, J.H. et al. 1991. Electrochemiluminescence detection for development of immunoassays and DNA probe assays for clinical diagnostics. *Clin. Chem.* 37: 1534–1539.

Bolleta, F., Ciano, M., Balzani, V., and Serpone, N. 1982. Polypyridine transition metal complexes as light emission sensitizers in the electrochemical reduction of the persulfate ion. *Inorg. Chim. Acta* 62: 207–213.

Bottini, M., Balasubramanian, C., Dawson, M.I., Bergamaschi, A., Bellucci, S., and Mustelin, T. 2006. Isolation and characterization of fluorescent nanoparticles from pristine and oxidized electric arc-produced single-walled carbon nanotubes. *J. Phys. Chem. B* 110: 831–836.

Bourlinos, A.B., Stassinopoulos, A., Anglos, D., Zboril, R., Karakassides, M., and Giannelis, E.P. 2008. Surface functionalized carbogenic quantum dots. *Small* 4: 455–458.

Butler, J. and Henglein, A. 1980. Elementary reactions of the reduction of Tl^+ in aqueous solution. *Radiat. Phys. Chem.* 15: 603–612.

Cao, L., Wang, X., Meziani, M.J. et al. 2007. Carbon dots for multiphoton bioimaging. *J. Am. Chem. Soc.* 129: 11318–11319.

Chang, G., Zhang, J., Oyama, M., and Hirao, K. 2005. Silver-nanoparticle-attached indium tin oxide surfaces fabricated by a seed-mediated growth approach. *J. Phys. Chem. B* 109: 1204–1209.

Chang, M.M., Saji, T., and Bard, A.J. 1977. Electrogenerated chemiluminescence. 30. Electrochemical oxidation of oxalate ion in the presence of luminescers in acetonitrile solutions. *J. Am. Chem. Soc.* 99: 5399–5403.

Chang, Y.L., Palacios, R.E., Fan, F.R.F., Bard, A.J., and Barbara, P.F. 2008. Electrogenerated chemiluminescence of single conjugated polymer nanoparticles. *J. Am. Chem. Soc.* 130: 8906–8907.

Chang, Z., Zhou, J., Zhao, K., Zhu, N., He, P., and Fang, Y. 2006. Ru (bpy)$_3^{2+}$-doped silica nanoparticle DNA probe for the electrogenerated chemiluminescence detection of DNA hybridization. *Electrochim. Acta* 52: 575–580.

Chen, D., Tang, L., and Li, J. 2010. Graphene-based materials in electrochemistry. *Chem. Soc. Rev.* 39: 3157–3180.

Chen, J., Lin, Z., and Chen, G. 2007a. An electrochemiluminescent sensor for glucose employing a modified carbon nanotube paste electrode. *Anal. Bioanal. Chem.* 388: 399–407.

Chen, X.M., Lin, Z.J., Cai, Z.M., Chen, X., Oyama, M., and Wang, X.R. 2009. Electrochemiluminescence of luminol on a platinum-nanoparticle-modified indium tin oxide electrode in neutral aqueous solution. *J. Nanosci. Nanotechnol.* 9: 2413–2420.

Chen, Y., Lin, Z., Chen, J., Sun, J., Zhang, L., and Chen, G. 2007b. New capillary electrophoresis-electrochemiluminescence detection system equipped with an electrically heated Ru (bpy)$_3^{2+}$/multi-wall-carbon-nanotube paste electrode. *J. Chromatogr. A* 1172: 84–91.

Chen, Y., Shen, Y., Sun, D. et al. 2011a. Fabrication of a dispersible graphene/gold nanoclusters hybrid and its potential application in electrogenerated chemiluminescence. *Chem. Commun.* 47: 11733–11735.

Chen, Z. and Zu, Y. 2007. Gold nanoparticle-modified ITO electrode for electrogenerated chemiluminescence: Well-preserved transparency and highly enhanced activity. *Langmuir* 23: 11387–11390.

Choi, H.N., Lee, J.Y., Lyu, Y.K., and Lee, W.Y. 2006. Tris (2,2'-bipyridyl) ruthenium (II) electrogenerated chemiluminescence sensor based on carbon nanotube dispersed in sol-gel-derived titania-Nafion composite films. *Anal. Chim. Acta* 565: 48–55.

Chu, H.H., Yan, J.L., and Tu, Y.F. 2011. Electrochemiluminescent detection of the hybridization of oligonucleotides using an electrode modified with nanocomposite of carbon nanotubes and gold nanoparticles. *Microchim. Acta* 175: 209–216.

Cole, C., Muegge, B.D., and Richter, M.M. 2003. Effects of poly (ethylene glycol) tert-octylphenyl ether on tris (2-phenylpyridine) iridium (III)-tripropylamine electrochemiluminescence. *Anal. Chem.* 75: 601–604.

Cui, H. and Dong, Y.P. 2006. Multichannel electrogenerated chemiluminescence of lucigenin in neutral and alkaline aqueous solutions on a gold nanoparticle self-assembled gold electrode. *J. Electroanal. Chem.* 595: 37–46.

Cui, H., Xu, Y., and Zhang, Z.F. 2004. Multichannel electrochemiluminescence of luminol in neutral and alkaline aqueous solutions on a gold nanoparticle self-assembled electrode. *Anal. Chem.* 76: 4002–4010.

Dai, H., Wang, Y., Wu, X., Zhang, L., and Chen, G. 2009. An electrochemiluminescent sensor for methamphetamine hydrochloride based on multiwall carbon nanotube/ionic liquid composite electrode. *Biosens. Bioelectron.* 24: 1230–1234.

Díez, I., Pusa, M., Kulmala, S. et al. 2009. Color tunability and electrochemiluminescence of silver nanoclusters. *Angew. Chem. Int. Ed.* 48: 2122–2125.

Ding, Z.F., Quinn, B.M., Haram, S.K., Pell, L.E., Korgel, B.A., and Bard, A.J. 2002. Electrochemistry and electrogenerated chemiluminescence from silicon nanocrystal quantum dots. *Science* 296: 1293–1297.

Dodeigne, C., Thunus, L., and Lejeune, R. 2000. Chemiluminescence as diagnostic tool. A review. *Talanta* 51: 415–439.

Dong, Y.P. 2010. Electrogenerated chemiluminescence of luminol at a carbon nanotube-perfluorosulfonate polymer (Nafion) modified gold electrode. *J. Lumin.* 130: 1539–1545.

Dong, Y.P., Cui, H., and Wang, C.M. 2006. Electrogenerated chemiluminescence of luminol on a gold-nanorod-modified gold electrode. *J. Phys. Chem. B* 110: 18408–18414.

Du, D., Wang, L., Shao, Y., Wang, J., Engelhard, M.H., and Lin, Y. 2011. Functionalized graphene oxide as a nanocarrier in a multienzyme labeling amplification strategy for ultrasensitive electrochemical immunoassay of phosphorylated p53 (s392). *Anal. Chem.* 83: 746–752.

Du, D., Zou, Z., Shin, Y. et al. 2010. Sensitive immunosensor for cancer biomarker based on dual signal amplification strategy of graphene sheets and multienzyme functionalized carbon nanospheres. *Anal. Chem.* 82: 2989–2995.

Du, Y., Qi, B., Yang, X., and Wang, E. 2006. Synthesis of PtNPs/AQ/Ru $(bpy)_3^{2+}$ colloid and its application as a sensitive solid-state electrochemiluminescence sensor material. *J. Phys. Chem. B* 110: 21662–21666.

Du, Y., Wei, H., Kang, J. et al. 2005. Microchip capillary electrophoresis with solid-state electrochemiluminescence detector. *Anal. Chem.* 77: 7993–7997.

Dufford, R., Nightingale, D., and Gaddum, L. 1927. Luminescence of Grignard compounds in electric and magnetic fields, and related electrical phenomena. *J. Am. Chem. Soc.* 49: 1858–1864.

Factor, B., Muegge, B., Workman, S., Bolton, E., Bos, J., and Richter, M.M. 2001. Surfactant chain length effects on the light emission of tris (2,2′-bipyridyl) ruthenium (II)/tripropylamine electrogenerated chemiluminescence. *Anal. Chem.* 73: 4621–4624.

Fähnrich, K.A., Pravda, M., and Guilbault, G.G. 2001. Recent applications of electrogenerated chemiluminescence in chemical analysis. *Talanta* 54: 531–559.

Fan, F.R.F., Park, S., Zhu, Y., Ruoff, R.S., and Bard, A.J. 2008. Electrogenerated chemiluminescence of partially oxidized highly oriented pyrolytic graphite surfaces and of graphene oxide nanoparticles. *J. Am. Chem. Soc.* 131: 937–939.

Fang, Y.M., Song, J., Li, J. et al. 2011. Electrogenerated chemiluminescence from Au nanoclusters. *Chem. Commun.* 47: 2369–2371.

Forster, R.J., Bertoncello, P., and Keyes, T.E. 2009. Electrogenerated chemiluminescence. *Ann. Rev. Anal. Chem.* 2: 359–385.

Frehill, F., Vos, J.G., Benrezzak, S. et al. 2002. Interconnecting carbon nanotubes with an inorganic metal complex. *J. Am. Chem. Soc.* 124: 13694–13695.

Fu, C.C., Lee, H.Y., Chen, K. et al. 2007. Characterization and application of single fluorescent nanodiamonds as cellular biomarkers. *Proc. Natl. Acad. Sci. USA* 104: 727.

Gao, L., Fan, L., and Zhang, J. 2009. Selective growth of Ag nanodewdrops on Au nanostructures: A new type of bimetallic heterostructure. *Langmuir* 25: 11844–11848.

Guerra, J. and Herrero, M.A. 2010. Hybrid materials based on Pd nanoparticles on carbon nanostructures for environmentally benign C–C coupling chemistry. *Nanoscale* 2: 1390–1400.

Guo, J.Z., Cui, H., Xu, S.L., and Dong, Y.P. 2007. A new electrogenerated chemiluminescence peak of lucigenin in the hydrogen-evolution region induced by platinum nanoparticles. *J. Phys. Chem. C* 111: 606–611.

Guo, Z. and Dong, S. 2004. Electrogenerated chemiluminescence from Ru $(bpy)_3^{2+}$ ion-exchanged in carbon nanotube/perfluorosulfonated ionomer composite films. *Anal. Chem.* 76: 2683–2688.

Guo, Z., Shen, Y., Wang, M., Zhao, F., and Dong, S. 2004. Electrochemistry and electrogenerated chemiluminescence of SiO_2 nanoparticles/tris (2,2′-bipyridyl) ruthenium (II) multilayer films on indium tin oxide electrodes. *Anal. Chem.* 76: 184–191.

Haapakka, K.E. and Kankare, J.J. 1982. The mechanism of the electrogenerated chemiluminescence of luminol in aqueous alkaline solution. *Anal. Chim. Acta* 138: 263–275.

Haghighi, B., Bozorgzadeh, S., and Gorton, L. 2011. Fabrication of a novel electrochemiluminescence glucose biosensor using Au nanoparticles decorated multiwalled carbon nanotubes. *Sensor Actuat. B-Chem.* 155: 577–583.

Harvey, N. 1929. Luminescence during electrolysis. *J. Phys. Chem.* 33: 1456–1459.

Hercules, D.M. 1964. Chemiluminescence resulting from electrochemically generated species. *Science* 145: 808–809.

Hu, L. and Xu, G. 2010. Applications and trends in electrochemiluminescence. *Chem. Soc. Rev. 39*: 3275–3304.

Huang, R.F., Wei, M.Y., and Guo, L.H. 2011. Enhanced electrogenerated chemiluminescence of $Ru(bpy)_3^{2+}$/tripropylamine system on indium tin oxide nanoparticle modified transparent electrode. *J. Electroanal. Chem. 656*: 136–139.

Jafri, R.I., Arockiados, T., Rajalakshmi, N., and Ramaprabhu, S. 2010. Nanostructured Pt dispersed on graphene-multiwalled carbon nanotube hybrid nanomaterials as electrocatalyst for PEMFC. *J. Electrochem. Soc. 157*: B874.

Jiang, H. and Ju, H. 2007a. Electrochemiluminescence sensors for scavengers of hydroxyl radical based on its annihilation in CdSe quantum dots film/peroxide system. *Anal. Chem. 79*: 6690–6696.

Jiang, H. and Ju, H. 2007b. Enzyme–quantum dots architecture for highly sensitive electrochemiluminescence biosensing of oxidase substrates. *Chem. Commun. 4*: 404–406.

Jie, G., Huang, H., Sun, X., and Zhu, J.J. 2008. Electrochemiluminescence of CdSe quantum dots for immunosensing of human prealbumin. *Biosens. Bioelectron. 23*: 1896–1899.

Jie, G. and Yuan, J. 2012. A novel magnetic Fe_3O_4@ CdSe composite quantum dot-based electrochemiluminescence detection of thrombin by multiple DNA cycle amplification strategy. *Anal. Chem. 84*: 2811–2817.

Jie, G.F., Liu, B., Miao, J.J., and Zhu, J.J. 2007a. Electrogenerated chemiluminescence from CdS nanotubes and its sensing application in aqueous solution. *Talanta 71*: 1476–1480.

Jie, G.F., Liu, B., Pan, H.C., Zhu, J.J., and Chen, H.Y. 2007b. CdS nanocrystal-based electrochemiluminescence biosensor for the detection of low-density lipoprotein by increasing sensitivity with gold nanoparticle amplification. *Anal. Chem. 79*: 5574–5581.

Kang, X., Wang, J., Wu, H., Aksay, I.A., Liu, J., and Lin, Y. 2009. Glucose oxidase–graphene–chitosan modified electrode for direct electrochemistry and glucose sensing. *Biosens. Bioelectron. 25*: 901–905.

Khairoutdinov, R.F., Doubova, L.V., Haddon, R.C., and Saraf, L. 2004. Persistent photoconductivity in chemically modified single-wall carbon nanotubes. *J. Phys. Chem. B 108*: 19976–19981.

Kim, D.J., Lyu, Y.K., Choi, H.N., Min, I.H., and Lee, W.Y. 2005. Nafion-stabilized magnetic nanoparticles (Fe_3O_4) for $[Ru(bpy)_3]^{2+}$(bpy = bipyridine) electrogenerated chemiluminescence sensor. *Chem. Commun.* 2966–2968.

Kuwana, T., Epstein, B., and Seo, E.T. 1963. Electrochemical generation of solution luminescence. *J. Phys. Chem. 67*: 2243–2244.

Lei, J. and Ju, H. 2011. Fundamentals and bioanalytical applications of functional quantum dots as electrogenerated emitters of chemiluminescence. *TrAC-Trend. Anal. Chem. 30*: 1351–1359.

Leland, J.K. and Powell, M.J. 1990. Electrogenerated chemiluminescence: An oxidative-reduction type ECL reaction sequence using tripropyl amine. *J. Electrochem. Soc. 137*: 3127.

Li, F. and Zu, Y. 2004. Effect of nonionic fluorosurfactant on the electrogenerated chemiluminescence of the tris (2,2'-bipyridine) ruthenium (II)/tri-n-propylamine system: Lower oxidation potential and higher emission intensity. *Anal. Chem. 76*: 1768–1772.

Li, H., Chen, J., Han, S., Niu, W., Liu, X., and Xu, G. 2009. Electrochemiluminescence from tris (2,2'-bipyridyl) ruthenium (II)-graphene-Nafion modified electrode. *Talanta 79*: 165–170.

Li, H., He, X., Kang, Z. et al. 2010. Water-soluble fluorescent carbon quantum dots and photocatalyst design. *Angew. Chem. Int. Ed. 49*: 4430–4434.

Li, J., Xu, Y., Wei, H., Huo, T., and Wang, E. 2007a. Electrochemiluminescence sensor based on partial sulfonation of polystyrene with carbon nanotubes. *Anal. Chem. 79*: 5439–5443.

Li, L., Li, M., Sun, Y. et al. 2011a. Electrochemiluminescence resonance energy transfer between an emitter electrochemically generated by luminol as the donor and luminescent quantum dots as the acceptor and its biological application. *Chem. Commun. 47*: 8292–8294.

Li, L., Liu, H., Shen, Y., Zhang, J., and Zhu, J.J. 2011b. Electrogenerated chemiluminescence of Au nanoclusters for the detection of dopamine. *Anal. Chem. 83*: 661–665.

Li, L.L., Liu, K.P., Yang, G.H., Wang, C.M., Zhang, J.R., and Zhu, J.J. 2011c. Fabrication of graphene-quantum dots composites for sensitive electrogenerated chemiluminescence immunosensing. *Adv. Funct. Mater. 21*: 869–878.

Li, Y., Qi, H., Fang, F., and Zhang, C. 2007b. Ultrasensitive electrogenerated chemiluminescence detection of DNA hybridization using carbon-nanotubes loaded with tris (2,2'-bipyridyl) ruthenium derivative tags. *Talanta 72*: 1704–1709.

Liu, X., Jiang, H., Lei, J., and Ju, H. 2007. Anodic electrochemiluminescence of CdTe quantum dots and its energy transfer for detection of catechol derivatives. *Anal. Chem. 79*: 8055–8060.

Liu, X., Niu, W., Li, H., Han, S., Hu, L., and Xu, G. 2008. Glucose biosensor based on gold nanoparticle-catalyzed luminol electrochemiluminescence on a three-dimensional sol–gel network. *Electrochem. Commun. 10*: 1250–1253.

Lyu, Y.K., Kyung, K.J., and Lee, W.Y. 2009. Functionalized magnetic nanoparticle with poly (3-thiopheneacetic acid) and its application for electrogenerated chemiluminescence sensor. *Synth. Met. 159*: 571–575.

Miao, J.J., Ren, T., Dong, L., Zhu, J.J., and Chen, H.Y. 2005. Double-template synthesis of CdS nanotubes with strong electrogenerated chemiluminescence. *Small 1*: 802–805.

Miao, W. 2008. Electrogenerated chemiluminescence and its biorelated applications. *Chem. Rev. 108*: 2506.

Miao, W. and Bard, A.J. 2004a. Electrogenerated chemiluminescence. 77. DNA hybridization detection at high amplification with [Ru(bpy)$_3$]$^{2+}$-containing microspheres. *Anal. Chem. 76*: 5379–5386.

Miao, W. and Bard, A.J. 2004b. Electrogenerated chemiluminescence. 80. C-reactive protein determination at high amplification with [Ru(bpy)$_3$]$^{2+}$-containing microspheres. *Anal. Chem. 76*: 7109–7113.

Miao, W., Choi, J., and Bard, A. 2002. Electrogenerated chemiluminescence 69: The tris (2,2'-bipyridine) ruthenium(II) (Ru(bpy)$_3$$^{2+}$)/tri-n-propylamine (TPrA) system revisited—A new route involving TPrA^{*+} cation radicals. *J. Am. Chem. Soc. 124*: 14478–14485.

Myung, N., Ding, Z.F., and Bard, A.J. 2002. Electrogenerated chemiluminescence of CdSe nanocrystals. *Nano Lett. 2*: 1315–1319.

Myung, N., Lu, X.M., Johnston, K.P., and Bard, A.J. 2004. Electrogenerated chemiluminescence of Ge nanocrystals. *Nano Lett. 4*: 183–185.

Noffsinger, J.B. and Danielson, N.D. 1987. Generation of chemiluminescence upon reaction of aliphatic amines with tris (2,2'-bipyridine) ruthenium (III). *Anal. Chem. 59*: 865–868.

Omer, K.M. and Bard, A.J. 2009. Electrogenerated chemiluminescence of aromatic hydrocarbon nanoparticles in an aqueous solution. *J. Phys. Chem. C 113*: 11575–11578.

Palacios, R.E., Fan, F.R.F., Grey, J.K., Suk, J., Bard, A.J., and Barbara, P.F. 2007. Charging and discharging of single conjugated-polymer nanoparticles. *Nat. Mater. 6*: 680–685.

Ren, T., Xu, J.Z., Tu, Y.F., Xu, S., and Zhu, J.J. 2005. Electrogenerated chemiluminescence of CdS spherical assemblies. *Electrochem. Commun. 7*: 5–9.

Richter, M.M. 2004. Electrochemiluminescence (ECL). *Chem. Rev. 104*: 3003–3036.

Rubinstein, I. and Bard, A.J. 1981. Electrogenerated chemiluminescence. 37. Aqueous ecl systems based on tris (2,2'-bipyridine) ruthenium (2+) and oxalate or organic acids. *J. Am. Chem. Soc. 103*: 512–516.

Santhanam, K. and Bard, A.J. 1965. Chemiluminescence of electrogenerated 9, 10-diphenylanthracene anion radical. *J. Am. Chem. Soc. 87*: 139–140.

Shan, C., Yang, H., Song, J., Han, D., Ivaska, A., and Niu, L. 2009a. Direct electrochemistry of glucose oxidase and biosensing for glucose based on graphene. *Anal. Chem. 81*: 2378–2382.

Shan, Y., Xu, J.J., and Chen, H.Y. 2009b. Distance-dependent quenching and enhancing of electrochemiluminescence from a CdS: Mn nanocrystal film by Au nanoparticles for highly sensitive detection of DNA. *Chem. Commun.*: 905–907.

Shan, Y., Xu, J.J., and Chen, H.Y. 2010. Opto-magnetic interaction between electrochemiluminescent CdS: Mn film and Fe$_3$O$_4$ nanoparticles and its application to immunosensing. *Chem. Commun. 46*: 4187–4189.

Shen, L., Cui, X., Qi, H., and Zhang, C. 2007. Electrogenerated chemiluminescence of ZnS nanoparticles in alkaline aqueous solution. *J. Phys. Chem. C 111*: 8172–8175.

Suk, J., Zhiyong, W., Wang, L., and Bard, A.J. 2011. Electrochemistry, electrogenerated chemiluminescence, and excimer formation dynamics of intramolecular π-stacked 9-naphthylanthracene derivatives and organic nanoparticles. *J. Am. Chem. Soc. 133*: 14675–14685.

Sun, X., Du, Y., Dong, S., and Wang, E. 2005. Method for effective immobilization of Ru(bpy)$_3^{2+}$ on an electrode surface for solid-state electrochemiluminescence detection. *Anal. Chem. 77*: 8166–8169.

Sun, Y.P., Zhou, B., Lin, Y. et al. 2006. Quantum-sized carbon dots for bright and colorful photoluminescence. *J. Am. Chem. Soc. 128*: 7756–7757.

Tang, D., Yuan, R., Chai, Y. et al. 2005. Potentiometric immunosensor based on immobilization of hepatitis B surface antibody on platinum electrode modified silver colloids and polyvinyl butyral as matrixes. *Electroanalysis 17*: 155–161.

Tang, L., Feng, H., Cheng, J., and Li, J. 2010. Uniform and rich-wrinkled electrophoretic deposited graphene film: A robust electrochemical platform for TNT sensing. *Chem. Commun. 46*: 5882–5884.

Tang, L., Wang, Y., Li, Y., Feng, H., Lu, J., and Li, J. 2009. Preparation, structure, and electrochemical properties of reduced graphene sheet films. *Adv. Funct. Mater. 19*: 2782–2789.

Tao, Y., Lin, Z.J., Chen, X.M., Chen, X., and Wang, X.R. 2007. Tris (2,2'-bipyridyl) ruthenium (II) electrochemiluminescence sensor based on carbon nanotube/organically modified silicate films. *Anal. Chim. Acta 594*: 169–174.

Tao, Y., Lin, Z.J., Chen, X.M. et al. 2008. Functionalized multiwall carbon nanotubes combined with bis (2,2'-bipyridine)-5-amino-1, 10-phenanthroline ruthenium (II) as an electrochemiluminescence sensor. *Sensor Actuat. B-Chem. 129*: 758–763.

Tokel, N.E. and Bard, A.J. 1972. Electrogenerated chemiluminescence. IX. Electrochemistry and emission from systems containing tris (2,2'-bipyridine) ruthenium (II) dichloride. *J. Am. Chem. Soc. 94*: 2862–2863.

Van Houten, J. and Watts, R. 1976. Temperature dependence of the photophysical and photochemical properties of the Tris (2,2'-bipyridyl) ruthenium (II) ion in aqueous solution. *J. Am. Chem. Soc. 98*: 4853–4858.

Visco, R.E. and Chandross, E.A. 1964. Electroluminescence in solutions of aromatic hydrocarbons. *J. Am. Chem. Soc. 86*: 5350–5351.

Wan, Y., Lin, Z., Zhang, D., Wang, Y., and Hou, B. 2011. Impedimetric immunosensor doped with reduced graphene sheets fabricated by controllable electrodeposition for the non-labelled detection of bacteria. *Biosens. Bioelectron. 26*: 1959–1964.

Wang, C., Yifeng, E., Fan, L., Yang, S., and Li, Y. 2009a. CdS-Ag nanocomposite arrays: Enhanced electro-chemiluminescence but quenched photoluminescence. *J. Mater. Chem. 19*: 3841–3846.

Wang, C.M. and Cui, H. 2007. Electrogenerated chemiluminescence of luminol in neutral and alkaline aqueous solutions on a silver nanoparticle self-assembled gold electrode. *Luminescence 22*: 35–45.

Wang, G., Jin, F., Dai, N. et al. 2011a. Signal-enhanced electrochemiluminescence immunosensor based on synergistic catalysis of nicotinamide adenine dinucleotide hydride and silver nanoparticles. *Anal. Biochem. 422*: 7–13.

Wang, H., Zhang, C., Li, Y. and Qi, H. 2006. Electrogenerated chemiluminescence detection for deoxyribonucleic acid hybridization based on gold nanoparticles carrying multiple probes. *Anal. Chim. Acta 575*: 205–211.

Wang, J., Shan, Y., Zhao, W.W., Xu, J.J., and Chen, H.Y. 2011b. Au nanoparticle enhanced electrochemiluminescence of CdS thin films for ultrasensitive thrombin detection. *Anal. Chem. 83*: 4004–4011.

Wang, L., Tian, Y., Ran, Q. et al. 2009b. Covalent grafting nitrophenyl group on Au surface via click reaction: Assembling process and electrochemical behaviors. *Electrochem. Commun. 11*: 339–342.

Wang, X.F., Zhou, Y., Xu, J.J., and Chen, H.Y. 2009c. Signal-on electrochemiluminescence biosensors based on CdS-carbon nanotube nanocomposite for the sensitive detection of choline and acetylcholine. *Adv. Funct. Mater. 19*: 1444–1450.

Wang, Y., Lu, J., Tang, L., Chang, H., and Li, J. 2009d. Graphene oxide amplified electrogenerated chemiluminescence of quantum dots and its selective sensing for glutathione from thiol-containing compounds. *Anal. Chem. 81*: 9710–9715.

White, H.S. and Bard, A.J. 1982. Electrogenerated chemiluminescence. 41. Electrogenerated chemiluminescence and chemiluminescence of the Ru(2,2′-bpy)$_3$$^{2+}$-S$_2O_8$$^{2-}$ system in acetonitrile-water solutions. *J. Am. Chem. Soc. 104*: 6891–6895.

Wu, M.S., Shi, H.W., Xu, J.J., and Chen, H.Y. 2011. CdS quantum dots/Ru (bpy)$_3$$^{2+}$ electrochemiluminescence resonance energy transfer system for sensitive cytosensing. *Chem. Commun. 47*: 7752–7754.

Wu, X., Hu, Y., Jin, J. et al. 2010. Electrochemical approach for detection of extracellular oxygen released from erythrocytes based on graphene film integrated with laccase and 2,2-azino-bis (3-ethylbenzothiazoline-6-sulfonic acid). *Anal. Chem. 82*: 3588–3596.

Xu, S., Liu, Y., Wang, T., and Li, J. 2010. Highly sensitive electrogenerated chemiluminescence biosensor in profiling protein kinase activity and inhibition using gold nanoparticle as signal transduction probes. *Anal. Chem. 82*: 9566–9572.

Xu, S., Liu, Y., Wang, T., and Li, J. 2011. Positive potential operation of a cathodic electrogenerated chemiluminescence immunosensor based on luminol and graphene for cancer biomarker detection. *Anal. Chem. 83*: 3817–3823.

Xu, X., Ray, R., Gu, Y. et al. 2004. Electrophoretic analysis and purification of fluorescent single-walled carbon nanotube fragments. *J. Am. Chem. Soc. 126*: 12736–12737.

Yang, H., Leland, J.K., Yost, D., and Massey, R.J. 1994. Electrochemiluminescence: A new diagnostic and research tool. *Nat. Biotechnol. 12*: 193–194.

Yin, X.B., Dong, S., and Wang, E. 2004. Analytical applications of the electrochemiluminescence of tris (2,2′-bipyridyl) ruthenium and its derivatives. *TrAC-Trend. Anal. Chem. 23*: 432–441.

Yin, X.B., Qi, B., Sun, X., Yang, X., and Wang, E. 2005. 4-(Dimethylamino) butyric acid labeling for electrochemiluminescence detection of biological substances by increasing sensitivity with gold nanoparticle amplification. *Anal. Chem. 77*: 3525–3530.

Yu, Y., Zhou, M., Shen, W., Zhang, H., Cao, Q., and Cui, H. 2012. Synthesis of electrochemiluminescent graphene oxide functionalized with a ruthenium (II) complex and its use in the detection of tripropylamine. *Carbon 50*: 2539–2545.

Yuan, Y., Li, H., Han, S. et al. 2012. Immobilization of tris (1, 10-phenanthroline) ruthenium with graphene oxide for electrochemiluminescent analysis. *Anal. Chim. Acta 720*: 38–42.

Zhang, L. and Dong, S. 2006. Electrogenerated chemiluminescence sensors using Ru(bpy)$_3$$^{2+}$ doped in silica nanoparticles. *Anal. Chem. 78*: 5119–5123.

Zhang, L., Liu, B., and Dong, S. 2007a. Bifunctional nanostructure of magnetic core luminescent shell and its application as solid-state electrochemiluminescence sensor material. *J. Phys. Chem. B 111*: 10448–10452.

Zhang, L., Xu, Z., Sun, X., and Dong, S. 2007b. A novel alcohol dehydrogenase biosensor based on solid-state electrogenerated chemiluminescence by assembling dehydrogenase to Ru(bpy)$_3$$^{2+}$-Au nanoparticles aggregates. *Biosens. Bioelectron. 22*: 1097–1100.

Zhang, L. and Zheng, X. 2006. A novel electrogenerated chemiluminescence sensor for pyrogallol with core-shell luminol-doped silica nanoparticles modified electrode by the self-assembled technique. *Anal. Chim. Acta 570*: 207–213.

Zhang, Z.F., Cui, H., Lai, C.Z., and Liu, L.J. 2005. Gold nanoparticle-catalyzed luminol chemiluminescence and its analytical applications. *Anal. Chem. 77*: 3324–3329.

Zhao, Q.L., Zhang, Z.L., Huang, B.H., Peng, J., Zhang, M., and Pang, D.W. 2008. Facile preparation of low cytotoxicity fluorescent carbon nanocrystals by electrooxidation of graphite. *Chem. Commun.* 5116–5118.

Zheng, L., Chi, Y., Dong, Y., Lin, J., and Wang, B. 2009. Electrochemiluminescence of water-soluble carbon nanocrystals released electrochemically from graphite. *J. Am. Chem. Soc. 131*: 4564–4565.

Zhou, J., Booker, C., Li, R. et al. 2007. An electrochemical avenue to blue luminescent nanocrystals from multiwalled carbon nanotubes (MWCNTs). *J. Am. Chem. Soc. 129*: 744–745.

Zhou, M., Zhai, Y., and Dong, S. 2009. Electrochemical sensing and biosensing platform based on chemically reduced graphene oxide. *Anal. Chem. 81*: 5603–5613.

Zhu, Y., Hill, C.M., and Pan, S. 2011. Reductive-oxidation electrogenerated chemiluminescence (ECL) generation at a transparent silver nanowire electrode. *Langmuir 27*: 3121–3127.

Zou, G. and Ju, H. 2004. Electrogenerated chemiluminescence from a CdSe nanocrystal film and its sensing application in aqueous solution. *Anal. Chem. 76*: 6871–6876.

Zu, Y. and Bard, A.J. 2000. Electrogenerated chemiluminescence. 66. The role of direct coreactant oxidation in the ruthenium tris (2,2′) bipyridyl/tripropylamine system and the effect of halide ions on the emission intensity. *Anal. Chem. 72*: 3223–3232.

Zu, Y. and Bard, A.J. 2001. Electrogenerated chemiluminescence. 67. Dependence of light emission of the tris (2,2′) bipyridylruthenium (II)/tripropylamine system on electrode surface hydrophobicity. *Anal. Chem. 73*: 3960–3964.

Section II

Electrical Biosensors

10

Nanocrystalline Diamond Biosensors

Prabhu U. Arumugam, Shabnam Siddiqui, Hongjun Zeng, and John A. Carlisle

CONTENTS

10.1 Introduction

Biosensors that can reliably detect target analytes in minimally prepared complex samples in real time represent one of the greatest challenges for remote environmental monitoring, point-of-use diagnostics, personalized medicine, and national security. Considerable progress has already been made to engineer stable antibodies that remain functional in harsh storage and operating conditions and to use advanced fabrication methods that can precisely pattern micro- and nanoscale electrode architectures for higher sensitivity and throughput. Much of this work utilizes detection signal amplification, processing, and other strengths of microelectronics in order to lower costs and integrate the sensor into sample preparation modules such as filtration, pre-concentration, lysing, amplification,

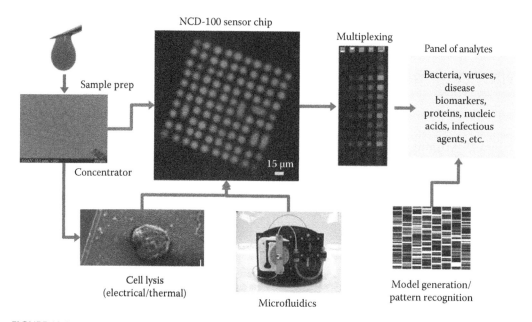

FIGURE 10.1

(See color insert.) A generic biosensor product concept showing the various modules required for a portable, rapid, automated, high-throughput system for detecting a suite of analytes in environmental monitoring and point-of-care diagnostics. NCD-100 sensor chip can be micro spotted with different capture molecules (antibodies, aptamers, AMPs, DNA, RNA) and here we illustrate the micro spotting of fluorescent tagged anti-*E. coli*.

microfluidics, etc. However, there is clearly more room for progress in several critical areas of integrated biosensor development to facilitate field deployability and to encourage the transition from laboratory to market. Figure 10.1 shows a generic systems concept showing the essential subcomponents required to achieve the ultimate goal of rapid turnaround "sample-in, answer-out" biosensors. The two principal areas of research and development are the achievement of highly stable active bio-interfaces that interact with and measure analytes of interest, and the engineering of highly robust transducer materials. This second goal is even more challenging when the sensor also fulfills the desired objectives of being ultra-small in size, versatile in immobilizing a wide range of bio-layers, uses simple chemistries in functionalizing biomolecules, promotes long-term functional stability of bio-layers, and is amenable to scale-up and large volume manufacturing.

Among the various biosensor transducer technologies (electrochemical, optical, acoustical, mechanical, calorimetric), electrochemical transducers have recently become popular because of their adaptability to automation and portability (Oleinikov et al. 2003, Bakker 2004, Wang 2006), high sensitivity, small dimensions, low cost, and compatibility with microfabrication techniques (Drummond et al. 2003, Fritzsche and Taton 2003, He et al. 2005, Liepold et al. 2005). The key advancement is the fabrication of electrochemical microelectrode and nanoelectrode array technology, which affords a superior combination of spatial, temporal, and analyte signal resolution (Heller 2002, Li 2003, Arumugam et al. 2009, Kiran et al. 2012), detects multiple analytes (i.e., multiplexing), and assays large numbers of samples in a matter of minutes or less (Ewalt et al. 2001). A wide variety of assays can be accomplished with electrochemical microarrays including gene expression analysis (Chiem 1997), genotyping (Gilles et al. 1999), DNA sequencing (Woolley and Mathies 1995), immunoassays (Arenkov et al. 2000, Yun et al. 2007, Arumugam et al. 2009), and cell sorting

(Cheng et al. 1998, Arumugam et al. 2007). It presents several advantages over previous electrochemical methods of detection using larger electrodes. First, it offers a higher signal-to-noise (S/N) ratio resulting from lower charging currents as a consequence of the smaller electrode areas (Wightman 1988). Second, it can be used for analysis of ultralow conductivity samples, small volumes, and at very low analyte concentrations (Cousino et al. 1997). In addition, detection at a microelectrode is useful for assay applications for which a rapid measurement is desired. They exhibit high current densities with low total currents and permit steady-state current in resistive media that are not possible with larger electrodes (Brett and Brett 1993). Third, it can be used to generate a response that is far less affected or unaffected by the sample turbidity that is prevalent in optical based assays (Heineman and Halsall 1985, Foulds et al. 1990, Clancy et al. 1999). These advantages are best demonstrated by the elegant studies that detected DNA label-free in real time down to femtomolar (fM) limit of detection (Hahm and Lieber 2004, Ghindilis et al. 2009). Electrochemical arrays are clearly well suited for state-of-the-art biological and chemical monitoring, but much work still remains, particularly in the area of engineering new, more robust electrode interfaces.

The current gold standard microarray electrode materials are the noble metals (Au, Pt, Pd, Ni), which exhibit fast electron-transfer kinetics and adequate sensitivity (Strein and Ewing 1993, Paeschke et al. 1995, Gerwen et al. 1998, Evans et al. 2002). Unfortunately, the increased sensitivity of metal arrays is tempered by increased background noise (Bruce et al. 1994, Nebel et al. 2007, Yang et al. 2008, Hu et al. 2009, Siddiqui et al. 2010) and the increased surface oxidation and surface fouling, which result in a loss of analyte signal. In addition, most microelectronic-compatible materials like silicon and gold show degradation of their bio-interfaces in electrolyte solutions, which add significant complexity to the design and selection of electrode material (Yang et al. 2002, Nebel et al. 2007). The most promising alternative is to use carbon materials that often offer superior electrochemical properties to those of noble metals. The well-known allotropes of carbon include glassy carbon, carbon nanotubes, HOPG, and diamond, each of which can be integrated with a variety of substrate materials and deposition formats with differing electrochemical properties. Most common are those based on the graphite structure, consisting of stacked sheets of "graphene" in parallel. The carbon atoms in graphite are all sp^2 hybridized. Diamond films are sp^3 hybridized and tetrahedral, and they are doped with boron or nitrogen to provide sufficient electrical conductivity for electrochemistry.

In recent years, carbon nanomaterials have attracted a considerable attention due to novel material synthesis options, the applications of scalable micro-nanofabrication techniques, and newly available size-dependent material properties. Carbon nanotubes (Lee et al. 2004), carbon nanofibers (Arumugam et al. 2009, Siddiqui et al. 2010, Koehne et al. 2011), microcrystalline diamond (Hupert et al. 2003, Fischer et al. 2004, Muna et al. 2004, Swain 2004), nanocrystalline and ultrananocrystalline diamond (Gruen et al. 1996, Haymond et al. 2002, Carlisle 2004, Show et al. 2003, Auciello et al. 2004, Lasseter et al. 2004, Williams et al. 2008, Auciello and Sumant 2010, Williams 2011), and graphene (Robinson et al. 2008, Shao et al. 2010), have been extensively studied to engineer highly stable biolayer–transducer interfaces. Among them, boron-doped diamond (BDD) exhibits excellent electronic, chemical, and biological properties (Yang et al. 2002, 2005, 2008, Nebel et al. 2007, Wang et al. 2007, Radadia et al. 2011, Siddiqui et al. 2012). Hu et al. (2009) estimated that the background current density of BDD ultra micro electrodes (UME, i.e., <25 μm in diameter) is about 30 times smaller than that of the Pt UME background current density and about five times smaller than the carbon fiber UME background current density. One of the reasons for observing the high sensitivities on diamond is due to weak surface adsorption of biomolecules such as proteins (Yang et al. 2002), nicotinamide adenine dinucleotide (NADH), a cofactor in a large number of dehydrogenese-based biosensors (Rao 1999), and oxidation reaction products in HPLC ECD systems (Acworth et al. 2008). The high surface stability of BDD finds application in HPLC–EC systems to detect analytes of high oxidation potentials that require high (over) potentials (e.g., +1.4 V for disulfide) without mobile phase oxidation and high background noise levels.

BDD is broadly classified into three types based on its crystallite (grain) size: microcrystalline (MCD), nanocrystalline (NCD), and ultrananocrystalline (UNCD). MCD and NCD surfaces are generally rough (R_a of ~500 to 1000 nm and 5 to 100 nm rms, respectively) and might increase nonspecific binding, which is undesirable for biosensing. Researchers at Argonne National Laboratory, USA, developed a near atomic-scale smooth ultrananocrystalline diamond UNCD® (e.g., R_a of ~5 to 8 nm rms) (Birrell et al. 2005). UNCD films have been proven to be (1) very smooth and the surface roughness is independent of thickness (i.e., they do not roughen) (Naguib et al. 2006). This surface characteristic leads to less adsorption of biomolecules and thus can solve surface fouling problem that plaques other electrode materials. (2) deposited over an extended temperature range (~350°C to 800°C) (Xiao et al. 2004), and thus can be more easily integrated with other thin film processes. (3) highly electrically insulating or conducting (up to ~1500 Ω^{-1} cm^{-1}) by changing the gas mixture used (Bhattacharyya et al. 2001); and (4) deposited with very low residual stress of ~50 MPa or less on silicon substrates. In spite of these many advantages, commercial fabrication of diamond films is greatly hindered by the general incompatibility of diamond with wafer-scale microfabrication technologies. There are several reasons for this: (1) deposition of diamond on micro-patterned metals commonly used in microfabrication (e.g., Au, Al, Pt, Cr, Cu) is difficult because of thermal expansion coefficient mismatches and the difficulty in forming carbides of those metals during diamond deposition; (2) it requires careful surface preparation to seed the surface selectively with diamond nanoparticles for excellent film adhesion; and (3) achieving films that are continuous and pinhole free is challenging due to the low renucleation rate associated with diamond growth chemical reactions. Because of these scientific and engineering challenges, only a few companies are developing commercial scale diamond thin films and these include Advanced Diamond Technologies, Inc. (ADT), sp^3 Diamond Technologies, Condias, Adamant, Element Six, Sumitomo, and a few others. Some of the exciting applications pursued in authors' laboratory are microarray biosensors, neurochemical sensors, scanning tip-based probes, biocompatible and low-friction coatings, electrodes for water disinfection and oxidative destruction of organic pollutants, ultra-hard surfaces for chemical mechanical polishing, pump seals, and many others (Figure 10.2).

This review will focus on providing a review of NCD film processing, characterization, and electrochemical properties and NCD electrochemical impedance spectroscopy (EIS) biosensors. Readers are encouraged to refer other reviews related to this topic (Nebel et al. 2007, Williams 2011, McCreery 2008).

10.2 Nanocrystalline Diamond Nucleation, Deposition, and Characterization

Diamond is one of the most precious materials in the world with unmatched physical and chemical properties, such as the hardness, extreme chemical stability, high thermal conductivity, very high acoustic speed, very low friction coefficient, etc. It is made

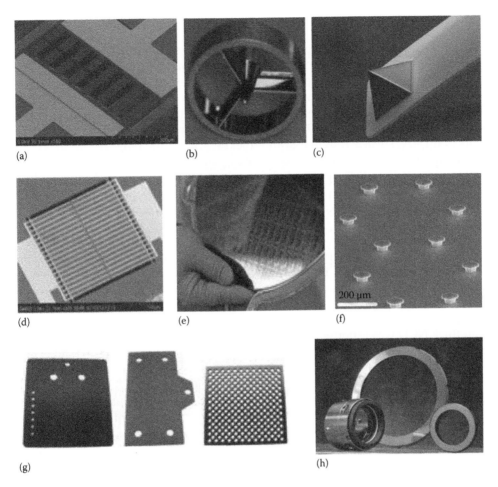

FIGURE 10.2
Applications development based on UNCD films at ADT, Inc. (a) Cantilever biosensors, (b) heart valve biomedical coatings, (c) AFM probes, (d) RF filters, (e) diamond wafers, (f) chemical mechanical polishing pads, (g) electrochemical water purification, and (h) mechanical seals.

of pure carbon element, which is intrinsically biocompatible and is ideal for biological applications. In the past several decades (Hall 2004), synthetic diamond has been realized, commercialized, and applied in multiple fields, with 3-D (cubic stones), 2-D (films), and 1-D (powders and nanoparticles) geometries, which is usually synthesized by high pressure and high temperature methods (HPHT) (Bundy et al. 1955), chemical vapor deposition (CVD) methods (Matsumoto et al. 1982, Kamo et al. 1983), and detonation methods (Decarli and Jamieson 1961). CVD diamond has two basic forms: single crystalline and polycrystalline. Single crystalline diamond's performance in many aspects such as thermal conductivity, carrier mobility, optical transparency, etc. is superior to those of polycrystalline diamond (PCD), but its prohibitive cost and its requirement for diamond-only substrates seriously limits its application and commercialization prospects (Hammersberg et al. 2002). This chapter focuses on PCD grown by CVD method because of their widespread use in biosensors.

10.2.1 NCD Definition

Films with large grain size (i.e., high surface roughness), low diamond purity, or large stress are undesirable for device integration and performance. In the 1990s, a new class of diamond material, nanocrystalline diamond (NCD) emerged (Butler and Sumant 2008). It is essentially a thin version of conventional MCD and its surface is composed of the facets of the largest crystals that survived during the nucleation process. Such a Van De Drift growth mechanism leads to NCD surface roughness proportional to the film thickness. With its grain size, surface roughness, and thickness, all in the range of 10s–100s of nanometers, it became easy to microfabricate and integrate than MCD films. NCD was reported to contain greater than 99% sp^3 bonded carbon representing very high diamond purity (Williams et al. 2008). The most important parameter that affects this purity is the ratio of C/H precursor gases. For example, in the popular CH_4/H_2 feedstock gas mixture, high purity NCD is achieved if CH_4/H_2 ratio is below 5%. When the growth occurs in a carbon-lean environment, for example, <0.3%, the purity can be >99.9% (Philip et al. 2003). Besides the difference in gas chemistry, the growth mechanism of UNCD film is substantially distinct from conventional NCD (Gruen et al. 1994). Renucleation occurs very frequently, that is, every 3–5 nm length scales during the growth. Such repeated nucleation enables the UNCD surface to possess extremely low roughness, of only several nanometers, and the roughness doesn't significantly increase as the film thickness increases, for example, 150 nm thick NCD was reported to be rougher than a 2 μm UNCD (Williams et al. 2006). From SEM images (Figure 10.3a and b) one observes facets only on NCD. In Raman spectra (Figure 10.3c and d), a single 1333 cm^{-1} peak represents a sp^3 diamond signature, which dominates in single crystal and microcrystalline diamond. As grain size becomes smaller, 1333 cm^{-1} peak becomes less obvious and the spectrum becomes more complicated. At the same time, peaks at 1360, 1480, and 1550 cm^{-1} emerge, representing graphite-related D band, trans-polyacetylene, and graphite-related G band, respectively (Popov et al. 2004). In UNCD, the peaks at 1480 and 1550 cm^{-1} become equal to or higher than D band peak. Particularly, the peak at 1159–1190 cm^{-1} appears as a featured UNCD signature. There is no consensus about the origin of this peak because some consider it to come from the nanodiamond grains, while the others believe it comes from the sp^2-rich grain boundary (Ferrari and Robertson 2001). The position of these peaks may shift due to different exciting wavelength, substrate temperature, and diamond gas chemistry in deposition. Figure 10.3c and d are typical spectra of NCD and UNCD on Si substrate, excited by a 532 nm laser. UNCD is an emerging material and there is a lot of new science being conducted at the current time (Jiao 2001, Auciello et al. 2004, Wang 2006). There is tradeoff between NCD and UNCD films in their application to biosensors. While conventional NCD addresses the issue of diamond purity and its effect on background current, UNCD addresses the issue of smoothness. The primary goal here is not to replace conventional NCD materials, but to fill in the application map with UNCD. For example, NCD is more suitably employed for optical devices (Kreuzer et al. 2008) and electronic thermal management (Gray and Windischmann 1999), while UNCD is more suitable for tribology (Kim et al. 2005) and biotechnology applications (Yang et al. 2002, Carlisle 2004).

10.2.2 Nanodiamond Seeding Process

Seeding is an essential pretreatment process for CVD diamond growth. Without seeding, it would take an extremely long time for diamond nucleation and hence lateral growth of the diamond at the beginning of the deposition cycle. Major seeding methods include

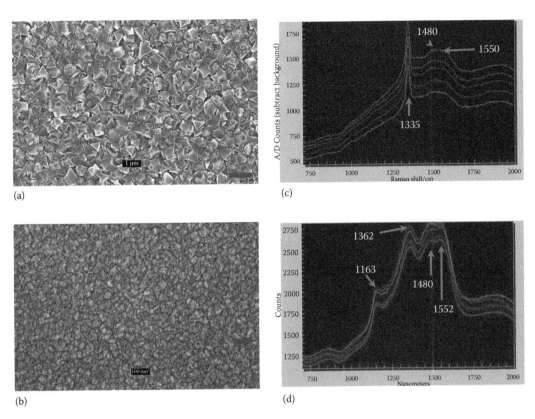

FIGURE 10.3
Typical SEM image of (a) NCD, (b) UNCD and Raman spectra of (c) NCD and (d) UNCD. The Raman exciting laser wavelength is 532 nm. Five spectra on (c) and (d) are sampled 5 points on each of a 4 in. wafer. The scale bar is 1 μm (a) and 100 nm (b).

surface scratching (Ascarelli and Fontana 1993, Bucka and Deuerlerb 1998), diamond particle attachment (Geis 1989, Arnault et al. 2008), electrical biasing (Zhu 1995, Das and Singh 2007), and interlayer pre-coating (Michau et al. 1993). Surface scratching is one of the earliest seeding methods. It uses small diamond or other hard powders to polish the substrates' surface, which minimizes the interfacial energy and exposes dangling bonds of the substrate at the scratched (defect) spots and the scratches "bite" or hold the diamond debris or seeds with a strong bond, which provides high seed density ($10^6–10^{10}$ cm^{-2}) and reliable nucleation sites for the deposition. For the diamond particle attachment methods, slurries of diamond particles are sprayed or spin-coated on a substrate, or the substrate is dipped into the slurries and/or treated with ultrasonic agitation. These methods take advantage of the simplicity of the process, and some of them can process complex 3-D substrates. Particularly, with the introduction of ultra-dispersed diamond (UDD), the seed density on the substrate can be as high as 10^{11} cm^{-2} (Shenderova et al. 2010). In the electrical biasing seeding method, positive or negative voltage is applied on the substrate to either accelerate the diamond precursors onto the surface or excite the substrate surface and break carbon (or other substrate) molecules by electron bombardment. This method is usually not a separate step but combined with the CVD process itself. Interlayer pre-coating describes a process that occurs before the diamond coating, in which the substrate is coated with a carbon-rich layer such as that provided by certain specific polymers (Bulychev et al. 2010), or a carbide forming layer such as W, C, or Si (Michau et al. 1993, Naguib et al. 2006). These layers either assist the nucleation reaction or enhance the bond between the substrate and incoming diamond precursors (such as methyl groups).

10.2.3 Choice of Substrate

CVD diamond coating requires relatively low pressure (10^{-2} to 10^2 torr) and a temperature in the range of 400°C–950°C except when using certain special techniques (Tsugawa et al. 2010), and therefore substrates with a high degas rate, high vapor pressure, low melting points, Curie or firing point material cannot be used as substrates. Given these restrictions, there are a few substrate types suitable for diamond growth: (1) Diamond deposition–compatible materials such as Si and SiC, and refractory metals such as Ti, Ta, and Mo (Yarbrough 1990, Haubner et al. 1996). Carbide can be easily formed on these materials, which ensures high quality diamond deposition with strong adhesion; (2) Materials with little or no carbon solubility. Au and Cu belong to this group. Diamond can be deposited on these materials, but the adhesion and/or growth rate is usually an issue; (3) Materials catalyzing graphite or having heavy C dissolution (carbon diffuses in the metal to form Me(C) mixed crystals), resulting in serious graphitizing, which can disturb diamond growth. Pt, Rh, Pd, Fe, Co, and Ni are in this group (Ramesham et al. 1996, Kalss et al. 1997, Kellermann et al. 2008). Usually substrate material from groups two and three requires a passivation layer or adhesion promoting layer in order to facilitate diamond film growth. A proper interlayer material can often be chosen from group one, if the chemistry between the substrate and the interlayer material is compatible and their thermal expansion coefficients are similar.

10.2.4 Chemical Vapor Deposition

CVD is the principal technology for manufacturing diamond films (May 2010). This technology also takes advantage of apparatus simplicity, large area coatings, flexibility of substrate choices, and a less critical requirement on the synthesis conditions such as higher pressure and high temperature compared with HPHT methods. The first practical CVD diamond coatings deposited from a gaseous mixture of CH_4 and H_2 were developed in the early 1980s, and the major techniques, plasma assisted CVD (PACVD) and hot filament CVD (HFCVD) were introduced at the same time (Matsumoto et al. 1982, Kamo et al. 1983). The essential difference between PACVD and HFCVD is the mechanism by which the gaseous and generated ionized species react to form deposition precursors. PACVD can be divided into direct current plasma (Suzuki et al. 1987) and microwave enhanced plasma (MWPECVD) methods, while MWPECVD dominates plasma methods of diamond deposition with applied reactor powers usually between 300 and 1200 W (Kamo et al. 1983, Butler and Sumant 2008). Hot filament temperatures for HFCVD are typically in the range of 2000°C–2400°C (Wei and Tzeng 1993, Polo et al. 1994). Both principal CVD techniques usually require substrate surface temperatures of 400°C–950°C to maintain high crystal quality for the deposited diamond films and practical deposition rates (Wang et al. 2004, Potocky et al. 2006). Efforts at low-temperature diamond deposition have continued and room temperature deposition has been reported (Tsugawa et al. 2010) but the quality of the films, deposition rate, stress, film adhesion, etc., still need significant improvements to approximate those deposited at higher temperatures.

A general understanding of CVD diamond deposition mechanisms has been gained over the years (Liu and Dandy 1995, Chhowalla et al. 2000, May et al. 2007, 2010). From these studies it is theorized that reacting gases enter an actuating space (plasma and/or high temperature zone) and gain energy through the actuation. As a result, the gases are converted into a mixture of atoms, radical molecules, ions, and electrons. These highly energetic species react with each other and diffuse to the substrate, are absorbed by and react with the substrate *via* dangling bonds, or they bounce back and participate in additional reactions in the reactor volume. Among the many types of reactions on the substrate surface, CH_x (x=0,1, 2, 3) radicals react to form sp^2 and sp^3 bonds simultaneously, and usually the sp^2 bond dominates. It is believed that high temperature atomic hydrogen plays the key role to extract hydrogen from the CH bond on the surface to form H_2, which usually leaves a C–dangling bond so that the next C atom from a precursor can react to continue the growth of the lattice. At the same time, atomic hydrogen preferentially etches the sp and sp^2 sites, thus freeing up sites for sp^3 carbon reaction and growth, that is, it suppresses the growth of graphite and enhances the growth of diamond. Hydrogen rich gas chemistry was quoted as a featured part of NCD synthesis ($CH_4/H_2 < 5\%$), which differs from that of UNCD initialized with Ar-rich H_2-lean/free gas chemistry ($CH_4/Ar = 1\%$) (Gruen et al. 1994). Another key point to note is that CH_4 is not the only carbon source that can be used, and there are actually several carbon based organics, such as ethanol and methanol that can also be used for diamond synthesis.

10.2.5 NCD Doping

P-type doped NCD can be deposited when boron compounds such as gaseous trimethylborane (Jiang et al. 2002, Gajewski et al. 2009), diborane (Liao et al. 1997), or vaporized liquid trimethyl borate are added to the gas chemistry during deposition (Wang et al. 1997). In earlier publications, methanol solutions of boron trioxide were also used as a boron doping source (Okano et al. 1989). N-type NCD can be deposited by adding nitrogen as a dopant (Baranauskas et al. 1999, Dipalo et al. 2006) and also phosphine (Koizumi et al. 2000). Vaporized liquid Tertiarybutylphosphine (TBP) was reported as an alternative to phosphine (Kociniewski et al. 2006). At lower doping levels, that is, below 10^{17} cm^{-3}, the carrier mobility is 10–90 $cm^2/V/s$. At high doping levels, that is, >10^{21} cm^{-3}, NCD has been reported to exhibit superconducting properties at 1.66 K (Mareš et al. 2007). For n-type NCD, the resistivity of nitrogen doped films was reported to be 0.005 $\Omega\cdot cm$ (Dipalo et al. 2006), but literature about the electronic properties of nitrogen-doped conventional NCD is still very sparse. Phosphine and TBP doped films have been reported with a doping level of 3–5×10^{18} cm^{-3}; the Hall mobility reaches 240 $cm^2/V/s$ at room temperature and 110 $cm^2/V/s$ at 350 K respectively. On the contrary, p-type UNCD has been rarely reported while n-type UNCD has been reported from several groups. With a 1% $CH_4/20\%N_2/79\%$ H_2 gas chemistry, nitrogen doped UNCD has a doping level, resistivity, and carrier mobility of 1.5×10^{20} cm^{-3}, 143 $\Omega\cdot cm$, and 10 $cm^2/V/s$ respectively (Bhattacharyya et al. 2001). Generally it was believed that dopant incorporation occurs in both grains and grain boundaries of conventional NCD, while it mainly or only occurs in the grain boundaries of UNCD (Zapol 2001, Williams et al. 2008). However, little or no experimental evidence has been obtained to support such a theory (Butler and Sumant 2008).

10.2.6 NCD Characterization

Basic characterization parameters for biosensor fabrication include diamond chemistry, film thickness, roughness, resistivity, and film stress. Defining the NCD chemistry is complicated because other forms of carbon can accompany the diamond's growth at various levels. A complete study of a NCD film for biosensor applications requires a Raman spectrum, a scanning electron microscopy (SEM) or atomic force microscopy (AFM) image, Transmission electron microscopy (TEM) image, a near-edge x-ray absorption fine-structure spectrum (NEXAFS), energy-dispersive x-ray spectrum (EDX), and secondary ion mass spectrum (SIMS). Raman spectroscopy reveals phonon vibration modes of diamond and other carbon forms. Since different phonons require different excitation energy, the wavelength of the incident light for an NCD Raman spectrum can range from UV to the infrared (Ferrari and Robertson 2001). SEM, AFM, and TEM reveal the morphology of various features, including grain and cluster sizes on different diamond surfaces. TEM is especially useful for the analysis of NCD grains and grain boundaries. NEXAFS can quantitatively provide the ratio of sp^2 and sp^3-bonded carbon, which directly measures the film quality. EDX is used to analyze the elemental composition of the sample. SIMS is a versatile composition analysis tool that specifically characterizes the dopant concentration in the film (May et al. 2007). It is expensive and time consuming to access many of these tools as well as sample preparation. Usually, Raman spectroscopy combined with a SEM can adequately determine diamond film chemistry and they are relatively more available and less expensive. Thickness measurement usually employs an optical tool such as an interferometer or ellipsometer if the film does not absorb (too opaque) or scatter (too rough) the incident light from the tool. If the thickness of a film cannot be measured *via* an optical tool, it can be measured by a profilometry at the edge of the film or an exposed substrate, or the film can be cleaved and measured by its cross section with a microscope or SEM. Many of today's CVD reactors are installed with a real-time thickness monitor with a mass sensitive device or an optical interferometer. Contact profilometry, optical profilometry, and AFM are used for the roughness measurement. Measurement of a contact profilometry is fast and scans very large scale up to several inches, but when the grain size of a film is below 100 nm, the stylus of the profilometry would be too rough to provide an accurate measurement. Optical profilometry is also fast and the measurement is noncontact, but limited to samples with sufficient optical reflectivity. AFM is mostly used to measure samples with a roughness of less than 10s of nanometer. Noncontact mode or diamond probes are recommended to scan a diamond surface due to the extreme hardness of diamond surface. Resistivity is usually characterized by a four-point probe tool. Stress affects the film-coated wafer's radius of curvature, so measuring this radius change before (R_{pre}) and after (R_{post}) the film deposition can be used to calculate the film stress *via* Stoney's formula:

$$\sigma = \frac{1}{6}\left(\frac{1}{R_{post}} - \frac{1}{R_{pre}}\right)\frac{E}{(1-\upsilon)}\frac{d^2}{t}$$

provided that the substrate's Young's Modulus E, Poisson's ratio υ, thickness d, and film thickness t are known accurately. Either an optical curvature measurement or a stylus profilometry can measure the wafer's curvature radius.

10.3 Electrochemical Properties of NCD

Carbon materials have significantly more complex surface chemistry than metals, because they form a wider variety of surface bonds and functional groups. Since electrochemistry is based fundamentally on interfacial phenomena the carbon electrode's surface reactivity, chemistry, and termination are important in reproducibly controlling the electrode's physicochemical properties (McCreery 2008). Several groups have contributed to the understanding of the factors that influence the electrochemical response of diamond materials including those of Swain, Hamers, Carlisle, Garrido, Angus, Butler, Martin, Fujishima, Nebel, May, Panizza, Comninellis, and Compton.

10.3.1 Cyclic Voltammetry of NCD Films

Cyclic voltammetry (CV) technique is generally useful for examining the diamond film quality because the electrochemical response is highly sensitive to physicochemical properties of the electrode surface. In CV technique, the potential E between the working electrode and a reference/counter electrode is swept with time and recording the current (i) vs. E. Usually the potential is varied linearly with time (i.e., applied signal is a voltage ramp) with sweep rates ranging from 10 mV/s to about 10^6 V/s and switching the direction of potential scan at a certain time. Two measured parameters of interest on these i–E curves (cyclic voltammograms) are the ratio of forward and reverse peak currents and the separation of peak potentials (ΔE_p). The magnitude of the background current, the working potential window, and the voltammetric features present within the working potential window are all important CV parameters and are sensitive to (1) the presence of nondiamond carbon (amorphous or graphitic) impurity phases (Martin et al. 1996, Xu 1998, Swain et al. 1998, Granger et al. 1999); (2) the surface termination (H vs. O) (Angus et al. 2004); (3) the dopant type, level, and distribution; (4) grain boundaries and other morphological defects; (5) the primary crystallographic orientation (Granger et al. 2000, Kondo et al. 2002); and (6) the relative structural perfection of the PCD (Pleskov et al. 1998). Depending on the deposition and post-deposition conditions, nondiamond carbon impurities can exist (1) as a reconstructed layer on the surface, (2) as an extended defect within the diamond lattice, and/or (3) in the intercrystalline grain boundaries. Typically, high-quality films have a flat and featureless, low and stable CV response in the potential range from −500 to +1000 mV vs. SCE (acidic or neutral pH), with a background current density (per geometric area) 10 times lower than polished glassy carbon (Xu et al. 1998, Granger et al. 1999, Show et al. 2003). Surface nondiamond impurities are more reactive (e.g., intercalation, surface oxidation, and gasification to CO and CO_2) than diamond, and this increased reactivity causes a larger background current. For single-crystal BDD, positive potentials as high as +2.5 V vs. normal hydrogen electrode are accessible in water before large anodic currents are observed (Martin et al. 1999). For PCD, a background oxidation is normally observed at +1.83 V on the first scan, and this has been attributed to irreversible oxidation of sp^2 impurities along grain boundaries. The wide working potential window in aqueous electrolyte solutions is due to slow kinetics of surface oxidation and hydrogen evolution. Studies have shown those larger potential windows are achieved in part by lowering the fraction of exposed grain boundaries and by tuning the boron-doping level, which would alter the density of electronic states. BDD electrodes are electrically heterogeneous, with both conductivity and heterogeneous electron-transfer rate constants varying across the BDD surface. Typical heterogeneous rate constants range from 0.02 to 0.2 cm/s for redox systems such as $Fe(CN)_6^{-3/-4}$, $Ru(NH_3)_6^{+3/+2}$, $IrCl_6^{-2/-3}$, and methyl viologen ($MV^{+2/+3}$) (Show et al. 2003, Fischer et al. 2004). For comparison, more commonly reported values on other electrodes in cm/s are 0.6–1.0 (metals), 0.06–0.1 (HOPG edge plane), 0.5 (Glassy Carbon, GC-fractured), 0.005 (GC-conventional polish), and 0.46 (GC-polish-laser) (McCreery 2008). Most studies used boron doping to make diamond electrically conductive. UNCD films are also doped with nitrogen. The electrochemical behavior in nitrogenated diamond is mainly determined by the N-containing amorphous carbon matrix, rather than the properties of the diamond nanocrystallites (Chen et al. 2001).

10.3.2 Electrochemical Properties of UNCD Microelectrode Arrays

Diamond microelectrode arrays (MEAs) are gaining attention for biological and chemical sensing because of their high sensitivity and selectivity, multiplexing capability, and low cost (Cvacka et al. 2003, Simm et al. 2005, Hu et al. 2009, Siddiqui et al. 2012). UNCD MEAs are now commercially available for researchers from ADT, Inc. They consist of nine individually addressable microelectrodes (diameters ranging from 10 to 200 µm), which permits multiple analytes to be assayed. The details of the microfabrication sequence and its performance characteristics are described in Siddiqui et al. (2012). UNCD MEAs were successfully used to detect a wide range of analytes including bacteria, neurochemicals, hormones, and heavy metals (Figure 10.4). Unlike other carbon electrodes that require elaborate, time-consuming surface cleaning steps, diamond electrodes require a simple 10 min sonication in isopropanol prior to use. It showed minimal variation in current peak separation in cyclic voltammograms from the array (<5%) demonstrating highly uniform, reliable microelectrodes with excellent electrochemical behavior: a quasi-reversible electrode process (the separation between oxidation and reduction peaks, $\Delta E_p \sim 110$ mV); two-Q (constant phase element, CPE) behavior; high S/N ratios of greater than 300, and

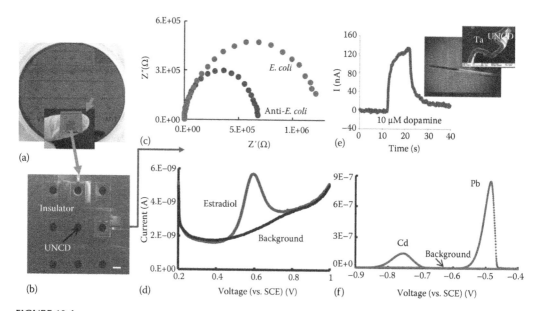

FIGURE 10.4

Biological and chemical sensing applications of UNCD microelectrodes: (a) Optical image of UNCD planar 3×3 microelectrode array (MEA) fabricated in a 4 in. silicon wafer. (b) SEM image of one of the chips showing the nine individually addressable microelectrodes (scale bar: 200 µm). (c) Electrochemical detection of *E. coli* K12 bacteria: Nyquist plot obtained after antibodies and after bacteria capture. (d) Differential Pulse Voltammetry (DPV) detection of 17-estradiol (3 ppm), a hormone in pharmaceutical water waste stream. (e) Flow Injection Analysis of dopamine (10 µM) on a UNCD coated tantalum microwire (Inset, SEM image). (f) DPV detection of heavy metals (Cd, Pb), 5 ppm each.

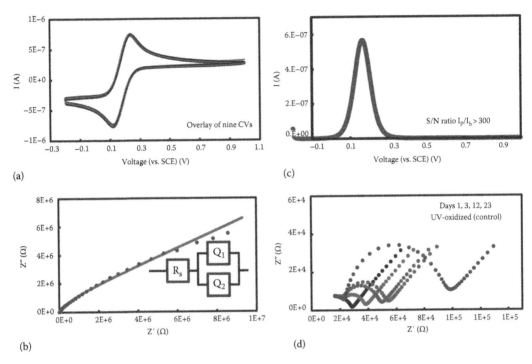

FIGURE 10.5
Electrochemical properties of 200 μm diameter UNCD microelectrodes. (a) Cyclic voltammograms of all nine microelectrodes in a UNCD microchip. Scan rate is 100 mV/s. (b) Nyquist plot of one of the microelectrodes with data fitted to [$R_s(Q_1Q_2)$] circuit model (inset) (dotted curve-experimental and solid curve-fitted). The electrolyte is 5 mM Fe(CN)$_6^{3-/4-}$ in 0.01 M PBS buffer. (c) Differential Pulse Voltammogram showing the extremely low background current I_b, which translates to signal-to-noise ratio of >300. I_p is peak current in amperes. (d) Comparison of EIS spectra of microelectrode stored in air for more than 3 weeks. The blue spectrum is a control surface that was air oxidized in UV for 60 min. The EIS spectra were recorded between 100 kHz and 100 mHz at 10 mV ac signal amplitude (rms value) at a 0 DC voltage. All measurements were carried out in a solution of 5 mM Fe(CN)$_6^{3-/4-}$ in 0.01 M phosphate buffered saline (pH7.4). (a,b: Reprinted with permission from S. Siddiqui et al., *Biosens. Bioelectron.*, 35(1), 284. Copyright 2012.)

minimal surface oxidation (Figure 10.5). The UNCD microelectrode experimental data fit well to an equivalent circuit model [R_s (Q_1Q_2)] that has two CPEs (Q_1, Q_2), where R_s is uncompensated resistance. The presence of CPE is indicative of time-constant or capacitive dispersion. CPE behavior could arise from surface heterogeneities such as grain boundaries, crystal faces on a PCD, or other variations in surface properties, for example, surface conductivity or surface roughness. Even though several groups have characterized diamond films using impedance spectroscopy (Ramesham and Rose 1997, Juttner and Becker 2007), the actual causes for CPE behavior of diamond is not well understood. Since UNCD is composed of phase pure sp^3-bonded grains separated by sp^2 grain boundaries (Gruen et al. 1996), the two values of Q are presumably due to these two phases. It is well-known that the crystalline diamond surface is more homogeneous in surface morphology than grain boundaries (Kondo 2003, Hernando et al. 2009); therefore higher N values, that is, a homogeneous surface morphology can be attributed to grains, and lower N values to grain boundaries. For N = 1, Q represents pure capacitance, for N = 0,

Q behaves as a resistor, for $N = -1$, Q behaves as an inductor, and for $0 < N < 1$, Q represents CPE behavior. The value of Q corresponding to grains is lower than that of grain boundaries. While higher Q corresponds to low impedance, grain boundaries are more conductive than grains. Similar observations were reported by Swain's group (Holt et al. 2004) as they showed that the concentration of boron dopants is higher in grain boundaries than in grains causing higher conductivity. This observation of unique "two-Q behavior" of UNCD surface shows that time-constant dispersion arising from grains can be distinguished from that of grain boundaries. This $[R_s(Q_1Q_2)]$ model could be very helpful in understanding the structural and electrical conductivity changes occurring at grain–grain boundary level in PCD films under different electrochemical environments, for example, bio-functionalized electrodes stored in buffers for several weeks, advanced oxidation of organics, etc.

10.3.3 NCD Surface Termination and Stability

The electrochemical properties of diamond electrodes were found to be quite sensitive to the surface termination (H vs. O) allowing further optimization of electronic properties of these electrodes. It is typical that at oxygen plasma treated diamond electrodes, ΔE_p increases on negatively charged redox species, indicating a large decrease in the heterogeneous electron transfer rate constant (Yagi et al. 1999). The diamond growth using hot filament CVD normally has an atomic hydrogen treatment post-deposition step that effectively removes the surface nondiamond carbon impurity phases and terminates the surface with hydrogen and is therefore highly hydrophobic. UNCD surfaces consist of 5%–10% sp^2 carbon and having a greater understanding of its surface stability is important. UNCD films exposed to air at room temperature for more than 3 weeks were characterized on different days using EIS technique. The solution resistance (R_s) and film resistance (R_f) were compared to a UV-oxidized UNCD control sample ($R_s \sim 18.5$ kΩ and $R_f \sim 85$ kΩ). R_s increased from 7 to 13 kΩ and R_f increased from 15 to 45 kΩ during the 3 week period (Figure 10.5d). Surface pretreatments such as hydrogen plasma treatment, hot filament treatment, or electrochemical cathodic treatment will be effective for reactivating (i.e., re-hydrogenating) the surface, when necessary, because hydrogen terminated diamond surfaces exhibit optimized electron transfer. The investigation using hydrogen plasma showed improvements in cyclic voltammograms, that is, faster electron kinetics and higher electroactive areas (Figure 10.6a). The ΔE_p increased from ~110 mV (as-deposited UNCD) to ~1100 mV after CF_4/O_2 plasma treatment. The kinetics improved when the same surface is treated in hydrogen plasma where the ΔE_p decreased to ~240 mV. Wet chemically oxidized NCD surfaces were H-terminated electrochemically by applying a −35.0 V in 2M hydrochloric acid for 1–5 min (Hoffmann et al. 2010). The treated surface showed a highly hydrophobic behavior with water wetting angles of more than 90° and the ΔE_p reduced from 243 mV to ~60 mV. At ADT, UNCD samples that were initially oxidized electrochemically by applying positive voltages (e.g., +25 V) in an acid mixture (solid curve, Figure 10.6b) were re-activated by applying −5 V, in standard electrolytes. Generally, the electrode kinetics improved similar to those for hydrogen plasma treatment (dashed curve, Figure 10.6b). Interestingly, the ability to reactivate the surface over several anodic and cathodic treatment cycles demonstrates the high stability of the UNCD surface and its attractiveness for real-time biosensing. Detailed studies are required to fully understand the long-term surface reactivity before it becomes viable for advanced applications, for example, continuous biomonitoring.

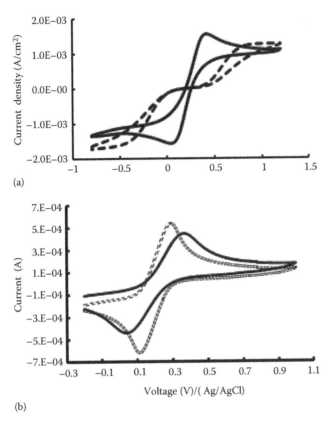

FIGURE 10.6
Effect of UNCD surface terminations on electrochemical properties. Cyclic voltammograms of (a) UNCD microarray after a 10 min oxygen (dashed curve) and hydrogen (solid curve) plasma treatments and (b) unpatterned UNCD after anodic (solid curve) and cathodic (dashed curve) treatments. The electrolyte used is 5 mM $Fe(CN)_6^{3-/4-}$ in 0.01 M PBS buffer. Scan rate is 100 mV/s.

10.4 Surface Functionalization of NCD

The key challenge in biosensor development is covalently immobilizing biomolecules on the inorganic transducer surface while retaining their function for extended time periods (several weeks to months). Physisorption based functionalization is not suitable for long-term use. Covalent surface chemistry is essential when longer liquid exposure times are required, which is mostly true for continuous biosensing applications. It is well-known that the stability of immobilized biomolecules is poor on SiO_2, glass, or gold at physiological conditions. In the case of diamond surfaces, its high chemical inertness poses challenges in covalently linking organic molecules. With H-rich CVD recipes, usually as-deposited NCD is H-terminated, hydrophobic, and chemically inert. The increased hydrophobicity prevents the stabilization of many biomolecules directly at the surface and the lack of chemically reactive groups precludes attachment of biomolecules to the as-grown surface. Thus, surface modification of NCD is required in order to promote a means of covalently coupling biomolecules to the surface, while preserving its otherwise favorable biomaterial properties. Covalent attachment of biomolecules on NCD is mostly accomplished using the UV–alkene chemistry (photochemical) and reduction of diazonium salts (electrochemical) or a one-step direct amination using plasmas. The most important properties for the choice of one of these methods are the identification of which chemistry yields the best combination of capture yield, selectivity, and stability.

10.4.1 Photochemical Surface Functionalization

Takahashi et al. in 2000 first introduced a photochemical chlorination/amination/carboxylation process of the initially H-terminated diamond surface, an important step toward diamond bio-functionalization. In 2002, Hamers and coworkers used the photochemical grafting of organic olefins to chemically modify clean, H-terminated NCD surfaces grown on silicon substrates, producing a homogeneous layer of amine groups that serve as sites for DNA attachment. It involves formation of a surface amine with trifluoroacetamide-protected 10-aminodec-1-ene (TFAAD) followed by coupling to DNA through a cross-linker sulfosuccinimidyl-4-(N-maleimidomethyl) cyclohexane-1-carboxylate (SSMCC). The stability of BDD electrodes modified by covalent monolayers was found to be superior to alternative bonding schemes such as silane and Au/thiol reactions in biosensor applications due to the thermal and hydrolytic stability of the C–C bond (Yang et al. 2002, Carlisle 2004). After linking DNA to the amine groups, hybridization reactions with fluorescently tagged complementary and non-complementary oligonucleotides showed no detectable nonspecific adsorption, with extremely good selectivity between matched and mismatched sequences even at elevated temperatures. Later on, numerous groups used this selective functionalization protocol as a basis for creating biologically sensitive transistor capable of detecting antibodies in real time as well as impedimetric antibody sensors (Yang et al. 2007, Siddiqui et al. 2012). Figure 10.7a shows the photochemical functionalization scheme to functionalize antibodies to NCD surfaces. XPS and fluorescent microscopy techniques are used to characterize the attachment efficiency. Figure 10.7b shows regions of XPS spectra taken after TFAAD/dodecane grafting (bottom) and TFAAD deprotection (top). The area under the CF_3 C1s peak was used to calculate deprotection efficiency, which was greater than 90% deprotection and adequate for antibody attachment. Radadia et al. (2011) used this attachment chemistry to demonstrate that anti-*E. coli O157:H7* functionalized UNCD substrates are more stable and selective and resist nonspecific binding as compared to Corning® glass substrates (GAPSII). Antibodies were found to be stable over UNCD over longer periods of time, that is, 7–10 days for UNCD as compared to 1–2 days for GAPSII. Molecular dynamics simulation studies indicate the possible reasons for antibody stability on UNCD are decreased water- and protein-surface interactions compared to glass surface and less unfolding of antibodies due to minimal antibody-surface interactions. It also reveals that the oxygenation of unfunctionalized UNCD carbon atoms due to carboxylation or hydroxylation will cause increased water pockets and protein-surface interactions and are detrimental for long-term use. Yang et al. (2002) demonstrated UNCD's superior bio-interface stability by regenerating the surface up to 30 times (Figure 10.8), which could be an important aspect for reducing the cost of expensive one-time use biosensors. Photochemical approaches developed for DNA immobilization suffer from several drawbacks, including reproducibility and the fact that it takes up to 24 h to complete the reaction. Recently Siddiqui et al. (2012) used this chemistry to demonstrate that anti-*E. coli K12* functionalized EIS based UNCD MEAs significantly improve bacteria capture signal reproducibility and increase sensitivity by four orders of magnitude (Figure 10.9a and b). However, large variations in charge transfer resistance

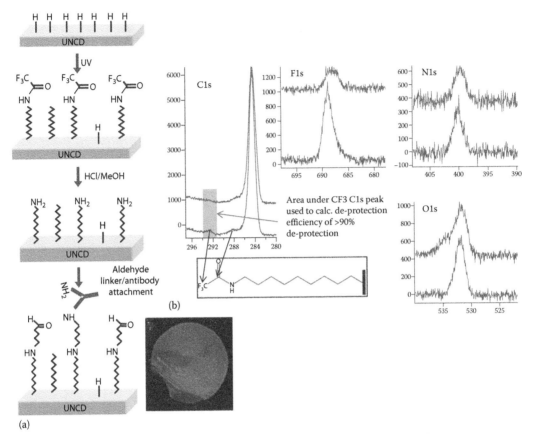

FIGURE 10.7
UV photochemical method for UNCD surface functionalization. (a) Schematic showing the functionalization steps involved in selectively capturing bacteria on UNCD. (Inset) fluorescent image of anti-*E. coli* (w/fluoresin). (b) XPS analysis of UNCD-surface functionalization. Regions of XPS spectra taken after TFAAD/dodecane grafting (bottom) and TFAAD Deprotection (top).

were observed on the microelectrodes after antibody attachment. The possible reasons for such variations are chemical and thermal instability of TFAAD–dodecene monolayers and their nonuniform arrangement on the electrode surface and inconsistencies in antibody density on microelectrodes within an array and from one array to another. This could be improved by optimizing incubation conditions and by using micro spotting techniques for consistent delivery of antibodies to microelectrodes in an array. To further advance the NCD MEA-EIS platform for label-free biosensing, new immobilization chemistries that are more efficient and robust and easy to implement on diamond microarrays are required. One alternative is the use of electrochemical reduction of diazonium salts (Wang et al. 2004).

10.4.2 Electrochemical Surface Functionalization

The electrochemical approach is comparatively easy with respect to previous approaches based on plasma treatments, wet chemical, and photochemical approaches. It also allows spatial and selective binding of aryldiazonium compounds to produce patterned chemical

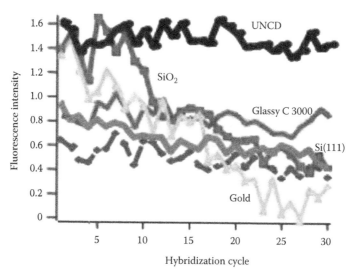

FIGURE 10.8
Stability of DNA binding to ultra-nano-crystalline diamond, Au, Si and glassy carbon as detected during 30 successive cycles of hybridization and denaturation. In each case the substrates were amine-modified and then linked to thiol-terminated DNA. (Reprinted with permission from W. Yang et al., *Nat. Mater.*, 1(4), 253, 2002. Copyright 2002.)

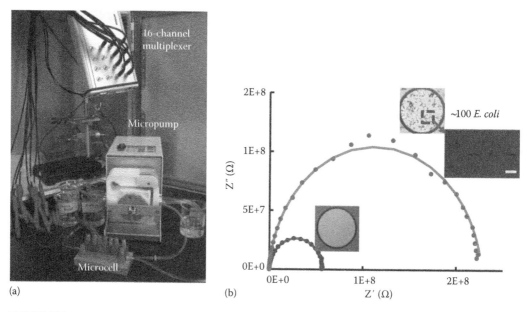

FIGURE 10.9
(a) A benchtop setup of EIS diamond MEA biosensor with a multiplexer module, peristaltic micropump and the microcell. (b) Impedance spectra of *bare* and *modified* UNCD microelectrodes, respectively, i.e., after antibody (50 μg/mL) and *E. coli K12* (<1.1E-07 cfu/mL) attachment. The increase in charge transfer resistance (R_{ct}) demonstrates binding event of the bacteria. The scale bar is 4 μm. The EIS spectra were recorded between 100 kHz and 100 mHz at 10 mV ac signal amplitude (rms value) at a 0 DC voltage. All measurements were carried out in a solution of 5 mM $Fe(CN)_6^{3-/4-}$ in 0.01 M phosphate buffered saline (pH7.4). (b: Reprinted with permission from S. Siddiqui et al., *Biosens. Bioelectron.*, 35(1), 284. Copyright 2012.)

groups that can serve as anchor points for biomolecules of interest and yields a high surface coverage of functional groups and very stable surface modifications and will also support electron transport more readily than other chemistries. The electrochemical reduction of phenyl diazonium ions at a carbon electrode to form a covalently modified surface was first reported by Delamar et al. in 1992 and was recently reviewed (Pinson and Podvorica 2005). The surface coverage of tethered aryl derivatives, estimated from both electrochemical and XPS measurements, is as high as 80% of a compact monolayer. The grafted organic layer is also hydrolytically stable, as no loss of the surface coverage was observed during months of soaking tests in phosphate buffer solutions. The process is shown schematically in Figure 10.10a for the case of a generic aromatic amine. Figure 10.10b and c shows the cyclic voltammograms during the two-step reduction process on UNCD. The surface modification may be patterned at the microscale using individually addressable microelectrodes similar to UNCD MEAs, "soft" lithography with PDMS molds, or at the nanoscale using scanning probe lithography. This method has been shown to yield very good biomolecular recognition properties and extremely good stability, both for storage and for repetitive use. This approach was successfully used to achieve an enzymatic biosensor to detect level of glucose *via* electrochemical reduction of H_2O_2 generated by the GOx enzyme tethered covalently to the diamond (Wang 2006). Hamers and coworkers have used this chemistry to produce electrically addressable arrays of DNA oligonucleotides on conductive diamond (Wang 2005, Hamers et al. 2007). Zhang et al. demonstrated the third approach, a one-step chemical modification to produce amine groups directly

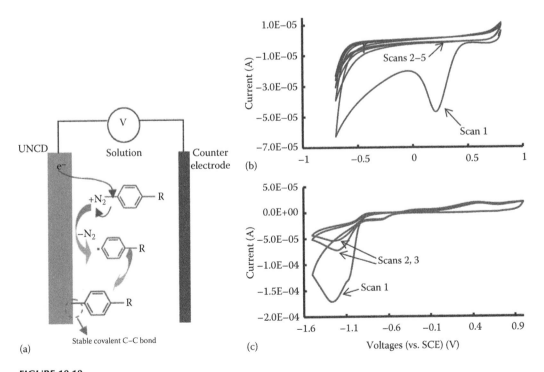

FIGURE 10.10
(a) Electrochemical surface functionalization of BD UNCD based on reduction of 4-nitrobenzene diazonium salt. (b) Cyclic voltammograms of 5 scans in 40 mM salt in 0.1M TBABF$_4$. The salt is reduced at <+0.2 V to covalently attach nitrophenyl groups to UNCD. (c) Cyclic voltammogram of 3 scans in 0.1M KCl in EtOH/H$_2$O TBABF$_4$ shows further reduction of the surface attached nitro group to amine at <–1.2 V.

on hydrogen-terminated PCD for patterning oligonucleotides with a fluorine-terminated surface as a passivation layer (Zhang et al. 2006). Amination time was found to be the main variable and the fluorescence intensity on 20 μm DNA micropatterns was highest at 2.5 h. The negligible loss of mean fluorescence intensity over the 20 hybridization and denaturation cycles demonstrates the high stability of the surface bound oligonucleotides on the directly aminated diamond.

10.5 EIS-Based NCD Biological Sensors

For the last several decades electrochemical impedance spectroscopy (EIS) has been used extensively to measure double-layer capacitance and study electrode processes and complex interfaces of numerous materials such as polymers, single crystal or amorphous semiconductors, glasses, solid and liquid electrolytes, fused salts, and biological membranes. EIS is also used to study fuel cells, rechargeable batteries, and corrosion. In the field of biosensing it is considered as a potential technique to attain label-free, low cost, and real-time sensing. It is a simple, sensitive technique but not quite well understood. In this technique, a small sinusoidal voltage perturbation is applied to the sample, and the current response is measured. Thus, by measuring the response of the electrode-interface (sample) to a signal, the processes taking place at the electrode surface can be easily determined. Since impedance is both an intrinsic and an extrinsic property of the material any change in the impedance of electrode surface such as bio-functionalization of the transducer surface or any change in material property such as the doping level must appear as a change in the measured signal. This extraordinary capability of the EIS technique to detect both extrinsic and intrinsic changes in impedance makes it highly sensitive. However, one of the main difficulties is in interpreting the measured response and understanding the causes for the change in impedance. For this, the technique does not have an established theory that can explain the observed response, and therefore requires the use of other techniques to validate experimental data.

10.5.1 Basic Principles of EIS

In impedance spectroscopy, a sinusoidal voltage with small amplitude is applied to the electrode surface and the resulting current response is measured. The impedance (Z) of the electrode is defined as the ratio of voltage and current and is given as $Z = V(t)/I(t) = V_o Sin(\omega t)/I_o Sin(\omega t + \phi)$, where V_o, I_o is the maximum voltage and current, ω is angular frequency, t is time, and ϕ is phase shift between current and voltage. As can be seen mathematically from this equation impedance is a complex quantity because the current can differ from voltage not only in terms of amplitude but also in terms of phase. It can be written in a simplified form as follows:

$$Z = Z_{re} + iZ_{im}$$

where Z_{re} and Z_{im} are real and imaginary parts of the impedance. Thus, the impedance data can be described in terms of real and imaginary parts. The plot of Z_{re} and Z_{im} is called a Nyquist plot, and the plot of modulus of impedance $|Z|$ and phase shift ϕ is called a Bode plot. The impedance data is obtained at different frequencies, rather than just one, and thus the name impedance spectrum. The spectrum is analyzed by fitting a circuit model to the data, and values of each element of the circuit are used to provide quantitative information about the properties of the surfaces, membranes, exchange current, and diffusion processes. The simplest circuit that is used is RC circuit in which the real part of the impedance represents resistance, and is given as $Z_{re} = R$, and imaginary part represent capacitance, $Z_{im} = 1/\omega C$ and the magnitude of Z is written as $|Z|^2 = |Z_{re}|^2 + |Z_{im}|^2 = R^2 + 1/\omega^2 C^2$ (Bard and Faulkner, 2nd edition). Thus, from the real and imaginary parts of the impedance, the values of resistance and capacitance can be obtained. However, for complex system, more complicated circuit called as equivalent circuit consisting of resistors (R), capacitors (C), Warburg element (Z_W), and inductors (I) is fitted to the experimental impedance data and information about the various elements of the system is derived. The most commonly used circuit to represent and to analyze an electrochemical cell/system is called Randles equivalent circuit (Figure 10.11a). It consists of elements such as a capacitor due to double-layer capacitance (C_{dl}), resistor due to charge transfer resistance (R_{ct}), and a resistor due to electrolyte solution resistance (R_s). However, these circuits cannot be directly correlated to the physical system and there is always more than one circuit model that fits well to impedance data. For this, either a best fit criterion is used or another technique is used to identify the right circuit model. In today's impedance analyzers, software is used to identify an equivalent circuit model that fits well to experimental data. The frequency (f) range that is used for collecting impedance data depends on the system under study. At low frequencies (f < 1 mHz) the DC

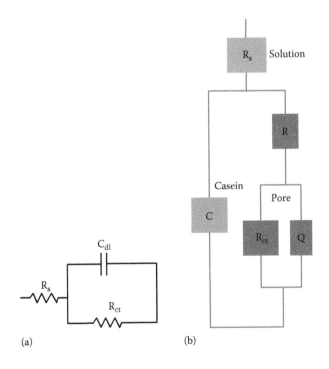

(a)   (b)

FIGURE 10.11
(a) Randles equivalent circuit model. (b) The equivalent circuit model fitted to experimental data of UNCD surface modified with antibody and bacteria capture. The origin of the various circuit parameters is as follows: uncompensated solution resistance; capacitance from casein layer and [$R(R_{ct}Q)$]—from pores. (b: Reprinted with permission from S. Siddiqui et al., *Biosens. Bioelectron.*, 35(1), 284. Copyright 2012.)

conductivity of the electrolyte solution determines the impedance. At high frequencies (f > 100 kHz) inductance of the electrochemical cell and connecting wires contribute to the impedance spectra. Thus, the analytically meaningful impedance spectra are usually recorded at frequencies where they are mainly controlled by the interfacial properties of the modified electrodes (Katz and Willner 2003).

10.5.2 Impedimetric Biosensor

Among the various classes of biosensors, molecular biosensors based on EIS have received widespread attention because of their potential for label-free detection. In this technique, a sensing biomolecule such as antibody or DNA is immobilized on the conductive electrode surface. The change in impedance due to binding of target such as antigen to sensing biomolecule is rendered as detection. The sensitivity of detection depends on material property of electrode surface, immobilization process, and interaction between sensing biomolecule and target. There are two types of detection processes: *non-faradaic* and *faradaic*. In non-faradaic process, the impedance change is mainly due to change in capacitance or dielectric properties of the double-layer and no redox molecule is used. This approach is particularly useful when the conductivity of the functionalized surface is changed by the specific binding event and is more suitable for on-site diagnostic (Lisdat and Schafer 2008). In faradaic process, the impedance change is due to change in charge transfer resistance from a redox molecule (e.g., $Fe(CN)_6^{-3/-4}$) present in the solution. To attain high sensitivity, usually a DC potential equal to that of open circuit potential (OCP) is applied to the electrode along with a sinusoidal voltage of small amplitudes. However, for some systems, OCP may be high enough to cause the breaking of covalent bonds between conductive surface of electrode and biolayer. In order to prevent breaking of covalent bonds, one can apply 0 V DC potential. Using these approaches, several researchers have demonstrated detection of DNA, antigens, and antibodies. However, there remain several issues that need to be resolved before a commercial biosensor can be built. Among them, the two most challenging issues are selectivity and nonspecific adsorption. Selectivity is one of the most common challenges for all label-free biosensors irrespective of the readout technique. The difficulty of detecting one or more targets in the presence of large concentrations of non-target material without labeling or using any additional technique has limited progress in this field. Such an issue can be resolved by developing models that can help to distinguish between the data sets of targets from non-targets of the EIS experimental data. The second challenge is to minimize nonspecific binding to the electrode surface to obtain a strong detection signal that does not need amplification. This issue can be resolved either by using electrode material that inhibits nonspecific adsorption or by chemical modification of the electrode surface in a way that shows strong detection signal even in the presence of huge concentrations of nonspecific interferents. Therefore, tremendous research efforts are needed along these directions to build a reliable label-free EIS biosensor.

10.5.3 UNCD MEA Impedimetric Biosensor

In a recent study, the authors (Siddiqui et al. 2012) used boron-doped UNCD MEAs and the EIS technique to demonstrate high selectivity and minimal nonspecific adsorption. They presented an electrochemical pore circuit model to explain the EIS detection mechanism, along with demonstration of improved signal reproducibility and increased sensitivity. By showing improvements for the earlier key issues, the potential of UNCD for a label-free EIS biosensing was realized. The sp^3 bonded carbon atom in UNCD prevents bonding of interferents and thus minimizes nonspecific adsorption. The differences in surface conductivities and bond structure of UNCD, that is, less conductive, homogenous grains and more conductive, heterogeneous grain boundaries ensure that the functionalization of such surfaces with TFAAD–dodecene monolayers and antibodies takes place only with certain carbon bonds of diamond. After functionalization, the electrode surface consists of two regions, one where the monolayers are formed with carbon atoms of diamond and to which antibodies are attached, and the other area surrounding the antibodies that is covered with casein blocker and acts as an insulator. Thus, pore-like structure is formed and antibodies reside inside the pores. It is inside this region where some part of the electrode surface is exposed to the electrolyte and exchange of electron "charge" between electrode and electrolyte takes place. This exchange of electrons takes place only inside the pores, because the remaining surface acts as an insulator. The addition of monolayers to the electrode surface reduces the electrochemically active surface, slows interfacial electron kinetics, and reduces exchange current (I_0). The Nyquist plot of impedance spectra of such a modified surface was found to be a semi-circle, which indicates a highly resistive interface. The high resistance is due to reductions in exchange current and increases in charge transfer resistance (R_{ct}). The relationship between I_0 and R_{ct} for such a surface at non-equilibrium condition is given by $R_{ct} = (1/\alpha f I_0) \text{Log}(I_0/I_{0eq})$, where F is the Faraday constant, α is the transfer coefficient, and I_{0eq} is the exchange current at equilibrium. As can be seen from this equation, charge transfer resistance is inversely proportional to exchange current. Therefore as the exchange current decreases, the impedance of the electrode surface is controlled by interfacial processes and no diffusional characteristic is observed in impedance spectra. It was found that the data from the impedance spectrum fits well to a pore circuit model (Figure 10.11b). The different elements of the circuit provide quantitative information on important parameters such as the coverage and density of immobilized antibody, the uniformity of casein coverage, electrolyte resistance inside and outside the pores, and charge transfer resistance. The values of these parameters are then used to distinguish between positive detection signals and false positive ones. The current research is geared toward collecting large data sets to optimize the parameters for high detection reliability. It is notable that due to the unique properties of the UNCD interface such as its chemical stability, ultra-smooth surface morphology that facilitates the deposition of more uniform, dense, and conformal monolayers and casein, and minimum nonspecific binding that a constant value of these parameters can be observed repeatedly, which may not be possible with other electrode materials.

10.6 Future Directions

NCD could emerge as the next best electrode material for biosensing because of its numerous advantages discussed in the chapter. Much progress is still needed in the areas of integrating sensors and components across length scales such as wafer-scale bonding (to achieve microfluidic handling functionality) and extensive field testing to validate the sensor stability and performance and its readiness to detect analytes in field water samples in real-time. More data need to be collected to fully quantify the stability of capture biomolecules on NCD surfaces when stored in different fluids for several weeks to months. Some of the key questions that we believe are essential in bringing the diamond biosensors to their full potential include the following: How does doping control the oxygenation of surface carbon atoms of NCD? How can growth parameters to deposit diamond films be optimized at low temperatures to allow integration into established CMOS technology and low-cost glass and polymer substrates? What are the effects of different storage conditions on surface oxidation rates of NCD grains and grain boundaries? What are the advantages of using 3D porous electrodes (pyramids, wires) in terms of increases in analyte diffusion and limits of detection? How can MEAs be functionalized at length scales ranging from submicron to tens-of-microns with distinct recognition agents to achieve high array-to-array reproducibility and repeatability, selectivity, and throughputs? How to rapidly develop, validate, and deploy robust electrical models that accurately detect analytes with few experiments? How effectively we answer these questions decides when this precious biosensor will be available for the common good.

Acknowledgments

The authors are grateful to ADT staff particularly Dr. Nicolaie Moldovan, Charles West, Ian Wylie, and Grace Catausan for their support over the years in developing UNCD film that was used for the various applications mentioned here. We thank Dr. Hamers Group, University of Wisconsin, Madison for XPS data; Dr. Radadia's Lab at Louisiana Tech University for the micro spotting image, and Dr. Paul Garris lab at Illinois State University, Normal for FIA dopamine detection data. The biosensor development work was supported by the Defense Threat Reduction Agency (DTRA) under contract HDTRA1–09-C-0007. We acknowledge the financial support from EPA, NIH, and NSF to continue working on developing UNCD based applications. The microfabrication work was performed in part at the Center for Nanoscale Materials (CNM), Argonne National Laboratory, IL, and University of Illinois at Chicago's Nanotechnology Core Facility, IL. The use of the CNM was supported by the U.S. Department of Energy, Office of Science, Office of Basic Energy Sciences, under Contract No. DEAC02-06CH11357.

References

Acworth, I. N., Bailey, B., Asa, D., Christensen, J., Goodall, E., and Waraska, J. 2008. A "Global" method for the determination of tissue thiols, disulfides and thioethers using an HPLC system incorporating a novel boron-doped diamond detector. *Pittcon Conference*, March 2–7, New Orleans, LA.

Angus, J. C., Pleskov, Y. V., and Eaton, S. C. 2004. *Electrochemistry of Diamond Thin Film Diamond: II (Semiconductors and Semimetals)* eds. C. E. Nebel and J. Ristein, Amsterdam, the Netherlands: Elsevier, Vol. 77, p. 97.

Arenkov, P. et al. 2000. Protein microchips: Use for immunoassay and enzymatic reactions. *Anal. Biochem.* 278, 123–131.

Arnault, J. C. et al. 2008. Diamond nanoseeding on silicon: Stability under H2 MPCVD exposures and early stages of growth. *Diam. Relat. Mater.* 17, 1143–1149.

Arumugam, P. U., Chen, H., Cassell, A. M., and Li, J. 2007. Dielectrophoretic trapping of single bacteria at carbon nanofiber nanoelectrode arrays. *J. Phys. Chem. A* 111(49), 12772–12777.

Arumugam, P. U., Chen, H., and Siddiqui, S. 2009. Wafer-scale fabrication of patterned carbon nanofiber nanoelectrode arrays: A route for development of multiplexed, ultrasensitive disposable biosensors. *Biosens. Bioelectron.* 24, 2818–2824.

Ascarelli, P., and Fontana, S. 1993. Dissimilar grit-size dependence of the diamond nucleation density on substrate surface pretreatments. *Appl. Surf. Sci.* 64, 307–311.

Auciello, O. et al. 2004. Materials science and fabrication processes for a new MEMS technology based on ultrananocrystalline diamond thin films. *J. Phys. Condens. Matter*, 16, R539–R552.

Auciello, O., and Sumant, A. V. 2010. Status review of the science and technology of ultrananocrystalline diamond (UNCD™) films and application to multifunctional devices. *Diam. Relat. Mater.* 19, 699–718.

Bakker, E. 2004. Electrochemical sensors. *Anal. Chem.* 76, 3285–3298.

Baranauskas, V., Li, B. B., Peterlevitz, A., Tosin, M. C., and Durrant, S. F. 1999. Nitrogen-doped diamond films. *J. Appl. Phys.* 85, 7455–7458.

Bard, A. J., and Faulkner, L. R. 2001. *Electrochemical Methods: Fundamentals and Applications* (2nd edn.). New York: John Wiley & Sons. p. 368.

Bhattacharyya, S. et al. 2001. Synthesis and characterization of highly-conducting nitrogen-doped ultrananocrystalline diamond films. *Appl. Phys. Lett.* 79, 1441–1443.

Birrell, J. et al. 2005. Interpretation of the Raman spectra of ultrananocrystalline diamond. *Diam. Relat. Mater.* 14(1), 86–92.

Brett, C. M. A., and Brett, A. M. O. 1993. *Electrochemistry Principles, Methods, and Applications*. Oxford, U.K.: Oxford University Press.

Bruce, P. G., Oleksiak, A. L., Los, P., Vincent, C. A. 1994. Electrochemical impedance spectroscopy at an ultramicroelectrode. *J. Electroanal. Chem.* 367, 279–283.

Bucka, V., and Deuerlerb, F. 1998. Enhanced nucleation of diamond films on pretreated substrates. *Diam. Relat. Mater.* 7, 1544–1552.

Bulychev, B. M. et al. 2010. Poly(naphthalenehydrocarbyne): Synthesis, characterization, and application to preparation of thin diamond films. *Russ. Chem. Bull.* 59, 1724–1728.

Bundy, F. P., Hall, H. T., Strong, H. M., and Wentorf, R. H. 1955. Man-made diamonds. *Nature* 176, 51–55.

Butler, J. E., and Sumant, A. V. 2008. The CVD of nanodiamond materials. *Chem. Vap. Deposition* 14, 145–160.

Carlisle, J. A. 2004. Precious biosensors. *Nat. Mater.* 3, 668–669.

Chen, Q. et al. 2001. The structure and electrochemical behavior of nitrogen-containing nanocrystalline diamond films deposited from CH/N/Ar mixtures. *J. Electrochem. Soc.* 148, E44.

Cheng, J. et al. 1998. Preparation and hybridization analysis of DNA/RNA from E. coli on microfabricated bioelectronic chips. *Natl. Biotechnol.* 16, 541–546.

Chhowalla, M., Ferrari, A. C., Robertson, J., and Amaratunga, G. A. J. 2000. Evolution of sp^2 bonding with deposition temperature in tetrahedral amorphous carbon studied by Raman spectroscopy. *Appl. Phys. Lett.* 76, 1419–1421.

Chiem, N., and Harrison, D. J. 1997. Micro-chip-based capillary electrophoresis for immunoassays: An integrated immunoreactor with electrophoretic separation for serum theophylline determination. *Clin. Chem.* 44, 591–598.

Clancy, J. L., Bukhari, Z., McCuin, R. M., Matheson, Z., and Fricker, C. R. 1999. USEPA Method 1622. *J. Am. Water Works A* 91, 60–68.

Cousino, M. A., Jarbawi, T. B., Halsall, H. B., Heineman, W. R. 1997. Pushing down the limits of detection: Molecular needles in a haystack. *Anal. Chem.* 69(17), 545A–549A.

Cvacka, J., Quaiserova, V., Park, J., Show, Y., Muck, A., and Swain, G. M. 2003. Boron-doped diamond microelectrodes for use in capillary electrophoresis with electrochemical detection. *Anal. Chem.* 75, 2678–2687.

Das, D., and Singh, R. N. 2007. A review of nucleation, growth and low temperature synthesis of diamond thin films. *Int. Mater. Rev.* 52, 29–64.

Decarli, P., and Jamieson, J. 1961. Formation of diamond by explosive shock. *Science* 133, 1821–1822.

Delamar, M., Hitmi, R., Pinson, J., and Saveant, J. M. J. 1992. Covalent modification of carbon surfaces by grafting of functionalized aryl radicals produced from electrochemical reduction of diazonium salts. *J. Am. Chem. Soc.* 114, 5883–5884.

Dipalo, M., Kusterer, J., Janischowsky, K., and Kohn, E. 2006. N-type doped nano-diamond in a first MEMS application. *Phys. Status Solidi A.* 203, 3036–3041.

Drummond, T. G., Hill, M. G., and Barton, J. K. 2003. Electrochemical DNA sensors. *Nat. Biotechnol.* 21(10), 1192–1199.

Evans, U., Colavita, P. E., Doescher, M. S., Schiza, M., and Myrick, M. L. 2002. Construction and characterization of a nanowell electrode array. *Nano Lett.* 2 (6), 641–645.

Ewalt, K. L., Haigis, R. W., Rooney, R., Ackley, D., and Krihak, M. 2001. Detection of biological toxins on an active electronic microchip. *Anal. Biochem.* 289, 162–172.

Ferrari, A. C., and Robertson, J. 2001. Origin of the 1150-cm^{-1} Raman mode in nanocrystalline diamond. *Phys. Rev. B* 63, 121405.

Fischer, A. E., Show, Y., and Swain, G. M. 2004. Electrochemical performance of diamond thin-film electrodes from different commercial sources. *Anal. Chem.* 2004, 76(9), 2553–2560.

Foulds, N. C., Frew, J. E., and Green, M. J. 1990. Immunoelectrodes. In *Biosensors a Practical Approach,* Ed., Cass, A. E., Oxford, U.K.: IRL Press, pp. 97–124.

Fritzsche, W., and Taton, T. A. 2003. Metal nanoparticles as labels for heterogeneous, chip-based DNA detection. *Nanotechnology* 14, R63–R73.

Gajewski, W. et al. 2009. Electronic and optical properties of boron-doped nanocrystalline diamond films. *Phys. Rev. B* 79, 045206.

Geis, M. W. 1989. Growth of textured diamond films on foreign substrates from attached seed crystals. *Appl. Phys. Lett.* 55, 550–552.

Gerwen, P. V., Laureyn, W., and Laureys, W. 1998. Nanoscaled interdigitated electrode arrays for biochemical sensors. *Sensor Actuat. B Chem.* 49(1–2), 73–80.

Ghindilis, A. L. et al. 2009. Sensor array: Impedimetric label-free sensing of DNA hybridization in real time for rapid, PCR-based detection of microorganisms. *Electroanalysis* 21(13), 1459–1468.

Gilles, P. N., Wu, D. J., Foster, C. B., Dillon, P. J., and Chanock, S. J. 1999. Single nucleotide polymorphic discrimination by an electronic dot assay on semiconductor microchips. *Nat. Biotechnol.* 17, 365–370.

Granger, M. C., Witek, M., and Swain, G. M. 2000. Standard electrochemical behavior of high-quality, boron-doped polycrystalline diamond thin-film electrodes. *Anal. Chem.* 72, 3793–3804.

Granger, M. C., Xu, J., Strojek, J. W., and Swain, G. M. 1999. Polycrystalline diamond electrodes: Basic properties and applications as amperometric detectors in flow injection analysis and liquid chromatography. *Anal. Chim. Acta* 397, 145–161.

Gray, K. J., and Windischmann, H. 1999. Free-standing CVD diamond wafers for thermal management by d.c. arc jet technology. *Diam. Relat. Mater.* 8, 903–908.

Gruen, D. M. et al. 1996. Characterization of nanocrystalline diamond films by core-level photoabsorption. *Appl. Phys. Lett.* 68(12), 1640–1642.

Gruen, D. M., Liu, S., Krauss, A. R., Luo, J., and Pan, X. 1994. Fullerenes as precursors for diamond film growth without hydrogen or oxygen additions. *Appl. Phys. Lett.* 64, 1502–1504.

Hahm, J.-I., and Lieber, C. M. 2004. Direct ultrasensitive electrical detection of DNA and DNA sequence variations using nanowire nanosensors. *Nano Lett.* 4(1), 51–54.

Hall, H. T. 2004. The transformation of graphite into diamond. In *50 Years Progress in Crystal Growth: A Reprint Collection.* Ed. Feigelson, R. S., pp. 194–198, Amsterdam, the Netherlands: Elsevier Inc.

Hamers, R. J. et al. 2007. Direct electrical detection of antigen-antibody binding on diamond and silicon substrates using electrical impedance spectroscopy. *Analyst* 132, 296–306.

Hammersberg, J. et al. 2002. High carrier mobility in single-crystal plasma-deposited diamond. *Science* 267, 1670–1672.

Haubner, R., Lindlbauer, A., and Lux, B. 1996. Diamond nucleation and growth on refractory metals using microwave plasma deposition. *Int. J. Refract. Met. Hard Mater.* 14, 119–125.

Haymond, S., Babcock, G. T., and Swain, G. M. 2002. Direct electrochemistry of cytochrome c at nanocrystalline boron-doped diamond. *J. Am. Chem. Soc.* 124(36), 10634–10635.

He, W., Yang, Q., Liu, Z., Yu, X., and Xu, D. 2005. DNA array biosensor based on electrochemical hybridization and detection. *Anal. Lett.* 38, 2567–2578.

Heineman, W. R., and Halsall, H. B. 1985. Strategies for electrochemical immunoassay. *Anal. Chem.* 57, 1321A–1331A.

Heller, M. J. 2002. DNA Microarray technology: Devices, systems, and applications. *Annu. Rev. Biomed. Eng.* 4, 129–153.

Hernando, J., Lud, S. Q., Bruno, P., Gruen, D. M., Stutzmann, M., and Garrido, J. A. 2009. Electrochemical impedance spectroscopy of oxidized and hydrogen-terminated nitrogen-induced conductive ultrananocrystalline diamond. *Electrochim. Acta* 54, 1909–1910.

Hoffmann, R., Kriele, A., and Obloh, H. 2010. Electrochemical hydrogen termination of boron-doped diamond. *Appl. Phys. Lett.* 97, 052103-1–052103-3.

Holt, K. B., Bard, A. J., Show, Y., and Swain, G. M. 2004. Scanning electrochemical microscopy and conductive probe atomic force microscopy studies of hydrogen-terminated boron-doped diamond electrodes with different doping levels. *J. Phys. Chem. B* 108(39), 15117–15127.

Hu, J., Holt, K. B., and Foord, J. S. 2009. Focused ion beam fabrication of boron-doped diamond ultra-microelectrodes. *Anal. Chem.* 81, 5663–5670.

Hupert, M., Muck, A., and Wang, J. 2003. Conductive diamond thin-films in electrochemistry. *Diam. Relat. Mater.* 12(10–11), 1940–1949.

Jiang, X., Au, F. C. K., and Lee, S. T. 2002 Ultrahigh boron doping of nanocrystalline diamond films and their electron field emission characteristics. *J. Appl. Phys.* 92, 2880–2883.

Juttner, K., and Becker, D. 2007. Characterization of boron-doped diamond electrodes by electrochemical impedance spectroscopy. *J. Appl. Electrochem.* 37(1), 27–32.

Kalss, W., Haubner, R., and Lux, B. 1997. Diamond deposition on noble metals. *Diam. Relat. Mater.* 6, 240–246.

Kamo, M., Sato, Y., Matsumoto, S., and Setaka, N. 1983. Diamond synthesis from gas phase in microwave plasma. *J. Cryst. Growth* 62: 642–644.

Katz, E., and Willner, I. 2003. Probing biomolecular interactions at conductive and semiconductive surfaces by impedance spectroscopy: Routes to impedimetric immunosensors, DNA-sensors, and enzyme biosensors. *Electroanalysis* 15(11), 913–947.

Kellermann, K., Barei, C., Rosiwal, S. M., and Singer, R. F. 2008. Well adherent diamond coatings on steel substrates. *Adv. Eng. Mater.* 10, 657–660.

Kim, K. H. et al. 2005. Novel ultrananocrystalline diamond probes for high resolution low-wear nanolithographic techniques. *Small* 1, 866–874.

Kiran, R. et al. 2012. Multichannel boron doped nanocrystalline diamond ultramicroelectrode arrays: Design, fabrication and characterization. *Sensors* 12, 7669–7681.

Kociniewski, T. et al. 2006. N-type CVD diamond doped with phosphorus using the MOCVD technology for dopant incorporation. *Physica Status Solidi A*. 203, 3136–3141.

Koehne, J. E., Marsh, M., Boakye, A., Douglas, B., and Kim, I. Y. 2011. Carbon nanofiber electrode array for electrochemical detection of dopamine using fast scan cyclic voltammetry. *Analyst* 136, 1802–1805.

Koizumi, S., Teraji, T., Kanda, H. 2000. Phosphorus-doped chemical vapor deposition of diamond. *Diam. Relat. Mater.* 9, 935–940.

Kondo, T., Einaga, Y., Sarada, B. V., Rao, T. N., Tryk, D. A., and Fujishima, A. 2002. Homoepitaxial single-crystal boron-doped diamond electrodes for electroanalysis. *J. Electrochem. Soc.* 149, E179–E184.

Kreuzer, C., Riedrich-Möller, J., Neu, E., and Becher, C. 2008. Design of photonic crystal microcavities in diamond films. *Opt. Express* 16, 1632–1644.

Lasseter, T. L., Clare, B. H., Abbott, N. L., and Hamers, R. J. 2004. Covalently modified silicon and diamond surfaces: Resistance to nonspecific protein adsorption and optimization for biosensing. *J. Am. Chem. Soc.* 126(33), 10220–10221.

Lee, C. S. et al. 2004. Electrically addressable biomolecular functionalization of carbon nanotube and carbon nanofiber electrodes. *Nano Lett.* 4(9), 1713–1716.

Li, J., Ng, H. T., and Cassell, A. 2003. Carbon nanotube nanoelectrode array for ultrasensitive DNA detection. *Nano Lett.* 3(5), 597–602.

Liao, X. Z., Zhang, R. J., Lee, C. S., Lee, S. T., and Lam, Y. W. 1997. The influence of boron doping on the structure and characteristics of diamond thin films. *Diam. Relat. Mater.* 6, 521–525.

Liepold, P., Wieder, H., Hillebrandt, H., Friebel, A., and Hartwich, G. 2005. DNA-arrays with electrical detection: A label-free low cost technology for routine use in life sciences and diagnostics. *Bioelectrochemistry* 67, 143–150.

Lisdat, F., and Schafer, D. 2008. The use of electrochemical impedance spectroscopy for biosensing. *Anal. Bioanal. Chem.* 391, 1555–1567.

Liu, H., and Dandy, D. S. 1995. Studies on nucleation process in diamond CVD: An overview of recent developments. *Diam. Relat. Mater.* 4, 1173–1188.

Mareš, J. J., Nesládek, M., Hubík, P., Kindl, D., and Krištofik, J. 2007. On unconventional superconductivity in boron-doped diamond. *Diam. Relat. Mater.* 16, 1–5.

Martin, H. B., Argoitia, A., Angus, J. C., and Landau, U. 1999. Voltammetry studies of single-crystal and polycrystalline diamond electrodes. *J. Electrochem. Soc.* 146(8), 2959–2964.

Martin, H. B., Argoitia, A., Landau, U., Anderson, A. B., and Angus, J. C. 1996. Hydrogen and oxygen evolution on boron-doped diamond electrodes. *J. Electrochem. Soc.* 143, L133–L136.

Matsumoto, S., Sato, Y., Tsutsumi, M., and Setaka, N. 1982. Growth of diamond particles from methane-hydrogen gas. *J. Mater. Sci.* 17, 3106–3112.

May, P. W. 2010. Chemical vapor deposition-a route to microcrystalline, nanocrystalline, ultrananocrystalline and single crystal diamond. In *Carbon Based Nanomaterials, Materials Science Foundation*. Chapter 6, Eds. Ali, E. N., Öchsner, A., and Ahmed, W., pp. 145–176, Zurich, Switzerland: Tans Tech.

May, P. W., Ashfold, M. N. R., and Mankelevich, Y. A. 2007. Microcrystalline, nanocrystalline, and ultrananocrystalline diamond chemical vapor deposition: Experiment and modeling of the factors controlling growth rate, nucleation, and crystal size. *J. Appl. Phys.* 101, 053115.

May, P. W., Harvey, J. N., Allan, N. L., Richley, J. C., and Mankelevich, Y. A. 2010. Simulations of chemical vapor deposition diamond film growth using a kinetic Monte Carlo model and two-dimensional models of microwave plasma and hot filament chemical vapor deposition reactors. *J. Appl. Phys.* 108, 114909.

May, P. W., Ludlow, W. J., Hannaway, M., Heard, P. J., Smith, J. A., and Rosser, K. N. 2007. Raman and conductivity studies of boron doped microcrystalline diamond, facetted nanocrystalline diamond and cauliflower diamond films. *Chem. Phys. Lett.* 446, 103–108.

McCreery, R. L. 2008. Advanced carbon electrode materials for molecular electrochemistry. *Chem. Rev.* 108, 2646–2687.

Michau, D., Tanguy, B., Demazeau, G., Couzi, M., and Cavagnat, R. 1993. Influence on diamond nucleation of the carbon concentration near the substrate surface. *Diam. Relat. Mater.* 2, 19–23.

Muna, G. W., Tasheva, N., and Swain, G. M. 2004. Electro-oxidation and amperometric detection of chlorinated phenols at boron-doped diamond electrodes: A comparison of microcrystalline and nanocrystalline thin films. *Environ. Sci. Technol.* 38(13), 3674–3682.

Naguib, N. N., Elam, J. W., and Birrell, J. 2006. Enhanced nucleation, smoothness and conformality of ultrananocrystalline diamond (UNCD) ultrathin films *via* tungsten interlayers. *Chem. Phys. Lett.* 430, 345–350.

Nebel, C. E., Rezek, B., Shin, D., Uetsuka, H., and Yang, N. 2007. Diamond for bio-sensor applications. *J. Phys. D Appl. Phys.* 40, 6443–6466.

Nebel, C. E., Shin, D., Rezek, B., Tokuda, N., Uetsuka, H., and Watanabe, H. 2007. Diamond and biology. *J. R. Soc. Interface* 4, 439–461.

Okano, K. et al. 1989. Characterization of boron-doped diamond film. *Jpn. J. Appl. Phys.* 28, 1066–1071.

Oleinikov, A. V., Gray, M. D., Zhao, J., and Montgomery, D. D. 2003. Self-assembling protein arrays using electronic semiconductor microchips and in vitro translation. *J. Proteome Res.* 2, 313–319.

Paeschke, M., Wollenberger, U., and Köhler, C. 1995. Properties of interdigital electrode arrays with different geometries. *Anal. Chim. Acta* 305(1–3), 126–136.

Philip, J. et al. 2003. Elastic, mechanical, and thermal properties of nanocrystalline diamond films. *J. Appl. Phys.* 93, 2164–2171.

Pinson, J., and Podvorica, F. 2005. Attachment of organic layers to conductive or semiconductive surfaces by reduction of diazonium salts. *Chem. Soc. Rev.* 34, 429–439.

Pleskov, Y. V., Evstefeeva, Y. E., Krotova, M. D., Elkin, V. V., Mazin, V. M., Mishuk, V. Y., Varnin, V. P., and Teremetskaya, I. G. 1998. Synthetic semiconductor diamond electrodes: The comparative study of the electrochemical behaviour of polycrystalline and single crystal boron-doped films. *J. Electroanal. Chem.* 455, 139–146.

Polo, M. C., Cifre, J., Puigdollers, J., and Esteve, J. 1994. Comparative study of trimethylboron doping of hot filament chemically vapour deposited and microwave plasma chemically vapour deposited diamond films. *Thin Solid Films* 253, 136–140.

Popov, C., Kulisch, W., Gibson, P. N., Ceccone, G., and Jelinek, M. 2004. Growth and characterization of nanocrystalline diamond/amorphous carbon composite films prepared by MWCVD. *Diam. Relat. Mater.* 13, 1371–1376.

Potocky, S. et al. 2006. Growth of nanocrystalline diamond films deposited by microwave plasma CVD system at low substrate temperatures. *Physica Status Solidi A* 203, 3011–3015.

Radadia, A. D. et al. 2011. Control of nanoscale environment to improve stability of immobilized proteins on diamond surfaces. *Adv. Funct. Mater.* 21, 1040–1050.

Ramesham, R., and Rose, M. F. 1997. Electrochemical characterization of doped and undoped CVD diamond deposited by microwave plasma. *Diam. Relat. Mater.* 6 (1), 17–26.

Ramesham, R., Rose, M. F., and Askew, R. F. 1996. Growth of diamond thin films on nickel-base alloys. *Surf. Coat. Tech.* 79, 55–66.

Rao, T. N., Yagi, I., Miwa, T., Tryk, D. A., and Fujishima, A. 1999. Electrochemical oxidation of NADH at highly boron-doped diamond electrodes. *Anal. Chem.* 71, 2506–2511.

Robinson, J. T., Perkins, F. K., Snow, E. S., Wei, Z., and Sheehan, P. E. 2008. Reduced graphene oxide molecular sensors. *Nano Lett.* 8(10), 3137–3140.

Shao, Y., Wang, J., Wu, H., Liu, J., Aksay, I.A., and Lin, Y. 2010. Graphene based electrochemical sensors and biosensors: A review. *Electroanalysis* 22, 1027–1036.

Shenderova, O., Hens, S., and McGuire, G. 2010. Seeding slurries based on detonation nanodiamond in DMSO. *Diam. Relat. Mater.* 19, 260–267.

Show, Y., Sonthalia, P., Swain, and G. M. 2003. Characterization and electrochemical responsiveness of boron-doped nanocrystalline diamond thin-film electrodes. *Chem. Mater.* 15, 879–888.

Siddiqui, S. et al. 2012. A quantitative study of detection mechanism of a label-free impedance biosensor using ultrananocrystalline diamond microelectrode array. *Biosens. Bioelectron.* 35(1), 284–290.

Siddiqui, S., Arumugam, P. U., Chen, H., Li, J., and Meyyappan, M. 2010. Characterization of carbon nanofiber electrode arrays using electrochemical impedance spectroscopy: Effect of scaling down electrode size. *ACS Nano* 4(2), 955–961.

Simm, A. O. et al. 2005. Boron-doped diamond microdisc arrays; electrochemical characterization and their use as a substrate for the production of microelectrode arrays of diverse metals (Au, Au, Cu) *via* electrodeposition. *Analyst* 130, 1303–1311.

Strein, T. G., and Ewing, A. G. 1993. Characterization of small noble metal microelectrodes by voltammetry and energy-dispersive x-ray analysis. *Anal. Chem.* 65(9), 1203–1209.

Suzuki, K., Sawabe, A., Yasuda, H., and Inuzuka, T. 1987 Growth of diamond thin films by dc plasma chemical vapor deposition. *Appl. Phys. Lett.* 50, 728–729.

Swain, G. M. 2004. Electroanalytical applications of diamond electrodes. *Semiconduct. Semimet.* 77, 121–148.

Swain, G. M., Anderson, A., and Angus, J. C. 1998. Applications of diamond thin films in electrochemistry. *MRS Bull.* 23(99), 56–60.

Takahashi, K., Tanga, M., Takai, O., and Okamura, H. 2000. DNA bonding to diamond. *Bio Indust.* 17, 44–51.

Tsugawa, K., Ishihara, M., Kim, J., Koga, Y., and Hasegawa, M. 2010. Nanocrystalline diamond film growth on plastic substrates at temperatures below 100°C from low-temperature plasma. *Phys. Rev. B* 82, 125460.

Wang, J. 2006. Electrochemical biosensors: Towards point-of-care cancer diagnostics. *Biosens. Bioelectron.* 21(10), 1887–1892.

Wang, J. et al. 2004. Surface functionalization of ultrananocrystalline diamond films by electrochemical reduction of aryldiazonium salts. *Langmuir* 20(26), 11450–11456.

Wang, J., and Carlisle, J. A. 2006. Covalent immobilization of glucose oxidase on conducting ultrananocrystalline diamond thin films. *Diam. Relat. Mater.* 15(2), 279–284.

Wang, T., Xin, H. W., Zhang, Z. M., Dai, Y. B., and Shen, H. S. 2004b. The fabrication of nanocrystalline diamond films using hot filament CVD. *Diam. Relat. Mater.* 13, 6–13.

Wang, W. L., Jiang, X., Taube, K., and Klages, C.-P. 1997. Piezoresistivity of polycrystalline p-type diamond films of various doping levels at different temperatures. *J. Appl. Phys.* 82, 729–732.

Wang, X. et al. 2007. Direct photopatterning and SEM imaging of molecular monolayers on diamond surfaces: Mechanistic insights into UV-initiated molecular grafting. *Langmuir* 23(23), 11623–11630.

Wei, J., and Tzeng, Y. 1993. Growth of diamond by sequential deposition and etching process using hot filament CVD. *J. Cryst. Growth.* 128, 413–417.

Wightman, M. 1988. Microvoltammetric electrodes. *Science* 240, 415–420.

Williams, O. A. 2011. Nanocrystalline diamond. *Diam. Relat. Mater.* 20, 621–640.

Williams, O. A., Daenena, M., and D'Haen, J. 2006. Comparison of the growth and properties of ultrananocrystalline diamond and nanocrystalline diamond. *Diam. Relat. Mater.* 15, 654–658.

Williams, O. A., Nesladek, M., and Daenen, M. 2008. Growth, electronic properties and applications of nanodiamond. *Diam. Relat. Mater.* 17, 1080–1088.

Woolley, A. T., and Mathies, R. A., 1995. Ultra-high-speed DNA sequencing using capillary electrophoresis chips. *Anal. Chem.* 67, 3676–3680.

Xiao, X. et al. 2004. Low temperature growth of ultrananocrystalline diamond. *J. Appl. Phys.* 96(4), 2232–2239.

Xu, J., Chen, Q., and Swain, G. M. 1998. Anthraquinonedisulfonate electrochemistry: A comparison of glassy carbon, hydrogenated glassy carbon, highly oriented pyrolytic graphite, and diamond electrodes. *Anal. Chem.* 70, 3146.

Yagi, I., Notsu, H., Kondo, T., Tryk, D. A., and Fujishima, A. 1999. Electrochemical selectivity for redox systems at oxygen-terminated diamond electrodes. *J. Electroanal. Chem.* 473, 173–178.

Yang, N. et al. 2007. Photochemical amine layer formation on H-terminated single-crystalline CVD diamond. *Chem. Mater.* 19(11), 2852–2859.

Yang, N., Uetsuka, H., Osawa, E., and Nebel, C. E. 2008. Vertically aligned diamond nanowires for DNA sensing. *Angew. Chem. Int. Ed.* 47, 5183–5185.

Yang, W. et al. 2002. DNA-modified nanocrystalline diamond thin films as stable, biologically active substrates. *Nat. Mater.* 1(4), 253–257.

Yang, W. S. et al. 2005. Electrically addressable biomolecular functionalization of conductive nanocrystalline diamond thin films. *Chem. Mater.* 17(5), 938–940.

Yarbrough, W., and Messier, R. 1990. Current issues and problems in the chemical vapor deposition of diamond. *Science*, 247, 688–696.

Yun, Y., Bange, A., and Heineman, W. R. 2007. A nanotube array immunosensor for direct electrochemical detection of antigen-antibody binding. *Sensor Actuat. B* 123, 177–182.

Zapol, P., Sternberg, M., Curtiss, L. A., Frauenheim, T., and Gruen, D. M. 2001. Tight-binding molecular-dynamics simulation of impurities in ultrananocrystalline diamond grain boundaries *Phys. Rev. B* 65, 045403.

Zhang, G.-J. et al. 2006. DNA micropatterning on polycrystalline diamond *via* one-step direct amination. *Langmuir*, 22, 3728–3734.

Zhao, H. X., Galligan, J. J., and Swain, G. M. 2010. Electrochemical measurements of serotonin (5-HT) release from the guinea pig mucosa using continuous amperometry with a boron-doped diamond microelectrode. *Diam. Relat. Mater.* 19, 182–185.

Zhu, W., Sivazlian, F. R., Stoner B. R., and Glass, J. T. 1995. Nucleation and selected area deposition of diamond by biased hot filament chemical vapor deposition. *J. Mater. Res.* 10, 425–430.

11

Carbon Nanotube–Based Electrochemical Biosensors

Feng Du, Lin Zhu, and Liming Dai

CONTENTS

11.1 Introduction

Owing to the large specific surface area as well as unusual electrical, thermal, and mechanical properties [1–3], carbon nanotubes are useful for various measurement devices, including electrochemical biosensors. However, it is essential to align and/or pattern the carbon nanotubes for device fabrication. In this regard, various carbon nanotubes (both multiwalled and single-walled carbon nanotubes, MWNTs and SWNTs) have been made either perpendicularly or horizontally aligned to the substrate surface, along with micropatterned carbon nanotubes with a sub-micrometer resolution [4–6]. The perpendicularly aligned carbon nanotube arrays, either in a patterned or non-patterned form, prepared by pyrolysis can be transferred to various other substrates of particular interest (e.g., polymer films for flexible organic optoelectronic devices or metal substrates for electrochemistry). The aligned structure facilitates surface functionalization of carbon nanotubes while largely retaining their structural integrity. By electrochemically depositing a concentric layer of an appropriate conducting polymer with trapped enzymes (e.g., glucose oxidizer) onto the individual aligned carbon nanotubes, we have prepared electrochemical biosensors based on the aligned conducting polymer–carbon nanotube coaxial nanowires with a high sensitivity [7,8]. The aim of this chapter is to provide a brief overview on the progress toward the synthesis and construction of aligned and micropatterned carbon nanotubes for electrochemical sensors by spotlighting some important work in the field.

11.2 Controlled Growth of Carbon Nanotubes

11.2.1 Nonaligned Carbon Nanotubes

There are mainly three different methods for carbon nanotube synthesis: arc discharge, laser ablation, and chemical vapor deposition (CVD) [9–15]. In an arc discharge method, either single- or multi-walled CNTs can be produced by applying a high DC voltage onto two graphite electrodes embedded with metal catalysts in a helium atmosphere [9]. For instance, Chen et al. [10,11] used Ni, Y metal, and metal oxide powders as catalysts to produce high-yield SWNTs with controlled length, bundle size, and purity. On the other hand, a pulsed laser was used in the laser ablation process to vaporize a graphite target to form carbon nanotubes in a high-temperature reactor under inert gas. SWNTs up to a yield around 70% are normally produced by the laser ablation method [12]. The formation of CNTs in both arc discharge and laser ablation methods requires a very high energy input [13–15], and the resultant CNTs are always nonaligned with a limited production capacity. Therefore, chemical vapor deposition (CVD) methods were developed for large-scale production of nonaligned and aligned CNTs (both MWNTs and SWNTs) [16–18].

11.2.2 Vertically Aligned Carbon Nanotubes

By performing pyrolysis of acetylene on cobalt catalyst within an alumina membrane template, Li et al. [19] prepared vertically aligned carbon nanotubes (VA-CNTs). As schematically shown in Figure 11.1, cobalt or nickel catalyst particles were pre-deposited at the bottom of the alumina membrane pores, followed by deposition of aligned carbon nanotubes in the pores through pyrolysis of appropriate hydrocarbon gases (e.g., acetylene). With a properly fabricated alumina template, the diameter, packing density, and even length of carbon nanotubes could be tuned.

Later the CVD method was used to prepare VA-CNTs even without the involvement of a template. For instance, Dai and coworkers [4] have prepared large-scale aligned carbon nanotubes perpendicularly aligned on the substrate surface via pyrolysis of iron (II) phthalocyanine (FePc) while Rao et al. [20] and Ajayan et al. [21] produced well-aligned CNTs from ferrocene in xylene solution by CVD. Apart from the VA-MWNT arrays, VA-SWNTs have also been prepared by CVD under appropriate conditions (e.g., specific

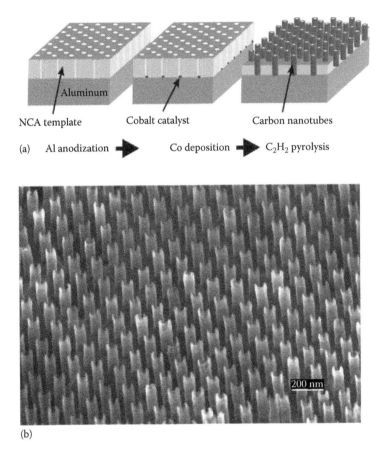

FIGURE 11.1
(a) Schematic of carbon nanotube growth process. (b) SEM image of the carbon nanotubes array. (From Li, J. et al., *Appl. Phys. Lett.*, 75, 367, 1999. With permission.)

catalyst, growth temperature). VA-SWNT arrays with a high percentage (96%) of semiconducting SWNTs have also been prepared by using the combined plasma-enhanced CVD and fast heating method [22].

11.3 Micropatterning of Vertically Aligned Carbon Nanotubes

For many applications (e.g., sensor chips), it is highly desirable to produce VA-CNTs into micropatterned structures. In this regard, Fan et al. [23] reported the synthesis of regular arrays of oriented nanotubes on Fe-patterned porous silicon by pyrolysis of ethylene.

In an independent study, Yang et al. [24] developed a photolithographic micropatterning method for patterned growth of VA-CNTs. Figure 11.2 shows the scheme of the photolithographic process (Figure 11.2a), together with a typical SEM image of the resultant VA-MWNT micropattern (Figure 11.2b) [25].

Soft-lithographic techniques, including the micro-contact printing and micro-molding, have also been used to prepare micropatterns of VA-CNTs [5]. The micro-contact printing

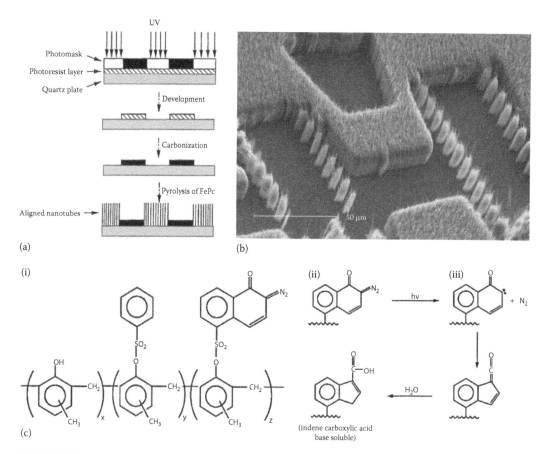

FIGURE 11.2

(a) Schematic representation of the micropattern formation of VA-MWNTs by photolithographic process. (b) Typical SEM micrographs of patterned films of VA-MWNTs prepared by the pyrolysis of FePc onto a photolithographically prepatterned quartz substrate. (c) (i) Molecular structure of the DNQ-Novolak photoresist, and (ii) photochemical reactions of the DNQ-Novolak photoresist. (From March, J., *Advanced Organic Chemistry*, 4th edn., 1992. Copyright Wiley-VCH Verlag GmbH & Co. KGaA; From Yang, Y. et al., *J. Am. Chem. Soc.* 121, 10832, 1999. With permission.)

process involves transferring monolayers of alkylsiloxane onto a quartz substrate in a patterned region by using a PDMS (polydimethylsiloxane) elastomer stamp (Figure 11.3a) while the micro-molding method [26] allows the formation of polymer patterns in the non-PDMS stamp region (Figure 11.3b). Compared with photolithographic patterning, the soft-lithography could lead to micropatterns of a resolution down to submicron and provide possibility to produce micro-/nanopatterns on curved surfaces [27,28] and even flexible substrates [26,29–33].

Besides, plasma patterning technique has also been used for patterned growth of VA-CNT arrays. For example, Chen and Dai [34] have performed region-specific plasma polymerization of n-hexane polymer onto a quartz substrate (Figure 11.4a), followed with VA-MWNTs growth by pyrolysis of FePc in the plasma-polymer-free regions (Figure 11.4b). Owing to the generic nature of the plasma polymerization, many other organic vapors can also be used to efficiently generate plasma polymer patterns for the region-specific growth of aligned carbon nanotubes.

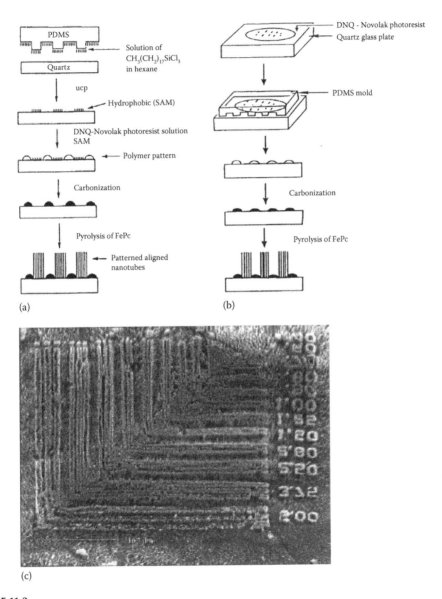

FIGURE 11.3
Schematic illustration of the procedure for fabricating patterns of VA-MWNTs by (a) microcontact printing, (b) solvent-assisted micromolding, and (c) a typical SEM image of a VA-MWNT micropattern prepared by the pyrolysis of FePc onto the quartz substrate prepatterned with photoresist by micromolding technique. (Adapted from Huang, S. et al., *J. Phys. Chem. B.*, 104, 2193, 2000. With permission.)

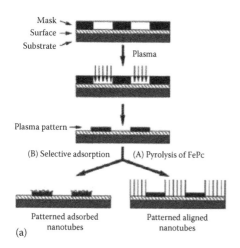

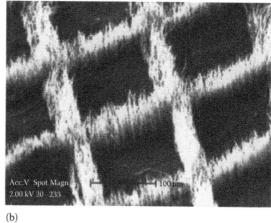

FIGURE 11.4

(a) Schematic illustration of the procedure for fabricating patterns of carbon nanotubes by (A) plasma polymerization followed by aligned nanotube growth, and (B) plasma activation followed by region-specific adsorption of nanotubes. (b) SEM images of VA-MWNT arrays growing out from the plasma-polymer-free regions on an n-hexane plasma-polymer-patterned quartz plate. (Adapted from Chen, Q. and Dai, L., *Appl. Phys. Lett.*, 76, 2719, 2000. With permission.)

11.4 Functionalization of Carbon Nanotubes

VA-CNT arrays, either in a patterned or nonpatterned form, with a well-defined large surface area can be easily incorporated into device architectures for various potential applications, including electrochemical sensing. Just like all other materials, however, it is very rare for VA-CNTs with desirable bulk properties to also possess the surface characteristics required for certain specific applications. Therefore, surface functionalization is essential. Although various covalent and noncovalent chemistries have been devised for functionalization of nonaligned CNTs, simple application of these solution chemistries to VA-CNTs could destroy the alignment structure [35]. Consequently, several innovative approaches have been developed for chemical modification of VA-CNTs while largely retaining their structural integrity. Examples include *in situ* functionalization during the nanotube growth, post-functionalization by chemical doping, plasma modification, and electrochemical and physical deposition of polymers.

11.4.1 Functionalization of Vertically Aligned Carbon Nanotubes by Chemical Doping during the Nanotube Growth

Recently, vertically aligned nitrogen containing carbon nanotubes have been prepared by pyrolysis of FePc (iron phthalycyanine) in either the presence or absence of additional ammonia gas [4,36]. The resultant N-doped VA-CNTs were demonstrated to act as metal-free electrocatalysts to replace platinum for oxygen reduction reaction (ORR) in fuel cells [36]. VA-CNTs co-doped with N and B or N and P have also been prepared for ORR applications (Figure 11.5) [37,38].

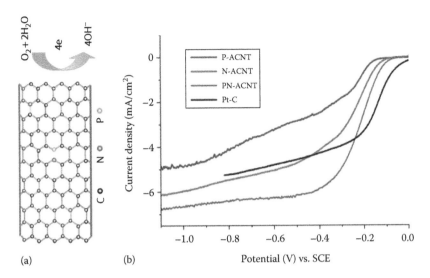

FIGURE 11.5
(a) Schematic representation of ORR on the N and P co-doped VA-CNTs and (b) the rotating-disk electrode (RDE) voltammograms of the P-ACNT/GC, N-ACNT/GC, PN-ACNT/GC, and Pt-C/GC electrodes in an oxygen-saturated, 0.10 M KOH solution at a rotation rate of 1600 rpm. Scan rate: 10 mV/s. (Adapted from Yu, D. et al., *J. Phys. Chem. Lett.*, 3, 2863, 2012. With permission.)

11.4.2 Functionalization of Vertically Aligned Carbon Nanotubes by Plasma Modification

Plasma treatment involves the gas/solid interface reaction, which is an ideal technique for surface modification of VA-CNTs while keeping the alignment unchanged. In this context, Chen et al. [39] have developed a novel approach for modifying VA-CNTs by using a plasma treatment method, followed by reactions characteristic of the plasma induced surface groups. In particular, they have demonstrated the attachment of polysaccharide chains (e.g., amino-dextran) onto acetaldehyde-plasma polymer coated VA-CNTs through the Schiff-base formation in the presence of sodium cyanoborohydride (Figure 11.6). The resultant VA-CNTs functionalized with polysaccharide chains became highly water-soluble and biocompatible, attractive for potential biomedical applications. Plasma activation has also been used to graft single-strand DNA chains (ss-DNAs) with an amine group at the 5′-phosphate end onto acetic-acid plasma treated VA-CNTs through the amide formation reaction with EDC as the coupling reagent [40]. As we will see in Section 11.5.3, the ss-DNA attached VA-CNT arrays can act as a highly sensitive DNA sensor for probing the sequences of a complementary DNA chain. Along with the plasma activation and functionalization, plasma etching has also been used to open VA-CNT tips for membrane- and energy-related applications [41,42].

11.4.3 Functionalization of Vertically Aligned Carbon Nanotubes by Electrochemical Deposition

VA-CNTs, particularly vertically aligned multi-walled CNTs, are electrically conductive. As such, they can be transferred to an electrode for direct electrochemical deposition of functional coatings onto the nanotube surface for various applications, ranging from sensors to energy storage devices. Specifically, Gao et al. [7] have used VA-CNTs as nanoelectrodes for

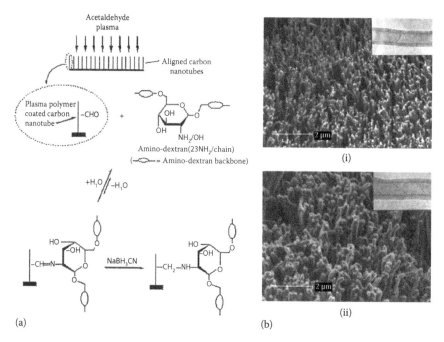

FIGURE 11.6

(a) Schematic representation of grafting polysaccharide chains onto plasma activated aligned CNTs through Schiff-base formation, followed by reductive stabilization of the Schiff-base linkage with sodium cyanoborohydride. (b) SEM images of the VA-CNTs (i) before and (ii) after the plasma polymerization of acetaldehyde. The insets show TEM images of an individual nanotube (i) before and (ii) after being coated with a layer of the acetaldehyde-plasma-polymer. Note that the micrographs shown in (i) and (ii) were not taken from the same spot due to technical difficulties. (Adapted from Chen, Q. et al., *J. Phys. Chem. B.*, 105, 618, 2001. With permission.)

electrochemically depositing an appropriate conducting polymer (e.g., polypyrrole) layer onto each of the constituent aligned nanotubes to form the vertically aligned conducting polymer coated CNT coaxial nanowires (CP-NTs) (Figure 11.7). They have also demonstrated the potential sensing applications for the vertically aligned CP-CNT coaxial nanowires [8]. Due to its good mechanical stability, intimate thermal/electrical contact, and large surface/interface area, the coaxial structure has unique advantages for optoelectronic and sensing applications.

11.4.4 Functionalization of Vertically Aligned Carbon Nanotubes by Polymer Masking

Composite materials with VA-CNT arrays partially or fully covered by polymer along the nanotube length could be useful for many multifunctional applications, ranging from advanced chemical and biological sensors [43–45], through smart membranes [46,47], to flexible electronics [48]. A few different polymers, including poly (dimethylsiloxane) (PDMS) [48], polystyrene (PS) [46], poly(methyl methacrylate) (PMMA) [44], and polydiene rubber [49], have been used for embedding VA-CNTs. By simply heating a thin polymer film on the top of VA-CNTs, Qu and Dai [50] successfully demonstrated the controllable polymer masking (Figure 11.8). After replacement of a PS thin film on the top of a VA-CNT array and upon heating the SiO_2/Si substrate by an underlying hot plate to a temperature above the melting temperature T_m (180°C) and below the decomposition temperature T_c (350°C), the melted PS film slowly penetrated into the nanotube forest through a capillary

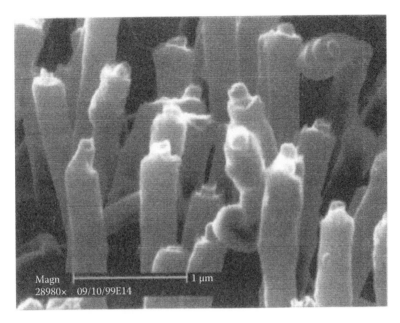

FIGURE 11.7
Typical SEM images of the CP-NT coaxial nanowires produced by cyclic voltammetry on the VA-CNT electrode, showing a thin layer of conducting polymer (polypyrrole) coating surrounding each of the constituent aligned CNTs. (From Gao, M. et al., *Angew. Chem. Int. Ed.*, 39, 3664, 2000. With permission.)

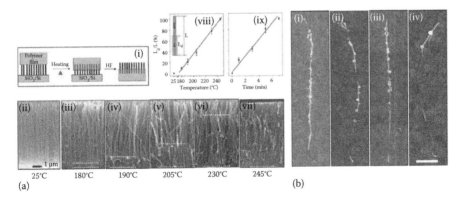

FIGURE 11.8
(See color insert.) (a) (i) Schematic representation of the VA-CNTs embedded into a polymer matrix by thermal infiltrating the melted polymer into the nanotube forest; (ii–vii) SEM images of (ii) the pristine VA-CNT array and (iii–vii) the VA-CNT array after being embedded into PS films by heating at different temperatures for 1 min. The dashed-line gaps crossing the polymer coated regions show the approximate embedment length for each of the PS-embedded VA-CNTs; (viii, ix) temperature and time dependence of the embedment length for VA-CNTs embedded into the PS matrix (L: the nanotube length (6 μm), L$_d$: the embedment length, which was estimated from the distance between the two dashed lines in each of the images shown in (iii–vii)). (b) SEM images of individual CNTs released out from the PS-embedded VA-CNTs by THF washing after the Au nanoparticle deposition by SEED. (i–iv) correspond to samples (iii–vi) in (a), respectively. Scale bar: 1 μm. (Adapted from Qu, L. and Dai, L., *Chem. Commun.*, 2007, 3859, 2007; Peng, Q. et al., *ACS Nano.*, 2, 1833, 2008. With permission.)

(continued)

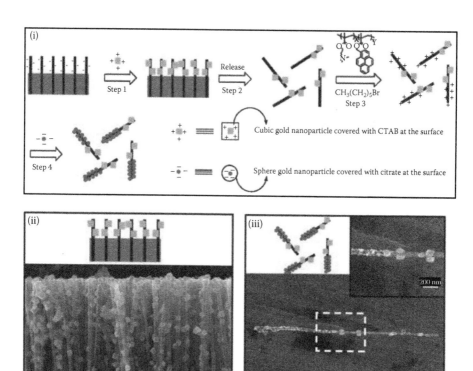

FIGURE 11.8 (continued)
(See color insert.) (c) Asymmetric functionalization of CNTs with opposite charges. (i) A schematic representation of procedures for asymmetric functionalization of CNTs with opposite charges, followed by tube-length-specific deposition of gold nanoparticles via electrostatical interactions; (ii) a schematic representation and SEM image of the CNT array partially functionalized with cubic gold nanoparticles; and (iii) a schematic representation and SEM image of the resultant asymmetrically sidewall-functionalized CNTs with half of the nanotube length covered by gold nanocubes and the other half by spherical gold nanoparticles through electrostatical assembly (inset shows a higher magnification SEM image for the squared area). Scale bars (ii,iii): 1 μm; Scale bar (right inset of iii): 200 nm. (Adapted from Qu, L. and Dai, L., *Chem. Commun.*, 2007, 3859, 2007; Peng, Q. et al., *ACS Nano.*, 2, 1833, 2008. With permission.)

force, together with gravity effect (Figure 11.8ai). Depending on the temperature and heating time, the carbon nanotube embedded length can be controlled to be directly proportional to the temperature and PS filtration heating time (Figure 11.8aviii and ix). Therefore, the VA-CNT array could be half functionalized along the nanotube length with the other half protected by a polymer matrix. Subsequently dissolving the polymer mask, the other half VA-CNTs could be further modified by different moieties, leading to asymmetrically functionalized VA-CNTs (Figure 11.8b and c) [51].

In addition to the asymmetric functionalization of VA-CNTs, the polymer masking concept can be used for making flexible devices based on the VA-CNT and polymer composites. As schematically shown in Figure 11.9a, flexible chemical vapor sensor chips have indeed been constructed by partially infiltrating poly(vinyl acetate)/polyisoprene (PVAc/PI) into the VA-CNT forest [43]. Figure 11.9bi and ii shows good responses to both cyclohexane and ethanol vapors with a high sensitivity and reliability. This is because the absorption and

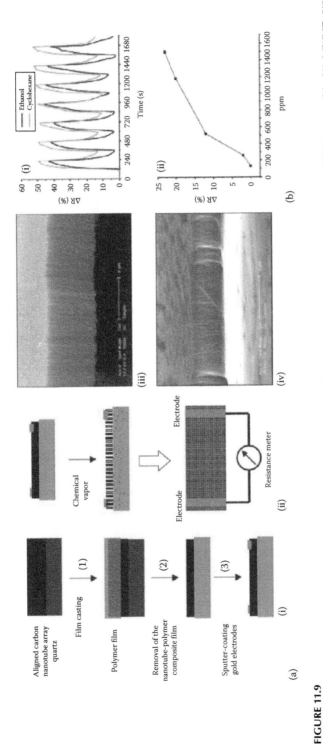

FIGURE 11.9

(a) Schematic illustration for (i) fabricating and (ii) characterizing the VA-CNT-polymer composite chemical vapor sensors. SEM images of the VA-MWNTs (iii) before and (iv) after being partially coated with a polymer (PVAc) film on top and turned upside down (Scale bars: 5 μm). (b) ΔR for a vertically aligned CNT-PVAc/PI film during (i) cyclohexane–air and ethanol–air cycles, and (ii) its equilibrium resistance peak height versus the partial cyclohexane vapor pressure. ΔR = (R$_{vapor}$ − R$_0$)/ R$_0$ × 100%, where R$_0$ and R$_{vapor}$ are the resistances of the aligned carbon nanotube-polymer composite film before and after exposure to a chemical, respectively. (Adapted from Wei, C. et al., *J. Am. Chem. Soc.* 128, 1412, 2006. With permission.)

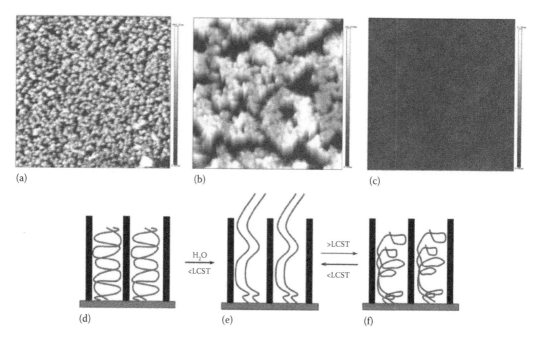

FIGURE 11.10
Tapping mode AFM images of (a) the pristine VA-CNT array; and the PNIPAAm/VA-CNT nanocomposite film: (b) in the dry state and (c) in the wet state. xy-Scale: (a–c) 5×5 μm, z-scale: (a) 445 nm; (b) 667 nm; (c) 17 nm. A schematic representation of the PNIPAAm/VA-MWNT film: (d and e) in the dry and wet state, respectively, at room temperature (20°C), and (f) in the wet state at a temperature above the LCST (32°C). For clarity, the infiltrated polymer mesh is represented by a few long polymer chains. (Adapted from Chen, W. et al., *Chem. Commun.*, 2008, 163, 2008. With permission.)

desorption of chemical vapors by the PVAc/PI matrix cause the volume swelling of supporting substrate, accompanied by a concomitant change in the CNT inter-tube distance and hence the surface resistance.

By infiltration of temperature responsive polymers (e.g., poly(*N*-isopropylacrylamide), PNIPAAm) into VA-CNT forests, Chen et al. [52] have also developed flexible polymer CNT composites with temperature-induced self-cleaning, sensing, and controlled release capabilities. Figure 11.10 shows AFM images for the pristine VA-CNT (Figure 11.10a) and the PNIPAAm/VA-CNTs nanocomposite films in both a dry (Figure 11.10b) and wet state (Figure 11.10c). As can be seen, the VA-CNTs extrude out from the polymer surface with a ~300 nm height in the dry state. In the wet state, the polymer absorbs water and swells to flat on the nanotube top surface, which shows a reduced roughness of ~10 nm. These results suggest potential biomedical applications for the VA-CNT and responsive polymer composites.

11.5 Biosensors Based on Vertically Aligned Carbon Nanotubes

Among many potential applications [53,54], CNTs have been demonstrated to be promising for the development of advanced biosensors. It was found that electron-transfers associated with various redox active proteins, ranging from glucose oxidase [55,56] with a deeply embedded redox center to cytochrome *c* [57,58] and horseradish peroxidase [59,60] with surface redox centers, could be significantly promoted by CNT electrodes. Carbon nanotubes functionalized with biological species, such as DNA, proteins, and enzymes [61–63] have further facilitated the development of advanced nanotube biosensors. Although many electrochemical biosensors have been reported based on randomly entangled carbon nanotubes [63–66], the use of VA-CNTs [67], coupled with well-defined chemical functionalization, should offer additional advantages for advanced electrochemical biosensors with a high sensitivity and good selectivity. Therefore, we will focus on VA-CNT electrochemical biosensors in the following sections.

11.5.1 Vertically Aligned Carbon Nanotube Glucose Sensors

Dai and coworkers [8] have developed electrochemical biosensors based on the aforementioned conducting polymer–carbon nanotube coaxial nanowires (CP-NTs, Figure 11.7). The coaxial structure allows the nanotube framework to provide mechanical stability and efficient thermal/electrical conduction [68,69] for the conducting polymer layer. The large surface area of the nanotube support facilitates efficient immobilization of glucose oxidase into the polymer coating layer by electropolymerization of pyrrole (0.1 M) in the presence of glucose oxidase. As a result, the glucose oxidase containing CP-NT coaxial nanowires can be used as a highly sensitive electrode to monitor concentration change of hydrogen peroxide (H_2O_2) from glucose oxidation reaction induced by the immobilized glucose oxidase, as shown later.

Figure 11.11 shows an almost linear dependence of the electrooxidation current on glucose concentration up to 20 mM, which is higher than the 15 mM typical limit used for the detection of blood glucose in practice [8]. The CP-NT nanowire sensors were also demonstrated to be highly selective and reliable.

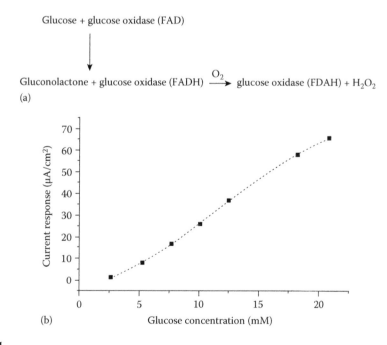

FIGURE 11.11
(a) Process of glucose oxidation reaction induced by the immobilized glucose oxidase, (b) The dependence of electrooxidation current at the oxidative potential of H_2O_2 on the glucose concentration for the CP-NT coaxial nanowire sensor. (From Gao, M. et al., *Electroanalysis*, 15, 1089, 2003. With permission.)

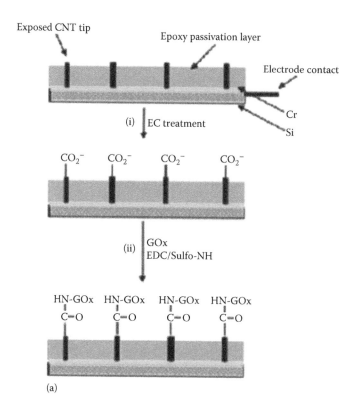

(a)

FIGURE 11.12

(a) Fabrication of a glucose biosensor based on CNT nanoelectrode ensembles: (i) Electrochemical treatment of the CNT-NEE for functionalization (ii) coupling of the enzyme (GOx) to the functionalized CNT-NEE. (Adapted from Lin, Y. et al., *Nano Lett.*, 4, 191, 2004. With permission.)

11.5.2 Vertically Aligned Carbon Nanotube Protein and Enzyme Sensors

By covalently immobilizing glucose oxidase onto a VA-CNT nanoelectrode ensemble (CNT-NEE) through the amide formation between the GOx and carboxylic acid groups on the aligned CNT tips (Figure 11.12a), Ren and coworkers [70–72] developed a glucose biosensor with a high sensitivity and selectivity for electrochemical analysis of glucose (Figure 11.12b).

Yu and coworkers [73] have also used the amide linkage to covalently graft myoglobin and horseradish peroxidase onto an aligned SWNT electrode for the detection of iron heme enzymes, myoglobin and horseradish peroxidase while Patolsky and coworkers [56] studied the long-range electron transfer from redox enzymes chemically bound onto the aligned SWNT structure.

11.5.3 Vertically Aligned Carbon Nanotube DNA Sensors

Nanotube DNA sensors of a high sensitivity and selectivity have also been developed by grafting single-strand DNA (ssDNA) chains onto aligned carbon nanotubes generated from FePc [40]. In this study, He and Dai [40] first treated aligned carbon nanotubes supported by gold substrate with acetic acid-plasma to introduce the surface carboxylic acid groups for grafting ssDNA chains with an amino group at the 5-phosphate end (i.e.,

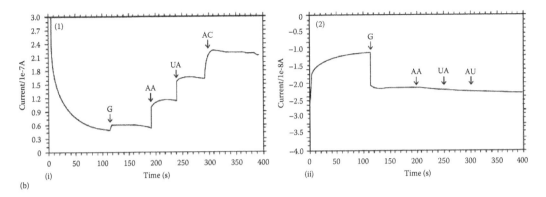

FIGURE 11.12 (continued)
(b) Amperometric responses of the CNT-NEE glucose biosensor to glucose (G), ascorbic acid (AA), uric acid (UA), and acetaminophen (AC) at potentials of +0.4 V (i) and −0.2 V (ii). (Adapted from Lin, Y. et al., *Nano Lett.*, 4, 191, 2004. With permission.)

[AmC6]TTGACACCAGACCAACTGGT-3, I). Complementary DNA (cDNA) chains labeled with ferrocenecarboxaldehyde, FCA (i.e., [FCA-C6]ACCAGTTGGTCTGGTGTCAA-3, II) were then used for hybridizing with the surface-immobilized oligonucleotides to form the double-strand DNA (dsDNA) helices on the aligned carbon nanotube electrodes (Figure 11.13).

Figure 11.14 shows a strong oxidation peak at 0.29 V attributable to ferrocene, which indicates the occurrence of hybridization of FCA-labeled cDNA(II) chains with the nanotube-supported ssDNA(I) chains to generate a long-range electron transfer from the FCA probe to the nanotube electrode through the DNA duplex. In contrast, the addition of FCA labeled non-complementary DNA chains (i.e., [FCA-C6] CTCCAGGAGTCGTCGCCACC-3, III) under the same conditions did not show any redox response of FCA (curve b of Figure 11.14). Subsequent addition of target DNA chains (i.e., 5-GAGGTCCTCAGCAGCGGTGGACCAGTTGGTCTGGTGTCAA-3, IV) into the aforementioned solution, however, led to a strong redox response from the FCA labeled DNA (III) chains (curve c of Figure 11.14) because the target DNA (IV) contains complementary sequences for both DNA (I) and DNA (III) chains.

Meyyappan and coworkers [74–76] have developed a more advanced micropatterned ultrasensitive DNA biosensor based on aligned carbon nanotubes (Figure 11.15a) by directly growing aligned MWNTs on individual metal microcontacts, followed by encapsulating the MWNT arrays and the substrate surface with a spin-on glass (SOG) layer to only expose the nanotube ends at the surface. Each of the SOG-encapsulated individual MWNTs acts as a nanoelectrode with about 100 MWNT nanoelectrodes or more on each microcontact. Electrochemical etching was used to generate carboxylic acid groups at the end of MWNTs, which were then used to functionalize with specific oligonucleotide probes through the amide formation. The mechanisms of the MWNT nanoelectrode array for the DNA detection were schematically shown in Figure 11.15b and c. In that study, a specific probe [Cy3]5-CTIIATTTCICAIITCCT-3-[AmC7-Q] containing the sequence of the normal allele of the BRCA1 gene associated with the occurrence of several cancers was used.

Figure 11.15d shows the electrophoresis results of a DNA molecular weight standard (ΦX174RFDNA-HaeIII digest) and the two PCR amplicons, respectively. By shaking the sample in each of the solutions at 40°C for 15 min, the nonspecific binding is removed

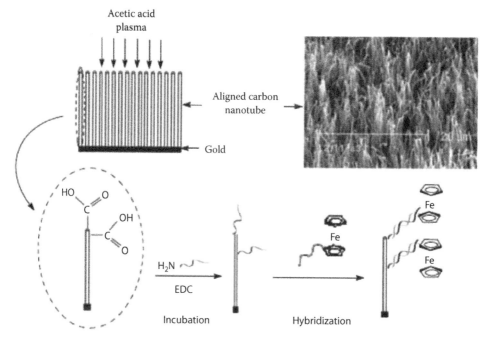

FIGURE 11.13
A schematic illustration of the aligned nanotube–DNA electrochemical sensor. The upper-right SEM image shows the aligned carbon nanotubes after having been transferred onto a gold foil. For reasons of clarity, only one of the many carboxyl groups is shown at the nanotube tip and wall, respectively. (From He, P. and Dai, L., *Chem. Commun.*, 2004, 348, 2004. With permission.)

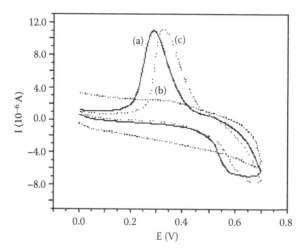

FIGURE 11.14
Cyclic voltammograms of the ssDNA (I)-immobilized aligned carbon nanotube electrode after hybridization with FCA-labeled complementary DNA (II) chains (a), in the presence of FCA-labeled noncomplementary DNA (III) chains (b), and after hybridization with target DNA (IV) chains in the presence of the FCA-labeled non-complementary DNA (III) chains (c). All the cyclic voltammograms were recorded in 0.1 M H_2SO_4 solution with a scan rate of 0.1 V/s. The concentration of the FCA-labeled DNA probes is 0.05 mg/mL. (From He, P. and Dai, L., *Chem. Commun.*, 2004, 348, 2004. With permission.)

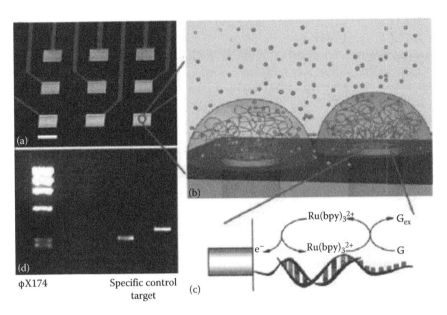

FIGURE 11.15
(See color insert.) (a) An SEM image of an individually addressable 3×3 microcontact array with an MWNT nanoelectrode array on each site. The scale bar is 200 μm. (b) Schematic of the mechanism to detect DNA hybridization using an MWNT nanoelectrode array. The long single-stranded DNA PCR amplicons are hybridized to the short oligonucleotide probes, which are functionalized at the very end of the MWNTs. $Ru(bpy)_3^{2+}$ mediators are used to transfer electrons from the guanine groups to the MWNT nanoelectrode for all target molecules within the hemispherical diffusion layer of the nanoelectrodes. (c) The schematic mechanism for the guanine oxidation amplified with $Ru(bpy)_3^{2+}$ mediators. (d) The gel electrophoresis. The lanes from left to right are DNA molecular weight standard (ΦX174RFDNA-HaeIII digest), a specific PCR amplicon target with ~300 bases, and a control sample with an unrelated PCR amplicon with ~400 bases, respectively. (Adapted from Koehne, J. et al., *Nanotechnology*, 14, 1239, 2003. With permission.)

through stringent washing in three steps using $2 \times$ SSC/0.1%SDS, $1 \times$ SSC, and 0.1% SSC, respectively. $Ru(bpy)_3^{2+}$ mediators were used to efficiently transport electrons from the guanine bases to the MWNT nanoelectrode and to provide an amplified guanine oxidation signal as long as target DNA molecules are within the three-dimensional diffusion layer.

11.6 Concluding Remarks

Carbon nanotubes, particularly vertically aligned carbon nanotube arrays (VA-CNTs), have been demonstrated to be useful for the development of various electrochemical biosensors, including glucose, protein, enzyme, and DNA sensors as well as biosensor chips. However, it is essential to functionalize and/or micropattern VA-CNTs for biosensing applications. Several innovative functionalization approaches, including *in situ* functionalization during the nanotube growth, post-functionalization by chemical doping, plasma modification, and electrochemical and physical deposition of polymers, have been developed for chemical modification of VA-CNTs while largely retaining their structural integrity. We have provided a brief overview on the progress toward the synthesis and construction of aligned and micropatterned carbon nanotubes for electrochemical sensors by spotlighting some important work in the field. As can be seen, aligned/patterned nanotube growth, in conjunction with controlled functionalization of the resultant carbon nanotubes, could provide various vertically aligned carbon nanotube arrays with tailor-made surface characteristics useful for construction of many advanced electrochemical biosensors.

Acknowledgments

The authors are grateful for the financial support from NSF, NSF-NSFC, AFOSR, DoD-MURI, DoD-Army, DOE, DAGSI, AFOSR-Korea NBIT, and UNIST-WCU, and also thank colleagues and collaborators for their work cited in this chapter.

References

1. Lu, X. and Chen, Z. 2005. Curved Pi-conjugation, aromaticity, and the related chemistry of small fullerenes (<C_{60}) and single-walled carbon nanotubes. *Chem. Rev.* 105(10):3643–3696.
2. Pop, E., Mann, D., Wang, Q., Goodson, K., and Dai, H. 2005. Thermal conductance of an individual single-wall carbon nanotube above room temperature. *Nano Lett.* 6(1):96–100.
3. Yu, M., Lourie, O., Dyer, M., Moloni, K., Kelly, T., and Ruoff, R. 2000. Strength and breaking mechanism of multiwalled carbon nanotubes under tensile load. *Science* 287(5453):637–640.
4. Huang, S., Dai, L., and Mau, A. 1999. Patterned growth and contact transfer of well-aligned carbon nanotube films. *J. Phys. Chem. B* 103:4223–4227.
5. Huang, S., Mau, A., Turney, T., White, P., and Dai, L. 2000. Patterned growth of well-aligned carbon nanotubes: A soft-lithographic approach. *J. Phys. Chem. B* 104:2193–2196.
6. Huang, S., Cai, X., and Liu, J. 2003. Growth of millimeter-long and horizontally aligned single-walled carbon nanotubes on flat substrates. *J. Am. Chem. Soc.* 125(19):5636–5637.
7. Gao, M., Huang, S., Dai, L., Wallace, G., Gao, R., and Wang, Z. 2000. Aligned coaxial nanowires of carbon nanotubes sheathed with conducting polymers. *Angew. Chem. Int. Edn.* 39:3664–3667.
8. Gao, M., Dai, L., and Wallace, G. 2003. Biosensors based on aligned carbon nanotubes coated with inherently conducting polymers. *Electroanalysis* 15:1089–1094.
9. Iijima, S. 1991. Helical microtubules of graphitic carbon. *Nature* 354:56–58.
10. Lv, X., Du, F., Ma, Y., Wu, Q., and Chen, Y. 2005. Synthesis of high quality single-walled carbon nanotubes at large scale by electric arc using metal compounds. *Carbon* 43:2020–2022.
11. Du, F., Ma, Y., Lv, X., Huang, Y., Li, F., and Chen, Y. 2006. The synthesis of single-walled carbon nanotubes with controlled length and bundle size using the electric arc method. *Carbon* 44:1327–1330.
12. Collins, P. and Avouris, P. 2000. Nanotubes for electronics. *Sci. Am.* 283:62–69.
13. Farhat, S. and Scott, C. 2006. Review of the arc process modeling for fullerene and nanotube production. *J. Nanosci. Nanotechnol.* 6:1189–1210.
14. Baddour, C. and Briens, C. 2005. Carbon nanotube synthesis: A review. *Int. J. Chem. Reactor Eng.* 3(1):1279.
15. Dupuis, A. 2005. The catalyst in the CCVD of carbon nanotubes-a review. *Prog. Mater. Sci.* 50:929–961.

16. Nikolaev, P., Bronikowski, M., Bradley, R., Rohmund, F., Colbert, D., Smith, K., and Smalley, R. 1999. Gas-phase catalytic growth of single-walled carbon nanotubes from carbon monoxide. *Chem. Phys. Lett.* 313:91–97.

17. Zhang, Q., Huang, J., Zhao, M., Qian, W., and Wei, F. 2011. Carbon nanotube mass production: Principles and processes. *Chem. Sus. Chem.* 4(7):864–889.

18. Cassell, A., Raymakers, J., Kong, J., and Dai, H. 1999. Large scale CVD synthesis of single-walled carbon nanotubes. *J. Phys. Chem. B.* 103:6484–6492.

19. Li, J., Papadopoulos, C., Xu, J., and Moskovits, M. 1999. Highly ordered carbon nanotube arrays for electronics applications. *Appl. Phys. Lett.* 75:367–369.

20. Rao, C., Sen, R., Satishkumar, B., and Govindaraj, A. 1998. Large aligned-nanotube bundles from ferrocene pyrolysis. *Chem. Commun.* 1998:1525–1526.

21. Wei, B., Vajtai, R., Jung, Y., Ward, J., Zhang, R., Ramanath, G., and Ajayan, P. 2002. Microfabrication technology: Organized assembly of carbon nanotubes. *Nature* 416:495–496.

22. Qu, L., Du, F., and Dai, L. 2008. Preferential syntheses of semiconducting vertically aligned single-walled carbon nanotubes for direct use in FETs. *Nano Lett.* 8(9):2682–2687.

23. Fan, S., Chapline, M., Franklin, N., Tombler, T., Cassell, A., and Dai, H. 1999. Self-oriented regular arrays of carbon nanotubes and their field emission properties. *Science* 283:512–514.

24. Yang, Y., Huang, S., He, H., Mau, A., and Dai, L. 1999. Patterned growth of well-aligned carbon nanotubes: A photolithographic approach. *J. Am. Chem. Soc.* 121:10832–10833.

25. March, J. 1992. *Advanced Organic Chemistry*, 4th edn., John Wiley, New York.

26. Zheng, G., Zhu, H., Luo, Q., Zhou, Y., and Zhao, D. 2001. Chemical vapor deposition growth of well-aligned carbon nanotube patterns on cubic mesoporous silica films by soft lithography. *Chem. Mater.* 13(7):2240–2242.

27. Xia, Y. and Whitesides, G. 1998. Soft lithography. *Angew. Chem. Int. Edn.* 37(5):550–575.

28. Jackman, R. and Whitesides, G. 1999. Electrochemistry and soft lithography: A route to 3-D microstructures. *Chem. Tech.* 29(5):18–30.

29. Khosla, A. and Gray, B. 2009. Preparation, characterization, and micromoulding of multiwalled carbon nanotube polydimethylsiloxane conducting nanocomposite polymer. *Mater. Lett.* 63:1203–1206.

30. Mazzoldi, A., Tesconi, M., Tognetti, A., Rocchia, W., Vozzi, G., Pioggia, G., Ahluwalia, A., and Rossi, D. 2008. Electroactive carbon nanotube actuators: Soft-lithographic fabrication and electro-chemical modeling. *Mater. Sci. Eng. C* 28(7):1057–1064.

31. Ng, H., Foo, M., Fang, A., Li, J., Xu, G., Jaenicke, S., Chan, L., and Li, S. 2001. Soft-lithography-medicated chemical vapor deposition of architecture carbon nanotube networks on elastomeric polymer. *Langmuir* 18:1–5.

32. Ng, H., Fang, A., Li, J., and Li, S. 2001. Flexible carbon nanotube membrane sensory system: Ageneric platform. *J. Nanosci. Nanotechnol.* 1(4):375–379.

33. Bennett, R., Hart, A., Miller, A., Hammond, P., Irvine, D., and Cohen, R. 2006. Creating patterned carbon nanotube catalysts through the microcontact printing of block copolymer micellar thin films. *Langmuir* 22(20):8273–8276.

34. Chen, Q. and Dai, L. 2000. Plasma patterning of carbon nanotubes. *Appl. Phys. Lett.* 76:2719–2721.

35. Futaba, D., Hata, K., Yamada, T., Hiraoka, T., Hayamizu, Y., Kakudate, Y., Tanaike, O., Hatori, H., Yumura, M., Iijima, S. 2006. Shape-engineerable and highly densely packed single-walled carbon nanotubes and their application as super-capacitor electrodes. *Nat. Mater.*, 5:987–994.

36. Gong, K., Du, F., Xia, Z., Dustock, M., and Dai, L. 2009. Nitrogen-doped carbon nanotube arrays with high electrocatalytic activity for oxygen reduction. *Science* 323:760–764.

37. Iyyamperumal, E., Wang, S., and Dai, L. 2012. Vertically aligned BCN nanotubes with high capacitance. *ACS Nano* 6(6):5259–5265.

38. Yu, D., Xue, Y., and Dai, L. 2012. Vertically aligned carbon nanotube arrays Co-doped with phosphorus and nitrogen as efficient metal-free electrocatalysts for oxygen reduction. *J. Phys. Chem. Lett.* 3:2863–2870.

39. Chen, Q., Dai, L., Gao, M., Huang, S., and Mau, A. 2001. Plasma activation of carbon nanotubes for chemical modification. *J. Phys. Chem. B* 105:618–622.

40. He, P. and Dai, L. 2004. Aligned carbon nanotube-DNA electrochemical sensors. *Chem. Commun.* 2004:348–349.

41. Lu, W., Qu, L., Henry, K., and Dai, L. 2009. High performance electrochemical capacitors from aligned carbon nanotube electrodes and ionic liquid electrolytes. *J. Power Source.* 189:1270–1277.

42. Lu, W., Goering, A., Qu, L., and Dai, L. 2012. Lithium-ion batteries based on vertically aligned carbon nanotube electrodes and ionic liquid electrolytes. *Phys. Chem. Chem. Phys.* 14:12099–12104.

43. Wei, C., Dai, L., Roy, A., and Tolle, T. 2006. Multifunctional chemical vapor sensors of aligned carbon nanotube and polymer composites. *J. Am. Chem. Soc.* 128:1412–1413.

44. Raravikar, N., Schadler, L., Vijayaraghavan, A., Zhao, Y., Wei, B., and Ajayan, P. 2005. Synthesis and characterization of thickness-aligned carbon nanotube-polymer composite films. *Chem. Mater.* 17:974–983.

45. Nguyen, C., Delzeit, L., Cassell, A., Li, J., Han, J., and Meyyappan, M. 2002. Preparation of nucleic acid functionalized carbon nanotube arrays. *Nano Lett.* 2(10):1079–1081.

46. Hinds, B., Chopra, N., Rantell, T., Andrews, R., Gavalas, V., and Bachas, L. 2004. Aligned multiwalled carbon nanotube membranes. *Science* 303:62–65.

47. Majumder, M., Chopra, N., Andrews, R., and Hinds, B. 2005. Nanoscale hydrodynamics: Enhanced flow in carbon nanotubes. *Nature* 438:44.

48. Jung, Y., Kar, S., Talapatra, S., Soldano, C., Viswanathan, G., Li, X., Yao, Z. et al. 2006. Aligned carbon nanotube-polymer hybrid architectures for diverse flexible electronic applications. *Nano Lett.* 6(3):413–418.

49. Li, L., Yang, J., Vaia, R., and Dai, L. 2005. Multicomponent micropatterns or carbon nanotubes. *Synth. Met.* 154:225–228.

50. Qu, L. and Dai, L. 2007. Polymer-masking for controlled functionalization of carbon nanotubes. *Chem. Commun.* 2007(37):3859–3861.

51. Peng, Q., Qu, L., Dai, L., Park, K., and Vaia, R. 2008. Asymmetrically charged carbon nanotubes by controlled functionalization. *ACS Nano* 2:1833–1840.

52. Chen, W., Qu, L., Chang, D., Dai, L., Ganguli, S., and Roy, A. 2008. Vertically aligned carbon nanotubes infiltrated with temperature-responsive polymers: Smart nanocomposite films for self-cleaning and controlled release. *Chem. Commun.* 2008(2):163–165.

53. Harris, P. 2001. *Carbon Nanotubes and Related Structures—New Materials for the Twenty-First Century*, Cambridge University Press, Cambridge, U.K.

54. Dai, L. 2004. *Intelligent Macromolecules for Smart Devices: From Materials Synthesis to Device Applications*, Springer-Verlag, London, U.K.

55. Yamamoto, K., Shi, G., Zhou, T., Xu, F., Xu, J., Kato, T., Jin, J., and Jin, L. 2003. Study of carbon nanotubes-HRP modified electrode and its application for novel on-line biosensors. *Analyst* 128:249–254.

56. Patolsky, F., Weizmann, Y., and Willner, I. 2004. Long-range electrical contacting of redox enzymes by SWCNT connectors. *Angew. Chem. Int. Edn.* 43:2113–2117.

57. Davis, J., Coles, R., Allen, H., and Hill, O. 1997. Protein electrochemistry at carbon nanotube electrodes. *J. Electroanal. Chem.* 440:279–282.

58. Wang, J., Li, M., Shi, Z., Li, N., and Gu, Z. 2002. Direct electrochemistry of cytochrome c at a glassy carbon electrode modified with single-wall carbon nanotubes. *Anal. Chem.* 74:1993–1997.

59. Wang, G., Xu, J., and Chen, H. 2002. Interfacing cytochrome c to electrodes with a DNA-carbon nanotube composite film. *Electrochem. Commun.* 4:506–509.

60. Zhao, Y., Zhang, W., Chen, H., Luo, Q., and Li, S. 2002. Direct electrochemistry of horseradish peroxidase at carbon nanotube powder microelectrode. *Sens. Actuators B* 87:168–172.

61. Tsang, S., Davis, J., Green, M., Hill, H., Leung, Y., and Sadler, P. 1995. Immobilization of small proteins in carbon nanotubes: High-resolution transmission electron microscopy study and catalytic activity. *Chem. Commun.* 1995(17):1803–1804.

62. Davis, J., Coleman, K., Azamian, B., Bagshaw, C., and Green, M. 2003. Chemical and biochemical sensing with modified single walled carbon nanotubes. *Chem. Eur. J.* 9:3732–3739.

63. Gooding, J., Wibowo, R., Liu, J., Yang, W., Losic, D., Orbons, S., Mearns, F., Shapter, J., and Hibbert, D. 2003. Protein electrochemistry using aligned carbon nanotube arrays. *J. Am. Chem. Soc.* 125:9006–9007.

64. Britto, P., Santhanam, K., and Ajayan, P. 1996. Carbon nanotube electrode for oxidation of dopamine. *Bioelectrochem. Bioenerg.* 41:121–125.

65. Luo, H., Shi, Z., Li, N., Gu, Z., and Zhuang, Q. 2001. Investigation of the electrochemical and electrocatalytic behavior of single-wall carbon nanotube film on a glassy carbon electrode. *Anal. Chem.* 73:915–920.

66. Zhao, Q., Gan, Z., and Zhuang, Q. 2002. Electrochemical sensors based on carbon nanotubes. *Electroanalysis* 14(23):1609–1613.

67. Dai, L., Patil, A., Gong, X., Guo, Z., Liu, L., Liu, Y., and Zhu, D. 2003. Aligned nanotubes. *Chem. Phys. Chem.* 4:1150–1169.

68. Frank, S., Poncharal, P., Wang, Z., and de Heer, W. 1998. Carbon nanotube quantum resistors. *Science* 280:1744–1746.

69. Odom, T., Huang, J., Kim, P., and Lieber, C. 2002. Structure and electronic properties of carbon nanotubes. *J. Phys. Chem. B* 104:2794–2809.

70. Lin, Y., Lu, F., Tu, Y., and Ren, Z. 2004. Glucose biosensors based on carbon nanotube nanoelectrode ensembles. *Nano Lett.* 4:191–195.

71. Tu, Y., Lin, Y., and Ren, Z. 2002. Nanoelectrode arrays based on low site density aligned carbon nanotubes. *Nano Lett.* 3:107–109.

72. Tu, Y., Huang, Z., Wang, D., Wen, J., and Ren, Z. 2002. Growth of aligned carbon nanotubes with controlled site density. *Appl. Phys. Lett.* 80:4018–4021.

73. Yu, X., Chattopadhyay, D., Galeska, I., Papadimitrakopoulos, F., and Rusling, J. 2003. Peroxidase activity of enzymes bound to the ends of single-wall carbon nanotube forest electrodes. *Electrochem. Commun.* 5:408–411.

74. Koehne, J., Chen, H., Li, J., Cassell, A., Ye, Q., Ng, H., Han, J., and Meyyappan, M. 2003. Ultrasensitive label-free DNA analysis using an electronic chip based on carbon nanotube nanoelectrode arrays. *Nanotechnology* 14:1239–1245.

75. Chen, J., Rao, A., Lyuksyutov, S., Itkis, M., Hamon, M., Hu, H., Cohn, R. et al. Dissolution of full-length single-walled carbon nanotubes. *J. Phys. Chem. B* 105:2525–2528.

76. Li, J., Ng, H., Cassell, A., Fan, W., Chen, H., Ye, Q., Koehne, J., Han, J., and Meyyappan, M. 2003. Carbon nanotube nanoelectrode array for ultrasensitive DNA detection *Nano Lett.* 3:597–602.

12

Vertically Aligned Carbon Nanofibers for Biointerfacing

Ryan Pearce, Timothy E. McKnight, and Anatoli Melechko

CONTENTS

12.1 Introduction

Vertically aligned carbon nanofibers (VACNFs), stacked cylinders of graphitic carbon, possess many properties that make them attractive structures for implementation as interfaces to biological systems on a cellular level or subcellular level. Their geometric dimensions, from tens to hundreds of nanometers in diameter, and from a few hundred nanometers to a hundred micrometers long, along with their mechanical properties facilitate their use as nanoneedles, suitable for insertion into tissue or single cells. Their electrical conductivity renders them suitable as nanoelectrodes. The electron transfer rates at the sidewall surfaces make VACNFs suitable for electrochemical probes. There are structural differences between VACNFs and carbon nanotubes (CNTs) though in literature, the two are often conflated (Figure 12.1). The exposed graphitic edge planes of VACNFs have been shown to exhibit ~30 times better capacitance and orders of magnitude, better electron transfer rates than carbon basal planes, which are present in CNTs [1,2]. Finally, the surface of VACNFs is amenable to a range of chemistries that allow their functionalization with desirable chemical or biochemical species.

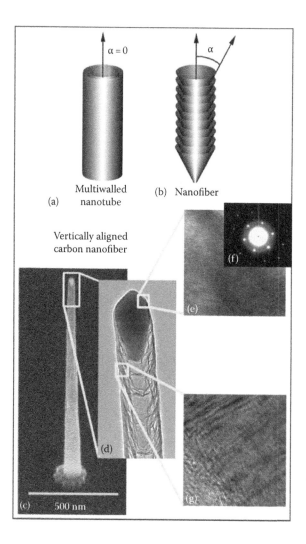

FIGURE 12.1

(a) Schematic structure of a carbon nanotube, made up of concentric cylindrical graphene sheets; (b) schematic structure of a VACNF composed of stacked graphene "cones" at some angle α with respect to the fiber axis; (c) tilted SEM image of a VACNF; (d) TEM image of the tip of a VACNF; (e) HRTEM lattice image of the nickel catalyst particle with face centered cubic symmetry; (f) diffraction pattern of catalyst particle from (e); (g) HRTEM image of fiber's graphitic sidewalls. (Reprinted with permission from Klein, K.L. et al., Surface characterization and functionalization of carbon nanofibers, *J. Appl. Phys.*, 103(6), 61301. Copyright 2008, American Institute of Physics.)

In biosensing both selectivity, that is, the ability to distinguish between molecular species, and sensitivity, that is, the signal amplitude, are important for signal detection. The selectivity of graphitic carbon can be achieved in two ways. The first is to use carbon nanostructures as electrochemical probes where selectivity is achieved via observation of a distinct signature in electrochemical spectra (redox). The second route is to utilize surface chemistry of graphitic carbon in enhancing sensitivity via attachment of biomolecules. Utilization of nanostructures can directly enhance sensitivity via increase in surface area. However, this route typically involves use of large numbers of nanostructures, such as a forest of carbon nanofibers [3]. If individual nanostructures are used, signals can be very small. However, this drawback is traded for another advantage of using nanostructures as highly localized probes. In this case, each individual nanostructure is connected to one channel of the measurement system. When interfacing to a single cell with a carbon nanofiber, such a local probe can provide access to one billionth of the volume of a cell. In this chapter, we explore another modality of using carbon nanofibers in biointerfacing, that is, via mechanical properties. Since VACNFs are extremely sharp needles with subcellular dimensions they can be inserted inside a cell. With proper insulation a nanofiber can serve as an intracellular electrochemical probe. Alternatively it can serve as a delivery vehicle of biochemical functionality if its surface is coated with biomolecules. One particular application of such biointerfacing is gene delivery. In this case, DNA coding for a particular exogenous gene is attached to a nanofiber surface and then inserted inside a cell nucleus.

12.2 Synthesis

12.2.1 Catalyst Particles and Growth Mechanism

VACNFS are synthesized using metal catalyst particles. Understanding of catalytic synthesis has seen many advances [4] since early TEM images of Fe nanoparticles at the ends of the carbon fibers over 50 years ago [5,6]. The most commonly used catalyst nanoparticles are Ni, Fe, and Co. Other materials have been used successfully as catalysts, and a more exhaustive list can be found elsewhere [7]. The catalyst particles can either be patterned on the substrate via lithographic processes or a uniform film can be deposited. During growth, the film dewets into discrete particles that serve as individual nucleation sites for nanofiber growth. Individually patterned thin films may also dewet into smaller particles, resulting in clusters of fibers. It has been found that a smaller diameter catalyst particle will yield fewer fibers as shown in Figure 12.2.

The currently accepted model for the mechanism of VACNF growth is known as the diffusion/precipitation model, which is attributed to Baker et al. [8,9]. The model proposes that the metal particle catalyzes the dissociation of the hydrocarbon gas upon its adsorption onto the surface of the particle, followed by diffusion of the carbon through and around the particle, where it incorporates into graphene layers on the other side of the particle. During the formation of these graphene layers, there are two distinct growth modes: base-type and tip-type. In base-type growth, the catalyst particle remains adhered to the substrate and the graphene layers are added in an irregular and seemingly random fashion, leading to unaligned CNFs. Tip-type growth is generally preferred, due to its more controllable nature. In tip-type growth, the graphene layers precipitate only from the bottom surface of the catalyst particle, lifting the particle off of the substrate. Tip-type growth can be ensured through choice of catalyst, substrate, and most importantly, growth conditions [10].

There is disagreement over the driving force behind the carbon diffusion through the catalyst particle, with Baker et al. suggesting that the driving force is a temperature gradient caused by the exothermic decomposition reaction of the carbonaceous gas at the particle/gas interface and an endothermic reaction occurring at the precipitation interface [8]. This explanation however does not account for the growth of nanofibers using methane as the carbon source, the decomposition of which is endothermic. A possible explanation is that a concentration gradient drives the carbon diffusion through

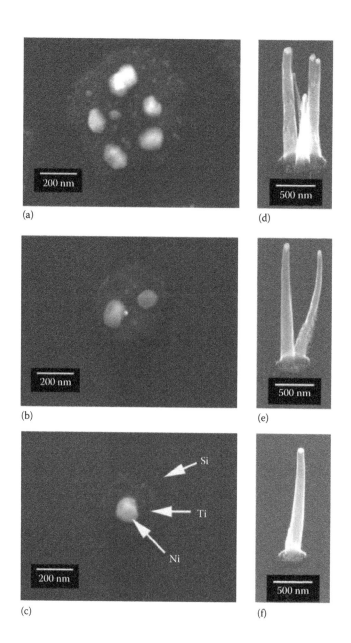

FIGURE 12.2

Multiple VACNFs can result from a single nanoparticle. Each particle was originally a 15 nm thick Ni dot patterned onto 10 nm Ti. (a–c) are images taken after dewetting and are ordered in decreasing diameter, while (d–f) are the corresponding resultant fibers. Larger initial dots dewetted into multiple nanoparticles, resulting in clusters of fibers. Once the catalyst dot was reduced to <350 nm, a single catalyst nanoparticle was formed, from which a single nanofiber grew, as can be seen in (f). (Adapted from Merkulov, V.I., Lowndes, D.H., Wei, Y.Y., Eres, G., and Voelkl, E. Patterned growth of individual and multiple vertically aligned carbon nanofibers, *Appl. Phys. Lett.*, 76(24), 3555–3557. Copyright 2000, American Institute of Physics.)

the catalyst particle, possibly involving surface carbides and differing carbon solubilities at the varying interfaces [11–14].

12.2.2 Controlling Synthesis through PECVD

Chemical vapor deposition allows for the growth of CNFs, but only PECVD has been demonstrated to obtain deterministically grown vertically aligned CNFs, necessary for most biological applications [7,15–18]. Through PECVD, control over size, position, chemical composition, and internal fiber structure is obtained through careful selection of the starting materials and the growth parameters. A number of PECVD power sources have been used for fiber growth (inductively coupled, radio frequency, microwave, etc.) [7]. The simplest of these systems is direct current (dc) PECVD. In dc-PECVD systems, the substrate heater doubles as the cathode, which was thought to necessitate a conducting substrate. Recent research however has discovered a technique for growing aligned fibers with dc-PECVD on insulating substrates by coating the substrate with a thin metallic layer, leaving thin (200–500 μm) "windows" of the underlying substrate uncovered [19]. The substrate is usually silicon or silicon dioxide for the ease of silicon-based processing, though many other substrates are of possible use, provided they can withstand the PECVD and metal deposition processes. After the sample is placed on the heater/cathode, the chamber is pumped down to a few milliTorr or less, followed by introducing a reducing gas (usually NH_3 or H_2) to pressurize the chamber to 1–20 Torr. The sample is heated to 500°C–700°C to ease plasma ignition. The plasma is then initiated, which causes the catalyst film/particles to dewet. After a few seconds, the carbonaceous gas is introduced to the chamber, which initiates the fiber growth.

The PECVD process adds some complexity to the diffusion/precipitation growth model. Figure 12.3 shows schematically these additional processes. Referring to Figure 12.3, (A) shows the arrival of excited carbonaceous species, which then (B) catalytically

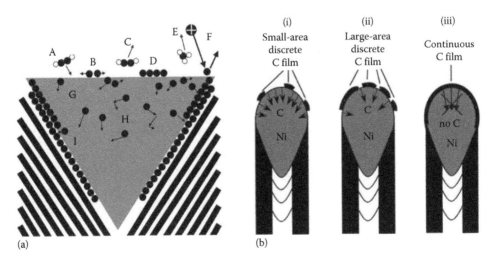

FIGURE 12.3
Processes at the metal catalyst particle during PECVD synthesis: (a) at the atomic level and (b) at the nanoscale. (Adapted from Melechko, A.V., Merkulov, V.I., McKnight, T.E. et al., Vertically aligned carbon nanofibers and related structures: Controlled synthesis and directed assembly, *Journal of Applied Physics*, 97(4), Artn 041301. Copyright 2005; Merkulov, V.I., Hensley, D.K., Melechko, A.V. et al., Control mechanisms for the growth of isolated vertically aligned carbon nanofibers, *J. Phys. Chem. B*, 106(41), 10570–10577. Copyright 2002, American Institute of Physics.)

dissociate on the surface. The undissociated species are then (C) desorbed while the remaining carbon species can either (D) form a carbon film on the surface of the particle, (G) go into solution with the catalyst particle, or (H) diffuse through/around the particle to become (I) incorporated into the growing graphene layer. The carbon film that forms on top of the catalyst particle inhibits any further carbon from incorporating into the growing fiber. This film is removed by (E) chemical etching and (F) ion bombardment. The underlying fiber is protected to a large extent from these removal processes by the catalyst nanoparticle.

The variables that can be controlled in the dc-PECVD process are pressure, total gas flow rate, substrate temperature, plasma current, and carbonaceous gas to etchant gas ratio. In dc systems, current and voltage cannot be changed independently of each other. It is possible to have several sets of parameters that result in roughly similar fibers. Selecting proper parameters depends greatly on the catalyst pattern (dots or film), catalyst material, and gas selection. The growth rate of VACNFs is linked primarily to total pressure, gas flow ratio, and temperature. Figure 12.4 shows the trends between these variables and the growth rate. Interestingly, the growth rate of fibers is relatively constant over the growth time, meaning that fibers can be grown to specified lengths simply by adjusting growth time [18,20]. There is a near linear correlation between growth rate and P up to 10 Torr [18]. The gas ratio is not as straightforward, with a peak growth rate appearing in the mid-range. This relationship can be explained by the relative amounts of carbon and etchant. If there is too much carbon source, then the catalyst particle will become coated faster than the etchant can remove the film, slowing growth, or even halting it completely. Temperature exhibits a similar curve to the gas ratio, with a peak in growth rate around 700°C. This behavior is

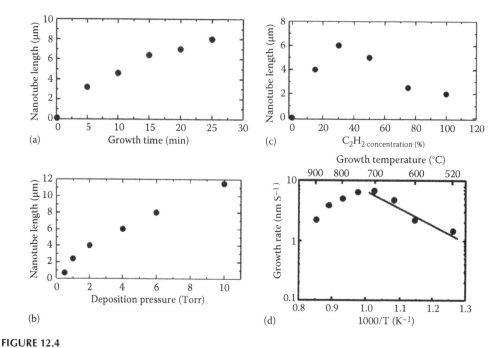

FIGURE 12.4
Trends in VACNF growth rate based on (a) growth time, (b) chamber pressure, (c) carbonaceous gas to etchant gas ratio, and (d) temperature. (Adapted from Chhowalla, M., Teo, K.B.K., Ducati, C. et al., Growth process conditions of vertically aligned carbon nanotubes using plasma enhanced chemical vapor deposition, *J. Appl. Phys.*, 90(10), 5308–5317. Copyright 2001, American Institute of Physics.)

due to increased carbon diffusion rate with temperature while simultaneously decreasing the sticking coefficient of carbon to the catalyst.

The shape of VACNFs can be controlled to either be conical or cylindrical, depending largely on the gas ratio and the catalyst pattern. With higher ratios of carbon gas to etchant, amorphous carbon is deposited onto the sidewalls of the catalytically grown fiber structure, leading to a conical shape. Conical fibers can also occur from deposition of volatilized silicon from the substrate, which then reacts with N if ammonia is being used, resulting in fiber sidewalls with a SiN_x composition [21–24]. Interestingly, using ammonia as an etchant does not dope the fibers with N. Merkulov et al. analyzed fibers with energy dispersive x-ray spectroscopy (EDS) and saw a high nitrogen content that disappeared after immersion in an SF_6 plasma that selectively removes silicon and silicon nitrides, indicating that nitrogen is only present in the sidewall coating [25]. Cylindrical shapes occur if the gas ratio is tuned to remove carbon that is unprotected by the catalyst particle at the same rate as the carbon is deposited. A forest of fibers will still be cylindrical even in a high carbon regime due to crowding, preventing the deposition of carbon to the sidewalls.

Alignment can also be controlled during synthesis of VACNFs. Vertical alignment, which is necessary for many applications, can be achieved with thermal CVD through a "crowding effect" caused by van der Waal's interactions between densely packed CNFs during growth [26]. Thermal CVD is limited though due to its inability to create spatially separated VACNFs. With PECVD, alignment can be achieved with any CNF density. A strong correlation has been observed between the direction of the electric field and the alignment of the fibers [27,28]. This phenomenon was noticed by observing tilted fibers grown at the edge of the cathode in dc PECVD, where the electric field was no longer perpendicular to the substrate. It had been suggested that the mechanism for alignment involved electrostatic forces on the nanofibers. One proposed hypothesis stated that the electrostatic forces created differential stresses at the nanoparticle/nanofiber interface, controlling mass transport distribution and providing negative feedback to self-correct any deviation from the direction of the electric field [27]. Recently experiments have shed more light on the alignment mechanism that contradicts this hypothesis. The recent evidence suggests that the direction of the ion flux is the determining factor in fiber alignment, as carbon will only diffuse through the catalyst particle where the carbon film has been removed by ion bombardment [19]. Thus by controlling the direction of the ionic flux through locally altering the electric fields, it was possible to control the alignment of the fibers.

The synthesis of VACNFs can be controlled to a large extent, a critical factor in their implementation. By tweaking the multidimensional parameter space, the height, diameter, location, composition, morphology, structure, and chemistry of the fibers can be deterministically chosen.

12.3 Biochemical Functionalization of VACNFs

The ability to attach biologically active molecules to VACNFs in a controlled fashion is critical to many of their biological applications. In this section, the attachment chemistry for DNA, proteins, and antibodies will be discussed. The fibers frequently undergo some form of surface treatment prior to any attachment. One example of a common pretreatment for VACNFs is a wet etch or an oxygen plasma etch, the result of which is production of COO^- groups on the surface, which can then be further modified with carbodiimide chemistry.

The presence of native H groups on the fiber surfaces allows for electrochemical or photochemical reactions to produce COO⁻ or amine terminated surfaces that can be useful with various cross-linking or adsorption strategies. The biochemicals that fibers are most commonly functionalized with are DNA, proteins, and antibodies. A few functionalization strategies that have been previously used will be discussed for each of these biochemicals.

12.3.1 DNA Functionalization

There are a number of strategies for attachment of DNA to VACNFs. Baker et al. have two methods of attachment that they have compared [29]. The first relies on a photochemical reaction between the nanofibers and linker molecules that have terminal olefin groups in addition to a protected amine group. A subsequent reaction results in a free primary amine, which is then attached to a thio-terminated oligonucleotide. In the second approach, a reaction between an aryldiazonium salt with the fibers is followed by an electrochemical reduction to the primary amine, which is linked to thio-terminated DNA oligonucleotides. Comparatively, the diazonium approach links amino groups to nanofibers via an aromatic ring, while the photochemical method generally links through an alkyl chain. The diazonium functionalization also allows for electrically addressable functionalization by selectively reducing the nitro group to an amino under electrochemical control.

After amino group attachment, thio-modified DNA can be linked covalently to the fibers. This addressable functionalization has been demonstrated by modifying discrete VACNF forest electrodes with two separate DNA probe sequences. The selectivity of hybridization that resulted from the different implementation methods was established through hybridization studies using complementary and non-complementary DNA. Quantitative measurements of the amount of DNA that hybridized to DNA attached to VACNFs were done using fluorescence measurements and fluorescence wash-off methods. Baker et al. found an eightfold increase in DNA attachment to VACNFs as opposed to the underlying planar footprint [29]. Other DNA attachment schemes have also been developed [30,31].

12.3.2 Protein and Antibody Functionalization

Several attachment chemistries have been used for protein functionalization of VACNFs. The simplest of these methods relies on biotin/avidin affinity. In one study, Baker et al. had avidin (50 Å diameter) bind to biotin (1 nm), which was then attached to VACNFs via a disulfide bond-bearing linker [29]. McKnight et al. used a slightly different biotin/avidin attachment chemistry, starting with a carboiimide cross-linking reaction to covalently bond gold-conjugated streptavidin to VACNFs [32]. Baker et al. have also functionalized VACNFs with the protein cytochrome *c* (cyt *c*) [33]. Figure 12.5 shows their approach schematically. The results of this study suggest that proteins can retain their functionality, post-functionalization. It has also been shown by Naguib et al. that phycoerythrin conjugated anti-CD3 antibodies can be adsorbed onto pyrolitically stripped CNFs and that protein adsorption can be drastically increased through pretreatment with poly-L-lysine [34].

It should be noted that the VACNF surface does not remain unchanged over time. It is speculated that the atoms on the edge planes of the fibers are hydrogen terminated immediately after growth in a highly reducing hydrogen environment, but that over time in ambient conditions these sites may degrade. This information is relevant to functionalization as Baker et al. reported that the functionalization yield of VACNFs exposed to ambient for extended periods is decreased.

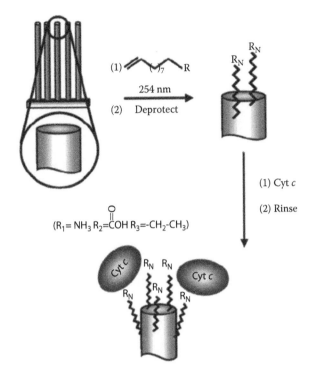

FIGURE 12.5
A schematic representation of VACNF functionalization with the protein cytochrome *c*. (Adapted from Baker, S.E., Colavita, P.E., Tse, K.Y., and Hamers, R.J. Functionalized vertically aligned carbon nanofibers as scaffolds for immobilization and electrochemical detection of redox-active proteins, *Chem. Mater.*, 18(18), 4415–4422. Copyright 2006 American Chemical Society.)

Functionalization of VACNFs extends beyond DNA, proteins, and antibodies. There are many molecules of biological relevance that can be attached to VACNF surfaces through traditional carbon chemistry strategies. It has also been demonstrated that click chemistry can be applied to VACNFs, with large potential for biological applications [35].

12.4 Cellular Interfacing of VACNFs for Gene/Material Delivery

Gene delivery to individual mammalian cells via a physical impalement process was one of the earliest demonstrations of VACNF utility in biointerfacing [36]. The aspect ratio of a VACNF is similar to the extreme tip of conventional, pulled-glass microcapillaries, with a 10–20 μm long nanofiber having a submicron base diameter and a tip diameter typically less than 100 nm. As with microinjection pipettes, the sharp tip and high aspect ratio enables the nanofiber to penetrate into the interior of a eukaryotic cell using a variety of techniques, and to deliver either physisorbed or covalently linked cargo during the penetration event (Figure 12.6). One of the earliest demonstrations achieved cellular penetration and delivery of an impermeant dye via a centrifugation process, whereby a VACNF array was positioned within a microcentrifuge tube such that the nanofibers were positioned to impale cells as they were pelleted from suspension. Subsequent developments

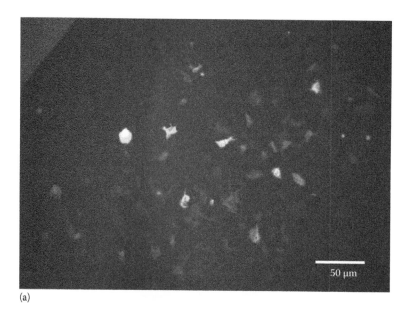

(a)

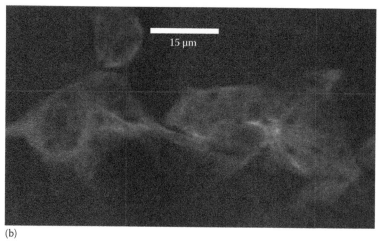

(b)

FIGURE 12.6
(See color insert.) Images of impalefected U2OS osteosarcoma cells resident upon a 2.2 mm square VACNF array following multiplexed delivery of plasmids encoding GFP-tubulin and dsRed-monomer H2B. (a) Widefield view (100×) with field of view approximately 1/4 of the VACNF array chip. (b) Laser scanning confocal micrograph of a 40×70 μm region showing individual nanofibers as a periodic array of red dots, and the interaction of cytoplasmic GFP-tubulin and nuclear dsRed-H2B with cell-penetrant nanofibers.

have simplified the approach, whereby small chips of nanofiber arrays are first modified with molecular cargo and then pressed into pellets of suspended cells, fragments of intact tissue, and even directly into intact tissue [37]. As with microinjection, a sharp, impulsive process is typically required to achieve intracellular/intranuclear penetration. Unlike microinjection, however, arrays of nanofibers alleviate the necessity of microscopic visualization of the process, as the array density can be such that every cell encounters one or several nanofiber spikes (Figure 12.6).

Gene delivery via this impalement process has been demonstrated with both physisorbed and covalently linked DNA immobilization strategies. For the former, DNA is suspended in water or stabilizing buffer solutions at very low concentration, and dispensed and dried onto small "chips" of VACNF arrays, typically at coverages of between 1 and 20 ng/μm^2. Choice of solvent is important, as conventional DNA stabilizing solutions such as 1× tris-edta (TE) will produce solid crystals during the drying process, the presence of which diminishes the ability of the deployed chip to effectively interact with individual cells and to achieve nanofiber intracellular residence. DNA modified chips are then prewetted immediately before cellular interfacing and pressed into pellets of cells or tissue.

Covalent strategies have also been demonstrated for effective gene delivery. Here, DNA is tethered to the nanofiber using a variety of strategies as outlined earlier. Early examples used a carbodiimide coupling to link plasmid DNA to nanofibers putatively via DNA-guanine amines and carboxylic acid sites native or generated upon the nanofiber surface. Subsequent methods have demonstrated effective gene expression from linear fragments of DNA generated using either restriction digest or PCR with high fidelity polymerases and primers chosen to provide coupling affinity to the nanofiber surface [31,38]. This includes amine-terminated primers for carbodiimide coupling, biotin-terminated fragments for binding to streptavidin-modified nanofibers, and the incorporation of disulfide linkages to promote intracellular release of the bound DNA fragment via reduction of the disulfide bridge.

Chip planarity is an important consideration for cellular and tissue interfacing. Conventionally, nanofibers are grown on a silicon wafer as vertical elements upon an otherwise planar, solid substrate. To promote handling, the silicon wafer is diced into small chips with a single, 100 mm diameter wafer yielding hundreds to thousands of millimeter scale gene delivery devices. The size of these chips is arbitrary, but the planarity of the resultant structure must be considered as the nanofibers only extend tens of microns from the surface. The target surface of tissue or a pellet of cells must therefore be very compliant such that the nanofiber elements across the expanse of the chip can extend into the tissue in order to deliver their cargo intracellularly. The surface of the chip must also be clear of debris and micro-/macroscopic contaminants. Dust particles, debris remaining from the dicing process, and other solid particulates can keep large regions of the chip from interacting with targeted tissue. Previous efforts have typically been conducted with chips diced to a size of 2–5 mm on a side. Protective coatings of photoresist can be used during the dicing process such that any debris generated from the process can be lifted off using conventional photoresist solvents, such as acetone/isopropanol/water or *n*-methyl pyrrolidone/water washes. The protective layer of photoresist may be patterned such that DNA solutions placed on the chips prior to photoresist liftoff are adsorbed or covalently attached only in localized regions of the chip [32]. Post-liftoff handling of the chips must be conducted in a way that minimizes accumulation of solid particulates prior to the cellular interfacing event. For example, as mentioned earlier, the solvent of DNA spotting solutions must be chosen to avoid the formation of large solid crystals of the solvent solution during the drying process. For this reason, conventional strength DNA buffering solutions such as 1× tris-edta (TE) should be avoided. Lower concentrations of TE can be used, as can pure water, with the recognition that these solutions should not be used for long-term storage of the DNA prior to experimentation, as they will result in hydrolytic decomposition of the DNA and reduced expression efficiency. By contrasting argument, it should be noted that once DNA is dried onto the array, it can remain active and intact for long periods of time provided it remains dark and dry similar to long-term storage of DNA as dried spots on blotter paper. DNA-modified nanofiber arrays thus provide a unique opportunity as a "reagentless" gene delivery method. All that is required for transgene expression is removal of the DNA-spotted array from dry storage and integration of the array with targeted cells or tissue.

One of the more effective methods for interfacing cultured cells onto nanofiber arrays employs a solid pellet of a cellular suspension as the interfacing target. Here, adherent cells are passed using conventional trypsination or chelation methods to release the adherent cell layer, and the resultant cell suspension is spun in a swinging bucket centrifuge to form a pellet. This pellet is then carefully dislodged from the centrifuge tube, and dispensed onto a concavity slide under a small volume of media. DNA-modified nanofiber arrays can be pressed directly into the pellet to achieve cellular penetration and gene delivery. When using planar, silicon-based nanofiber arrays, the concavity slide presents a surface, which does not allow the cell pellet to be completely sandwiched beneath the nanofiber array. Rather, cells within the pellet are impaled and loose enough with respect to one another to come away with the chip when the chip is withdrawn from the pellet. A subsequent wash step, whereby the chip is agitated in fresh media, serves to remove the bulk of unpenetrated cells, leaving behind a monolayer of cells impaled upon the chip surface. Subsequent culture of the chip results in very rapid transgene expression, due to a high potential for nuclear penetration of the nanofiber and its DNA cargo during the penetration event. Using time-lapse fluorescent microscopy of cells impaled upon a nanofiber array spotted with the pd2eYFP-n1 plasmid, Hensley reported visual fluorescence of transgene yellow fluorescent protein within 55 min of the impalement event [39].

Flexible films of nanofiber arrays have been developed as an interface capable of interacting with large areas of non-planar tissue. By embedding the nanofibers in a thin film of ultraviolet cross-linked epoxy, Fletcher demonstrated that intact arrays of vertically aligned nanofibers could be peeled from their silicon growth substrate and remained freestanding and vertical within the flexible epoxy film [40]. Further development of this approach, using a variety of spun-cast, vapor-deposited, or dimerization deposition techniques is anticipated to provide flexible films of nanofibers with tailored mechanical properties for a variety of tissue interfacing applications.

While it is not too surprising that carbon nanofibers are capable of penetrating soft mammalian tissues or cells in a cell matrix, it has been recently shown that they are sufficiently resilient to cross dermal tissue as well. Figure 12.7 shows results of impaling pig skin, which has been stripped of stratum corneum. This opens up a possibility of using carbon nanofibers for construction of transdermal sensors.

12.5 VACNF Biosensors

This section will contain case studies of VACNFs that have been implemented as biosensors, combining information from the previous sections to discuss how the fibers were grown, how the device was made, the fibers functionalized, etc.

12.5.1 Ricin Detector

Meyyappan et al. recently used a nanoelectrode array (NEA) consisting of VACNFs to detect the protein ricin [41]. Ricin detection is of interest due to its potential use as a

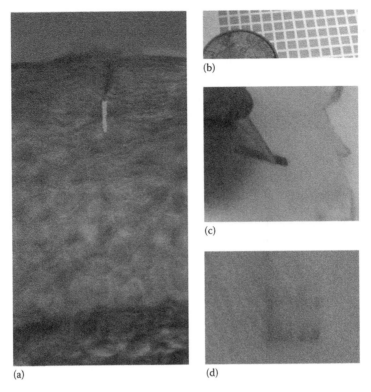

FIGURE 12.7
Application of an array of nanofibers to porcine skin for gene delivery. (a) A laser scanning confocal micrograph of a nanofiber spanning a portion of epidermis. This nanofiber is 32 μm long tilted with respect to a scan slice (its tip pointing out of the plane). Si$_3$N$_4$ coating on a nanofiber provides fluorescent label. The tissue is unstained and imaged in DIC mode. The stratum corneum was reduced by tape stripping. (b) A photograph showing a portion of a silicon wafer with nanofiber arrays. (c) A chip with nanofibers (up to 50 μm long) is laid down and then repeatedly pressed against a skin slice to insert and leave nanofibers in the tissue (d). The darkness of the squares corresponds to nanofiber density (5, 10, 20, and 50 μm in periodicity from dark to light). The experiments were performed in collaboration with Dr. Monteiro-Riviere, NCSU.

biowarfare agent. The authors bound ricin-A antibody or ricin aptamer to the NEAs to detect the presence of ricin. To create the array, a silicon wafer was coated with 200 nm of chromium with 500 nm thick thermal oxides, and a 30 nm nickel catalyst layer. The fibers were grown as a "forest" using a dc-PECVD system with 125 sccm acetylene and 444 sccm of ammonia at 4.73 Torr and 180 W of power. This recipe resulted in ~3 μm tall fibers after a growth time of 15 min. This forest of fibers was then completely encapsulated by CVD deposition of SiO$_2$. Chemical mechanical polishing left a smooth SiO$_2$ layer and only the tips of the VACNFs protruding from the surface.

After fabrication the chips were chemically activated by a HNO$_3$ soak followed by a wash with sterile water, which served to introduce –COOH groups for covalent binding of the antibody or aptamer probe for the biosensor. Functionalization with the antibody was carried out by combining 5 μL of ricin-A antibody in 50 μL phosphate buffered saline containing 1 mM MgCl mixed with a coupling reagent of 0.5 g *N*-(3-dimethylaminopropyl-*N*'-ethylcarbodiimide hydrochloride (EDC) and 0.25 mg *N*-hydroxysulfosuccinimide sodium salt (NHS). This mixture was then placed on the VACNF NEA and incubated at room temperature for 2 h. During incubation, the primary amine groups of the Ricin A antibody formed amide bonds with the carboxyl-groups on the VACNF tips. To remove any non-specific binding, the authors performed a stringent wash. The antibody binding and functional activity was evaluated by cyclic voltammetry (CV) and electrochemical impedance spectroscopy (EIS). The capture binding was performed by first incubating the antibody-functionalized chip in ricin protein or collagen, which served as a control protein, mixed with PBS buffer for 1 h. The incubation was followed by another rinsing phase. Target capture binding was determined with CV and EIS as well.

To detect the protein using ricin aptamer, an anti-ricin RNA aptamer with a specific sequence in a PBS buffer that contained magnesium chloride was mixed with a coupling reagent consisting of EDC and NHS. This solution was allowed to incubate on the VACNF chip for 2 h at 40°C. A stringent wash procedure was followed again to remove the possibility of nonspecific binding. Target binding was performed by incubation of the chip in ricin protein–PBS buffer solution. The control was a nonspecific DNA aptamer. The authors found that the ricin-A antibody probe did not bind sufficiently to the VACNFs, but the aptamer probe was stable and could be regenerated multiple times for a reusable biosensor.

12.5.2 Glucose Biosensor

Glucose is considered to be one of the most important biosignatures due to its use in identifying some bacteria, eukaryotes, and archaea. VACNFs could potentially replace CNTs for glucose biosensors, since VACNFs have better sensitivity and responsiveness than CNTs [42]. Islam et al. have created a mediator free amperometric bienzymatic glucose biosensor made with VACNFs that can detect concentrations as low as 0.4 μM [43]. The authors use an enzyme wiring technique, which improves the electrical contact between the electrode surfaces and the glucose oxidase, with VACNFs used as the working electrode. Their amperometric bienzymatic glucose biosensor is based on glucose oxidase (GO_x) and horseradish peroxidase (HRP).

Fabrication of the electrode began with creating a ∼500 nm thick silicon oxide layer on a silicon substrate followed by deposition and patterning of nickel catalyst arrays using photolithography. After growth of the VACNF clusters, a ∼200 nm thick chromium electrode layer was sputter deposited and patterned to create five individually addressable electrode pads. After fabrication, the wafer was sonicated in sulfuric acid to ensure the cleanliness of the fibers.

The next step is the chemical functionalization of the chips. To do this, the authors used the enzyme wiring technique where they carefully spread just enough HRP and GO_x to cover the entire surface area of the VACNF forest. When this sensor comes in contact with glucose, a reduction to gluconic acid occurs and the resulting current can be detected. HRP has the ability to react with other interfering molecules, but amperometric tests carried out by the authors revealed that even in the presence of these other molecules glucose can be detected due to its significantly higher response. They conclude that their sensor has a sensitivity of 89.035 μA/mM and has a dynamic range of 0.4–40 μM.

12.5.3 Ethanol Biosensor

A VACNF biosensor has been made for the detection of ethanol by immobilizing yeast alcohol dehydrogenase (YADH) and its coenzyme on the fibers by Weeks et al. [44]. YADH is an oxidoreductase enzyme that catalyzes the following redox reaction:

$$\text{Ethanol} + \text{NAD}^+ \leftrightarrow \text{Acetaldehyde} + \text{NADH}$$

YADH's coenzyme is the oxidized form of adenine dinucleotide NAD^+ that must be bound to the enzyme's active site in order for a reaction to occur. Thus, when ethanol is present in the biosensor, a reaction takes place.

The working electrode containing the nanofibers was created on silicon dioxide. Small regions of the wafer (0.5×0.5 mm) had catalyst deposited on them for growth of fiber forests. After dc-PECVD, the fibers were approximately 4 µm tall and 100 nm in diameter. A thin titanium wire lead was connected electrically to the electrode area. Following growth, the fibers were sonicated in sulfuric acid to clean the fibers.

Two different immobilization techniques were used to attach the enzyme and coenzyme to the nanofibers. The first method used was adsorption where the VACNF electrode was first immersed in the solution containing YADH followed by a rinse to remove excess enzyme. Afterward, the electrode was immersed in a solution of NAD^+ followed by another rinse. The second method used was covalent bonding through diimide-activated amidation. Reactive intermediates can be formed at the carboxylic acid sites on the nanofibers by 1-ethyl-3-(3-dimethylaminopropyl) carbodiimide (EDAC), which can then couple with amines to form amides. The subsequent reaction was stabilized by N-hydroxysuccinimide (NHS). The electrode was allowed to soak in a mixture of EDAC and NHS with a buffer. After this soak, the electrode was transferred to a solution of YADH, followed by rinsing. The electrode then underwent immersion in NAD^+ and a final rinse.

Drops of 0.1 mL of ethanol were introduced into the electrochemical cell every 20 s and amperometric measurements were made with both attachment schemes. The results were obtained from electrodes on which the enzyme is adsorbed and covalently attached. The initial current increase seen upon each injection of ethanol slightly over-shoots and then approaches a steady state after ~5 s. The linear concentration range for the adsorbed electrode was 1.75–10 mM while the covalent electrode was 2–8 mM. The electrodes were also tested after storage for 1–7 days and it was found that both electrodes only lost 1.5% of electrical current in amperometric analysis after a full week. Reusability tests also showed that after 10 tests the current decreased by 75% and 60% for 20 tests. The study concluded that both electrodes were effective after multiple uses and week-long storage periods.

12.5.4 Neuronal Interfacing

The ability to stimulate and record signals from multiple neurons simultaneously has the potential to increase our understanding of neuronal network physiology. In this section, several studies using VACNF arrays to record and/or stimulate hippocampal slices will be reviewed.

Zhe Yu et al. were the first to report the use of VACNFs for stimulation and extracellular recording of spontaneous and evoked neuroelectrical activity in hippocampal slices [45]. They created a 40-element linear array of VACNFs by insulating n-type silicon wafers with 1 µm of silicon dioxide, after which metal buffer layers and 100 µm thick, 2 µm diameter nickel catalyst pucks with 15 µm spacing were patterned and deposited. Each puck resulted in a cluster of nanofibers ~10 µm tall after PECVD. Interconnects were then defined lithographically and generated by reactive ion refractory metal etch. A passivation layer was then deposited upon the entire wafer and then removed from the contact pads

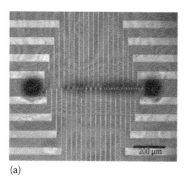

(a)

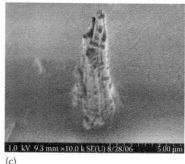

(c)

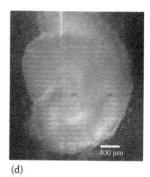

(d)

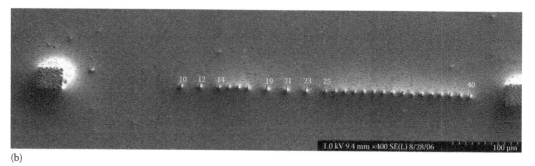

(b)

FIGURE 12.8

(a) Light microscopy image of the array prior to use. (b) SEM image of the VACNF array after several record-ings had taken place. The missing electrodes (1–9, 11, 13, 18, 20, 22, 24) were absent before testing, as can be seen in (a), indicating that the fibers were not shorn from the mechanical stress of testing. (c) SEM image of a single electrode from (b). (d) Light micrograph of a hippocampal slice impaled upon the VACNF array chip. (Adapted with permission from Yu, Z., McKnight, T.E., Ericson, M.N. et al., Vertically aligned carbon nanofiber arrays record electrophysiological signals from hippocampal slices, *Nano Lett.*, 7(8), 2188–2195. Copyright 2007 American Chemical Society.)

and the electrode tips. This step was followed by an HF buffered oxide etch to remove the exposed silicon oxide coating from the contact pads and the portion of the nanofibers above the passivation layer. Figure 12.8 shows optical and SEM micrographs of the VACNF arrays used.

Before performing recordings, the VACNF chips were cleaned by an air plasma treatment for 30 s before being coated with a poly-L-lysine and laminin in water mixture overnight followed by three water rinses. The hippocampal slices were obtained from a postnatal 8–11 day rat pup and were sectioned to be 400 µm thick.

Spontaneous electrical activity of hippocampal slices was recorded by aligning the tis-sue with the electrode array crossing the hilus of the hippocampus, with electrode 1 of the linear array in the CA3 pyramidal cell layer and electrode 40 in the dentate gyrus (DG) granule cell layer. Other measurements required various alignments of the slices with the fiber electrodes, which could be reused with multiple tissue slices and align-ments. Spontaneous complex spikes were recorded and were easily distinguishable from the background noise of 25 μV_{rms}. Nanofibers could also be used to evoke responses by applying current through individual VACNF electrodes and then recording the responses at other electrodes in the linear array.

The authors conclude that the VACNF electrodes are capable of performing the same functions as other microelectrode arrays (MEAs) despite being much smaller and having sufficient charge injection capacity to stimulate the tissue. The electrodes were capable of a maximal stimulus of 100 µA for 100 µs, passing 10 nC of charge to the tissue without damaging it. The theoretical maximum charge injection of the VACNF electrodes is 8 mC/cm^2. The VACNF electrodes also have an advantage over planar MEAs due to their ability to penetrate the tissue. Penetration of slices may provide improved means of interrogating the native condition of acute tissue slices rather than requiring extended culture periods required for tissue recovery at the surface of the slice.

In the second study, Nguyen-Vu et al. compared the function of a plain VACNF electrode to the one coated with polypyrrole. It has been shown that electrically conductive polymer coatings on CNFs can improve the biocompatibility of the electrodes and potentially prevent electrolysis from occurring [46–48]. The electrodes are fabricated by first defining and depositing the electrode pads and interconnects, followed by deposition of a 30 nm thick catalyst layer on the electrode area. The nickel particles left at the tips of the VACNFs after growth were then removed by a nitric acid etch. The authors then electrochemically deposited polypyrrole using an Autolab potentiostat. They found that the polypyrrole coated arrays were the only electrodes they tested capable of evoking a large amplitude, short duration field potential, with lower latency and able to function at lower voltage, preventing electrolysis. Additionally the polymer coated arrays did not induce a toxic extracellular pH change that were observed with metallic MEAs and unmodified VACNF electrodes.

A follow-up of the Yu study demonstrated VACNF neural interfaces being used to monitor the dynamic behavior of neuronal network activity [49]. Neuronal cells sat randomly on the electrode and some electrode tips were engulfed via endocytosis by the cells, which is thought to be minimally invasive or noninvasive. Paired-pulse facilitation and depression (PPF/D) ratios were generated in the cells by two successive stimuli of equal intensity with different inter-stimulus intervals. PPF/D is an example of short-term neuroplasticity that is thought to be involved with temporal cognitive abilities. These ratios were simultaneously recorded by all the electrodes.

VACNF electrodes are very promising for use in neuronal interfacing since they can record and stimulate signals in and around single cells without any apparent damage. Further, the spatial characteristics of both individual nanofiber electrodes and arrays of these electrodes can provide enhanced spatiotemporal information of tissue response.

12.5.5 Neurotransmitter Sensor

The ability to measure neural transmitter dynamics is critical to further develop our understanding of neural network physiology. Lamprecht et al. measured dopamine concentrations in the nanomolar range using VACNF arrays coated with over-oxidized polypyrrole [50]. The dopamine concentration was measured by attaching a small well to a typical nanofiber array through which a constant flow of artificial cerebral spinal fluid was introduced for baseline measurements. After 2 min, artificial cerebral spinal fluid with a known concentration of dopamine was introduced and electrochemical measurements were recorded using a potentiostat and an Ag/AgCl electrode for both the reference and counter electrodes in three-electrode amperometry mode. The over-oxidized polypyrrole was synthesized on the electrodes by filling the well with KCl and pyrrole and then cycled from 0–1 V at 10 V/s followed by another 10 cycles while placed in NaOH. This entire process was performed three times for three coats of over-oxidized polypyrrole. The purpose of this coating was to increase the limit of detection of the electrodes due to the high background capacitive current that resulted from the large surface area of the

VACNF electrodes. This coating increased the limit of detection from 100 to 10 nM while simultaneously improving the sensitivity from 17.5 to 57.1 pA/µM. It has also been shown in a similar manner that VACNF arrays are sensitive to other easily oxidized neurotransmitters such as norepinephrine and 5-hydroxytyramide [51].

12.6 Future Challenges and Conclusions

The true potential of VACNFs as elements in biosensor platforms is yet to be fully realized. There are several challenges that have to be overcome in order to make them attractive for large scale sensor manufacturing. The first is the high temperature of catalytic synthesis. Reduction of nanofiber synthesis temperature is essential for *in situ* growth of nanofibers on substrates that cannot withstand high thermal load, such as plastics and underlying electronics. Among strategies that have been proposed is selective heating of catalyst, for example. The second challenge is control of nanofiber structure and geometry by precisely tuning plasma properties. For example, controlling ion flux without significant power dissipation into the substrate could be of high interest. Further development of spatially controlled functionalization strategies is essential in creating multiplexed sensors in which combinations of signals could significantly enhance selectivity and sensitivity of the sensor. Further developments in integration of VACNFs as microelectrodes require improvements in insulating sheathing. One of the possible solutions lies in utilization of atomic layer deposition and it has yet to be used in formation of such coatings.

References

1. Rice, R.J. and R.L. Mccreery, Quantitative relationship between electron-transfer rate and surface microstructure of laser-modified graphite-electrodes. *Analytical Chemistry*, 1989. **61**(15):1637–1641.
2. Robinson, R.S., K. Sternitzke, M.T. Mcdermott, and R.L. Mccreery, Morphology and electrochemical effects of defects on highly oriented pyrolytic-graphite. *Journal of the Electrochemical Society*, 1991. **138**(8):2412–2418.
3. McKnight, T.E., A.V. Melechko, M.A. Guillorn et al., Effects of microfabrication processing on the electrochemistry of carbon nanofiber electrodes. *Journal of Physical Chemistry B*, 2003. **107**(39):10722–10728.
4. Helveg, S., C. Lopez-Cartes, J. Sehested et al., Atomic-scale imaging of carbon nanofibre growth. *Nature*, 2004. **427**(6973):426–429.
5. Radushkevich, L.V. and V.M. Lukyanovich, On the structure of carbon, formed by thermal decomposition of carbon monoxide on iron surface, *Zh. Fiz. Khim.*, 1952. **26**:88–95.
6. Tesner, P.A., E.Y. Robinovi, I.S. Rafalkes, and E.F. Arefieva, Formation of carbon fibers from acetylene. *Carbon*, 1970. **8**(4):435–442.
7. Melechko, A.V., V.I. Merkulov, T.E. McKnight et al., Vertically aligned carbon nanofibers and related structures: Controlled synthesis and directed assembly. *Journal of Applied Physics*, 2005. **97**(4):Artn 041301.
8. Baker, R.T.K., Catalytic growth of carbon filaments. *Carbon*, 1989. **27**(3):315–323.

9. Baker, R.T.K., M.A. Barber, R.J. Waite, P.S. Harris, and F.S. Feates, Nucleation and growth of carbon deposits from nickel catalyzed decomposition of acetylene. *Journal of Catalysis*, 1972. **26**(1): 51–62.

10. Melechko, A.V., V.I. Merkulov, D.H. Lowndes, M.A. Guillorn, and M.L. Simpson, Transition between 'base' and 'tip' carbon nanofiber growth modes. *Chemical Physics Letters*, 2002. **356**(5–6):527–533.

11. Alstrup, I., A new model explaining carbon-filament growth on nickel, iron, and Ni-Cu alloy catalysts. *Journal of Catalysis*, 1988. **109**(2):241–251.

12. Kock, A., P.K. Debokx, E. Boellaard, W. Klop, and J.W. Geus, The formation of filamentous carbon on iron and nickel-catalysts. 2. Mechanism. *Journal of Catalysis*, 1985. **96**(2):468–480.

13. Nielsen, J.R. and D.L. Trimm, Mechanisms of carbon formation on nickel-containing catalysts. *Journal of Catalysis*, 1977. **48**(1–3):155–165.

14. Sacco, A., P. Thacker, T.N. Chang, and A.T.S. Chiang, The initiation and growth of filamentous carbon from alpha-iron in H_2, CH_4, H_2O, CO_2, and Co gas-mixtures. *Journal of Catalysis*, 1984. **85**(1):224–236.

15. Melechko, A.V., R. Desikan, T.E. McKnight, K.L. Klein, and P.D. Rack, Synthesis of vertically aligned carbon nanofibres for interfacing with live systems. *Journal of Physics D: Applied Physics*, 2009. **42**(19):193001.

16. Merkulov, V.I., D.H. Lowndes, Y.Y. Wei, G. Eres, and E. Voelkl, Patterned growth of individual and multiple vertically aligned carbon nanofibers. *Applied Physics Letters*, 2000. **76**(24):3555–3557.

17. Ren, Z.F., Z.P. Huang, D.Z. Wang et al., Growth of a single freestanding multiwall carbon nanotube on each nanonickel dot. *Applied Physics Letters*, 1999. **75**(8):1086–1088.

18. Chhowalla, M., K.B.K. Teo, C. Ducati et al., Growth process conditions of vertically aligned carbon nanotubes using plasma enhanced chemical vapor deposition. *Journal of Applied Physics*, 2001. **90**(10):5308–5317.

19. Pearce, R.C., A.V. Vasenkov, D.K. Hensley et al., Role of ion flux on alignment of carbon nanofibers synthesized by DC plasma on transparent insulating substrates. *Applied Materials & Interfaces*, 2011. **3**(9):3501–3507.

20. Merkulov, V.I., A.V. Melechko, M.A. Guillorn, D.H. Lowndes, and M.L. Simpson, Sharpening of carbon nanocone tips during plasma-enhanced chemical vapor growth. *Chemical Physics Letters*, 2001. **350**(5–6):381–385.

21. Cui, H., X. Yang, H.M. Meyer et al., Growth and properties of Si-N-C-O nanocones and graphitic nanofibers synthesized using three-nanometer diameter iron/platinum nanoparticle-catalyst. *Journal of Materials Research*, 2005. **20**(4):850–855.

22. Klein, K.L., A.V. Melechko, P.D. Rack et al., Cu-Ni composition gradient for the catalytic synthesis of vertically aligned carbon nanofibers. *Carbon*, 2005. **43**(9):1857–1863.

23. Melechko, A.V., T.E. McKnight, D.K. Hensley et al., Large-scale synthesis of arrays of high-aspect-ratio rigid vertically aligned carbon nanofibres. *Nanotechnology*, 2003. **14**(9): 1029–1035.

24. Yang, X.J., M.A. Guillorn, D. Austin et al., Fabrication and characterization of carbon nanofiber-based vertically integrated Schottky barrier junction diodes. *Nano Letters*, 2003. **3**(12):1751–1755.

25. Merkulov, V.I., D.K. Hensley, A.V. Melechko et al., Control mechanisms for the growth of isolated vertically aligned carbon nanofibers. *Journal of Physical Chemistry B*, 2002. **106**(41):10570–10577.

26. Fan, S.S., M.G. Chapline, N.R. Franklin et al., Self-oriented regular arrays of carbon nanotubes and their field emission properties. *Science*, 1999. **283**(5401):512–514.

27. Merkulov, V.I., A.V. Melechko, M.A. Guillorn, D.H. Lowndes, and M.L. Simpson, Alignment mechanism of carbon nanofibers produced by plasma-enhanced chemical-vapor deposition. *Applied Physics Letters*, 2001. **79**(18):2970–2972.

28. Merkulov, V.I., A.V. Melechko, M.A. Guillorn et al., Controlled alignment of carbon nanofibers in a large-scale synthesis process. *Applied Physics Letters*, 2002. **80**(25):4816–4818.

29. Baker, S.E., K.Y. Tse, E. Hindin et al., Covalent functionalization for biomolecular recognition on vertically aligned carbon nanofibers. *Chemistry of Materials*, 2005. **17**(20):4971–4978.
30. Mann, D.G.J., T.E. McKnight, A.V. Melechko, M.L. Simpson, and G.S. Sayler, Quantitative analysis of EDC-condensed DNA on vertically aligned carbon nanofiber gene delivery arrays. *Biotechnology and Bioengineering*, 2007. **97**(4):680–688.
31. Peckys, D.B., N. de Jonge, M.L. Simpson, and T.E. McKnight, End-specific strategies of attachment of long double stranded DNA onto gold-coated nanofiber arrays. *Nanotechnology*, 2008. **19**(43):435301.
32. McKnight, T.E., C. Peeraphatdit, S.W. Jones et al., Site-specific biochemical functionalization along the height of vertically aligned carbon nanofiber arrays. *Chemistry of Materials*, 2006. **18**(14):3203–3211.
33. Baker, S.E., P.E. Colavita, K.Y. Tse, and R.J. Hamers, Functionalized vertically aligned carbon nanofibers as scaffolds for immobilization and electrochemical detection of redox-active proteins. *Chemistry of Materials*, 2006. **18**(18):4415–4422.
34. Naguib, N.N., Y.M. Mueller, P.M. Bojczuk et al., Effect of carbon nanofibre structure on the binding of antibodies. *Nanotechnology*, 2005. **16**(4):567–571.
35. Landis, E.C. and R.J. Hamers, Covalent grafting of redox-active molecules to vertically aligned carbon nanofiber arrays via "Click" chemistry. *Chemistry of Materials*, 2009. **21**(4):724–730.
36. McKnight, T.E., A.V. Melechko, G.D. Griffin et al., Intracellular integration of synthetic nanostructures with viable cells for controlled biochemical manipulation. *Nanotechnology*, 2003. **14**(5):551–556.
37. McKnight, T.E., A.V. Melechko, D.K. Hensley et al., Tracking gene expression after DNA delivery using spatially indexed nanofiber arrays. *Nano Letters*, 2004. **4**(7):1213–1219.
38. Peckys, D.B., A.V. Melechko, M.L. Simpson, and T.E. McKnight, Immobilization and release strategies for DNA delivery using carbon nanofiber arrays and self-assembled monolayers. *Nanotechnology*, 2009. **20**(14):145304.
39. Hensley, D.K., A.V. Melechko, M.N. Ericson, M.L. Simpson, and T.E. McKnight. Transparent microarrays of vertically aligned carbon nanofibers as a multimodal tissue interface. in *Biomedical Sciences and Engineering Conference (BSEC), 2010*, Oak Ridge National Laboratory, Oak Ridge, TN. 2010.
40. Fletcher, B.L., T.E. McKnight, A.V. Melechko et al., Transfer of flexible arrays of vertically aligned carbon nanofiber electrodes to temperature-sensitive substrates. *Advanced Materials*, 2006. **18**(13):1689.
41. Periyakaruppan, A., P.U. Arumugam, M. Meyyappan, and J.E. Koehne, Detection of ricin using a carbon nanofiber based biosensor. *Biosensors and Bioelectronics*, 2011. **28**(1):428–433.
42. Jang, J., J. Bae, M. Choi, and S.H. Yoon, Fabrication and characterization of polyaniline coated carbon nanofiber for supercapacitor. *Carbon*, 2005. **43**(13):2730–2736.
43. Islam, A.B., F.S. Tulip, S.K. Islam, T. Rahman, and K.C. MacArthur, A mediator free amperometric bienzymatic glucose biosensor using vertically aligned carbon nanofibers (VACNFs). *IEEE Sensors Journal*, 2011. **11**(11):2798–2804.
44. Weeks, M.L., T. Rahman, P.D. Frymier, S.K. Islam, and T.E. McKnight, A reagentless enzymatic amperometric biosensor using vertically aligned carbon nanofibers (VACNF). *Sensors and Actuators B: Chemical*, 2008. **133**(1):53–59.
45. Yu, Z., T.E. McKnight, M.N. Ericson et al., Vertically aligned carbon nanofiber arrays record electrophysiological signals from hippocampal slices. *Nano Letters*, 2007. **7**(8):2188–2195.
46. Nguyen-Vu, T.D.B., H. Chen, A.M. Cassell et al., Vertically aligned carbon nanofiber arrays: An advance toward electrical-neural interfaces. *Small*, 2006. **2**(1):89–94.
47. Nguyen-Vu, T.D.B., C. Hua, A.M. Cassell et al., Vertically aligned carbon nanofiber architecture as a multifunctional 3-D neural electrical interface. *Biomedical Engineering, IEEE Transactions on*, 2007. **54**(6):1121–1128.
48. de Asis, E.D., T.D.B. Nguyen-Vu, P.U. Arumugam et al., High efficient electrical stimulation of hippocampal slices with vertically aligned carbon nanofiber microbrush array. *Biomedical Microdevices*, 2009. **11**(4):801–808.

49. Yu, Z., T.E. McKnight, M.N. Ericson et al., Vertically aligned carbon nanofiber as nano-neuron interface for monitoring neural function. *Nanomedicine-Nanotechnology Biology and Medicine*, 2012. **8**(4):419–423.
50. Lamprecht, M.R., T.E. McKnight, M.N. Ericson, and B. Morrison, VACNF arrays for recording dopamine concentrations in the brain. *2010 IEEE 36th Annual Northeast Bioengineering Conference*, Columbia, NY, March 26–28, 2010.
51. McKnight, T.E., A.V. Melechko, B.L. Fletcher et al., Resident neuroelectrochemical interfacing using carbon nanofiber arrays. *Journal of Physical Chemistry B*, 2006. **110**(31):15317–15327.
52. Klein, K.L., A.V. Melechko, T.E. McKnight et al., Surface characterization and functionalization of carbon nanofibers. *Journal of Applied Physics*, 2008. **103**(6):61301.

13

Graphene-Based Electrochemical Biosensors

Chun Xian Guo, Shu Rui Ng, and Chang Ming Li

CONTENTS

13.1 Introduction

Graphene is a single-atom-thick planar sheet of sp^2-bonded carbon atoms perfectly arranged in a honeycomb structure that forms a large polyaromatic molecule of semi-infinite size [1]. The unique structure endows graphene with interesting and extraordinary properties including room temperature high electron mobility, room temperature quantum Hall effect, a tunable bandgap, high transparency, strong mechanical strength, and good chemical/physical stability [2,3]. Owing to these prominent properties, graphene has quickly attracted tremendous interests in the fundamental science areas of materials, physics, and chemistry and their broad applications such as nanoelectronics, energy storage and conversion, biomedicine, and sensors [4–8].

Electrochemical biosensors constitute an interdisciplinary field that is currently one of the most active areas of research in analytical chemistry and sensor community [9]. They combine the sensitivity of electroanalytical methods with the selectivity of the biotransducer to recognize target molecule and further ultimately convert binding or interaction events to electrical signal by an electrocatalytic process for detections. Thus, the sensor performances are greatly influenced by the electrode architecture, surface area, and interface structure at nanoscales [10]. Much effort has been dedicated to the use of nanostructured materials with nanoscale size-dependent properties as electrode materials or to functionalize electrodes to develop high-performance electrochemical biosensors. Two-dimensional (2-D) graphene, with its unique structural property of single-atom-thick planar, large contact surface area, and high electron transfer/transport rate for high electrocatalytic activity, has become one of the best nanostructured materials to fabricate electrodes in electrochemical applications. Despite its recent debut, graphene has demonstrated its tremendous potentials in electrochemical biosensors [11–13].

In this chapter, we focus on the recent progress in graphene-based electrochemical biosensors. We begin by introducing the properties of graphene, paying particular attention to its unique surface chemistry and electrochemical properties. Subsequently, the electrochemistry of graphene most relevant to its performances as electrochemical biosensors is discussed. We then provide an overview on the latest advances in electrochemical biosensors utilizing graphene and its nanocomposites. Future prospects and directions in this exciting area are proposed.

13.2 Graphene Properties and Preparation

13.2.1 Electronic Structure and Properties

The electronic properties of a material are always determined by its electronic structure. The electron configuration of carbon atoms is $1s^2 2s^2 2p^2$, where the outer shell consisting of $2s^2 2p^2$ can hybridize to form different hybrid orbitals, resulting in various carbon nanomaterials [14]. Graphene has a sp^2 hybridization that adopts a hexagonal lattice configuration with two interpenetrating triangular sublattices while having an unhybridized z-axis-oriented orbital perpendicular to the plane of the 2-D sheet. Three sp^2 bonds between the adjacent atoms of graphene have a strong interaction and form π-bonds, leading to unique electronic properties. Two valence and conducting bands exist in graphene and are formed by the π- and π^*-states, respectively. These π valence bands and π^* conduction bands are indistinguishable at the Fermi energy located in the bandgap and remain equal in energy [15]. Therefore, the two bands touch each other at the K-point (K and K' valleys) in the Brillouin zone, leading to the formation of two cones, a top cone for the electrons and an inverse one for the holes (Figure 13.1). These K-points are referred to as Dirac points. This bandgap structure imparts graphene unique properties, as its charge carriers mimic

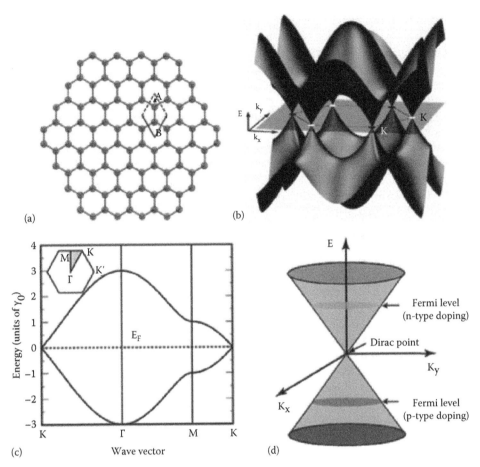

FIGURE 13.1
(a) Hexagonal honeycomb lattice of graphene with two atoms (A and B) per unit cell. (b) The 3-D band structure of graphene. (c) Dispersion of the states of graphene. (d) Approximation of the low energy band structure as two cones touching at the Dirac point. The position of the Fermi level determines the nature of the doping and the transport carrier. (With permission from Avouris, P., Graphene: Electronic and photonic properties and devices, *Nano Lett.*, 10(11), 4285–4294. Copyright 2010 American Chemical Society.)

relativistic particles and behave as massless and chiral fermions as opposed to conventional massive electrons in metals and semiconductors. Furthermore, the unique band-gap structure endows graphene with many superior electronic properties including an anomalous integer quantum Hall effect, a Klein tunneling effect, and an insensitivity to disorder-induced localization.

13.2.2 Electron Transport Behaviors

As a 2-D planar sheet of sp^2-bonded carbon atoms perfectly arranged in a defect-free honeycomb structure, graphene exhibits interesting electron transport behaviors. Experimental transport measurements show that graphene can achieve a carrier concentration of 10^{13} cm^{-2} and an electron mobility up to 20,000 cm^2 V^{-1} s^{-1} at low temperatures [1]. In addition, its mobility is nearly independent of temperatures between 10 and 100 K and the hole and electron mobilities are comparable [16]. In other words, it behaves like a metal with almost high constant mobility over a large range of temperatures. These observations indicate that the electron transport behavior of graphene is essentially ballistic on the micrometer-scale in its 2-D planar sheet. Not all graphene materials prepared in laboratories are single-layered and the number of layers affects the electron transport properties of graphene, producing fascinating properties in double-, few-, and multilayer graphene [13]. Double-layer graphene has a zero bandgap, which can be opened by applying an electric field axially toward the bilayer, resulting in interlayer electron hopping. Few-layer graphene (<10 layers) exhibits metal-like electron transport while multilayer graphene (10–100 layers) displays electron transport behavior similar to that of highly ordered pyrolytic graphite. In addition, edge structures, surface functionalization, and doping can affect the electron transport properties of graphene. Clearly, the electron transport properties of graphene can be tailored by improving the quality of graphene, controlling the number of layers, changing its dimensions, increasing the edge density, and eliminating defects and impurities.

13.2.3 Chemical Properties

The chemical properties of graphene are considered to be similar to those of benzene and polycyclic aromatic hydrocarbons as they share analogous structures [17]. Breaking and formation of conjugated sp^2 C–C bonds (basal plane) or sp^2 C–H bonds (edge) are important in the chemistry of graphene. Two approaches, doping and functionalization, are often utilized to achieve desired chemical properties of graphene. Doping substitutes carbon atoms in graphene with heteroatoms, producing novel graphene materials with either electrons or holes that exhibit n-type or p-type behaviors, respectively. Nitrogen doping is one of the most popular ways to generate n-type graphene. For example, during the chemical vapor deposition (CVD) process, ammonia gas or N-containing molecules such as pyridine are introduced into the growth system for the direct growth of nitrogen-doped graphene [18]. The chemical treatment of pristine graphene films can also produce nitrogen-doped graphene, such as exposing them to ammonia plasma [19] or annealing reduced graphene oxide in an ammonia gas atmosphere [20]. There are basically two types of functionalization approaches, covalent functionalization and noncovalent functionalization. Covalent functionalization offers high stability but the process is tedious and has low efficiency. On the other hand, noncovalent functionalization provides high efficiency and can retain the conjugated structure of graphene well but suffers from low stability. Relatively high energetic species are needed to break the sp^2 bonds of graphene to initiate its covalent functionalization reactions. In an initial attempt, hydrogenation was used to covalently functionalize mechanically exfoliated graphene, resulting in its p-type behavior [21]. Aryl diazonium salt, a moderately reactive species, was used to covalently functionalize graphene through a free radical mechanism (Figure 13.2a). Interestingly, graphene prepared from different chemical processes displayed varied reactivity toward aryl diazonium salts [22]. Noncovalent functionalization based on van der Waals forces or π–π stacking of aromatic molecules onto the surface of graphene is also a popular choice. Pyrene derivatives such as pyrene butanoic acid succidymidyl ester (PBASE) have strong affinity to the basal plane of graphene via π–π interactions (Figure 13.2b) and this helps to stabilize graphene in aqueous solutions and also tune the electron density on graphene [23]. Some polymers such as conducting polymer polyaniline can also form strong π–π interactions with graphene between their backbones and the surface of graphene (Figure 13.2c) [2]. Graphene/polyaniline can promote graphene solubility in water and enhance its stability and electrochemical activity [25]. Other molecules, including enzymes, DNA, surfactants, and even inorganic nanoparticles, can be used to noncovalently functionalize graphene for a wide range of applications [26].

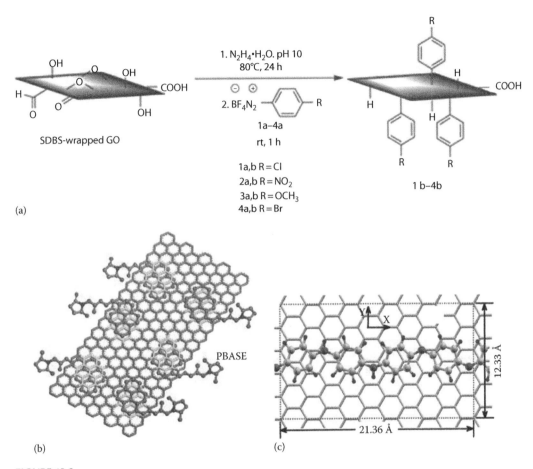

FIGURE 13.2
(a) Starting with sodium dodecylbenzenesulfonate (SDBS)-wrapped graphene oxide, reduction and functionalization of intermediate SDBS-wrapped chemically converted graphene with diazonium salts. (With permission from Lomeda, J.R. et al., Diazonium functionalization of surfactant-wrapped chemically converted graphene sheets, *J. Am. Chem. Soc.*, 130(48), 16201–16206. Copyright 2010 American Chemical Society.) (b) Noncovalent interactions between graphene and small molecules of pyrene butanoic acid succidymidyl ester (PBASE) and (c) graphene and conducting polymer polyaniline through π–π interactions. (With permission from Loh, K.P. et al., The chemistry of graphene, *J. Mater. Chem.*, 20(12), 2277–2289. Copyright 2010 Royal Society of Chemistry; From Wang, R.X., Huang, L.F., and Tian, X.Y., Understanding the protonation of polyaniline and polyaniline–graphene interaction, *J. Phys. Chem. C*, 116(24), 13120–13126. With permission of the Royal Society of Chemistry.)

13.2.4 Other Properties

Single-layer graphene is a highly transparent material with a transparency of 97.3%, independent of wavelength. Its optical transparency can be tailored through electrical gating [27]. Moreover, graphene displays remarkable photoluminescence (PL). Two different approaches are developed to enhance the PL of graphene, one to cut graphene into small pieces such as graphene nanoribbons and the other to use physical/chemical methods to reduce the connectivity of the electron network [28]. These remarkable optical properties make graphene a highly viable option for optoelectronic devices. In terms of its mechanical properties, graphene possesses a mechanical strength similar to that of the theoretical strength of a defect-free solid and a theoretical tensile strength as high as 150 GPa and

Young's modulus up to 1.0 TPa [29,30], making it the thinnest and strongest material. Other outstanding properties of graphene include its large specific surface area, good thermal qualities, storage capability, and magnetic properties. These interesting and exciting properties make graphene a fundamentally superior material with promising applications.

13.2.5 Preparation Methods

The properties of graphene are greatly affected by its synthesis routes. Various synthesis routes can be used to tailor graphene for specific applications. In this section, we briefly discuss graphene preparation methods that are frequently used for electrochemical biosensors. In general, there are two kinds of approaches to produce graphene. Graphene can be detached from a pre-existing graphite crystal via exfoliation, which includes mechanical cleavage of graphite, reduction of exfoliated graphene oxide (GO), and unzipping of carbon nanotubes (CNTs). Alternatively graphene can be grown directly on a substrate surface, which includes chemical vapor deposition (CVD) and epitaxial growth.

Mechanical cleavage of graphite can produce high quality single-layer graphene sheets, which has been a fascinating model system to reveal fundamental properties of this amazing material [31]. Mechanically exfoliated single-layer graphene is useful in development of nanoelectronic devices such as field emission transistors. The drawback of this method is its low throughput and difficulty in transferring the single-layer graphene, thus greatly limiting its practical applications in electrochemical biosensors. Compared to other graphene preparation methods, reduction of exfoliated GO (rGO) provides the advantage of low-cost mass-production of graphene [32,33]. Reported reduction methods include chemical [33], electrochemical [34], photochemical [35], and thermal reduction [36]. GO can also disperse well in water and many other solvents, making its reduced form, rGO, a prime material for further functionalization in solutions. Moreover, with abundant reactive sites at the edges and in a defective basal plane, rGO is much more electrochemically active than pristine graphene [12]. The properties of rGO are different from those of pristine graphene due to the existence of numerous defects in the carbon lattice. Nevertheless, its scalable preparation, facile functionalization, and electrochemically active nature make it the most attractive method to produce graphene for electrochemical biosensors. Another exfoliation approach to produce graphene (specifically, graphene nanoribbons) is unzipping CNTs. Hyper-manganate chemical oxidation of CNTs [37] or plasma etching of multiwalled CNTs [38] can open them up into graphene. Similarly, the unzipping of CNTs has potential for mass production. However, the resulted graphene materials may contain metallic impurities, leading to unpredictable electrochemical behavior. Unless the obtained graphene material is free of impurities, such methods are not suitable to produce graphene for electrochemical applications.

Graphene can grow on transition metal substrates such as nickel and copper using CVD [39]. An advantage of the CVD method is its capability for simultaneous doping of graphene by introducing heteroatoms such as nitrogen and boron into the carbon lattice during the growth of graphene. By selecting suitable substrates, the CVD method can also produce large-sized graphene films that can be easily incorporated into electronic devices. However, due to the existence of defects, impurities, and few-layered domains, CVD-grown graphene has properties, which deviate from those of pristine graphene. Other challenges to using CVD-grown graphene are its low throughput and difficulties in transferring the graphene from the growth substrate to the desired substrate [40]. These disadvantages limit the range of applications for CVD-grown graphene in electrochemical biosensors. Recently, a unique graphene material with a 3-D structure developed by growing graphene via CVD on 3-D nickel foams has been reported and might find applications as electrochemical sensors [41]. Epitaxial growth is another substrate growth approach to produce graphene [42]. One popular method is to decompose silicon carbide (SiC) to graphene at high temperatures. Since SiC is an insulator, the graphene on SiC can be directly used to build electronic devices. However, for applications in electrochemical biosensors, the transfer of epitaxially grown graphene from SiC to the desired substrate is required. This method also suffers from low throughput production and nonuniform thickness of the resulting graphene film that leads to deviated properties.

In brief, reduction of exfoliated graphene oxide and CVD are two favorable methods to prepare graphene for electrochemical biosensors. In comparison to CVD, the reduction of exfoliated graphene oxide offers more advantages such as mass production, facile functionalization/doping, solution-processible capability, and electrocatalytic activity. In fact, most of the graphene-based electrochemical biosensors reported up to date are fabricated using graphene prepared by the reduction approach.

13.3 Electrochemical Biosensors and Graphene Electrochemistry

13.3.1 Electrochemical Biosensors and Performance Evaluations

Based on the nature of the biological recognition process, electrochemical biosensors can be divided into two main categories: biocatalytic sensors and affinity sensors. Biocatalytic sensors utilize biotransducers that can recognize the target biomolecule and catalyze a reaction at the electrode to produce an electrical signal proportional to the biomolecule concentration. Electrochemical sensors for detection of redox or electroactive molecules that are related to biological processes are also considered as electrochemical biosensors. Affinity sensors rely on the selective binding between the analyte and a biological component such as an antibody, nucleic acid, or a receptor. Affinity sensors can be electrochemical ones if the binding event is detected by electrochemical methods such as impedimetry, amperimetry, and potentiometry. Electrochemical immunosensors and DNA hybridization biosensors are examples of electrochemical affinity sensors [25]. Like other sensors, electrochemical biosensors are usually experimentally evaluated based on the main parameters of selectivity, sensitivity, limit of detection, dynamic ranges, response time, and reproducibility. For practical applications, storage life, ease of use, and portability are also important. Online detection capability is required for sensors to continuously monitor the analytes in many clinical and national defense applications. In most cases, in order for several consecutive measurements to be made, the sensing surface should be regenerable. Nevertheless, for special applications such as personal blood glucose monitoring, single-use and disposable electrochemical biosensors are highly demanded.

13.3.2 Graphene Electrochemistry and Its Advantages in Electrochemical Biosensors

As discussed in Section 13.2.2, graphene has a ballistic electron transport behavior on the micrometer-scale in its 2-D planar sheet with a carrier concentration of 10^{13} cm^{-2} and an electron mobility up to 20,000 cm^2 V^{-1} s^{-1}. On the other hand, electron transfer (heterogeneous electron transfer, which is different from electron transport), is a critical process in electrochemical reactions and often refers to electron transfer at an interface between different materials or components. Electron transfer at graphene refers to electron transfer out of or into the graphene sheet from the surrounding environment. It has been reported that the edge plane of a graphene sheet exhibits a heterogeneous electron transfer rate constant (k) on the order of 0.01 cm s^{-1} while the basal plane is almost electrochemically inert with k lower than 10^{-9} cm s^{-1} [13]. Recently, it has been demonstrated that the rate of heterogeneous electron transfer at graphene increases systematically with the number of graphene layers, and the stacking in multilayers also has a subtle influence on the heterogeneous electron transfer kinetics [43]. Nevertheless, the aggregation of graphene sheets should be avoided, since it could make the unique electronic, chemical, and electrochemical properties of graphene reduced or even totally lost.

Graphene is not the only carbon material used in electrochemical biosensors. Other carbons including graphite, diamond, carbon nanocages, and carbon black have also been explored [10,44]. Particularly, CNTs, 1-D carbon materials, have dominated carbon-based electrochemical biosensors [45]. This trend, however, is gradually changing with the introduction of graphene, which offers several advantages while overcoming some weaknesses encountered by CNTs. Nonetheless, it should be noted that the advances in the development of graphene-based electrochemical biosensors are at least partially built on the basis of techniques and knowledge gained from decades of research on CNT-based ones. In this section, the advantages of graphene in electrochemical biosensors are discussed by using CNTs as a comparison.

It is difficult to answer if graphene or CNT is better for electrochemical biosensors as there are limited literatures for the comparison. Nevertheless, three differences in properties, which include surface functional groups, material structure, and material purity, suggest that graphene has a number of advantages over CNTs for some electrochemical biosensors. A major advantage of graphene derived from the reduction of graphene oxide is the presence of oxygen-containing groups at its edges or surface. These functional groups have a great influence on the electrochemical performance of graphene in terms of the heterogeneous electron transfer rate [46]. A recent study has reported that the selectivity and sensitivity of electrochemical biosensors toward some biomolecules such as uric acid and ascorbic acid can be achieved at reduced graphitic oxide fabricated by a microwave-assisted hydrothermal elimination method, which can retain the edge plane and control the density of oxygen-containing functional groups [47]. Such selectivity and sensitivity are attributed to the very distinct behavior of uric acid and ascorbic acid to form hydrogen bonds with oxygen-containing surface groups. Apart from its oxygenated groups, other active elements/components with controlled positive or negative charges can be easily introduced on the graphene surface because of its unique 2-D structure with large contact surface area. The functional groups on graphene can effectively act as anchoring sites to promote the growth and attachment of ultrasmall active elements/components with uniform distribution on the graphene surface for electrochemical biosensors. An example is the use of these oxygenated groups as the anchoring sites to attach glucose oxidase (GOD) for glucose biosensing [48]. Moreover, functional groups on graphene can greatly influence the adsorption/desorption of biomolecules that take place before and after an electrochemical reaction. However, the presence of functional groups may have the drawback of reduced charge transfer/transport rate on graphene and may also suppress the electrocatalytic activity. Fortunately, various methods including graphene reduction through various chemical, electrochemical, thermal, and photochemical approaches have been developed to control the functional groups on the surface of graphene targeting specific applications while blocking their negative effects. The unique 2-D structure of graphene is also superior to CNTs. The high-aspect-ratio and 1-D structure of CNTs are useful in many ways, but these characteristics make them difficult to be controllably assembled onto complicated sensing architectures. In contrast, the unique 2-D structure and larger contact surface area make graphene highly beneficial for incorporation into sensing transducers. Graphene is almost free of metallic impurities, while purity often plagues CNTs due to resulting unpredictable electrochemical signals.

13.4 Graphene-Based Electrochemical Biosensors

13.4.1 Direct Electrochemistry–Based Enzyme Electrochemical Biosensors

Direct electrochemistry (DET) of enzyme is known to have direct electron transfer between its active center and an electrode without the help from mediators or other reagents [49]. DET of enzyme-based electrochemical biosensors offer advantages of simplicity, less mediator-caused toxicity, high selectivity, and potential for miniaturization. However, enzyme is difficult to conduct DET on a plain electrode because its active sites are always deeply buried within electrically well-insulated prosthetic shells [50]. The remarkable characteristics of nanomaterials, in particular the enzyme-comparable sizes, high surface-to-volume ratio, fast charge mobility, and quantum-confined electronic properties could enable tunnel effects or/and pseudomediator for DET between them and enzymes. Various nanomaterials including CNTs, metal nanoparticles, metal oxide hollow spheres, and conducting polymer nanofilms have demonstrated DET ability of enzymes for high-performance electrochemical biosensors [44,51,52]. With excellent electron transport/transfer ability, functionalized surface chemistry, large contact surface area, abundant edge sites, and biocompatibility, graphene-based materials have demonstrated their superior capability to enable DET of enzymes for high-performance electrochemical enzyme-based biosensors.

13.4.1.1 Functionalization of Graphene for High-Performance DET-Based Enzyme Biosensors

One of the pioneering works reported the direct electron transfer of GOD on functionalized graphene followed GOD adsorption (Figure 13.3a) [53]. It is interesting that before the immobilization of GOD, the polyvinylpyrrolidone (PVP)-protected graphene shows good electrocatalytic activity toward reduction of oxygen and hydrogen peroxide, possibly due to the effect of the active sites of the functional groups or/and edges of graphene. The graphene–GOD electrode was coated on glassy carbon electrodes (GCEs) with a mixture of PVP-protected graphene and polyethylenimine (PEI)-functionalized ionic liquid, followed by GOD adsorption. The electrocatalytic behavior of graphite–GOD and graphene–GOD in PBS solution was compared and only graphene–GOD exhibited a pair of well-defined redox peaks with a formal potential (averaging the cathodic and anodic peak potentials) of ~–0.43 V (vs. Ag/AgCl in saturated KCl), peak-to-peak separation of ~69 mV, and also a ratio of cathodic to anodic current intensity close to 1, which is in good agreement with the reversible electron transfer process of the redox active center (flavin adenine dinucleotide, FAD) in GOD (Figure 13.3b). In addition, the plot of peak current against scan rate exhibited a linear relation, suggesting a surface-confined process. These results clearly indicate that graphene by functionalization is able to realize the direct electron transfer of GOD. The graphene–GOD electrode was utilized for electrochemical glucose sensing and showed a wide linear detection range of 2–14 mM (Figure 13.3c), which sufficiently covers the glucose level in human blood. The prepared biosensor also exhibited good reproducibility and stability.

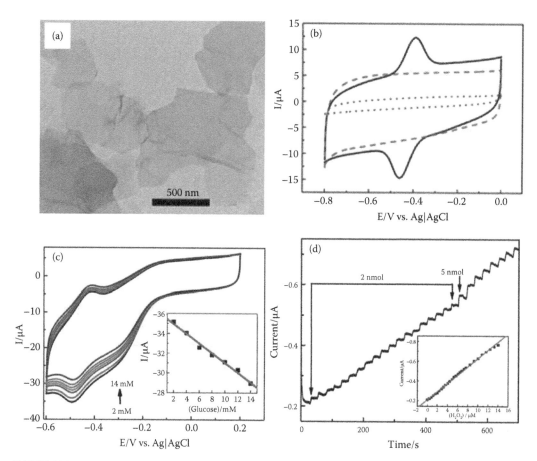

FIGURE 13.3

(a) TEM image of polyvinylpyrrolidone (PVP)-protected graphene. (b) CVs of graphene- polyethylenimine-functionalized ionic liquid (PFIL) (dashed), graphite-GOD-PFIL (dotted), and graphene-GOD-PFIL (solid) modified electrodes in 0.05 M PBS solution saturated with N_2. (c) CVs of the graphene-GOD-PFIL electrode in various concentrations of glucose PBS solution saturated with O_2. The inset of (c) is the calibration curve with current responses at −0.49 V. (With permission from Shan, C. et al., Direct electrochemistry of glucose oxidase and biosensing for glucose based on graphene, *Anal. Chem.*, 81(6), 2378–2382. Copyright 2009 American Chemical Society.) (d) Amperometric response of a Nafion/HRP/graphene/GC electrode to successive addition of H_2O_2 into a PBS. The working potential was −0.4 V. Inset: the calibration curve of I–C obtained by chrono-amperometry. (From *Electrochimica Acta*, 56(3), Li, M. et al., Direct electrochemistry of horseradish peroxidase on graphene-modified electrode for electrocatalytic reduction towards H_2O_2, 1144–1149. Copyright 2011, with permission from Elsevier.)

Graphene can be functionalized by noncovalent approach followed by covalently bonding protein for DET. As an example, electrochemically reduced single-layer graphene oxide nanosheets with negative charge were adsorbed on amino-group functionalized GCEs and used to covalently immobilize GOD, which realized DET. The resulting biosensor provides high sensitivity toward glucose oxidation [48].

Some unique surface modifications of graphene can lead to the DET. Hydrazine-reduced graphene oxide drop-cast on GCEs was utilized to immobilize horseradish peroxidase (HRP), which undergoes DET according to the electrochemical redox reaction between HRP-Fe(III) and HRP-Fe(II) (Figure 13.3d) [54]. The graphene–HRP electrode displayed an improved electrocatalytic reduction behavior toward H_2O_2 with a linear range of

0.33–14.0 μM, a detection limit of 0.11 μM, and good operational and storage stability. Many other functionalized graphene materials such as water-soluble sulfonated graphene film prepared by functionalizing $NaBH_4$-reduced graphene oxide with aryl diazonium for HRP DET toward the electrochemical sensing of H_2O_2 and $NaNO_2$ [55] have also been reported.

13.4.1.2 Graphene/Polymer Nanocomposites for DET-Based Enzyme Electrochemical Biosensors

Graphene can be well-mixed with polymers to form novel nanocomposites for synergistic properties of its components. These graphene–polymer nanocomposites have demonstrated their DET ability of enzymes for electrochemical sensing. Graphene–chitosan nanocomposite was fabricated and used for GOD DET and electrochemical glucose sensing [56]. The nanocomposite is designed to have synergistic properties of graphene with large contact surface area and high electron transfer/transport rate, and chitosan with positively charged primary amine and high solubility in aqueous solution. The graphene/chitosan nanocomposite was prepared by mixing thermally expanded graphene and chitosan solution with the help of ultra-sonication. The GOD–graphene–chitosan electrode was fabricated by sequentially drop-casting the graphene–chitosan mixture solution and GOD on GCE. CV curves of the GOD–graphene–chitosan electrode in N_2-saturated solution exhibited a pair of well-defined peaks with anodic and cathodic peak potential at −0.437 and −0.517 V (vs. Ag/AgCl) respectively, a peak potential separation of around 80 mV, and a formal potential of −0.477 V (vs. Ag/AgCl), which is very close to the standard electrode potential of −0.505 V (vs. Ag/AgCl) for $FAD/FADH_2$ of GOD at neutral pH, suggesting a good DET behavior. No such redox peak for the control electrodes of GOD–chitosan/GCE and GOD/GCE was observed, clearly demonstrating the effectiveness of graphene in facilitating the DET of GOD. The electron transfer rate constant of GOD in the GOD–graphene–chitosan is around 2.83 s^{-1}, which is much larger than that of GOD on CNTs, CNTs–chitosan, and CNTs–CTAB. The GOD–graphene–chitosan electrode provides a linear range from 0.08 to 12 mM for the electrochemical sensing of glucose, which is much wider than that of GOD–CNTs–chitosan and GOD–Au–carbon electrodes, making GOD–graphene–chitosan a promising material for GOD DET-based glucose biosensors.

Two polymer components, poly (3, 4-ethylenedioxythiophene) (PEDOT) and poly (diallyldimethylammonium chloride) (PDDA) have also been used together with graphene to prepare graphene nanocomposites for DET of enzyme-based electrochemical biosensors. The graphene–PEDOT (G–PEDOT) composite was synthesized by chemical oxidation of monomer EDOT on graphene oxide surface in the presence of poly(styrenesulfonic acid) as a charge balancing dopant, followed by the chemical reduction of GO to rGO [57]. Enzyme cytochrome c adsorbed on the G–PEDOT composite displayed excellent DET and retained its biocatalytic activity toward the reduction of H_2O_2, showing a linear response in the range of 5.0×10^{-7} to 4.0×10^{-4} M with a detection limit of 2.49×10^{-7} M. Another composite of graphene–PDDA (G–PDDA) was prepared by mixing GO and PDDA followed by the chemical reduction of GO to rGO and was further combined with ionic liquid (IL) [58]. The IL/G–PDDA nanocomposite displays an enhanced capability for the immobilization of hemoglobin to realize its DET, exhibiting excellent electrocatalytic activity for the detection of nitrate with a wide linear range from 0.2 to 32.6 μM and a calculated detection limit of 0.04 μM (S/N = 3). Many other composites including graphene–hexadecyltrimethylammonium bromide (CTAB)–IL for myoglobin DET and H_2O_2 sensing [59], graphene–chitosan for microperoxidase-11 DET and H_2O_2 sensing [60], and graphene–CTAB–chitosan for hemoglobin and nitric oxide sensing [61] have been reported. These works demonstrate that graphene-organic nanocomposites possess the synergistic properties of graphene and polymers with good biocompatibility, enhanced electric conductivity, and large specific surface area, and can greatly promote DET of enzymes for high-performance electrochemical biosensors.

13.4.1.3 Graphene/Inorganic Nanocomposites for DET-Based Enzyme Electrochemical Biosensors

Inorganic nanomaterials have advantages of well-designed nanostructures, good stability, and ease of fabrication and have recently been incorporated with graphene to prepare graphene/inorganic nanocomposites for DET-based enzyme electrochemical sensors. Zinc oxide (ZnO) is a metal oxide with advantages of non-toxicity, good interaction with enzymes, chemical stability, and high electron mobility and has been used to prepare a graphene/ZnO nanocomposite for GOD DET toward electrochemical glucose sensing [62]. The graphene/ZnO nanocomposite was fabricated by electrodepositing ZnO microflowers on rGO-modified GCE and the GOD electrode was prepared by drop-casting GOD solution on the prepared graphene/ZnO electrode. GOD molecules can strongly adsorb onto the graphene/ZnO nanocomposite via the electrostatic interaction between the negatively charged GOD and positively charged graphene/ZnO nanocomposite. CVs of the GOD/graphene/ZnO electrode showed a pair of stable and well-defined reversible redox peaks with a formal potential of -0.40 V (vs. Ag/AgCl) and a peak-to-peak separation of 70 mV, demonstrating the good DET behavior of GOD. The pH study indicated that the DET of $FAD/FADH_2$ at GOD on graphene/ZnO is a two-proton ($2H^+$) and two-electron ($2e^-$) process. The GOD/graphene/ZnO electrode exhibited a linear range from 0.02 to 6.24 mM and a detection limit of 0.02 mM for electrochemical glucose sensing. The strong electrostatic interactions between GOD and the graphene/ZnO nanocomposite also promoted the good stability of the electrode, as it retained 92% of its original response after 400 consecutive testing cycles.

TiO$_2$ is another commonly used metal oxide with better stability than ZnO, and has very recently been used to prepare a graphene/TiO$_2$ nanocomposite. The nanocomposite was fabricated using TiCl$_3$ and graphene oxide as the starting materials via a one-step approach, in which graphene oxide was reduced by the titanium(III) ion to form graphene while the titanium(III) ion was oxidized to titanium(IV) ion and further hydrolyzed to TiO$_2$ nanoparticles on the graphene sheets [63]. Structural characterizations illustrated that the anatase TiO$_2$ nanoparticles with an average size of 5 nm densely covered the graphene sheets. The graphene/TiO$_2$ nanocomposite provided a high surface coverage of hemoglobin (Hb) with a value of 2.15×10^{-9} mol cm^{-2}, even larger than that of theoretical monolayer Hb coverage (1.89×10^{-11} mol cm^{-2}), suggesting a good interaction between the Hb and the nanocomposite. Hb immobilized on the nanocomposite showed a pair of well-defined and quasi-reversible redox peaks at -0.297 and -0.402 V (vs. saturated calomel electrode) respectively, which are in good accordance with the characteristic Fe^{III}/Fe^{II} redox couple of Hb DET. The Hb–graphene/TiO$_2$ was applied for the electrochemical sensing of H$_2$O$_2$ and exhibited a good linear relationship with concentrations of H$_2$O$_2$ from 3 to 180 mM, an estimated detection limit of 1.5 mM, and an apparent Michaelis–Menten constant of 63.67 mM, which is smaller than those previously reported. This indicated that the immobilized Hb on graphene/TiO$_2$ possesses higher enzymatic activity and the Hb electrode has a higher affinity for H$_2$O$_2$. The nanocomposite plays a critical role in the enhanced Hb DET and improved H$_2$O$_2$ sensing, in which graphene provides high specific surface areas and establishes a fast electron transfer path to facilitate the DET of Hb, and

TiO_2 nanoparticles contribute more absorption sites and provide a good biocompatible microenvironment for the loading of Hb and retain its native bioactivity. Other graphene/inorganic nanocomposites such as graphene/Fe_3O_4 for Hb DET and H_2O_2 sensing [64] have also been demonstrated.

In summary, various graphene materials including functionalized graphene, graphene/polymer nanocomposites, graphene/inorganic nanocomposites, and even graphene/polymer/inorganic nanocomposites such as a graphene/chitosan/silver nanoparticle nanocomposite have demonstrated their capabilities in facilitating DET of enzyme and promoting the performances of these enzyme electrochemical biosensors. These works clearly highlight that graphene and its nanocomposites are promising candidates for the DET-based enzyme high-performance electrochemical biosensors.

13.4.2 Graphene for Electrocatalytic Small Biomolecule Sensors

Electrochemical reactions of small biomolecules such as hydrogen peroxide, nitric oxide, dopamine, and some aromatic molecules mainly involve three steps on electrode surface, adsorption from electrolytes to electrode surface, undergoing electrochemical reactions, and desorption from the electrode surface to the electrolyte. Thus, electrocatalysis plays a critical role for a sensitive detection of a specific small biomolecule and a highly electrocatalytic sensing layer is demanded. As discussed earlier, graphene has a unique structure of a 2-D planar sheet of sp2-bonded six-carbon rings and also large contact surface area, making it favorable as active material to adsorb small molecules via electron affinity/hydrogen bonding (with hydrogen peroxide and nitric oxide) or via π–π interaction (with dopamine). Moreover, graphene has high charge mobility, high electrocatalytic activity from its abundant edge sites/surface functional groups, and strong functionalization ability with bio- or chemical species for construction of electrochemically catalyzed sensing interface toward sensitive detection of small biomolecules.

13.4.2.1 Graphene for Electrocatalytic Sensing of Hydrogen Peroxide

Graphene has been used to construct high-performance electrochemical sensors for detection of hydrogen peroxide (H_2O_2) (Table 13.1). H_2O_2 is a reactive oxygen species, which can function as a secondary messenger and regulate gene expression through various intracellular signaling pathways [65]. It is also implicated in pathological processes such as carcinogenesis [66]. Being stable and small, H_2O_2 can easily diffuse across cell membranes and can form OH, leading to oxidative DNA damage. Thus, the selective, quantitative detection of H_2O_2 is important in understanding its physiological and pathological roles and could serve as a biomarker for diseases [67]. H_2O_2 can be directly detected by electrochemical oxidation or reduction at the electrode. The reduction of H_2O_2 is generally preferred as it can avoid interferences from species like ascorbic acid, uric acid, and dopamine that are oxidized at positive potentials. During reduction, H_2O_2 firstly gains a proton and electron and forms adsorbed OH^- on the electrode. The adsorbed OH^- is then rapidly converted to H_2O by gaining another proton and electron during the electrochemical step [68].

Nitrogen doped-graphene (N-graphene) has been used to build sensitive electrochemical biosensors toward detection of H_2O_2. The doping of nitrogen atom can induce charge enhancement of its adjacent carbon atom of graphene, making N-graphene favorable for the chemisorption of H_2O_2. Subsequently, the O–O bond of H_2O_2 could be weakened more easily, thereby facilitating H_2O_2 reduction. N-graphene prepared by the chemical reduction of graphene oxide by hydrazine has been applied for electrochemical sensing of H_2O_2

TABLE 13.1

Graphene-Based Electrochemical Sensors for the Detection of H_2O_2 and Their Performances[a]

Electrode	Sensitivity[b]/ $\mu A \, \mu M^{-1} \, cm^{-2}$	Detection Limit/μM	Linear Range	Response Time/s	Reference
Prussian blue nanocubes-graphene-PEI/GCE	—	0.045	50 nM to 0.12 mM	5	[81]
Nafion/Au NPs-PDDA-graphene-PVP/GCE	—	0.44	0.5 μM to 0.5 mM	<6	[70]
Ag NPs-graphene-polyelectrolyte/GCE	—	28.0	0.1–40 mM	2	[73]
(Laminin/Prussian blue/graphene)$_{10}$/ITO glass	4.50	0.10	0.1 μM to 0.1 mM	5	[67]
Ag NPs-graphene-benzylamine/GCE	—	31.3	0.1 mM to 0.1 M	2	[74]
Ag NPs-graphene-DMF/GCE	—	0.50	0.1 mM to 0.1 M	<2	[75]
erGO/IL-SPE	0.0535	0.08	0.15 μM to 1.8 mM	4	[84]
Pt NPs-graphene-PVP/GCE	0.141	0.50	2 μM to 0.71 mM	3	[78]
Hemin-graphene/GCE	0.285	0.20	0.5 μM to 0.4 mM	5	[82]
Ag NPs-graphene-aniline/GCE	—	7.10	0.1–80 mM	<2	[76]
Chitosan/Ag NPs-graphene-tannic acid/GCE	—	7.00	0.1 mM to 10 mM	<2	[77]
Chitosan-Fe$_3$O$_4$ NPs-graphene/AuE	0.688	3.20	0.1 6 mM	<5	[83]
Amphiphilic Au NPs/graphene paper	0.237	2.00	5 μM to 8.6 mM	—	[71]
Nitrogen-doped graphene/GCE	—	0.05	0.5 μM to 1.2 mM	<2	[69]
Au NPs-POM-graphene/GCE	0.0589	1.54	5 μM to 18 mM	3	[72]
Pt NPs-graphene/GCE	0.289	0.80	2.5 μM to 6.65 mM	<4	[79]
ZnO microflowers/erGO/GCE	13.5	0.02	1–22.5 μM	<5	[85]
Pt NPs/MnO$_2$ nanowires/graphene paper	0.130	1.00	2 μM to 13.3 mM	3	[80]

Note: "—" denotes a mixture or dispersion; "/" denotes a separate layer; "()" denotes a multilayer assembly and the number of layers is denoted by the number in subscript; AuE, gold electrode; DMF, dimethylformamide; erGO, electrochemically reduced graphene oxide; GCE, glassy carbon electrode; IL, ionic liquid; ITO, indium-doped tin oxide; NPs, nanoparticles; PDDA, poly(diallyldimethyl ammonium chloride); POM, poly(oxometalate); PVP, poly(N-vinyl-2-pyrrolidone); SPE, screen-printed electrode.

[a] The development of H_2O_2 electrochemical biosensors from 2010 to 2012 has been presented in chronological order.

[b] For general comparison, the sensitivity expressed in $\mu A \, \mu M^{-1} \, cm^{-2}$ was calculated by dividing the reported sensitivity in terms of $\mu A \, \mu M^{-1}$ by the apparent surface area of the working electrode if the electrode dimensions were stated.

and its performance was compared to N-free graphene produced by reducing graphene oxide with $NaBH_4$ [69]. The results showed that the N-graphene has better electrocatalytic performance toward H_2O_2 reduction than N-free graphene. The N-graphene sensor displayed a linear range of 0.5 μM to 1.2 mM, a detection limit around 0.05 μM (S/N = 3), and good selectivity for H_2O_2. Moreover, it exhibited good stability with only a slight decrease in responses after continuous catalysis (1000 s) at −400 mV.

A variety of graphene nanocomposites with synergistic properties arising from its components for electrochemical H_2O_2 biosensors have emerged over the last few years. Metal nanoparticles (NPs) such as Au NPs [70–72], Ag NPs [73–77], and Pt NPs [78–80] with well-defined cathodic peaks for H_2O_2 reduction have been incorporated with graphene to construct high-performance H_2O_2 electrochemical biosensors. A Pt NPs–graphene nano-composite was prepared by a photochemical method to deposit Pt NPs on glucose-reduced graphene sheets in the presence of poly(vinylpyrrolidone) [78]. The nanocomposite comprised a good dispersion of high density Pt NPs on a graphene sheet with well-preserved electrocatalytic activity across a large electrochemically active surface area and exhibited a high electrocatalytic performance with a cathodic peak corresponding to H_2O_2 reduction at 0.15 V (vs. Ag/AgCl). Other than metal NPs, the incorporation of materials that can mimic the enzymatic H_2O_2 catalysis, such as Prussian blue [67,81], hemin [82], and Fe_3O_4 NPs [83] into graphene is another smart approach to fabricate electrochemical sensors for highly sensitive and selective H_2O_2 sensing.

Highly sensitive graphene-based electrochemical sensors with low detection limits and fast response times for H_2O_2 detection have been developed and it is expected these sensors will be used for more biological studies and clinical diagnostic applications.

13.4.2.2 Graphene for Electrocatalytic Sensing of Nitric Oxide

Graphene has been utilized to fabricate high-performance nitric oxide (NO) electrochemical biosensors (Table 13.2). NO is a biological signaling molecule, which plays key roles in regulating cell function [86]. NO is produced by NO synthases in various cell types and can function as a neurotransmitter in the nervous system [87], modulate vasodilation in the vascular system [88], and regulate the action of macrophages in the immune system [89]. NO is also implicated in tumor angiogenesis [90] and Parkinson's disease [91] and it is therefore imperative to detect it with high sensitivity to begin studying how its temporal and spatial release profile changes between the physiological and pathological states of cells. It is particularly challenging to fabricate a NO biosensor with a fast response time to rapidly detect NO, which has a short half life of 5 s [92].

A three-dimensional (3-D) graphene-ionic liquid nanocomposite was reported by our group [93]. The 3-D nanocomposite has high specific surface area, superior conductivity, and high electrocatalytic activity for a highly sensitive NO sensor. The nanocomposite was fabricated as follows. Graphite oxide was heated to 150°C in vacuum for 45 min, then cooled to form the 3-D graphene powder. 1-Butyl-3-methylimidazolium hexafluorophosphate,

TABLE 13.2

Graphene-Based+ Electrochemical Sensors for the Detection of Nitric Oxide and Their Performances[a]

Electrode	Sensitivity[b]/ $\mu A \, \mu M^{-1} \, cm^{-2}$	Detection Limit/μM	Linear Range	Response Time/s	Reference
Nafion/3-D graphene-IL/GCE	11.2	0.016	16 nM to 16 μM	<4	[93]
Nafion/Graphene/GCE	—	0.2	0.72–78.4 μM	<3	[94]
RGD/Graphene-PB film	—	0.025	0.1–100 μM 200–800 μM	—	[95]

Note: "—", denotes a mixture or dispersion; "/" denotes a separate layer; 3-D, 3-dimensional; GCE, glassy carbon electrode; IL, ionic liquid; PB, pyrenebutyric acid; RGD, arginine-glycine-aspartic acid.

[a] The development of NO electrochemical biosensors from 2010 to 2012 has been presented in chronological order.

[b] For general comparison, the sensitivity expressed in $\mu A \, \mu M^{-1} \, cm^{-2}$ was calculated by dividing the reported sensitivity in terms of $\mu A \, \mu M^{-1}$ by the apparent surface area of the working electrode if the electrode dimensions were stated.

an ionic liquid (IL), was mixed together with the 3-D graphene, forming a porous nano-composite gel. This was cast onto a glassy carbon electrode (GCE), followed by a layer of Nafion to prevent leaching of the hydrophobic IL and to potentially prevent interfering species like ascorbic acid and nitrite. The Nafion/3-D graphene–IL/GCE behaved like a planar electrode at low scan rates but a thin-layer cell at high scan rates due to its porosity. NO could be electrocatalytically oxidized on the Nafion/3-D graphene–IL/GCE based on the following electrochemical–chemical reactions:

$$NO - e^- \rightarrow NO^+ \text{ (Electrochemical step)}$$

$$NO^+ + OH^- \rightarrow HNO_2 \rightarrow H^+ + NO_2^- \text{ (Chemical step)}$$

Our sensor achieved a high sensitivity of 11.2 μA μM^{-1} cm^{-2} and a low detection limit of 16 nM (S/N = 3) with a linear range up to 16 μM and fast response less than 4 s.

An electrochemically reduced graphene oxide (erGO) on GCE was reported for the detection of NO by electrochemical oxidation [94]. Graphene oxide was cast onto GCE and reduced to graphene by CV in PBS and Nafion was cast onto the graphene/GCE and prevented the interferences from nitrite and ascorbic acid. The sensor had a sensitivity of 0.299 μA μM^{-1}, detection limit of 0.2 μM (S/N = 3), linear range of 0.72–78.4 μM, and superior response time of less than 3 s. A biomimetic, flexible graphene film for the *in situ* detection of NO released by human umbilical vein endothelial cells (HUVECs) under drug stimulation has been recently developed by our group [95]. Graphene nanosheets were functionalized with pyrenebutyric acid (PB) and filtered to form the graphene–PB film. Arginine–glycine–aspartic acid (RGD) peptide, a cell adhesive ligand, was covalently grafted onto the graphene–PB film to endow it with biomimetic properties. The repro-ducibility of current responses following film bending was demonstrated. The film also showed good selectivity with negligible responses toward interfering species like NO$_2^-$, NO$_3^-$, and ascorbic acid due to the surface carboxylic groups that could repel these anions. The RGD/graphene–PB film exhibited two linear regions for logarithm plot of current against NO concentration and had a detection limit of 25 nM (S/N = 3) in cell culture medium and 80 nM with HUVECs cultured on the film.

Although NO is a very important biological signaling molecule with vital roles in vari-ous cell functions, there are currently only few reports on graphene-based electrochemical biosensors for NO. The hinterland of graphene-based NO biosensors remains much to be explored and we anticipate active developments in this area for *in situ* cell studies in the near future.

13.4.2.3 Graphene for Electrocatalytic Sensing of Dopamine

The graphene planar sheet structure composed of six-carbon rings has a similar structure to dopamine (DA), which is favorable for the adsorption of DA and its electro-oxidation. For the past few years we have witnessed an exponential growth of research works on graphene-based DA biosensors, which are summarized in Table 13.3. DA is an important neurotransmitter that primarily regulates the functions of the central nervous system [96]. Abnormal levels of DA are observed in Parkinson's disease [97] and schizophrenia [98] and also associated with drug addiction [99]. Administration of dopamine into patient serum is found to elicit changes in the immune [100], cardiovascular, and renal systems [101]. The accurate detection of DA would allow us to gain insights into its biological roles and

TABLE 13.3

Graphene-Based Electrochemical Sensors for the Detection of Dopamine and Their Performances[a]

Electrode	Selectivity	Sensitivity[b]/ µA µM⁻¹ cm⁻²	Detection Limit/µM	Linear Range	Reference
Graphene-chitosan/GCE	DA only, negligible response from AA	—	—	5 µM to 0.2 mM	[107]
Graphene-DMF/GCE	Simultaneous detection of DA, AA, ST	—	—	—	[103]
Graphene-DMF/alkanethiol SAM/AuE	Simultaneous detection of DA, AA, UA	—	—	—	[113]
Pt NPs-PFIL-graphene/GCE	Simultaneous detection of DA, AA, UA	—	—	—	[114]
β-cyclodextrin-graphene/GCE	Simultaneous detection of DA, AA	—	0.005	9 nM to 2.0 µM / 2.0 µM to 12.7 mM	[115]
Graphene-DMF/GCE	Simultaneous detection of DA, AA	0.932	2.64	4 µM to 0.1 mM	[116]
Nafion-EDTA-Graphene/GCE	DA only, negligible response from AA	—	0.01	0.2–25 µM	[105]
Nafion-DMF/Cu₂O-graphene/GCE	Simultaneous detection of DA, UA	—	0.01	0.1–10 µM	[117]
Graphene-DMF/carbon fiber microelectrode	Simultaneous detection of DA, UA	26.7	0.01	10 nM to 0.1 mM	[118]
Nafion-Pt NPs-graphene/GCE	Simultaneous detection of DA, AA, UA	4.94	0.03	30 nM to 8.13 µM	[119]
Polycyclodextrin- Graphene-MWCNTs/GCE	Simultaneous detection of DA, AA, NO₂⁻	0.318	0.05	0.15–21.7 µM	[120]
Over-oxidized PPy/graphene/GCE	DA only, negligible response from AA	1.33 / 0.212	0.10	0.5–10.0 µM / 25.0 µM to 1 mM	[121]
PABA/graphene-DMF/GCE	DA only, negligible response from AA	149 / 35.1	0.02	50 nM to 1 µM / 1–10 µM	[122]
Graphene nanosheets molecularly imprinted with DA/GCE	DA only, negligible response from AA, epinephrine	—	0.10	0.1 µM to 0.83 mM	[110]
Au NPs-β-cyclodextrin-graphene/GCE	Simultaneous detection of DA, AA, UA	—	0.15	0.5–4 µM / 4 µM to 0.15 mM	[108]
Graphene-IL SPE	Simultaneous detection of DA, AA, UA	1.08	0.12	0.5 µM to 2 mM	[123]
Au NPs/erGO/GCE	Simultaneous detection of DA, UA, negligible response from AA	—	0.04	0.1–10 µM	[124]

(continued)

TABLE 13.3 (continued)

Graphene-Based Electrochemical Sensors for the Detection of Dopamine and Their Performances[a]

Electrode	Selectivity	Sensitivity[b]/ μA μM⁻¹ cm⁻²	Detection Limit/μM	Linear Range	Reference
Graphene-porphyrin/GCE	Simultaneous detection of DA, AA, UA	19.8	0.01	10 nM to 5 μM	[109]
Nitrogen-doped graphene-DMF/GCE	Simultaneous detection of DA, AA, UA	0.452	0.25	0.5 μM to 0.17 mM	[125]
(Au NPs-PAMAM/Graphene-PSS)$_{20}$/ PDDA/GCE	Simultaneous detection of DA, UA, negligible response from AA	5.46	0.02	1–60 μM	[126]
DA aptamer/Graphene-PANI-DMF/GCE	DA only	—	1.98×10^{-6}	7 pM to 90 nM	[112]
Graphene–chitosan molecularly imprinted with DA/GCE	DA only, negligible responses from AA, UA, urea, creatinine, norepinephrine	2660 13.3	10×10^{-6}	1–80 nM 0.1 μM to 0.1 mM	[111]
Au NPs/erGO/ITO glass	DA only, negligible responses from AA, UA	0.0627	0.06	10 μM to 1 mM	[104]
3-D graphene foam	Simultaneous detection of DA, UA	0.620	0.025	25 nM to 25 μM	[127]
PVP/erGO/GCE	DA only, negligible responses from AA, UA	983	0.0002	0.5 nM to 1.13 mM	[106]

Note: "—" denotes a mixture or dispersion; "/" denotes a separate layer; "()" denotes a multilayer assembly and the number of layers is denoted by the number in subscript; 3-D, 3-dimensional; AA, ascorbic acid; DA, dopamine; DMF, dimethylformamide; erGO, electrochemically reduced graphene oxide; GCE, glassy carbon electrode; IL, ionic liquid; ITO, indium-doped tin oxide; MWCNTs, multi-walled carbon nanotubes; NPs, nanoparticles; PABA, poly(p-aminobenzoic acid); PAMAM, poly(amidoamine); PANI, poly(aniline); PDDA, poly(diallyldimethyl ammonium chloride); PFIL, polyelectrolyte-functionalized ionic liquid; Ppy, poly(pyrrole); PSS, poly(sodium-4-styrenesulfonate); PVP, poly(vinyl pyrrolindone); SAM, self-assembly monolayer; SPE, screen-printed electrode; ST: serotonin; UA, uric acid.

a   The development of dopamine electrochemical biosensors from 2009 to 2012 has been presented in chronological order.

b   For general comparison, the sensitivity expressed in μA μM⁻¹ cm⁻² was calculated by dividing the reported sensitivity in terms of μA μM⁻¹ by the apparent surface area of the working electrode if the electrode dimensions were stated.

could be predictor of such diseases or conditions while allowing the evaluation of drug efficacy for the development of more effective drugs. The electrochemical detection of DA provides advantages of simplicity, rapid detection, and great potential for portable devices. However, it requires very good selectivity as its oxidation peak can be easily masked by several biological compounds like ascorbic acid (AA) and uric acid (UA), which coexist with DA in high concentrations in biological systems and have similar oxidation potentials, making the discrimination of DA from these compounds challenging [102]. Graphene has some extraordinary properties including high electrocatalytic activity from its abundant edge sites/surface functional groups, large contact surface area, and in particular, a planar sheet composed of six-carbon rings that have a similar structure to DA.

Graphene dispersed in dimethylformamide (DMF) was cast onto a GCE for the detection of DA [103]. The graphene–DMF/GCE displayed a pair of well-defined redox peaks in its CV curve for DA oxidation, which occurs as a two-electron transfer process where DA loses two electrons and two protons and is oxidized to dopamine-o-quinone [104]. In comparison, single-walled carbon nanotubes (SWCNTs)–DMF/GCE shows a much smaller response. It was proposed that the much higher response on graphene–DMF/GCE could be because graphene possesses more sp^2-like domains and edge defects than SWCNTs. The sensitivity of DA biosensors is generally obtained from differential pulse voltammetry (DPV) measurements as DPV is a more sensitive electrochemical technique than cyclic voltammetry (CV). The DPV response of DA on graphene–DMF/GCE was recorded in a mixed sample of 0.1 mM DA, 1 mM AA, and 1 mM ST. The sensor could differentiate all three compounds with well-resolved peaks, which was possible because graphene possesses an appropriate amount of negative charge.

Graphene has also been combined with materials such as Nafion [105], PVP [106], and AuNPs [104] to fabricate graphene nanocomposites with good selectivity for DA detection. Graphene–chitosan (graphene–CS) was cast onto GCE for the detection of DA [107] and exhibited a pair of well-defined redox peaks for DA oxidation with negligible response for AA, demonstrating the good selectivity of the biosensor toward DA. The authors postulated that the good selectivity for graphene–CS toward DA might have arisen from the strong π–π interactions between the phenyl structure of DA and the 2-D planar hexagonal structure of graphene. Many other graphene nanocomposites including Au NPs–β-cyclodextrin–graphene [108] and graphene–porphyrin [109] have also been fabricated for high-performance DA electrochemical sensors. Notably, novel approaches like molecularly imprinted (MIP) matrices [110,111] and advanced functional materials such as aptamers [112] have been also used together with graphene to offer superior selectivity and high sensitivity.

The rapid growth of graphene and its nanocomposites has dramatically increased DA detection sensitivities by three orders of magnitude, significantly pushed down the limits to the nM and even pM, and widened linear ranges up to the mM while providing high selectivity. With the biocompatibility of graphene, the development of implantable and portable graphene-based DA electrochemical biosensors will be an exciting area that will greatly aids *in vivo* DA studies.

13.4.3 Graphene for Label-Free Electrochemical Immunosensors

Label-free electrochemical immunosensors allow facile, one-step detection of antigens compared to sandwich-type immunoassays that require labeling with secondary antibodies [128]. In principle, the highly specific binding of the antigen to the antibody can be easily monitored by electrochemical techniques such as CV [128–133] and DPV [134–137].

Typically, the binding of the antigen from the solution to the antibody immobilized on the electrode results in a decrease in current response as the antigen is nonconductive and increases the charge transfer resistance [137]. Graphene and its nanocomposites with desired properties have been used to fabricate highly sensitive electrochemical immuno-sensors. The use of graphene with electron mediators [128,131,134,136], metal nanoparticles [129,130,134–136], and polymers [132,133,137] can synergistically enhance the performances of these electrochemical immunosensors. The good electrical properties of these graphene nanocomposites allow the detection of the antigen with high sensitivity. Moreover, the large specific surface area of these graphene nanocomposites promotes high loading of antibodies and can improve the accessibility of binding sites to antigens by orienting the antibodies away from the electrode surface and into the solution [134]. These favorable characteristics allow the ng mL^{-1} and even pg mL^{-1} detection of biomarkers and some examples are given in Table 13.4.

Instead of measuring the binding-induced change in current response, another approach to monitor the response catalytically involves incorporating an enzyme into the graphene-based electrochemical immunosensor [134]. Thionine was electropolymerized on a GCE to form poly(thionine) (PTH), which acted as the electron mediator. Graphene–chitosan nanocomposite was cast on the PTH electrode, which was used as the matrix to immobilize

TABLE 13.4

Graphene Nanocomposites for Label-Free Electrochemical Immunosensors and Their Performances[a]

Electrode	Biomarkers	Detection Limit/pg mL^{-1}	Linear Range/ng mL^{-1}	Reference
Anti-AFP/graphene-thionine/GCE	α-Fetoprotein	5.77	0.05–2	[128]
HRP-anti-AFP/Au NPs/graphene-chitosan/PTH/GCE	α-Fetoprotein	700	1–10	[134]
Anti-AFP/Au NPs/Amine-functionalized graphene/IL-graphite paste electrode	α-Fetoprotein	100	1–250	[135]
Anti-PSA/Co NPs-graphene-PBSE/GCE	Prostate-specific antigen	10	0.02–2	[129]
Anti-hCG/nanoporous Au/Graphene/GCE	Human chorionic gonadotropin	34	0.5–40	[130]
Anti-CEA/Au NPs-graphene/Fc-chitosan-TiO$_2$/GCE	Carcinoembryonic antigen	3.4	0.01–80	[131]
Anti-CEA/AuNPs-graphene-thionine/GCE	Carcinoembryonic antigen	4.0	0.01–0.5	[136]
Anti-CEA/AuNPs/PLA/graphene-DMF/IL-graphite paste electrode	Carcinoembryonic antigen	30	0.5–200	[137]
Anti-PSA/graphene-methylene blue-chitosan/GCE	Prostate-specific antigen	13	0.05–5	[132]
Anti-TM/Ag-Ag$_2$O NPs/graphene-Nafion/AuE	Thrombomodulin	31.5	0.1–20	[133]

Note: "-" denotes a mixture or dispersion; "/" denotes a separate layer; AFP, α-fetoprotein; AuE, gold electrode; CEA, carcinoembryonic antigen; DMF, dimethylformamide; Fc, ferrocene; GCE, glassy carbon electrode; hCG, human chorionic gonadotropin; HRP, horseradish peroxidase; IL, ionic liquid; NPs, nanoparticles; PBSE, 1-pyrenebutanoic acid succinimidyl ester; PLA, poly(L-arginine); PSA, prostate specific antigen; PTH, poly(thionine); TM, thrombomodulin.

[a] The development of some electrochemical immunosensors from 2010 to 2012 has been presented in chrono-logical order.

Au NPs and subsequently horseradish peroxidase (HRP)–anti-α-fetoprotein. The remaining electrode surface was passivated with bovine serum albumin. In the presence of H_2O_2 but not the antigen α-fetoprotein, HRP catalyzed the reduction of H_2O_2 and a cathodic current peak corresponding to the regeneration of PTH at the electrode was produced. When α-fetoprotein was present along with H_2O_2, the binding of α-fetoprotein to the HRP–anti-α-fetoprotein caused a decrease in cathodic current, possibly because the active site of the HRP was blocked or H_2O_2 could no longer reach the enzyme.

For graphene-based label-free electrochemical immunosensors no matter the use of binding-induced changes in current response or monitoring the current response catalytically by incorporating an enzyme, the ability to detect trace amounts of biomarkers in one step makes them highly attractive for clinical applications and is very useful for early disease diagnosis and monitoring of disease progression.

13.4.4 Graphene-Based Electrochemical Living Cell Assays

As a superior dimensionally compatible, mechanically strong, electrically conductive, and highly electrocatalytic component, graphene could be used to build a smart biointerface for electrochemical living cell assays. Compared to the needle-like structures of CNTs, which risk penetrating membranes to damage cells, the 2-D flat structure of graphene with large contact surface area offers much better biocompatibility. In addition, graphene can be electrophoretically deposited onto substrates with well-controlled film thickness and easily functionalized with cell-adhesive ligands for cell adhesion [67]. It is very feasible to make free-standing, flexible biosensors [95].

A cell is the basic structural and functional unit of all known living organisms. Living cell analysis is not only fundamentally essential to understand various biological functions but also provides great potentials for a wide variety of practical applications. Cell–cell communication is facilitated by the release of biochemical messengers from a cell to its bonded target cell to trigger biological responses. Many biochemical messengers including H_2O_2, NO, and O_2 molecules are electroactive and can be detected by electrochemical biosensors. Therefore, real-time electrochemical living cell assays is highly significant in probing the biological processes of cells during responses to their biochemical environment. However, the release or uptake process of the triggers is very fast and the messenger molecules are often present in trace amounts. It is essential to use a high-performance sensing platform for high specificity, sensitivity, and fast response toward detection of a target molecule. Moreover, real-time living cell assays require an interface with good biocompatibility to promote cell growth and retain the cells in their native states without changing the physiochemical and biological properties of both the cells and their surrounding environment [50,67,138]. It is highly challenging to construct smart biosensors to electrochemically analyze living cells in real-time.

A nanolayered graphene-based smart multifunctional electrochemical biointerface has been built by layer-by-layer electrodeposition of graphene with Prussian blue (PB) and extracellular matrix protein (laminin) as building blocks on transparent conducting glass (Figure 13.4) [67]. In this interface, graphene acts as the basic scaffold to deposit PB and laminin and provides good electrical conductivity for electrochemical detection as well as a dimensionally compatible interface for the growth of MCF-7 (human breast endocarcinoma) cells. PB functions as an artificial peroxidase for the electrocatalytic reduction of H_2O_2 while laminin enhances cell adhesion and growth on the interface. This graphene-based nanolayered multifunctional sensing platform showed superior sensitivity and selectivity toward H_2O_2 and enabled excellent cell growth. With these extraordinary characteristics,

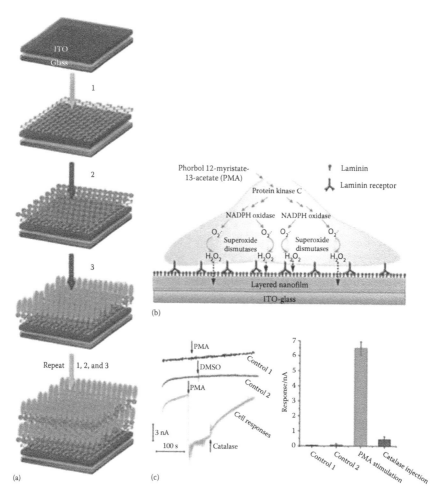

FIGURE 13.4

(See color insert.) (a) Fabrication process of nanolayered graphene-based film. (1) Electrophoretic deposition of graphene. (2) Electrochemical deposition of Prussian blue. (3) Dip coating of laminin. (b) Scheme showing the pathway of PMA-triggered H_2O_2 production from a MCF-7 cell and its detection by the nanolayered graphene-based film. (c) Amperometric responses obtained at nanolayered graphene-based film without cells (control 1) and with cultured cells under injection of DMSO, the solvent for PMA (control 2), and with cultured cells under PMA, followed by catalase injection. The corresponding current responses are shown on the right of (c). (From Guo, C.X. et al.: Biointerface by cell growth on layered graphene–artificial peroxidase–protein nanostructure for *in situ* quantitative molecular detection, *Adv. Mater.* 2010. 22. 5164–5167. Copyright Wiley-VCH Verlag GmbH & Co. KGaA. With permission.)

the multifunctional sensing platform was applied to the quantitative real-time detection of extracellular H_2O_2 released by the MCF-7 cells following phorbol 12-myristate-13-acetate (PMA) stimulation. Upon the injection of PMA, an increased cathodic current corresponding to the reduction of H_2O_2 was observed and 10^{11} H_2O_2 molecules were found to be released per cell. Other graphene-based platforms including a flexible Au NPs/graphene paper [71] and a flexible Pt NPs/MnO_2 nanowires/graphene paper [80] have also been recently reported for real-time electrochemical detection of H_2O_2 in living cells assays.

NO is a biological messenger that plays vital roles in regulating the cell functions of the nervous, vascular, and immune systems. However, live-cell NO detection is still a challenge because NO is rapidly metabolized and degraded under cell-culture conditions and its diffusion distance is also limited. To address this problem, a smart graphene-based functional biomimetic film sensor was constructed by covalently bonding RGD-peptide onto the graphene surface [95]. Graphene, with its high electrical conductivity, was employed as the basic building block to fabricate a biofilm for high sensitivity toward NO detection. Graphene oxide was reduced and functionalized with pyrenebutyric acid via π–π interactions and the solution was filtered to form the graphene biofilm. The bio-mimetic surface was achieved through the covalent bonding of graphene biofilm with the RGD-peptide via ethyl(dimethylaminopropyl) carbodiimide/hydrosulfosuccinimide (EDC/NHS) coupling. The peptide moiety of RGD mimics the cell-binding sequence of extracellular matrix proteins and can promote good cell adhesion via integrin ligation. The covalent bonding of the RGD-peptide to the biofilm provided excellent stability for immobilized molecules and the biofilm retained its surface carboxyl groups from chemi-cally reduced graphene oxide/pyrenebutyric acid. These negative charges could help repel negatively charged interfering species such as nitrite and ascorbic acid, resulting in good selectivity for NO. Human umbilical vein endothelial cells (HUVECs) were cul-tured on the biofilm and the detection of NO released by these cells under drug stimu-lation was used to demonstrate its real-time NO sensing capabilities. The NO release profile following acetylcholine stimulation was found to be dose-dependent and the release of NO was inhibited by N^G-nitro-L-arginine-methyl ester (L-NAME) as expected, demonstrating the ability of the biofilm for real-time *in situ* NO measurements and sug-gesting its potentials for monitoring drug therapy effects on live-cells. The applications of this graphene-based biofilm can also be extended to studying the real-time NO release behaviors of other cell types.

O$_2$ molecules participate in several important functions in cells, such as acting as an electron acceptor in the mitochondria. However, the stepwise reduction of O$_2$ produces a number of potentially harmful oxygen metabolites including H_2O_2, superoxide anion radicals, and hydroxyl radicals, which may be involved in many pathological events such as lipid peroxidation, organ injury, DNA damage, and tumor formation [139]. A selective and sensitive platform for the accurate determination of O$_2$ is required to gain a full under-standing of the role of oxygen in physiology and pathology. In order to detect extracellular O$_2$, a graphene film with enzyme laccase and 2,2-azino-bis(3-ethylbenzothiazoling-6-sulfonic acid) (ABTS) was developed [140]. Laccase is an enzyme that selectively catalyzes O$_2$ reduction. Being the mediator for laccase, ABTS with aromatic rings can assemble on graphene surface via π–π interactions while its negatively charged groups can inter-act electrostatically with the positively charged laccase for the immobilization of laccase onto graphene. The laccase–ABTS–graphene was successfully used to selectively monitor O$_2$ molecules released by the cell-packed pellet of erythrocytes following stimulation by NaNO$_2$. However, it was difficult to precisely determinate the number of O$_2$ molecules released from the erythrocytes as some O$_2$ molecules were inevitably released before the addition of NaNO$_2$. Nevertheless, this graphene-based platform provides a great potential in understanding the kinetics of O$_2$ release from cells, which might be helpful for physi-ological and pathological studies.

Although graphene and its nanocomposites have been successfully utilized in real-time electrochemical living cell assays and have helped us to understand more about the bio-logical processes of cells in real-time, the number of reported works for such an applica-tion is still limited. With the development of a myriad of graphene-based electrochemical biosensors, we anticipate increasing attention in this emerging research area and more exciting reports on electrochemical living cell assays in the near future.

13.5 Graphene Nanocomposites and Their Electrochemical Biosensors

Although graphene is an extraordinary material with various superior properties, its broad applications greatly rely on its further functionalization enhancement. Nanocomposites capitalize on the advantages of their individual components while totally or at least partially compensating for their weaknesses. The types of materials to compose with graphene can be divided into two categories, inorganic and organic. We survey the use of some inorganic and organic materials for graphene nanocomposites and their notable properties that contribute to high-performance electrochemical biosensors.

Inorganic materials such as metal and metal oxide nanoparticles (NPs) have been a largely popular choice for graphene nanocomposites. Au NPs, Ag NPs, and Pt NPs offer high surface area-to-volume ratio and are well-known for their good electrocatalytic performances. Graphene provides a large, flat surface for the high density loading of these NPs, increasing the number of electrocatalytic sites for the reactions to occur and improving charge transfer. Nanocomposites of graphene decorated with these NPs can be prepared by the chemical reduction or heating of precursors of these NPs with graphene either in one-pot techniques [77,79] or electrochemical reduction in a separate step [80]. The NPs can also be synthesized first and then allowed to be adsorbed onto graphene [135]. The use of graphene–metal NP nanocomposites has proved successful for establishing DET of different kinds of enzymes as well as the electrocatalytic detection of many small molecules such as H_2O_2 and dopamine and has also found applications in live-cell electrochemical biosensors. Au NPs are a good choice for high-performance electrochemical immunosensors because they help to immobilize the antibodies and can also aid in orienting the antibodies toward the solution to expose their binding sites [134]. Nanostructured metal oxides such as Fe_3O_4 NPs, TiO_2 NPs, MnO_2 nanowires, and ZnO microflowers have also been employed in graphene nanocomposites. ZnO microflowers with large surface areas and highly porous structure were used to prepare graphene–ZnO microflowers, which demonstrated a high performance for H_2O_2 sensing with a superior sensitivity of 13.5 μA μM^{-1} cm^{-2} over a linear range of 1 –22.5 μM, a detection limit of 20 nM, and fast response time of <5 s [85]. Graphene–metal oxide–metal nanocomposites have also been reported and used for electrochemical biosensors. MnO_2 nanowires deposited on graphene were used as a matrix to accommodate Pt NPs for creating a hierarchically structured nanocomposite of graphene–metal oxide–metal [80], which shows improved sensitivity and detection limits toward H_2O_2.

A wide range of organic materials such as polymers, polyelectrolytes, and aromatic molecules have also been incorporated with graphene to prepare graphene nanocomposites. Chitosan is biocompatible and positively charged and often used to prepare graphene–chitosan nanocomposites for the incorporation of negatively charged enzymes for enzyme-based electrochemical biosensors [141]. The use of polyelectrolytes to assemble layer-by-layer graphene nanocomposites has also been reported. Poly(vinyl pyrrolidone) (PVP), a neutral nonionic macromolecule, was combined with graphene to form a defect-free layer of graphene–PVP nanocomposite, which was highly selective for dopamine sensing [106]. Another notable organic compound is IL, which possesses high intrinsic ionic conductivity and electrochemical stability and can act as a binder to graphene through cationic–π and/or π–π interaction. Graphene–IL nanocomposites can be easily prepared by mixing the two together. A 3-D graphene–IL nanocomposite was prepared and used for the highly sensitive detection of NO [93]. Aromatic molecules can be combined with graphene via π–π interactions to prepare functionalized graphene. One such example is the graphene–pyrenebutyric acid nanocomposite, in which pyrenebutyric acid functionalization increases the number of carboxylic acid groups on graphene for the covalent attachment of cell-adhesive peptides to construct biomimetic cell surfaces, providing a biocompatible sensing platform for real-time living cell NO detection [95].

The synergistic combination of both inorganic and organic materials with graphene opens up endless possibilities for unique nanocomposites with interesting properties for electrochemical biosensor applications. With increasing attention and effort, we highly anticipate the development of novel graphene nanocomposites and their applications to take us forward in gaining a better understanding of cell biology and pathology and developing novel approaches for disease diagnosis and intervention.

13.6 Perspectives

As a building block to form different dimensional graphitic materials, graphene exhibits extraordinary properties of unique bandgap structure, specific electronic properties, high electron transfer/transport rate, excellent chemical properties, and well-defined optical and mechanical properties. As a 2-D planar sheet with sp^2-bonded carbon atoms perfectly arranged in a honeycomb structure with a large contact surface area, graphene has been further functionalized with different chemical functional groups or composed with many other materials to fabricate graphene nanocomposites with properties tailored to various applications. Graphene, graphene functionalization by surface modification, and its nanocomposites have demonstrated excellent performances in various electrochemical biosensors including the DET-based electrochemical enzyme biosensors, electrocatalytic small biomolecule sensors, label-free electrochemical immunosensors, and electrochemical living cell assays.

The development of graphene-based electrochemical biosensors has been fuelled up. The great challenges for further advances in graphene-related scientific research still remain. Drug monitoring is a new research area with great importance in pharmacology and disease therapy. Most drugs are aromatic molecules that have been widely utilized as components of therapeutic drugs effective against various diseases. Real-time monitoring aromatic drug molecules should be very useful in understanding their biological roles and therapeutic effects on diseases. With a similar structure to the aromatic drug molecules, graphene could absorb these aromatic drug molecules and can be used as active component to construct electrocatalytic or affinity biosensors for real-time monitoring of these drug molecules. For drugs without aromatic structures but with known antibodies, the designs of graphene-based label-free electrochemical immunosensors are also possible for real-time monitoring of these drugs.

A better understanding of the interactions between molecules/bimolecules with graphene at the interface can further advance graphene science and broaden the use of graphene for electrochemical biosensors. The interactions of graphene with different molecules include the adsorption mechanism, orientation of molecules/biomolecules on the graphene surface, and effects of these interactions on the charge transfer/transport behaviors of graphene. Theoretical studies, delicate experimental designs, and persistent investigations are important to understand the fundamental insights. One challenge of incorporating graphene into an electrochemical biosensor device is its ease of aggregation arising from its 2-D structure with single-atom thickness, resulting in weakened or even totally lost advantages. Moreover, due to insufficient binding sites, it is difficult to deposit or grow ultrasmall and uniformly distributed active components/materials on the graphene surface. Surface functionalization can provide rich surface chemistries for graphene to overcome the challenge. A suitable functional agent should be carefully chosen to modify graphene with required functionalization for its specific electrochemical biosensor application. Nevertheless, functionalization of graphene with designed components at a molecular level to control location and distribution of electroactive sites on the surface is still an arduous task. Doping graphene with heteroatoms such as nitrogen and boron is an effective approach to enhance the electrocatalytic properties and stability of doped graphene electrodes for high-performance electrochemical sensors. The successful doping strategies from CNTs can be utilized for graphene doping. However, it would be wise to avoid use of harsh conditions such as extremely high temperature, which makes graphene restack more easily. Alternatively, mild doping strategies are preferred. Functionalized/doped graphene can further be combined with other active materials to construct advanced graphene nanocomposites with novel properties, which might be beneficial for producing optimized graphene-based electrochemical sensors.

Finally, we envision more exciting developments of various nanostructured graphene materials, which are another promising research direction to achieve graphene-based high-performance electrochemical biosensors. Free-standing graphene films have been fabricated with different methods and explored in applications of electrochemical biosensors. However, the properties of these graphene films are primarily inherent in the 2-D graphene sheets. The fabrication of nanostructured graphene materials including hierarchical 3-D graphene materials with abundant edges and nanopores, 2-D graphene nanoribbons (GNRs) with quantum confinement in one of the two planar directions, and 0-D graphene quantum dots (GQDs) might provide unique advantages for specific electrochemical biosensors. Compared with 2-D graphene sheets, hierarchical 3-D graphene materials can provide several advantages such as high specific surface area, unique pore structures, multi-dimensional electron transport pathways, easy access to the solid-state electrolyte, and minimized transport distances between the bulk electrode and electrolyte. Currently, methods to prepare hierarchical 3-D graphene materials include low-temperature vacuum exfoliation of graphite oxide, template-directed CVD, and the fabrication of graphene aerogels. These hierarchical 3-D graphene materials provide immense potentials for high performance electrochemical biosensors. When one of its lateral dimensions shrinks to the nanoscale, graphene becomes GNRs, which may transform into a semiconductor with a large bandgap due to quantum confinement of the electron wave function. GNRs have similar functions to CNTs but provide large contact surface areas and are easy to manipulate. Several approaches including longitudinally unzipping CNTs, templated growth on SiC, surface-assisted bottom-up synthesis, and top-down lithographic fabrication have been reported to prepare GNRs. When both lateral dimensions shrink to the nanoscale, graphene forms GQDs, which exhibit unique optical and electronic properties due to their quantum confinement and edge effects. To date, methods developed to prepare GQDs include cutting large graphene oxide sheets via a hydrothermal route, electrochemical approach, mechanical grinding, exfoliation of natural graphite in a small quantity of ionic liquid, and carbonizing suitable organic precursors by thermal treatment. Despite their recent emergence, these nanostructured graphene materials including hierarchical 3-D graphene materials, 1-D GNRs, 0-D GQDs, and even porous graphene materials hold tremendous potentials for performance enhancement and the development of novel types of high-performance electrochemical biosensors.

References

1. Geim, A.K. and K.S. Novoselov, *The rise of graphene. Nature Materials*, 2007. **6**(3):183–191.
2. Rao, C.N.R. et al., Graphene: The new two-dimensional nanomaterial. *Angewandte Chemie International Edition*, 2009. **48**(42):7752–7777.
3. Guo, C.X. et al., A hierarchically nanostructured composite of MnO2/conjugated polymer/ graphene for high-performance lithium ion batteries. *Advanced Energy Materials*, 2011. **1**(5):736–741.
4. Guo, C.X., G.H. Guai, and C.M. Li, Graphene based materials: Enhancing solar energy harvesting. *Advanced Energy Materials*, 2011. **1**(3):448–452.
5. Zhu, Y. et al., Graphene and graphene oxide: Synthesis, properties, and applications. *Advanced Materials*, 2010. **22**(35):3906–3924.
6. Allen, M.J., V.C. Tung, and R.B. Kaner, Honeycomb carbon: A review of graphene. *Chemical Reviews*, 2009. **110**(1):132–145.
7. Guo, C.X. and C.M. Li, A self-assembled hierarchical nanostructure comprising carbon spheres and graphene nanosheets for enhanced supercapacitor performance. *Energy & Environmental Science*, 2011. **4**(11):4504–4507.
8. Wang, Y. et al., Hydrogen storage in a Ni-B nanoalloy-doped three-dimensional graphene material. *Energy & Environmental Science*, 2011. **4**(1):195–200.
9. Ronkainen, N.J., H.B. Halsall, and W.R. Heineman, Electrochemical biosensors. *Chemical Society Reviews*, 2010. **39**(5):1747–1763.
10. Chen, D., G. Wang, and J. Li, Interfacial bioelectrochemistry: Fabrication, properties and applications of functional nanostructured biointerfaces. *The Journal of Physical Chemistry C*, 2006. **111**(6):2351–2367.
11. Chen, D., L. Tang, and J. Li, Graphene-based materials in electrochemistry. *Chemical Society Reviews*, 2010. **39**(8):3157–3180.
12. Liu, Y., X. Dong, and P. Chen, Biological and chemical sensors based on graphene materials. *Chemical Society Reviews*, 2012. **41**(6):2283–2307.
13. Pumera, M., Graphene-based nanomaterials and their electrochemistry. *Chemical Society Reviews*, 2010. **39**(11):4146–4157.
14. Bonaccorso, F. et al., Graphene photonics and optoelectronics. *Nature Photonics*, 2010. **4**(9):611–622.
15. Avouris, P., Graphene: Electronic and photonic properties and devices. *Nano Letters*, 2010. **10**(11):4285–4294.
16. Chen, J.H. et al., Intrinsic and extrinsic performance limits of graphene devices on SiO2. *Nature Nanotechnology*, 2008. **3**(4):206–209.
17. Sun, Z., D.K. James, and J.M. Tour, Graphene chemistry: Synthesis and manipulation. *The Journal of Physical Chemistry Letters*, 2011. **2**(19):2425–2432.
18. Jin, Z. et al., Large-scale growth and characterizations of nitrogen-doped monolayer graphene sheets. *ACS Nano*, 2011. **5**(5):4112–4117.
19. Lin, Y.-C., C.-Y. Lin, and P.-W. Chiu, Controllable graphene N-doping with ammonia plasma. *Applied Physics Letters*, 2010. **96**(13):133110.
20. Li, X. et al., Simultaneous nitrogen doping and reduction of graphene oxide. *Journal of the American Chemical Society*, 2009. **131**(43):15939–15944.
21. Elias, D.C. et al., Control of graphene's properties by reversible hydrogenation: Evidence for graphane. *Science*, 2009. **323**(5914):610–613.
22. Lomeda, J.R. et al., Diazonium functionalization of surfactant-wrapped chemically converted graphene sheets. *Journal of the American Chemical Society*, 2008. **130**(48):16201–16206.
23. Xu, Y.X. et al., Flexible graphene films via the filtration of water-soluble noncovalent functionalized graphene sheets. *Journal of the American Chemical Society*, 2008. **130**(18):5856–5857.
24. Wang, R. X., Huang, L. F., and Tian, X. Y., Understanding the protonation of polyaniline and polyaniline–graphene interaction. *The Journal of Physical Chemistry C*, 2012. **116**(24):13120–13126.

25. Bai, H. et al., Non-covalent functionalization of graphene sheets by sulfonated polyaniline. *Chemical Communications*, **2009**(13):1667–1669.
26. Shao, Y. et al., Graphene based electrochemical sensors and biosensors: A review. *Electroanalysis*, 2010. **22**(10):1027–1036.
27. Nair, R.R. et al., Fine structure constant defines visual transparency of graphene. *Science*, 2008. **320**(5881):1308–1308.
28. Yao, J. et al., Chemistry, physics and biology of graphene-based nanomaterials: New horizons for sensing, imaging and medicine. *Journal of Materials Chemistry*, 2012. **22**(29):14313–14329.
29. Booth, T.J. et al., Macroscopic graphene membranes and their extraordinary stiffness. *Nano Letters*, 2008. **8**(8):2442–2446.
30. Bunch, J.S. et al., Electromechanical resonators from graphene sheets. *Science*, 2007. **315**(5811):490–493.
31. Novoselov, K.S. et al., Electric field effect in atomically thin carbon films. *Science*, 2004. **306**(5696):666–669.
32. Jiang, H.J., Chemical preparation of graphene-based nanomaterials and their applications in chemical and biological sensors. *Small*, 2011. **7**(17):2413–2427.
33. Li, D. et al., Processable aqueous dispersions of graphene nanosheets. *Nature Nanotechnology*, 2008. **3**(2):101–105.
34. Shao, Y. et al., Facile and controllable electrochemical reduction of graphene oxide and its applications. *Journal of Materials Chemistry*, 2010. **20**(4):743–748.
35. Li, X.-H. et al., A green chemistry of graphene: Photochemical reduction towards monolayer graphene sheets and the role of water adlayers. *ChemSusChem*, 2012. **5**(4):642–646.
36. Guo, C.X. et al., Ionic liquid–graphene composite for ultratrace explosive trinitrotoluene detection. *Electrochemistry Communications*, 2010. **12**(9):1237–1240.
37. Kosynkin, D.V. et al., Longitudinal unzipping of carbon nanotubes to form graphene nanoribbons. *Nature*, 2009. **458**(7240):872-U5.
38. Jiao, L.Y. et al., Narrow graphene nanoribbons from carbon nanotubes. *Nature*, 2009. **458**(7240):877–880.
39. Reina, A. et al., Large area, few-layer graphene films on arbitrary substrates by chemical vapor deposition. *Nano Letters*, 2009. **9**(1):30–35.
40. Mattevi, C., H. Kim, and M. Chhowalla, A review of chemical vapour deposition of graphene on copper. *Journal of Materials Chemistry*, 2011. **21**(10):3324–3334.
41. Chen, Z.P. et al., Three-dimensional flexible and conductive interconnected graphene networks grown by chemical vapour deposition. *Nature Materials*, 2011. **10**(6):424–428.
42. Al-Temimy, A., C. Riedl, and U. Starke, Low temperature growth of epitaxial graphene on SiC induced by carbon evaporation. *Applied Physics Letters*, 2009. **95**(23):231907.
43. Güell, A.G. et al., Structural correlations in heterogeneous electron transfer at monolayer and multilayer graphene electrodes. *Journal of the American Chemical Society*, 2012. **134**(17):7258–7261.
44. Guo, C.X. et al., Thin-walled graphitic nanocages as a unique platform for amperometric glucose biosensor. *ACS Applied Materials & Interfaces*, 2010. **2**(9):2481–2484.
45. Yang, W. et al., Carbon nanomaterials in biosensors: Should you use nanotubes or graphene? *Angewandte Chemie International Edition*, 2010. **49**(12):2114–2138.
46. Brownson, D.A.C. and C.E. Banks, Graphene electrochemistry: An overview of potential applications. *Analyst*, 2010. **135**(11):2768–2778.
47. Chang, J.L. et al., Improved voltammetric peak separation and sensitivity of uric acid and ascorbic acid at nanoplatelets of graphitic oxide. *Electrochemistry Communications*, 2010. **12**(4):596–599.
48. Wang, Z. et al., Direct electrochemical reduction of single-layer graphene oxide and subsequent functionalization with glucose oxidase. *The Journal of Physical Chemistry C*, 2009. **113**(32):14071–14075.
49. Guo, C.X. and C.M. Li, Direct electron transfer of glucose oxidase and biosensing of glucose on hollow sphere-nanostructured conducting polymer/metal oxide composite. *Physical Chemistry Chemical Physics*, 2010. **12**(38):12153–12159.

50. Guo, C.X. et al., in situ molecular detection of ischemic cells by enhanced protein direct electron transfer on a unique horseradish peroxidase-Au nanoparticles-polyaniline nanowires biofilm. *Chemical Communications*, 2011. **47**(9):2652–2654.

51. Liu, J. et al., Carbon-decorated ZnO nanowire array: A novel platform for direct electrochemistry of enzymes and biosensing applications. *Electrochemistry Communications*, 2009. **11**(1):202–205.

52. Guo, C. et al., Direct electrochemistry of hemoglobin on carbonized titania nanotubes and its application in a sensitive reagentless hydrogen peroxide biosensor. *Biosensors and Bioelectronics*, 2008. **24**(4):819–824.

53. Shan, C. et al., Direct electrochemistry of glucose oxidase and biosensing for glucose based on graphene. *Analytical Chemistry*, 2009. **81**(6):2378–2382.

54. Li, M. et al., Direct electrochemistry of horseradish peroxidase on graphene-modified electrode for electrocatalytic reduction towards H2O2. *Electrochimica Acta*, 2011. **56**(3):1144–1149.

55. Zhang, Q. et al., Direct electrochemistry and electrocatalysis of horseradish peroxidase immobilized on water soluble sulfonated graphene film via self-assembly. *Electroanalysis*, 2011. **23**(4):900–906.

56. Kang, X. et al., Glucose oxidase–graphene–chitosan modified electrode for direct electrochemistry and glucose sensing. *Biosensors and Bioelectronics*, 2009. **25**(4):901–905.

57. Wang, G.-X. et al., Direct electrochemistry of cytochrome c on a graphene/poly (3,4-ethylenedioxythiophene) nanocomposite modified electrode. *Electrochemistry Communications*, 2012. **20**:1–3.

58. Liu, K. et al., Direct electrochemistry and electrocatalysis of hemoglobin based on poly(diallyldimethylammonium chloride) functionalized graphene sheets/room temperature ionic liquid composite film. *Electrochemistry Communications*, 2010. **12**(3):402–405.

59. Liao, H.-g. et al., Direct electrochemistry and electrocatalysis of myoglobin immobilized on graphene-CTAB-ionic liquid nanocomposite film. *Electroanalysis*, 2010. **22**(19):2297–2302.

60. Zhou, Y. et al., Direct electrochemistry and bioelectrocatalysis of microperoxidase-11 immobilized on chitosan-graphene nanocomposite. *Electroanalysis*, 2010. **22**(12):1323–1328.

61. Wen, W. et al., A highly sensitive nitric oxide biosensor based on hemoglobin–chitosan/graphene–hexadecyltrimethylammonium bromide nanomatrix. *Sensors and Actuators B*, 2012. **166–167**:444–450.

62. Palanisamy, S. et al., direct electrochemistry of glucose oxidase at reduced graphene oxide/zinc oxide composite modified electrode for glucose sensor. *International Journal of Electrochemical Science*, 2012. **7**:2153–2163.

63. Shen, Q. et al., Anatase TiO2 nanoparticle-graphene nanocomposites: One-step preparation and their enhanced direct electrochemistry of hemoglobin. *Analytical Methods*, 2012. **4**(3):619–622.

64. He, Y. et al., Magnetite–graphene for the direct electrochemistry of hemoglobin and its biosensing application. *Electrochimica Acta*, 2011. **56**(5):2471–2476.

65. Rojkind, M. et al., Role of hydrogen peroxide and oxidative stress in healing responses. *Cellular and Molecular Life Sciences*, 2002. **59**(11):1872–1891.

66. Maynard, S. et al., Base excision repair of oxidative DNA damage and association with cancer and aging. *Carcinogenesis*, 2009. **30**(1):2–10.

67. Guo, C.X. et al., Biointerface by cell growth on layered graphene–artificial peroxidase–protein nanostructure for in situ quantitative molecular detection. *Advanced Materials*, 2010. **22**:5164–5167.

68. Katsounaros, I. et al., Hydrogen peroxide electrochemistry on platinum: towards understanding the oxygen reduction reaction mechanism. *Physical Chemistry Chemical Physics*, 2012. **14**:7384–7391.

69. Wu, P. et al., Facile synthesis of nitrogen-doped graphene for measuring the releasing process of hydrogen peroxide from living cells. *Journal of Materials Chemistry*, 2012. **22**:6402–6412.

70. Fang, Y. et al., Self-assembly of cationic polyelectrolyte-functionalized graphene nanosheets and gold nanoparticles: A two-dimensional heterostructure for hydrogen peroxide sensing. *Langmuir*, 2010. **26**(13):11277–11282.

71. Xiao, F. et al., Coating graphene paper with 2D-Assembly of electrocatalytic nanoparticles: A modular approach toward high-performance flexible electrodes. *ACS Nano*, 2012. **6**(1):100–110.

72. Liu, R. et al., Facile synthesis of Au-nanoparticle/polyoxometalate/graphene tricomponent nanohybrids: An enzyme-free electrochemical biosensor for hydrogen peroxide. *Small*, 2012. **8**(9):1398–1406.

73. Liu, S. et al., Stable aqueous dispersion of graphene nanosheets: Noncovalent functionalization by a polymeric reducing agent and their subsequent decoration with Ag nanoparticles for enzymeless hydrogen peroxide detection. *Macromolecules*, 2010. **43**(22):10078–10083.

74. Liu, S. et al., A method for the production of reduced graphene oxide using benzylamine as a reducing and stabilizing agent and its subsequent decoration with Ag nanoparticles for enzymeless hydrogen peroxide detection. *Carbon*, 2011. **49**:3158–3164.

75. Liu, S. et al., Microwave-assisted rapid synthesis of Ag nanoparticles/graphene nanosheet composites and their application for hydrogen peroxide detection. *Journal of Nanoparticle Research*, 2011:1–10.

76. Liu, S. et al., Aniline as a dispersing and stabilizing agent for reduced graphene oxide and its subsequent decoration with Ag nanoparticles for enzymeless hydrogen peroxide detection. *Journal of Colloid and Interface Science*, 2011. **363**(2):615–619.

77. Zhang, Y. et al., One-pot green synthesis of Ag nanoparticles-graphene nanocomposites and their applications in SERS, H2O2, and glucose sensing. *RSC Advances*, 2011. **2**(2):538–545.

78. Xu, F. et al., Graphene–Pt nanocomposite for nonenzymatic detection of hydrogen peroxide with enhanced sensitivity. *Electrochemistry Communications*, 2011. **13**(10):1131–1134.

79. Zhang, F. et al., Microwave-assisted synthesis of Pt/Graphene nanocomposites for nonenzymatic hydrogen peroxide sensor. *International Journal of Electrochemical Science*, 2012. **7**:1968–1977.

80. Xiao, F. et al., Growth of metal–metal oxide nanostructures on freestanding graphene paper for flexible biosensors. *Advanced Functional Materials*, 2012. **22**(12):2487–2494.

81. Cao, L. et al., in situ controllable growth of Prussian blue nanocubes on reduced graphene oxide: Facile synthesis and their application as enhanced nanoelectrocatalyst for H2O2 reduction. *ACS Applied Materials & Interfaces*, 2010. **2**(8):2339–2346.

82. Guo, Y., J. Li, and S. Dong, Hemin functionalized graphene nanosheets-based dual biosensor platforms for hydrogen peroxide and glucose. *Sensors and Actuators B: Chemical*, 2011. **160**(1):295–300.

83. Ye, Y. et al., Enhanced nonenzymatic hydrogen peroxide sensing with reduced graphene oxide/ferroferric oxide nanocomposites. *Talanta*, 2011. **89**:417–421.

84. Ping, J. et al., Direct electrochemical reduction of graphene oxide on ionic liquid doped screen-printed electrode and its electrochemical biosensing application. *Biosensors and Bioelectronics*, 2011. **28**(1):204–209.

85. Palanisamy, S., S.-M. Chen, and R. Sarawathi, A novel nonenzymatic hydrogen peroxide sensor based on reduced graphene oxide/ZnO composite modified electrode. *Sensors and Actuators B: Chemical*, 2012. **166–167**:372–377.

86. Calabrese, V. et al., Nitric oxide in the central nervous system: Neuroprotection versus neurotoxicity. *Nature Reviews Neuroscience*, 2007. **8**(10):766–775.

87. Zhou, L. and D.Y. Zhu, Neuronal nitric oxide synthase: Structure, subcellular localization, regulation, and clinical implications. *Nitric Oxide*, 2009. **20**(4):223–230.

88. Napoli, C. et al., Nitric oxide and atherosclerosis: An update. *Nitric Oxide*, 2006. **15**(4):265–279.

89. MacMicking, J., Q. Xie, and C. Nathan, Nitric oxide and macrophage function. *Annual Review of Immunology*, 1997. **15**(1):323–350.

90. Thejass, P. and G. Kuttan, Allyl isothiocyanate (AITC) and phenyl isothiocyanate (PITC) inhibit tumour-specific angiogenesis by downregulating nitric oxide (NO) and tumour necrosis factor-α (TNF-α) production. *Nitric Oxide*, 2007. **16**(2):247–257.

91. Kavya, R. et al., Nitric oxide synthase regulation and diversity: Implications in Parkinson's disease. *Nitric Oxide*, 2006. **15**(4):280–294.

92. Zhang, X., Chapter 1—Nitric oxide (NO) electrochemical sensors, in *Electrochemical Sensors, Biosensors and Their Biomedical Applications*. 2008, Academic Press: San Diego, CA. pp. 1–29.

93. Ng, S.R., C.X. Guo, and C.M. Li, Highly sensitive nitric oxide sensing using three-dimensional graphene/ionic liquid nanocomposite. *Electroanalysis*, 2011. **23**(2):442–448.

94. Wang, Y.L. and G.C. Zhao, Electrochemical sensing of nitric oxide on electrochemically reduced graphene-modified electrode. *International Journal of Electrochemistry*, 2012. **2012**:1–6.

95. Guo, C.X. et al., RGD-peptide functionalized graphene biomimetic live-cell sensor for real time detection of nitric oxide molecule. *ACS Nano*, 2012:doi: 10.1021/nn301974u.

96. Smeets, W.J.A.J. and A. González, Catecholamine systems in the brain of vertebrates: New perspectives through a comparative approach. *Brain Research Reviews*, 2000. **33**(2–3):308–379.

97. de la Fuente-Fernández, R. et al., Levodopa-induced changes in synaptic dopamine levels increase with progression of Parkinson's disease: Implications for dyskinesias. *Brain*, 2004. **127**(12):2747–2754.

98. Breier, A. et al., Schizophrenia is associated with elevated amphetamine-induced synaptic dopamine concentrations: Evidence from a novel positron emission tomography method. *Proceedings of the National Academy of Sciences*, 1997. **94**(6):2569–2574.

99. Berke, J.D. and S.E. Hyman, Addiction, dopamine, and the molecular mechanisms of memory. *Neuron*, 2000. **25**(3):515–532.

100. Beck, G.C. et al., Clinical review: Immunomodulatory effects of dopamine in general inflammation. *Critical Care*, 2004. 8(6):485–491.

101. Seri, I. et al., Effects of low-dose dopamine infusion on cardiovascular and renal functions, cerebral blood flow, and plasma catecholamine levels in sick preterm neonates. *Pediatric Research*, 1993. **34**:742–749.

102. Falat, L. and H. Cheng, Voltammetric differentiation of ascorbic acid and dopamine at an electrochemically treated graphite/epoxy electrode. *Analytical Chemistry*, 1982. **54**(12):2108–2111.

103. Alwarappan, S. et al., Probing the electrochemical properties of graphene nanosheets for biosensing applications. *The Journal of Physical Chemistry C*, 2009. **113**(20):8853–8857.

104. Yang, J., S. Gunasekaran, and R.J. Strickler, Indium tin oxide-coated glass modified with reduced graphene oxide sheets and gold nanoparticles as disposable working electrodes for dopamine sensing in meat samples. *Nanoscale*, 2012. **4**:4594–4602.

105. Hou, S. et al., Highly sensitive and selective dopamine biosensor fabricated with silanized graphene. *The Journal of Physical Chemistry C*, 2010. **114**(35):14915–14921.

106. Liu, Q. et al., Electrochemical detection of dopamine in the presence of ascorbic acid using PVP/graphene modified electrodes. *Talanta*, 2012:doi: 10.1016/j.talanta.2012.05.013.

107. Wang, Y. et al., Application of graphene-modified electrode for selective detection of dopamine. *Electrochemistry Communications*, 2009. **11**(4):889–892.

108. Tian, X. et al., Simultaneous determination of L-ascorbic acid, dopamine and uric acid with gold nanoparticles–β-cyclodextrin–graphene-modified electrode by square wave voltammetry. *Talanta*, 2012. **93**:79–85.

109. Wu, L. et al., Electrochemical detection of dopamine using porphyrin-functionalized graphene. *Biosensors and Bioelectronics*, 2012. **34**(1):57–62.

110. Mao, Y. et al., Electrochemical sensor for dopamine based on a novel graphene-molecular imprinted polymers composite recognition element. *Biosensors and Bioelectronics*, 2011. **28**(1):291–297.

111. Liu, B. et al., Dopamine molecularly imprinted electrochemical sensor based on graphene–chitosan composite. *Electrochimica Acta*, 2012. **75**:108–114.

112. Liu, S. et al., A novel label-free electrochemical aptasensor based on graphene–polyaniline composite film for dopamine determination. *Biosensors and Bioelectronics*, 2012. **36**:186–191.

113. Yang, S. et al., Controllable adsorption of reduced graphene oxide onto self-assembled alkanethiol monolayers on gold electrodes: Tunable electrode dimension and potential electrochemical applications. *The Journal of Physical Chemistry C*, 2010. **114**(10):4389–4393.

114. Li, F. et al., Synthesis of Pt/ionic liquid/graphene nanocomposite and its simultaneous determination of ascorbic acid and dopamine. *Talanta*, 2010. **81**(3):1063–1068.

115. Tan, L. et al., Nanomolar detection of dopamine in the presence of ascorbic acid at β-cyclodextrin/ graphene nanocomposite platform. *Electrochemistry Communications*, 2010. **12**(4):557–560.

116. Kim, Y.-R. et al., Electrochemical detection of dopamine in the presence of ascorbic acid using graphene modified electrodes. *Biosensors and Bioelectronics*, 2010. **25**(10):2366–2369.

117. Zhang, F. et al., One-pot solvothermal synthesis of a Cu$_2$O/Graphene nanocomposite and its application in an electrochemical sensor for dopamine. *Microchimica Acta*, 2011. **173**:103–109.

118. Zhu, M., C. Zeng, and J. Ye, Graphene-modified carbon fiber microelectrode for the detection of dopamine in mice hippocampus tissue. *Electroanalysis*, 2011. **23**(4):907–914.

119. Sun, C.-L. et al., The simultaneous electrochemical detection of ascorbic acid, dopamine, and uric acid using graphene/size-selected Pt nanocomposites. *Biosensors and Bioelectronics*, 2011. **26**(8):3450–3455.

120. Zhang, Y. et al., Simultaneous voltammetric determination for DA, AA and NO2– based on graphene/poly-cyclodextrin/MWCNTs nanocomposite platform. *Biosensors and Bioelectronics*, 2011. **26**(9):3977–3980.

121. Zhuang, Z. et al., Electrochemical detection of dopamine in the presence of ascorbic acid using overoxidized polypyrrole/graphene modified electrodes. *International Journal of Electrochemical Science*, 2011. **6**:2149–2161.

122. Huang, K.-J. et al., Enhanced sensing of dopamine in the presence of ascorbic acid based on graphene/poly(p-aminobenzoic acid) composite film. *Colloids and Surfaces B: Biointerfaces*, 2011. **88**(1):310–314.

123. Ping, J. et al., Simultaneous determination of ascorbic acid, dopamine and uric acid using high-performance screen-printed graphene electrode. *Biosensors and Bioelectronics*, 2012. **34**:70–76.

124. Li, S.J. et al., Electrochemical synthesis of a graphene sheet and gold nanoparticle-based nanocomposite, and its application to amperometric sensing of dopamine. *Microchimica Acta*, 2012. **177**:325–331.

125. Sheng, Z.-H. et al., Electrochemical sensor based on nitrogen doped graphene: Simultaneous determination of ascorbic acid, dopamine and uric acid. *Biosensors and Bioelectronics*, 2012. **34**(1):125–131.

126. Liu, S. et al., Layer-by-layer assembled multilayer films of reduced graphene oxide/gold nanoparticles for the electrochemical detection of dopamine. *Journal of Electroanalytical Chemistry*, 2012. **672**:40–44.

127. Dong, X. et al., 3D graphene foam as a monolithic and macroporous carbon electrode for electrochemical sensing. *ACS Applied Materials & Interfaces*, 2012. **4**(6):3129–3133.

128. Wei, Q. et al., A novel label-free electrochemical immunosensor based on graphene and thionine nanocomposite. *Sensors and Actuators B: Chemical*, 2010. **149**(1):314–318.

129. Li, T., M. Yang, and H. Li, Label-free electrochemical detection of cancer marker based on graphene–cobalt hexacyanoferrate nanocomposite. *Journal of Electroanalytical Chemistry*, 2011. **655**(1):50–55.

130. Li, R. et al., Label-free amperometric immunosensor for the detection of human serum chorionic gonadotropin based on nanoporous gold and graphene. *Analytical Biochemistry*, 2011. **414**(2):196–201.

131. Han, J. et al., Highly conducting gold nanoparticles–graphene nanohybrid films for ultrasensitive detection of carcinoembryonic antigen. *Talanta*, 2011. **85**(1):130–135.

132. Mao, K. et al., Label-free electrochemical immunosensor based on graphene/methylene blue nanocomposite. *Analytical Biochemistry*, 2012. **422**:22–27.

133. Yang, Y.C. et al., A label-free amperometric immunoassay for thrombomodulin using graphene/ silver-silver oxide nanoparticles as a immobilization matrix. *Analytical Letters*, 2012. **45**:724–734.

134. Su, B. et al., Graphene and nanogold-functionalized immunosensing interface with enhanced sensitivity for one-step electrochemical immunoassay of alpha-fetoprotein in human serum. *Electroanalysis*, 2010. **22**(22):2720–2728.

135. Huang, K.J. et al., An electrochemical amperometric immunobiosensor for label-free detection of [alpha]-fetoprotein based on amine-functionalized graphene and gold nanoparticles modified carbon ionic liquid electrode. *Journal of Electroanalytical Chemistry*, 2011. **656**:72–77.

136. Kong, F.-Y. et al., A novel label-free electrochemical immunosensor for carcinoembryonic antigen based on gold nanoparticles–thionine–reduced graphene oxide nanocomposite film modified glassy carbon electrode. *Talanta*, 2011. **85**(5):2620–2625.

137. Yu, S., X. Cao, and M. Yu, Electrochemical immunoassay based on gold nanoparticles and reduced graphene oxide functionalized carbon ionic liquid electrode. *Microchemical Journal*, 2012. **103**:125–130.

138. Zheng, X.T. et al., Bifunctional electro-optical nanoprobe to real-time detect local biochemical processes in single cells. *Biosensors & Bioelectronics*, 2011. **26**(11):4484–4490.

139. Halliwell, B. and J. Gutteridge, Oxygen toxicity, oxygen radicals, transition metals and disease. *Biochemical Journal*, 1984. **219**:1–14.

140. Wu, X. et al., Electrochemical approach for detection of extracellular oxygen released from erythrocytes based on graphene film integrated with laccase and 2, 2-azino-bis (3-ethylbenzothiazoline-6-sulfonic acid). *Analytical Chemistry*, 2010. **82**(9):3588–3596.

141. Wu, J.F., M.Q. Xu, and G.C. Zhao, Graphene-based modified electrode for the direct electron transfer of cytochrome c and biosensing. *Electrochemistry Communications*, 2010. **12**(1):175–177.

14

Bioelectronics on Graphene

Vikas Berry

CONTENTS

This chapter discusses the functioning of graphene-based electronic biosensors and the influence of graphene's chemical and structural properties on the sensitivity and specificity of these sensors.

14.1 Introduction

Since the 1990s, several studies have originated on the effect of interfacing nanomaterials with bio-components on their properties, with the goal of detecting bio-components or biological phenomena.[1–6] Until 2004, the primary focus had been on applying zero-dimensional (0-D) and one-dimensional (1-D) nanomaterials (semiconducting nanoparticles, silicon nanowires), which are excellent for interfacing with biomolecules (DNA, proteins) and nanoscale bio-components (viral particles, lipid micelles). These interfaces have led to the development of valuable tools and devices for bio-diagnostics and bio-medicine.[1,4–6]

The 2004 experiments on graphene[7]—a single-atom thick sheet of sp^2 hybridized carbon atoms arranged in honeycomb lattice—led to the evolution of 2-D nanotechnology. Other 2-D materials include boron nitride (αBN), molybdenum disulfide, tungsten sulfide, and niobium diselenide. Owing to a unique combination of its crystallographic and electronic structure,[8] graphene exhibits several superior and atypical properties, including weakly scattered ($\lambda_{scattering} > 300$ nm), ballistic transport of its charge-carriers at room temperature[7,9,10]; gate-tunable band-gap in bilayers[11]; a chemically[12,13] and geometrically[14] controllable band-gap; quantum Hall effect at room temperature[15,16];

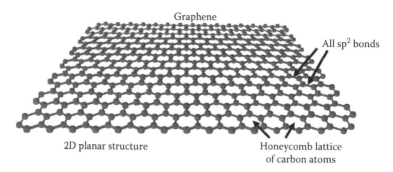

FIGURE 14.1
Graphene Lattice Structure: sp^2 hybridized carbon atoms arranged in a 2D honeycomb lattice.

quantum interference[17]; exceptional mechanical strength[18]; and megahertz character-istic frequency.[19] Due to these properties, graphene has emerged as an attractive can-didate for several unique applications, including ultrafast nano-electronic devices,[12,15] single molecule detectors,[20] ultra-capacitors,[21] opto-electronics,[22] and nano-mechanical devices.[19,23]

Graphene (Figure 14.1) exhibits ultrahigh sensitivity for detection[20] owing to (1) its atomic thickness resulting in lateral confinement of carriers,[7] (2) high quantum capacitance,[24] (3) its delocalized π–electrons[25] on crystalline surface, allowing scattering from molecular attachment (due to disruption of potential-continuum), and (4) a high carrier mobility,[25,26] and thus low noise in detection. Molecular attachment electrically gates the charge carri-ers on graphene[63] and/or introduces scattering sites, which can sensitively modulate its electrical properties. On the other hand, the lack of functionality on graphene significantly reduces its specificity to other molecular groups. This challenge can be addressed by func-tionalization of graphene. There are several methodologies to functionalize graphene, including (1) oxidation via Hummer's process, (2) π–π interfacing, (3) functionalization via activated plasma, (4) nanoparticle nucleation, and (5) electrochemical modification. Out of these techniques, π–π interfacing does not convert the sp^2 hybridized state of the carbon atoms of graphene. All the methods generally lead to modulation of carrier density and introduction of scattering sites due to formation of electron–hole puddles, lattice distor-tion, and/or breakage of potential-continuum. Currently, most studies on graphene bio-electronics have been focused on DNA, protein, virus, and cellular detection. This chapter provides an analysis of attributes, mechanisms, and properties of graphene-based biosen-sors and cellular bioactivity detection.

14.2 Graphene-Based Biocellular Sensors

Conclusively isolated for the first time in 2004, graphene (Figure 14.1) is a single-atom thick sheet of sp^2 bound carbon atoms arranged in a honeycomb lattice.[8,27–29] In compari-son to 0-D nanoparticles[1,2] and 1-D nanowires,[3–5] including their 2-D networks,[6] the 2-D graphene sheets possess a large and continuous sensing/interfacing area[2], which provides a stable interface for large-area microbes and biological cells (Figure 14.2). The large area also increases the analyte attachment probability. The mechanism of the graphene/cell

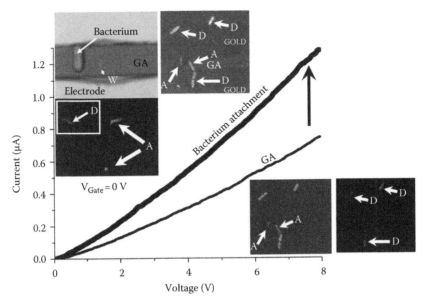

FIGURE 14.2
(See color insert.) Conductivity of the p-type AFG-device increases upon attachment of a single bacterial cell on the surface of AFG (top-inset). Further, the cells are alive when attached. The bacteria on graphene were found to sustain the current and did not die, while the bacteria on gold electrode died. (Reprinted and adapted with permission from Mohanty, N. and Berry, V., Graphene-based single-bacterium resolution biodevice and DNA transistor: Interfacing graphene derivatives with nanoscale and microscale biocomponents, *Nano Lett.*, 8, 4469–4476. Copyright 2008 American Chemical Society.)

detection system is based on carrier-doping via the cell wall's electronegativity or dipole moment.[30] The attributes that enhance the sensitivity of graphene include (1) quantum capacitance: The quantum-coupling of the cell-wall with graphene enhances the effective electric field due to the dipole moment of the interfacing cell wall.[24] The quantum capacitance of graphene is given by $C_q = 4e\pi^{1/2} / h\vartheta_F (n_l + n_g)^{1/2}$, where e is the electron charge, h is Planck's constant, ϑ_F is the Fermi velocity of the Dirac electron, and n_g and n_l are the carrier concentrations from the gate potential and the intrinsic carrier concentration of graphene, respectively. The effective gating potential (ΔV_G), therefore, translates from a change in dipole voltage (ΔV) of the cell wall to $\Delta V_G = (C_q / C_{tot})\Delta V$, which is much higher than ΔV. Here, $C_{tot} = \left(C_q^{-1} + C_g^{-1}\right)^{-1}$ and C_g is the gate capacitance. (2) Confined doping: The change in the carrier concentration of graphene due to the change in the chemical potential of the cell wall is amplified as a result of the confinement of the doped carriers within graphene's ultrathin structure. (3) Functionalization: Graphene can be functionalized with cell wall compatible biomolecules, to further strengthen the interfacing with the cell. The consortium of these properties makes it an ideal candidate for cellular detection.

In 2008, Berry et al. fabricated and studied bacteria-interfaced graphenic devices.[63] Here, the bacterial cells were detected on amide-functionalized graphene (AFG), synthesized by diaminization of the immobilized graphene oxide (GO) sheets to produce chemically modified graphene (CMG). These sheets were deposited on a silica substrate. The study was conducted for Gram-positive *Bacillus cereus* cells, which possess highly negatively charged surface due to polyteichoic acid molecules densely tethered on their cell wall.[31,32] The device construct was achieved by electrostatically assembling the negatively charged bacterial cells on positively charged AFG sheet.[31] Importantly, the deposited bacteria illustrated a strong binding with AFG, and did not detach from the surface when washed with DI water at room temperature.

The binding of a single bacterium on the AFG device exhibited a sharp 42% increase in conductivity, attributed to the p-type characteristic of AFG, where the interfacing of the highly electronegative polyteichoic acid doped a high density of holes on the AFG. Further, the resultant increase in the hole density was confined within the few-atom-thick structure, leading to a very sensitive response. The hole density increase due to the bacterium attachment on AFG was 3.53×10^{10} cm^{-2} ($R_1|_{GA} = 10.85 \pm 0.51$ MΩ, $R_2|_{Bacteria} = 6.3 \pm 0.4$ MΩ). This corresponds to a generation of $\sim$1400 holes per bacterium in the AFG. The electrical measurements did not have any visible effect on the integrity of the bacterium's structure as against the CNT-network devices.[6] The results showed a proof-of-concept of a highly sensitive graphene-based biodiagnostic tool with single-bacterium resolution.

In 2010, Zhang and Chen[33] demonstrated that reduced graphene oxide (RGO) devices can be applied for detection of cellular secretion. In this device, live neuroendocrine PC12 cells were cultured directly on top of poly-L-lysine-coated RGO transistor. This was followed by triggering the vesicular secretion of catecholamine molecules (dopamine, epinephrine, and norepinephrine). Here, the high K$^+$ solution was introduced into the recording chamber, which depolarized the cell membrane and allowed Ca^{2+} influx through the Ca^{2+} channels on the cell membrane. The change in the potential of the cellular membrane interfaced with the underlying RGO subsequently induced a device response shown by current spikes in the device. This was attributed to the vesicular release of catecholamines from a single PC12 cell. This study showed that graphene-based field effect transistor (FET) can be highly sensitive to the dynamic cellular bio-activities atop its surface.

Lieber and Fang et al.[35] showed that graphene devices can also be used to detect the change in the electrical potential (or "beating") of the cardiomyocyte cells (Figure 14.3). Here, graphene FET device was interfaced with embryonic chicken cardiomyocytes (Figure 14.3b, left) cultured under optimized conditions on thin poly(dimethylsiloxane) (PDMS) sheets and transferred over the device via an x-y-z manipulator. This brought a spontaneously "beating" cell into direct contact with graphene sheet (Figure 14.3b, left). The cardiomyocyte cell atop an active graphene device exhibited regulated change in cell potential, which led to an ordered modulation of graphene's electrical properties with the high-conductivity peaks spaced with a frequency of 1.1 Hz and a signal-to-noise of >4. The high signal-to-noise ratio was attributed to the large interfacial area between graphene and the cell. Further, the magnitude of the conductance peak was also controlled by varying the gate voltage (V_{wg}). This device operation clearly showed that graphene is excellent for interfacing with mammalian cells and is sensitive to the electrogenics or the biochemical activity of the interfaced cell. This reinforces the impact of quantum-capacitance induced enhancement of effective gating from the cell wall for these applications.

Hess and Garrido extended the aforementioned work by using large-area graphene grown by chemical vapor deposition (CVD).[34] Here, graphene device could detect electronic activity of the electrogenic cells[35] more sensitively due to the higher charge carrier mobility and chemical stability of CVD graphene. In the fabricated device, cardiomyocyte-like HL-1 cells were cultured live directly on an array of graphene-based solution gated transistors (G-SGFET). Here, the gate voltage was applied via electrolyte, thus controlling the Fermi level of graphene and changing the conductance across the device. The propagation of the surface potentials (action potential) across the cells exhibited the gate voltage spike signal of 900 µV and signal-to-noise of 70. Furthermore, the frequency of the voltage

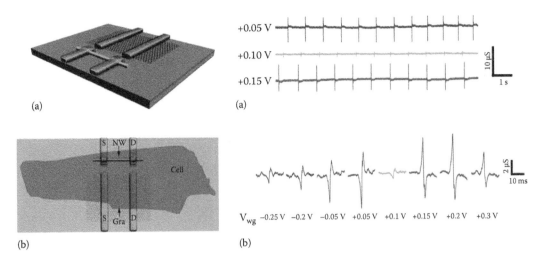

(a)

(a)

(b)

(b)

FIGURE 14.3
Left: (a) Schematic of the graphene chip design. (b) Representation of the cardiomyocyte cell interfaced to typical graphene devices. Right: (a) Temporal response of the graphene device at different water gate potentials (top, middle, and bottom traces are at +0.05, +0.10, and +0.15 V, respectively). The corresponding sensitivities are 2020, 398, and 2290 μS/V, respectively. (b) Representative expanded peaks. First four pulses represents p-type graphene polarity, last three pulses peaks represent n-type graphene polarity, and the middle ($V_{wg} = +0.1$ V) peak was recorded near the Dirac point. (Reprinted and adapted with permission from Cohen-Karni, T., Qing, Q., Li Q., Fang, Y., and Lieber, C.M., Graphene and nanowire transistors for cellular interfaces and electrical recording, *Nano Lett.*, 10, 1098–1102. Copyright 2010 American Chemical Society.)

spikes was modulated by controlling the amount of fight-or-flight hormone, norepinephrine, in the media used to grow the cells. This study clearly shows the superiority of graphene for cellular-interfaced sensing devices with applications in neuroprosthetic devices and recording electrogenics activity.

14.3 Importance of Functionalization in Detection

Functionalization is important because of two reasons: (1) it adds specificity to the event being detected, which enhances the magnitude of the desired signal, and (2) it improves the interface between the cell and graphene. Berry's group has shown that graphene functionalized with concanavalin–a pectin protein with high specific affinity to the bacterial cell wall (Gram-positive)–can cause it to hermetically wrap bacterial cells[36]. The functionalization dramatically improved graphene's interaction with the cell wall. Here, the graphenic wrapping acts as an impermeable, electron transparent encasement, allowing real wet imaging of the cells.

However, functionalization of graphene converts the sp^2 hybridized state of the carbon atoms to sp^3 and thus reduces its carrier mobility and sensitivity. This implies that a nondestructive functionalization, which does not convert the sp^2 hybridization state of the carbon atoms in graphene, can have significant impact on the cell-interfaced graphene devices. Traditional routes like Hummers method–based oxidation, plasma-induced functionalization, and nanoparticle incorporation lead to significant sp^3 hybridization, reduction in π?carrier density, and introduction of scattering sites.

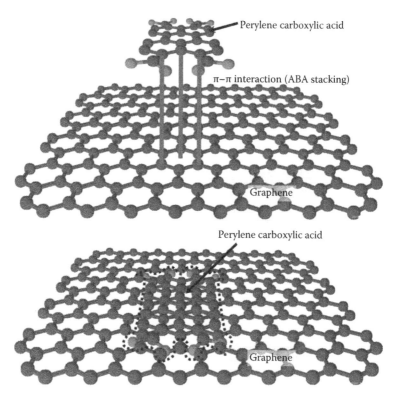

FIGURE 14.4

(See color insert.) *π–π Interfacing*: Model for π–π interfacing of PCA on graphene *via* ABA-type stacking.

One route for non-destructive functionalization of graphene is π–π interfacing (Figure 14.4). Here, π–π bonded molecules on graphene do not disturb the sp² hybridization state of the carbon atoms on graphene such that the high mobility of graphene is retained. Here, the π electrons on graphene enable π–π interfacing with π–activated polyaromatic molecules like anthracene, pyrelene, pyrene, coronene, etc. Polycyclic aromatic compounds can bond with one another via π–orbital overlapping to form π–π bond, which is stronger than hydrogen bond, van der Waals, and dipole–dipole interactions (not as strong as covalent). The higher the number of rings involved, the stronger the π–π bond. The π–π functionalization is a known technique for graphite,[38,39,60] (Figure 14.5) and Hersham,[40] Liu,[41] and Dai,[42] have shown perylene functionalization on graphene sheets. The major challenge with π–π bonds[40–42] (aromatic–aromatic) is that it is weak and can cause multiple stacking on graphene, while covalent bonding (discussed later) is self-limiting and produces only a monolayer of functional groups, and hence exhibits more control. The positive aspects of π–π functionalization are that it does not convert the sp² hybridized state of the carbon atoms, does not distort the planar graphene structure, and maintains the aromaticity and thus the carrier density in graphene. Currently, the most studied π–conjugated molecule to functionalize graphene is perylene tetracarboxylic dianhydride (PTCDA), since it produces a monolayer on graphene[40]. This implied that π–π functionalization not only retains the ultrahigh sensitivity of graphene but also functionalizes graphene to enhance specificity.

Covalent functionalization has been used widely[63] to chemically modify graphene. Here, the most common CMG is graphene oxide (GO),[43–53] where graphene sheet is functionalized with oxy-groups (Figure 14.6, bottom). These hydroxyl, epoxy, and carboxylic

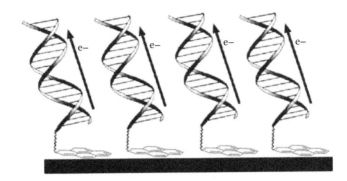

FIGURE 14.5
Pyrene–DNA attached on graphite layer. (Reprinted and adapted with permission from Gorodetsky, A.A. and Barton, J.K., Electrochemistry using self-assembled DNA monolayers on highly oriented pyrolytic graphite, *Langmuir*, 22, 7917–7922. Copyright 2006 American Chemical Society.)

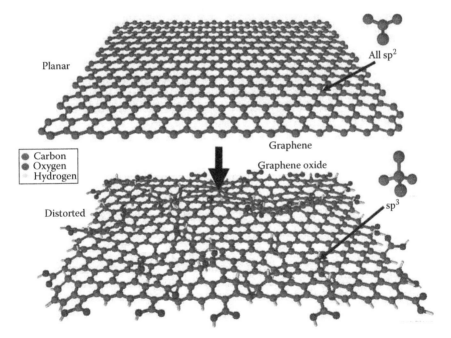

FIGURE 14.6
Oxy-functionalization of graphene to form graphene oxide (GO).

acid groups are then employed to further attach other molecular groups, like DNA[63] (Figure 14.7), antibodies,[63] amines,[63] and azo, via amide chemistry to graphene. Geim and Novoselov's team[54] covalently hydrogenated graphene, producing highly scattering sp^3 carbons resulting in loss of π–electrons; while Ishigami's group[55] atomically doped potassium on graphene lattice, which added scattering sites.

Covalent functionalization deteriorates graphene's superior electrical properties by (1) opening up a bandgap via removal of π–electrons and (2) increasing carrier scattering due to (a) the distorted structure (Figure 14.6, bottom) produced by conversion of planar sp^2 to tetrahedral sp^3 carbons, (b) the charged impurities introduced, and (c) the vacancy defects formed via removed carbon atoms (Figure 14.6, bottom). Kern et al.,[13,56]

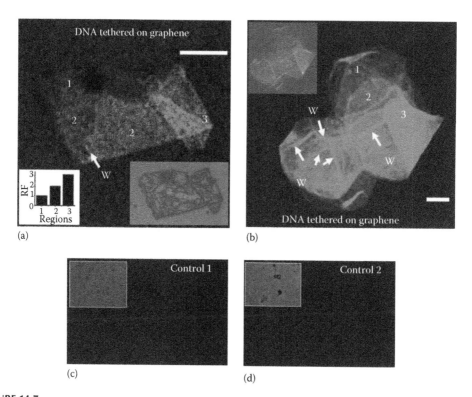

FIGURE 14.7
Covalent functionalization of graphene with DNA. (a, b) Confocal images of graphene–DNA with hybridized dye-labeled complementary DNA. (c, d) Control experiments with no DNA functionalization and with no complementary DNA hybridization. (Reprinted and adapted with permission from Mohanty, N. and Berry, V., Graphene-based single-bacterium resolution biodevice and DNA transistor: Interfacing graphene derivatives with nanoscale and microscale biocomponents, *Nano Lett.*, 8, 4469–4476. Copyright 2008 American Chemical Society.)

Kaner et al.,[12] and others[43,44,52,57–60] observed similar results for graphene oxide. These results clearly show a loss of graphene's superior properties after its covalent functionalization. Other methods to covalently functionalize graphene include aryl functionalization (Figure 14.8) enabled by reduction of phenyl diazonium salt. Haddon et al.[60] demonstrated this functionalization for graphene. Further, there is also an increase in the density of electron–hole puddles in graphene, which also increase the charge scattering.[61]

14.4 Effect of Structure on Detection Sensitivity

While the chemical modification improved specificity, structural modification of graphene can improve its sensitivity. For example, the opening-up of a bandgap with electrical gating in bilayer graphene[11] makes it a more sensitive system than single-layer graphene for bio-electronic sensors. It is expected that cellular interfaces with bilayer graphene will be

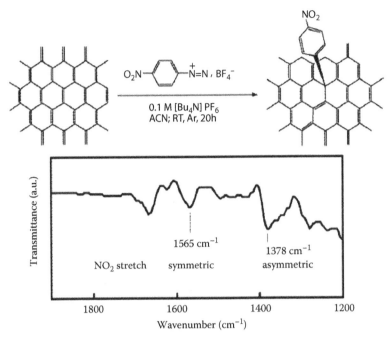

FIGURE 14.8
Covalent functionalization of graphene with aryl. FTIR spectrum shows the signal from the nitrogen attached to graphene. (Reprinted and adapted with permission from Bekyarova, E., Itkis, M.E., Ramesh, P., Berger, C., Sprinkle, M., de Heer, W.A., and Haddon, R.C., Chemical modification of epitaxial graphene: Spontaneous grafting of aryl groups, *J. Am. Chem. Soc.* 131, 1336. Copyright 2009 American Chemical Society.)

able to detect lower-order signals more effectively via bioelectrical gating. This is expected to improve the signal-to-noise ratio in the detection of electrogenic activity of cardiomyocytes. Further, thin films of graphene nanoribbons (GNRs) will also provide an important opportunity for bio-interfacing. Here, the bandgap due to quantum confinement will produce a barrier for the carriers, which will further increase the sensitivity of the device. Similarly, graphene with punched holes (or graphene nanomesh[62]) can also be used as a sensitive graphenic substrate with a bandgap for biocellular interfacing and detection. Graphene nanomesh can be fabricated via transferring the film morphology of block copolymers on graphene via lithography.

14.5 Single Molecule Detection

Geim et al. have demonstrated that graphene's electrical properties are sensitive to the interfacing of a single molecule (donor or acceptor), which can change the local carrier concentration of graphene one electron or hole at a time. This leads to the change in conductivity in quanta proportional to the number of molecules. This graphene sensor is therefore the only "electronic sensor" with molecular resolution. Further, gating analysis can distinguish between the electronegative and electropositive molecules.[20]

14.6 Biomolecular (DNA) Detection

Berry et al. have shown that graphene is an excellent candidate for robust and reversible detection of DNA by covalently interfacing DNA with graphene to form graphene–DNA (G–DNA) hybrid. Electrical characterization of the G–DNA hybrids was conducted to examine its viability and sensitivity as a biomolecular transistor. First, selective tethering of the single-stranded DNA (AAC TGC CAG CCT AAG TCC AA) on GO to form G–DNA was carried out (method explained earlier). This led to a 128% increase in the conductivity, partially attributed to the attachment of the negatively charged DNA on the p-type GO (Figure 14.9). Subsequently, hybridization with complementary DNA (TTG GAC TTA GGC TGG CAG TT) was conducted on the G–DNA device. This led to a 71% increase in conductivity ($R_1|_{DNA} = 9.86 \pm 0.24$ MΩ; $R_2|_{dsDNA} = 5.77 \pm 0.17$ MΩ) (Figure 14.9). The robustness of this device was tested by dehybridizing the complementary DNA from G–DNA, which resulted in the restoration of G–DNA's original conductivity. Further, multiple hybridization–dehybridization runs showed consistent increase and restoration of the conductivity. It was found that one quantum of hole is generated or removed by hybridization or dehybridization of ~ six DNA molecules. The generation of holes is attributed to the electronegativity of the interfacing DNA. The change in conductivity due to hybridization/dehybridization varied from 60% to 200% for different G–DNA samples.

Immersing the G–DNA device in a solution of non-complementary DNA did not change the conductivity. Although the DNA hybridization/dehybridization

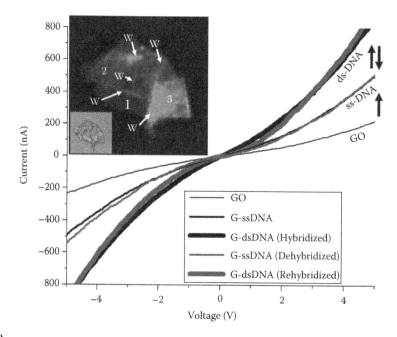

FIGURE 14.9
Conductivity of a p-type graphene device increases upon attachment of a single-stranded DNA probe and then hybridized with a complementary DNA target. (Reprinted and adapted with permission from Mohanty, N. and Berry, V., Graphene-based single-bacterium resolution biodevice and DNA transistor: Interfacing graphene derivatives with nanoscale and microscale biocomponents, *Nano Lett.*, 8, 4469–4476. Copyright 2008 American Chemical Society.)

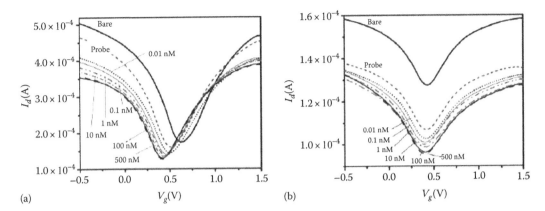

FIGURE 14.10

Transfer characteristics for the graphene transistors before adsorbing DNA, after immobilization with probe DNA, and after reaction with (a) complementary or (b) one-base mismatched DNA molecules with the concentration ranging from 0.01 to 500 nM. (From Dong, X., Shi, Y., Huang, W., Chen, P., and Li, L.J.: Electrical detection of DNA hybridization with single-base specificity using transistors based on CVD-grown graphene sheets. *Adv Mater.* 2010. 22. 1649–1653. Copyright Wiley-VCH Verlag GmbH & Co. KGaA. Reprinted and adapted with permission.)

measurements were made in dry-nitrogen conditions, they were effective in producing the negative-charge gating. These results further elucidate the high sensitivity of graphene biosensors, which function effectively as a label-free DNA detector and a molecular transistor.

In another study, Chen and Li developed a pristine graphene-based DNA detector.[62] Here, DNA is adsorbed on graphene device, which causes a shift of the Dirac point toward lower voltages (Figure 14.10). Upon interfacing the G–DNA device with complementary DNA, the resultant hybridization causes a further reduction in the Dirac point. Single pair mismatched DNA did not change the Dirac point (Figure 14.10). The shift was attributed to the charge transfer from DNA stacking. Further, DNA hybridization does not cause desorption of the adsorbed DNA. In fact, it leads to DNA hybridization. The device's sensitivity can be further increased by covalently attaching the DNA on graphene device by first attaching gold nanoparticles on graphene. The sensitivity of DNA detection was measured as 0.01 nM.

14.7 Ultrasensitivity of Graphene for Biosensing

A unique combination of the right structure and electronic configuration makes graphene ultrasensitive. Structurally, all the carbon atoms in graphene are surface-exposed and are arranged in a low-scattering honeycomb lattice enabling an ultrahigh mobility and low noise in detection. Electronically, graphene's carbon atoms are sp^2 hybridized, rendering its free electrons (π–electrons[7]) to be surface-bound, while being confined in one-atom-thick space (quantum confinement[7]) with a small bandgap. When a molecule interfaces with graphene, (1) it sensitively gates the carriers through its small bandgap, which allows even small molecules to excite carriers between conduction and valance bands[15,25]; or (2) the molecule scatters the high-speed, surface-bound carriers.

Further, graphene's highest carrier mobility measured to date[25,26] means more modulation of its electrical properties, which further increases sensitivity. The consortium of these properties along with the large detection areas and low electrical noise[20] in graphene makes graphene ultrasensitive. Graphene's large area[2] enables its stable interfacing with large microbes and mammalian cells (as discussed earlier), making graphene an excellent candidate for detection of large cells.

14.8 Graphene Bioelectronic Sensing Principles

In the graphene/biocellular or graphene/biomolecular devices, the generalized mechanism of modulation of graphene's carrier properties due to bio-entity interfacing follows five steps:

1. The bioentity (cell wall of the cellular or biomolecule analyte) interfaces with graphene leading to a change in the local dipoles around graphene, which generates a change in the surface potential. For cellular interfacing, a further change in the local dipoles can be caused by a change in cell wall chemistry or potential due to cellular biophysical phenomena.

2. The effective gating potential due to this change is amplified via the quantum capacitance of graphene $\left(\Delta V_G = (C_q/C_{tot})\Delta V\right)$, as mentioned earlier.

3. The density of carriers in graphene is modulated as a response (doping). The semi-metallic nature of graphene enables direct interface-dipole-induced doping of the carriers.[15,25]

4. The confinement of the π carriers within a few atoms[7] ensures that the change in the interfacial potential directly and efficiently modulates graphene's carrier density. This is because the modulation of the number of charge carriers is not distributed over a large thickness (or volume).

5. The transport of the carriers occurs. The π orbitals in graphene are atop its lattice plane, thus the carriers experience low scattering, exhibiting high mobility. Therefore, a highly amplified sensor signal ($\Delta I/V_{DS} \propto nA\mu$) is realized, which enables sensitive detection of the interfacial event.

   At molecular scale, the interfacial event on graphene's surface can also introduce scattering sites, and/or electrically gate the carriers on grapheme,[63] which can also modulate its electrical properties. The change in carrier density (Δq) can be measured by the difference in the resistivity before and after the interfacial event: $\mu_{Carrier} = (\Delta I_{DS}/\Delta V_G)/\left(C(l/w)V_{DS}\right), \Delta q = \left(R_2^{-1} - R_1^{-1}\right)/\left((l/w)\mu_{Carrier}\right); \Delta q = C\Delta V_{Dirac}$.

Effects of functionalization on graphene's structural and electronic properties include

1. Covalent functionalization induced conversion of the basal carbon's hybridization state (sp^2–sp^3):
   a. Distorts the lattice
   b. Disrupts the potential continuum

    c. Enhances electron–hole puddles

    d. Changes the density of electronic states

2. Interaction of the dipole moment of the bioentity with graphene or functionalized graphene:

    a. Enhanced doping due to quantum capacitance

    b. Increase in electron-hole puddles

    c. Disruption of potential

3. *Transport Mechanism:* Geim's group[7,8,10,25,28,65,66] and others[13,17,44,54,58,67–70] have shown that the conduction mechanism for pristine graphene follows Klein tunneling, while that for reduced graphene oxide (RGO) with some oxy-groups follows variable range hopping.[13,44,54,56,58,69,70,71] For biosensing applications graphene is most commonly functionalized with a probe molecule. This functionalization process creates regions on sp^3 hybridized states in graphene. These states will then lead to the electronic transport following the variable range hopping mechanism:

$$I = I_0 \exp\left(-\left(\frac{T_0}{T}\right)^{1/3}\right).$$

Factors that contribute to making graphene ultrasensitive for biodetection are

1. Atomic thickness resulting in lateral confinement of carriers, and a high quantum capacitance:

    a. Amplifies the influence of bioentity on changing the charge density in graphene

2. Delocalized π-electrons on crystalline surface that allow scattering from disruption of potential continuum due to interfacing with bioentity

3. High carrier mobility that

    a. Reduces the detection noise

    b. Amplifies the signal

Therefore, it is important that the functionalization of graphene be designed such that there the density of scattering sites remains low: for example via π–π functionalization.

14.9 Conclusion

This chapter outlines the phenomena and the principles associated with graphene-based electronic biosensors. The chapter describes the mechanism of detection, the various device functionalization routes, and the factors influencing the sensitivity and specificity of graphenebiosensors.

References

1. H. Cai, C. Xu, P. G. He, and Y. Z. Fang, Colloid Au-enhanced DNA immobilization for the electrochemical detection of sequence-specific DNA, *J Electroanal Chem* 510 (2001) 78–85.

2. J. D. Le, Y. Pinto, N. C. Seeman, K. Musier-Forsyth, T. A. Taton, and R. A. Kiehl, DNA-templated self-assembly of metallic nanocomponent arrays on a surface, *Nano Lett* 4 (2004) 2343–2347.

3. H. Cai, X. N. Cao, Y. Jiang, P. G. He, and Y. Z. Fang, Carbon nanotube-enhanced electrochemical DNA biosensor for DNA hybridization detection, *Anal Bioanal Chem* 375 (2003) 287–293.

4. Y. Cui, Q. Q. Wei, H. K. Park, and C. M. Lieber, Nanowire nanosensors for highly sensitive and selective detection of biological and chemical species, *Science* 293 (2001) 1289–1292.

5. F. Patolsky, G. F. Zheng, and C. M. Lieber, Nanowire-based biosensors, *Anal Chem* 78 (2006) 4260–4269.

6. H. M. So, D. W. Park, E. K. Jeon, Y. H. Kim, B. S. Kim, C. K. Lee, S. Y. Choi, S. C. Kim, H. Chang, and J. O. Lee, Detection and titer estimation of *Escherichia coli* using aptamer-functionalized single-walled carbon-nanotube field-effect transistors, *Small* 4 (2008) 197–201.

7. K. S. Novoselov, A. K. Geim, S. V. Morozov, D. Jiang, Y. Zhang, S. V. Dubonos, I. V. Grigorieva, and A. A. Firsov, Electric field effect in atomically thin carbon films, *Science* 306 (2004) 666–669.

8. K. S. Novoselov, D. Jiang, F. Schedin, T. J. Booth, V. V. Khotkevich, S. V. Morozov, and A. K. Geim, Two-dimensional atomic crystals, *Proc Natl Acad Sci USA* 102 (2005) 10451–10453.

9. S. Y. Zhou, G. H. Gweon, J. Graf, A. V. Fedorov, C. D. Spataru, R. D. Diehl, Y. Kopelevich, D. H. Lee, S. G. Louie, and A. Lanzara, First direct observation of Dirac fermions in graphite, *Nat Phys* 2 (2006) 595–599.

10. K. S. Novoselov, A. K. Geim, S. V. Morozov, D. Jiang, M. I. Katsnelson, I. V. Grigorieva, S. V. Dubonos, and A. A. Firsov, Two-dimensional gas of massless Dirac fermions in graphene, *Nature* 438 (2005) 197–200.

11. Y. Zhang, T. T. Tang, C. Girit, Z. Hao, M. C. Martin, A. Zettl, M. F. Crommie, Y. R. Shen, and F. Wang, Direct observation of a widely tunable bandgap in bilayer graphene, *Nature* 459 (2009) 820–823.

12. S. Gilje, S. Han, M. Wang, K. L. Wang, and R. B. Kaner, A chemical route to graphene for device applications, *Nano Lett* 7 (2007) 3394–3398.

13. C. Gomez-Navarro, R. T. Weitz, A. M. Bittner, M. Scolari, A. Mews, M. Burghard, and K. Kern, Electronic transport properties of individual chemically reduced graphene oxide sheets, *Nano Lett* 7 (2007) 3499–3503.

14. V. Barone, O. Hod, and G. E. Scuseria, Electronic structure and stability of semiconducting graphene nanoribbons, *Nano Lett* 6 (2006) 2748–2754.

15. K. S. Novoselov, Z. Jiang, Y. Zhang, S. V. Morozov, H. L. Stormer, U. Zeitler, J. C. Maan, G. S. Boebinger, P. Kim, and A. K. Geim, Room-temperature quantum hall effect in graphene, *Science* 315 (2007) 1379.

16. K. S. Novoselov, E. McCann, S. V. Morozov, V. I. Fal'ko, M. I. Katsnelson, U. Zeitler, D. Jiang, F. Schedin, and A. K. Geim, Unconventional quantum Hall effect and Berry's phase of 2 pi in bilayer graphene, *Nat Phys* 2 (2006) 177–180.

17. A. F. Young and P. Kim, Quantum interference and Klein tunnelling in graphene heterojunctions, *Nat Phys* 5 (2009) 222–226.

18. C. Lee, X. D. Wei, J. W. Kysar, and J. Hone, Measurement of the elastic properties and intrinsic strength of monolayer graphene, *Science* 321 (2008) 385–388.

19. J. S. Bunch, A. M. van der Zande, S. S. Verbridge, I. W. Frank, D. M. Tanenbaum, J. M. Parpia, H. G. Craighead, and P. L. McEuen, Electromechanical resonators from graphene sheets, *Science* 315 (2007) 490–493.

20. F. Schedin, A. K. Geim, S. V. Morozov, E. W. Hill, P. Blake, M. I. Katsnelson, and K. S. Novoselov, Detection of individual gas molecules adsorbed on graphene, *Nat Mater* 6 (2007) 652–655.

21. M. D. Stoller, S. Park, Y. Zhu, J. An, and R. S. Ruoff, Graphene-based ultracapacitors, *Nano Lett* 8 (2008) 3498–3502.
22. Q. Liu, Z. F. Liu, X. Y. Zhang, N. Zhang, L. Y. Yang, S. G. Yin, and Y. S. Chen, Organic photovoltaic cells based on an acceptor of soluble graphene, *Appl Phys Lett* 92 (2008).
23. M. Poot and H. S. J. van der Zant, Nanomechanical properties of few-layer graphene membranes, *Appl Phys Lett* 92 (2008).
24. J. Xia, F. Chen, J. Li, and N. Tao, Measurement of the quantum capacitance of graphene, *Nat Nanotechnol* 4 (2009) 505–509.
25. A. K. Geim and K. S. Novoselov, The rise of graphene, *Nat Mater* 6 (2007) 183–191.
26. J. C. Meyer, A. K. Geim, M. I. Katsnelson, K. S. Novoselov, T. J. Booth, and S. Roth, The structure of suspended graphene sheets, *Nature* 446 (2007) 60–63.
27. J. J. Wang, M. Y. Zhu, R. A. Outlaw, X. Zhao, D. M. Manos, B. C. Holloway, and V. P. Mammana, Free-standing subnanometer graphite sheets, *Appl Phys Lett* 85 (2004) 1265–1267.
28. M. H. Gass, U. Bangert, A. L. Bleloch, P. Wang, R. R. Nair, and A. K. Geim, Free-standing graphene at atomic resolution, *Nat Nanotechnol* 3 (2008) 676–681.
29. M. Ishigami, J. H. Chen, W. G. Cullen, M. S. Fuhrer, and E. D. Williams, Atomic structure of graphene on SiO2, *Nano Lett* 7 (2007) 1643–1648.
30. P. Nguyen and V. Berry, Graphene interfaced with biological cells: Opportunities and challenges, *J Phys Chem Lett* 3 (2012) 1024–1029.
31. V. Berry and R. F. Saraf, Self-assembly of nanoparticles on live bacterium: An avenue to fabricate electronic devices, *Angew Chem Int Ed* 44 (2005) 6668–6673.
32. V. Berry, A. Gole, S. Kundu, C. J. Murphy, and R. F. Saraf, Deposition of CTAB-terminated nanorods on bacteria to form highly conducting hybrid systems, *J Am Chem Soc* 127 (2005) 17600–17601.
33. Q. He, H. G. Sudibya, Z. Yin, S. Wu, H. Li, F. Boey, W. Huang, P. Chen, and H. Zhang, Centimeter-long and large-scale micropatterns of reduced graphene oxide films: Fabrication and sensing applications, *ACS Nano* 4 (2010): 3201–3208.
34. T. Cohen-Karni, Q. Qing, Q. Li, Y. Fang, and C. M. Lieber, Graphene and nanowire transistors for cellular interfaces and electrical recording, *Nano Lett* 10 (2010) 1098–1102.
35. L. H. Hess, M. Jansen, V. Maybeck, M. V. Hauf, M. Seifert, M. Stutzmann, I. D. Sharp, A. Offenhäusser, and J. A. Garrido, Graphene transistor arrays for recording action potentials from electrogenic cells, *Adv Mater* 23 (2011) 5045–5049.
36. N. Mohanty, M. Fahrenholtz, A. Nagaraja, D. Boyle, and V. Berry, Impermeable graphenic encasement of bacteria, *Nano Lett* 11 (2011) 1270–1275.
37. A. A. Gorodetsky and J. K. Barton, Electrochemistry using self-assembled DNA monolayers on highly oriented pyrolytic graphite, *Langmuir* 22 (2006) 7917–7922.
38. A. Hoshino, S. Isoda, H. Kurata, and T. Kobayashi, Scanning tunneling microscope contrast of perylene-3, 4, 9, 10-tetracarboxylic-dianhydride on graphite and its application to the study of epitaxy, *J Appl Phys* 76 (1994) 4113.
39. T. Schmitz-Hnbsch, F. Sellam, R. Staub, M. Torker, T. Fritz, C. Knbel, K. Mnllen, and K. Leo, Direct observation of organic-organic heteroepitaxy: perylene-tetracarboxylic-dianhydride on hexa-peri-benzocoronene on highly ordered pyrolytic graphite, *Surf Sci* 445 (2000) 358–367.
40. Q. H. Wang and M. C. Hersam, Room-temperature molecular-resolution characterization of self-assembled organic monolayers on epitaxial graphene, *Nat Chem*, 1 (2009): 206–211.
41. F. Li, H. Yang, C. Shan, Q. Zhang, D. Han, A. Ivaska, and L. Niu, The synthesis of perylene-coated graphene sheets decorated with Au nanoparticles and its electrocatalysis toward oxygen reduction, *J Mater Chem*, 19 (2009): 4022–4025.
42. X. Wang, S. M. Tabakman, and H. Dai, Atomic layer deposition of metal oxides on pristine and functionalized graphene, *J Am Chem Soc* 130 (2008) 8152–8153.
43. H. A. Becerril, J. Mao, Z. Liu, R. M. Stoltenberg, Z. Bao, and Y. Chen, Evaluation of solution-processed reduced graphene oxide films as transparent conductors, *Acs Nano* 2 (2008) 463–470.
44. G. Eda, G. Fanchini, and M. Chhowalla, Large-area ultrathin films of reduced graphene oxide as a transparent and flexible electronic material, *Nat Nanotechnol* 3 (2008) 270–274.

45. G. Eda, Y. Y. Lin, S. Miller, C. W. Chen, W. F. Su, and M. Chhowalla, Transparent and conducting electrodes for organic electronics from reduced graphene oxide, *Appl Phys Lett* 92 (2008).

46. M. Mermoux, Y. Chabre, and A. Rousseau, Ftir and C-13 NMR-study of graphite oxide, *Carbon* 29 (1991) 469–474.

47. W. W. Cai, R. D. Piner, F. J. Stadermann, S. Park, M. A. Shaibat, Y. Ishii, D. X. Yang et al., Synthesis and solid-state NMR structural characterization of C-13-labeled graphite oxide, *Science* 321 (2008) 1815–1817.

48. W. S. Hummers and R. E. Offeman, Preparation of graphitic oxide, *J Am Chem Soc* 80 (1958) 1339.

49. X. L. Li, G. Y. Zhang, X. D. Bai, X. M. Sun, X. R. Wang, E. Wang, and H. J. Dai, Highly conducting graphene sheets and Langmuir-Blodgett films, *Nat Nanotechnol* 3 (2008) 538–542.

50. J. I. Paredes, S. Villar-Rodil, A. Marti?ünez-Alonso, and J. M. D. Tascón, Graphene oxide dispersions in organic solvents, *Langmuir* 24 (2008) 10560–10564.

51. S. Park, J. H. An, I. W. Jung, R. D. Piner, S. J. An, X. S. Li, A. Velamakanni, and R. S. Ruoff, Colloidal suspensions of highly reduced graphene oxide in a wide variety of organic solvents, *Nano Lett* 9 (2009) 1593–1597.

52. Y. Hernandez, V. Nicolosi, M. Lotya, F. M. Blighe, Z. Y. Sun, S. De, I. T. McGovern et al., High-yield production of graphene by liquid-phase exfoliation of graphite, *Nat Nanotechnol* 3 (2008) 563–568.

53. S. Stankovich, D. A. Dikin, R. D. Piner, K. A. Kohlhaas, A. Kleinhammes, Y. Jia, Y. Wu, S. T. Nguyen, and R. S. Ruoff, Synthesis of graphene-based nanosheets via chemical reduction of exfoliated graphite oxide, *Carbon* 45 (2007) 1558–1565.

54. D. C. Elias, R. R. Nair, T. M. Mohiuddin, S. V. Morozov, P. Blake, M. P. Halsall, A. C. Ferrari et al., Control of graphene's properties by reversible hydrogenation: Evidence for graphane, *Science* 323 (2009) 610–613.

55 J. H. Chen, C. Jang, S. Adam, M. S. Fuhrer, E. D. Williams, and M. Ishigami, Charged-impurity scattering in graphene, *Nat Phys* 4 (2008) 377–381.

56. A. B. Kaiser, C. Gomez-Navarro, R. S. Sundaram, M. Burghard, and K. Kern, Electrical conduction mechanism in chemically derived graphene monolayers, *Nano Lett* 9 (2009) 1787–1792.

57. D. Dragoman and M. Dragoman, Giant thermoelectric effect in graphene, *Appl Phys Lett* 91 (2007) 203116.

58. I. Jung, D. A. Dikin, R. D. Piner, and R. S. Ruoff, Tunable electrical conductivity of individual graphene oxide sheets reduced at "low" temperatures, *Nano Lett* 8 (2008) 4283–4287.

59. Z. T. Luo, P. M. Vora, E. J. Mele, A. T. C. Johnson, and J. M. Kikkawa, Photoluminescence and band gap modulation in graphene oxide, *Appl Phys Lett* 94 (2009) 111909.

60. E. Bekyarova, M. E. Itkis, P. Ramesh, C. Berger, M. Sprinkle, W. A. de Heer, and R. C. Haddon, Chemical modification of epitaxial graphene: Spontaneous grafting of aryl groups, *J Am Chem Soc* 131 (2009) 1336.

61. J. Martin, N. Akerman, G. Ulbricht, T. Lohmann, J. H. Smet, K. von Klitzing, and A. Yacoby, Observation of electron-hole puddles in graphene using a scanning single-electron transistor, *Nat Phys* 4 (2008) 144–148.

62. J. Bai, X. Zhong, S. Jiang, Y. Huang, and X. Duan, Graphene nanomesh, *Nat Nano* 5 (2010) 190–194.

63. N. Mohanty and V. Berry, Graphene-based single-bacterium resolution biodevice and DNA transistor: Interfacing graphene derivatives with nanoscale and microscale biocomponents, *Nano Lett* 8 (2008) 4469–4476.

64. X. Dong, Y. Shi, W. Huang, P. Chen, and L. J. Li, Electrical detection of DNA hybridization with single-base specificity using transistors based on CVD-grown graphene sheets, *Adv Mater* 22 (2010) 1649–1653.

65. A. J. M. Giesbers, G. Rietveld, E. Houtzager, U. Zeitler, R. Yang, K. S. Novoselov, A. K. Geim, and J. C. Maan, Quantum resistance metrology in graphene, *Appl Phys Lett* 93 (2008).

66. M. I. Katsnelson, K. S. Novoselov, and A. K. Geim, Chiral tunnelling and the Klein paradox in graphene, *Nat Phys* 2 (2006) 620–625.

67. R. Nouchi, M. Shiraishi, and Y. Suzuki, Transfer characteristics in graphene field-effect transistors with Co contacts, *Appl Phys Lett* 93 (2008) 152104.
68. X. Du, I. Skachko, A. Barker, and E. Y. Andrei, Approaching ballistic transport in suspended graphene, *Nat Nanotechnol* 3 (2008) 491–495.
69. G. Eda and M. Chhowalla, Graphene-based composite thin films for electronics, *Nano Lett* 9 (2009) 814–818.
70. K. Kim, H. J. Park, B. C. Woo, K. J. Kim, G. T. Kim, and W. S. Yun, Electric property evolution of structurally defected multilayer graphene, *Nano Lett* 8 (2008) 3092–3096.
71. F. Guinea, A. H. Castro, and N. M. R. Peres, Electronic properties of stacks of graphene layers, *Solid State Commun* 143 (2007) 116–122.

15

Nanowire Field-Effect Transistor Biosensors

Fumiaki Ishikawa, Xiaoli Wang, Noppadol Aroonyadet, and Chongwu Zhou

CONTENTS

15.1 Introduction to Nanowire FET Biosensors

15.1.1 Basic Principles

Detection of chemical agents and biological species using nanostructured materials has shown significant progress in recent years, driven by the high demand for superior analytical tools in areas such as environmental monitoring, new drug screening, and disease diagnosis. Various detection techniques have been proposed and demonstrated using a wide variety of nanomaterials.[1–8]

Among such emerging technologies, detection of biomolecules using semiconducting nanowire and carbon nanotube (CNT) field-effect transistors (FETs) has attracted considerable interest. The device structure and the operation principle are analogous to a previously developed sensor technology, chemical and ion sensitive FET (ChemFET and ISFET).[9–11] An ISFET is a metal oxide FET (MOSFET) where the gate electrode is replaced by an aqueous solution. The schematic diagrams of a MOSFET and an ISFET are shown in

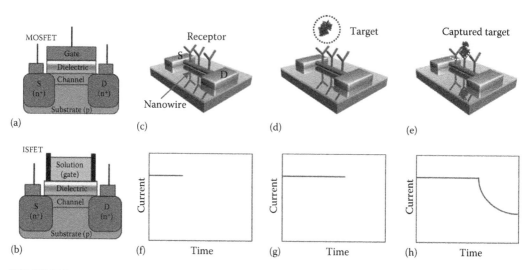

FIGURE 15.1
Schematic diagram of (a) a MOSFET and (b) an ISFET. (c–e) Schematic diagrams showing the operation principle of a nanobiosensor. (c) Start of the sensing. The sensor consists of nanowire/nanotube as the channel with source-drain electrodes for electrical read-out. Receptor molecules are attached on the sensor surface. (d) An analyte is introduced to the buffer, and approaches the sensor. (e) The analyte molecule is captured by the receptor molecule on the sensor. (f–h) Typical read-out of a nanobiosensor during a sensing experiment over time. (f) A baseline is established at the beginning of the sensing. (g) There is no change in the current read-out before the analyte molecule moves close to the sensor and is captured. (h) The current changes due to the interaction between the captured analyte molecule and the sensor.

Figure 15.1a and b, respectively. An ISFET can detect presence of ions in the solution as follows. When there is a change in the ionic concentrations in the solution, it induces a change in the solution gate potential. This leads to a change in the carrier concentration (or current) through the channel to produce signal, as a change in the metal gate in the MOSFET induces a carrier concentration (or current) change in the channel of the MOSFET. Using similar structure, such sensors were also applied to detect biomolecules that are either positively or negatively charged in aqueous solutions.[12,13]

This type of sensor has advantages such as compatibility with microfabricated electronics, real-time detection, and electrical signal read-out compared to other biosensing technologies. Especially, electrical readout is beneficial from a practical viewpoint since there is no need to have bulky and expensive optical setup that results in significantly reduced cost and spatial requirement of the system. Thus, with these advantages, this type of sensors has attracted significant attention. Conventionally, 2D bulk materials have been used as the active element, and significant improvement in sensitivity, selectivity, and the underlining physics has been made. However, the use of 2D bulk materials still limits the sensitivity of the sensors.

Use of 1D structured nanomaterials, such as NWs and CNTs, can further improve the sensitivity, since it offers significantly enhanced surface-to-volume ratios compared to the bulk 2D materials. By combining nanomaterial-based sensors with surface chemistry and biological reaction, a sensory system with high sensitivity, label-free detection, real-time sensing, integration capability, and apparatus simplicity (electrical readout) can be achieved. A schematic diagram of a nanobiosensor and the operation principle is shown in Figure 15.1c through h. A nanobiosensor is a transistor using nanotubes/nanowires as the channel (Figure 15.1c). The nanotube/nanowire surface is functionalized with receptor molecules to add selectivity to the sensor. In a typical biosensing experiment, the current through the channel is monitored over time. When the device is exposed to a sample containing the target, the target molecules approach the sensor surface (Figure 15.1d), and eventually get captured by the receptors (Figure 15.1e). Typical changes of the read-out through these consecutive events are shown in Figure 15.1f and g, presenting the current output plotted over time. At the beginning of the sensing (Figure 15.1c), a stable baseline is established as shown in Figure 15.1f. When the target molecule approaches the sensor as in Figure 15.1d, there is no change in the current since the distance between the molecule and sensor is far beyond the length over which the molecule can affect the conduction through the channel (Figure 15.1g). When the target molecule is captured by the receptor molecules (Figure 15.1c), the current output changes due to the interaction between the molecule and the sensor to result in a current output as shown in Figure 15.1h.

The aforementioned section and Figure 15.1 describe the basic operation of the nanobiosensor. However, the detailed physics behind the interaction between the molecule and the sensor that causes the change, or the signal, in a current output has been, and is still, a subject of an intense investigation.[14–17] The possible mechanisms of the biosensing include (1) gating of the channel (including electrostatic and chemical doping), (2) dielectric constant change, (3) mobility change, and (4) Schottky barrier height change. The difference of these mechanisms is well illustrated in Figure 15.2 made by Heller et al.[14] They simulated the I_{ds}–V_g curves of an ambipolar CNT device before/after the sensing for different mechanisms to compare with experiments and identify the sensing mechanism.

Figure 15.2a corresponds to a case where the sensing is done by gating of the channel (body) of the transistor by the biomolecules. Gating of the channel leads to a shift in the I_{ds}–V_g curves, and it is notable that the transconductance of each transport (n and p) branch stays constant before/after the sensing. Mechanisms of (1) electrostatic gating and (2) chemical gating fall into this gating category and give same changes in the I_{ds}–V_g curves.

Figure 15.2b shows the case of sensing by Schottky barrier height modulation. In this mechanism, for example, biomolecules increase the work function of the source-drain electrodes as shown in the inset of Figure 15.2b, leading to reduced conduction for p branch and enhanced conduction for n branch due to the increased/reduced Shottky barrier height for each transport. It is notable that threshold voltage stays constant, while transconductance changes before/after the sensing.

Figure 15.2c shows that the capacitance of the double layer was decreased before/after the sensing due to the different dielectric constants of H_2O and biomolecules. It was simulated to result in reduced transconductance for both transports, since it reduces the capacitive coupling efficiency for both carriers.

Lastly, as shown in Figure 15.2d, the mobility inside the channel (nanotube) was reduced. This is due to the disordered electrostatic field distribution around the nanotubes caused by unperiodically distributed biomolecules with charges. This mechanism leads to reduction in the transconductance for both transport branches.

In spite of the need for further investigation into the physics and mechanism of nanobiosensing, there has been a great amount of successful detection of various biological species with excellent performance, including short detection time, label-free sensing, and high sensitivity, using such NW/CNT-based devices.[6,8,16,18–25] For example, single virus detection has been demonstrated using a Si nanowire, and aM or fM sensitivity for protein detection has been demonstrated as well. These demonstrations open up the possibility of establishing the novel diagnostic system capable of performing rapid and cheap blood testing with portability, which is expected to greatly increase the quality of our life.

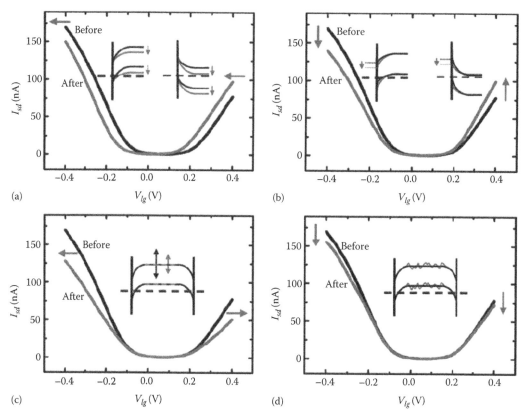

FIGURE 15.2

Calculated $I-V_{lg}$-curves before (bold line) and after (light line) protein adsorption for four different sensing mechanisms. The bias voltage is 10 mV. (a) Electrostatic gating effect corresponding to a 50 meV shift of the semiconducting bands downward. (b) Schottky barrier effect that corresponds to a change of the difference between metal and SWNT work functions of 30 meV. In panels a and b, left and right insets illustrate the corresponding changes in the band diagrams for hole and electron doping, respectively. (c) Capacitance mechanism for a 90% coverage of SWNT with protein. In panels c and d, the insets illustrate the corresponding changes in the band diagrams. (d) Mobility mechanism that corresponds to a mobility reduction to a mere 2% of the initial value. (Reprinted with permission from Heller, I., Janssens, A.M., Mannik, J., Minot, E.D., Lemay, S.G., and Dekker, C., Identifying the mechanism of biosensing with carbon nanotube transistors, *Nano Lett.*, 8(2), 2008, 591–595. Copyright 2008 American Chemical Society.)

In the following section, we will further introduce several key, basic concepts in the nanobiosensor field, after which we will discuss the major progress made in our research group to demonstrate the potential of such nanobiosensors. Finally, we will outline the remaining challenges toward the commercialization of the nanobiosensor technology for realizing clinically meaningful diagnostic systems.

15.1.2 Tutorial Materials

15.1.2.1 Device Fabrication

Device fabrication can be categorized into two methods: one is bottom up and the other is top down. Bottom up method normally starts from synthesizing nanowires using chemical vapor deposition (CVD) or laser assisted CVD, as shown in Figure 15.3a. Superlattice

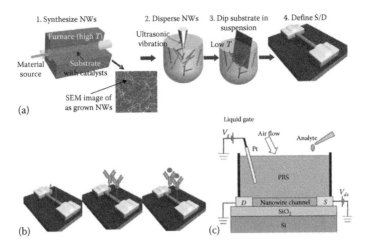

FIGURE 15.3
(See color insert.) (a) In_2O_3 nanowires are synthesized by laser ablation in a high temperature furnace. Next, they are dispersed onto a new substrate for fabrication. (b) Fabricated nanowire FETs are functionalized on the surface to bind to capture probes for biomolecule targets. (c) The sensor environment includes a solution gate, chamber for detection in liquid, and electrical connections for the nanowire FET biosensor.

nanowire pattern transfer (SNAP) method was also used to create nanosized wires.[21] After the nanowires are synthesized, they are deposited onto a substrate. Conventional, standard Si/SiO_2 substrate has been used, but it can be replaced by other functional substrates such as flexible polyethylene terephthalate (PET). After deposition of nanowire on the substrate, metal electrodes are deposited in lithographically defined areas on top of the nanowire film surface. This bottom up method is simple and inexpensive, but has the disadvantage that it is a probabilistic approach, and the resultant devices have relatively large device-to-device variation in the electrical performance.

Top down approaches do not suffer from such limitation, and they utilize the mature and developed silicon technology. Several groups have successfully demonstrated nanowire biosensor fabrication with such top down methods.[26–29] In the example of Stern et al.,[29] Si nanowire devices were fabricated by thinning/narrowing the wire thickness/width from the top silicon layer of silicon-on-insulator (SOI) wafers with oxidation and etching. Such sensors would have relatively uniform performance. However, in these top down approaches, the use of expensive SOI wafers puts a burden on the cost of the nanowire biosensors, and the process is relatively time-consuming and complicated. Those issues will be mentioned again in the last section of this review.

15.1.2.2 Device Functionalization

Device functionalization usually starts from depositing a linker molecule onto the sensor surface (Figure 15.3b). The linker molecule then conjugates with the antibody and immobilizes the antibody as the capture probe onto the sensor surface, by a well developed biochemistry process. The linker molecule should be designed in a way that it does not damage the nanowire's electrical property or change the structure of the antibody so that it may retain biochemical activity. Furthermore, the importance of the thickness of the linker molecule layer has been reported by Patolsky et al.[30] and other researchers.[31–33] The observation is that the thicker the linker molecule layer is, the less sensitive the devices are. Zhang et al.[33] also indicated that the distance between the probe molecule and the sensor surface plays an important role in defining sensitivity of nanobiosensors. These indicate that care must be taken to precisely control the functionalization chemistry to make full use of the sensor capability.

15.1.2.3 Sensing Environment

Many of the biosensing experiments have been carried out with the sensors and molecules submerged in a liquid environment. This is useful not only for eliminating washing and drying steps necessary for measurements done in air (dry sensing) but also for acquiring direct, real-time information, such as kinetics, from the biomolecules interacting with the sensor surface. Figure 15.3c shows the basic configuration of the sensing environment. The sensor is placed in a chamber filled with an aqueous medium, which is usually a phosphate-based buffer (PBS), and electrical contacts are made to the source and drain. Liquid gate electrode is inserted into the medium and serves to stabilize the liquid potential. The importance of the choice of the gate electrode will be presented in the following section. The chamber can be either a solid container or a microfluidic device designed to deliver the analyte solution.

15.1.3 Critical Issues

15.1.3.1 Debye Length

It was demonstrated that Debye length (λ_D) plays an important role in determining the magnitude of the sensor response, consistent with the electrostatic mechanism.[32] The Debye length of a thermally equilibrated system can be calculated as follows:

$$\lambda_D = \frac{1}{\sqrt{4\pi l_B \sum_i \rho_i z_i}} \tag{15.1}$$

where
  l_B is the Bjerrum length that is 0.7 nm
  ρ_i and z_i are the density and the valence of the ion, respectively

Following this model, the relative strength of the electrostatic potential created by a charged molecule as the function of distance can be calculated as follows:

$$\varphi(r) = \frac{Q}{4\pi\varepsilon_0 r} e^{-k_0 r} \tag{15.2}$$

where
  $\varphi(r)$ is the potential change at distance r
  Q is the charge
  ε_0 is the dielectric constant of the medium
  k_0 is $1/\lambda_D$

This is a solution for screened Poisson equation. It is clear from the equation that the effect of a charge is reduced dramatically beyond a certain Debye length. However, it was proposed that under the influence of an external flow of ions, the Debye length can be larger than the value calculated by the equation.[34] Intuitively speaking, this is due to the shift of the balance between diffusion of ions and localization of charges (ions) through electrostatic interaction to the diffusion side, since the diffusion is enhanced by the external flow of the ions. Indeed, in actual biosensing experiments, there can be flows of ions induced by potential difference between source, drain, and gate electrodes, or mechanical pressure when microfluidic channels are used to deliver the samples. This implies that, while it is apparent that Debye length plays an important role in nanobiosensors, further investigations are required to fully describe the experimental results.

15.1.3.2 Stability of Liquid Gate Electrode

During the sensing experiments, it is necessary to keep the potential of the liquid constant to prevent false signaling. Conventionally, a Pt electrode has been widely used as the gate electrode due to the stability of Pt in liquid (little electrochemical degradation).[17,18,22,25] However, a study by Minot et al.[35] revealed that the potential of a Pt electrode is unstable when proteins bind to the surface of the electrode. They monitored the open-circuit voltage of a Pt wire inserted in a buffer against an Ag/AgCl electrode as common, and exposed the Pt wire to BSA. The potential showed a rapid decrease upon exposure to BSA. Following this observation, they proposed that it is necessary to use an Ag/AgCl electrode as the liquid gate electrode where the interface potential drop is constant due to the inaccessibility of proteins to the surface by the slit and AgCl coating. It is worth noting that several groups including ours now use an Ag/AgCl electrode as the liquid gate.

15.2 Past Research

The following sections are based on past work done in our research group that were originally published in.[25,36,40,49,63,87]

15.2.1 Interaction of Proteins with In₂O₃ Nanowire FET

Our work started by investigating the potential of using our In_2O_3 nanowire devices as a biosensor. More specifically, lightly doped In_2O_3 nanowire transistors were used to investigate the chemical gating effect of small organic molecules and biomolecules with amine or nitro groups.[36] The electron-donating capability of amine groups and electron-withdrawing capability of nitro groups were found to induce dramatic changes in the nanowire conductance as well as significant shifts in the gate threshold voltages, as a result of the carrier concentration variation. In addition, adsorption of the nitro compound on partial lengths of the nanowires led to modulated chemical gating and intra-nanowire junctions exhibiting prominent rectifying behavior.[36]

A schematic diagram and a scanning electron micrograph (SEM) of an In_2O_3 nanowire bridging the source/drain electrodes are shown in Figure 15.4a inset. Figure 15.4a shows two *I–V* curves of an In_2O_3 nanowire transistor, with the gate biased at 0 V, before and after exposure to tert-butylamine.[36] Before chemical exposure, the device exhibited small conduction with a zero bias resistance of 250 MΩ, but it showed significantly enhanced conduction with a zero bias resistance of 17 MΩ after exposure to tert-butylamine.[36] In addition to the conductance variation, the sensing properties of devices can also be studied

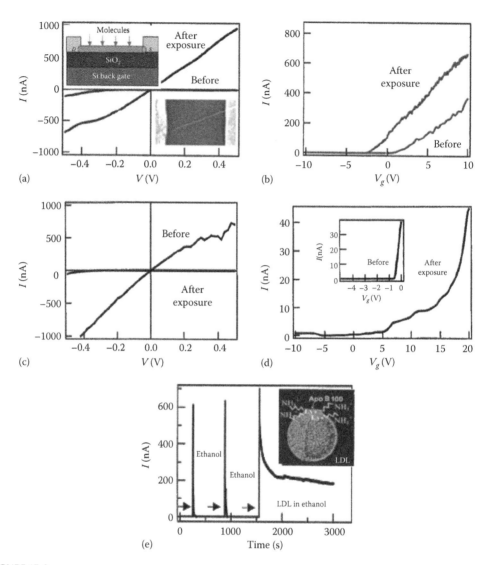

FIGURE 15.4

(a) I–V curves of an In_2O_3 device before and after exposure to butylamine. Inset: schematic for molecular absorption on an In_2O_3 nanowire device and SEM image of the device. (b) I–V_g curves recorded before and after molecular absorption with the drain–source bias $V = 0.1$ V (c) I–V curves of an In_2O_3 device before and after exposure to butyl nitrite. (d) I–V_g curve of the device after exposure. Inset: I–V_g curve of the device before exposure with $V = 50$ mV (e) Time domain measurement for a device after exposure to pure ethanol twice and then LDL in ethanol Inset: Schematic of an LDL particle. (Reprinted with permission from Li, C., Lei, B., Zhang, D., Liu, X., Han, S., Tang, T., Rouhanizadeh, M., Hsiai, T., and Zhou, C., Chemical gating of In_2O_3 nanowires by organic and biomolecules, *Appl. Phys. Lett.*, 83(19), 4014–4016. Copyright 2003, American Institute of Physics.)

by monitoring the current dependence on the gate bias. Figure 15.4b shows two I–Vg curves recorded before and after exposure to butylamine with a constant drain–source bias of $V = 0.1$ V. Both curves confirm In_2O_3 nanowires are n-type-doped semiconductors, and a −3 V shift in the threshold voltage (from 0.5 to −2.5 V) was observed after the exposure. This indicates an increase of electron concentration in the nanowire (n), which can be estimated to be 1.1×10^7 cm^{-1} from the equation ($n = C\Delta V_T/eL$), where C is the nanowire capacitance, ΔV_T is the shift in threshold voltage, e the electron charge, and L the channel length.[36,37] This increase in electron concentration and conductance is attributed to the chemical gating effect of the amino groups in butylamine, consistent with previous observation that lightly doped nanowires exhibited enhanced conduction upon NH_3 exposure.[38] Similar results were obtained with other In_2O_3 devices exposed to 3'-(aminopropyl) triethoxysilane (APTES), where a dramatic increase in conductance and a negative shift in the gate threshold voltage were consistently observed.[36] This further confirms the electron-donating effect of the amino groups. In sharp contrast to butylamine and APTES, In_2O_3 nanowire devices exhibited a very different behavior when exposed to butyl nitrite. Figure 15.4c shows two I–V curves recorded before and after the butyl nitrite adsorption at the fixed gate bias of $V_g = 0$ V. This device was relatively conductive before the exposure; however, after the exposure, the device showed a reduction in conductance around five orders of magnitude for $V = 0.3$ V. Furthermore, a significant positive shift in the gate threshold voltage from −0.6 V before the exposure (Figure 15.4d inset) to 5–10 V after the exposure (Figure 15.4d) was observed, indicating a decrease in the electron concentration. This can be understood as nitro groups are highly oxidative and are thus expected to withdraw electrons from the nanowires, subsequently leading to reduced conduction for n-type In_2O_3 nanowires.[36]

The electron transfer process described earlier illustrated the feasibility of using In_2O_3 nanowires as sensors for bio-species by binding the amino or nitro groups on biomolecules to the sensor surface. This was further demonstrated in the study of low density lipoprotein (LDL) cholesterol detection, as an average LDL particle contains a hydrophobic core and a protein called apolipoprotein B-100 (apoB-100), which has positively charged amino groups (NH_3^+) at the outer surface.[39] Electronic measurements were performed before and after applying one drop of the LDL suspension onto nanowire transistors under ambient conditions. As a control experiment, a drop of pure ethanol was applied to the device with the current monitored over time under $V = 0.1$ V and $V_g = 0$ V, and the results are shown in Figure 15.4e. The current increased immediately after the ethanol drop was introduced, and then returned to the original state once the ethanol drop evaporated away within 1 min. The current increased immediately after applying one drop of the LDL suspension to the device; however, instead of returning to the original state, the device stabilized in a highly conductive state after a slight drop in current related to the ethanol evaporation. This enhanced conductance is also evident in the I–V curve recorded after the LDL exposure that shows a zero-bias resistance of 0.7 MΩ as compared to a resistance of 118 MΩ before the exposure.[36] In addition to increase in conduction, the I–V_g curves recorded before and after the LDL exposure, where a negative shift in the gate threshold voltage can be clearly seen, corresponding to an increase in the electron concentration. Two factors may account for the increased electron concentration in the nanowires. The first is that the amino groups carried by the ApoB-100 protein in LDL particles may function as reductive species and hence donate electrons to the nanowires. The second concomitant factor is due to positive charges carried by the amino groups, which can function as a positive gate bias to nanowires, thus leading to the enhanced carrier concentration.[36]

15.2.2 Selective Functionalization Using Electrochemical Method

Sensitivity to a given analyte can be accomplished by anchoring an analyte specific recognition group to the surface of the nanowires. In addition, spatially selective functionalization of biosensors located within a small footprint is of importance since it enables multiplexed sensing of several analytes, which leads to more reliable and accurate diagnostics. We used 4-(1,4-dihydroxybenzene)butyl phosphonic acid (HQ-PA) as the linker. HQ-PA is an electrochemically active molecule containing a hydroquinone group that undergoes reversible oxidation/reduction at low potentials.[41] The use of electrochemically active HQ-PA eliminates the use of UV photoactivation and BBr$_3$, a very corrosive Lewis acid that attacks many metal oxide NWs.[40]

Self-assembled monolayer (SAM) of HQ-PA was generated on the In$_2$O$_3$ NW surface (Figure 15.5a). Oxidized HQ-PA (Q-PA) reacts with a range of functional groups, which can be easily incorporated into biomolecules and other materials, such as thiols, azides, cyclopentadienes, and primary amines as shown in Figure 15.5b where a thiol terminated DNA has been attached only on the desired NWs.[40]

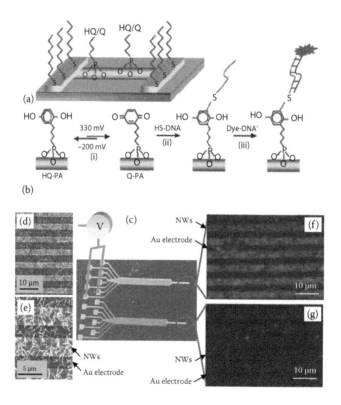

FIGURE 15.5

(a) Schematic representation of an In$_2$O$_3$ NW mat device (only one NW is shown for clarity). The NW is functionalized with a SAM of HQ-PA and is placed between two gold electrodes protected by a SAM of dodecane-1-thiol. (b) (i) The monolayer of HQ-PA, deposited on the In$_2$O$_3$ NW or ITO, can be reversibly oxidized to Q-PA in an electrochemical cell. (ii) Addition of the probe, thiol-terminated DNA (HS-DNA) to QPA. (iii) Attachment of complementary DNA strand (dye-DNA′) to the probe DNA (c) A photograph of a NW mat sample contacted by two groups of electrodes. Only the HQ-PA attached to the NWs between the upper electrodes was converted to Q-PA. (d) An SEM image of the In$_2$O$_3$ NWs before functionalization. The brighter stripes are gold electrodes covering the NW mat. (e) The same sample imaged at higher magnification, where the NW mat is clearly visible. (f) A fluorescence image of the NWs with Q-PA taken after DNA attachment. The gold electrodes, passivated with an alkanethiol, appear dark under the fluorescence microscope. (g) A fluorescence image of the NWs with HQ-PA after DNA incubation. The NWs appear dark, indicating no DNA attached to HQ-PA. (Reprinted with permission from Currell, M., Li, C., Sun, Y.H., Lei, B., Gundersen, M.A., Thompson, M.E., and Zhou, C.W., Selective functionalization of In2O3 nanowire mat devices for biosensing applications, *J. Am. Chem. Soc.*, 127(19), 2005, 6922–6923. Copyright 2005 American Chemical Society.)

A mat sample of In_2O_3 NWs was grown on a SiO_2/Si wafer, followed by photolithography and metal deposition to pattern an electrode array. The resultant device is shown in Figure 15.5c. Figure 15.5d and e show typical SEM images of the NW mat sample used in this study. Multiple nanowires were found bridging the Au electrodes. A SAM of HQ-PA was created on a freshly cleaned In_2O_3 NW mat sample. The In_2O_3 NW device was placed into the electrochemical cell and completely reduced to HQ-PA. In order to prevent the thiol terminated DNA from attaching to the gold electrodes, the sample was treated with dodecane-1-thiol after HQ-PA SAM formation. This resulted in the formation of a SAM of a C_{12} alkyl chain on the Au electrode surface (Figure 15.5a). The device was then placed into an electrochemical cell with both electrodes submerged in the electrolyte but with potential applied across only select Au electrodes (upper electrode in Figure 15.5c). The potential of the cell was held at +450 mV for 5 s. In this way, the monolayer of HQ-PA coating on specific NWs was oxidized to Q-PA. Then, the entire device was submerged in the thiol-terminated DNA (HS-DNA) solution for 2 h, resulting in the selective, covalent linkage of DNA to the NWs with Q-PA (Figure 15.5f). Fluorescence studies were used to confirm the selective functionalization of the In_2O_3 NWs array. Typical fluorescence images from similar nanowire devices with Q-PA and HQ-PA, which have been treated with the complementary DNA strand containing a fluorescent dye label, are shown in Figure 15.5f and g, respectively. In Figure 15.5f the gold electrodes appear as dark lines, whereas the NW mat-Q-PA, derivatized with DNA, appears as a bright network. In contrast the NWs with HQ-PA, which went through the same DNA treatment, do not show any fluorescence, as seen in Figure 15.5g. This demonstrates there is no DNA binding to the NWs with HQ-PA.[40]

15.2.3 Prostate-Specific Antigen Sensing Using In_2O_3 Nanowire Biosensor

Recent biosensing literature has reported the use of either CNTs or nanowires as successful sensors for a number of biological analytes;[8,18,42–46] however, combining these two nanomaterials may offer an interesting comparison and also novel sensing strategies. A complementary of *n*-type In_2O_3 nanowires and *p*-type CNTs was implemented to detect prostate-specific antigen (PSA), an oncological marker for the presence of prostate cancer. Combination of In_2O_3 NWs and SWNTs for the detection of PSA revealed complementary electrical response upon PSA binding. Detection of PSA in solution has been demonstrated to be effective as low as 5 ng/mL, a level useful for clinical diagnosis of prostate cancer.[47,48]

The device structure of nanowire/nanotube sensors is schematically shown in Figure 15.6a, where an active channel made up of nanowires or nanotubes bridges the source/drain electrodes, and the silicon substrate can be used as gate.[25] Both individual and mat nanowires/nanotubes have been used as the active channel. Key to selective detection of PSA is to functionalize the nanochannel surface with anti-PSA monoclonal antibody (PSA-AB), a specific ligand for PSA protein. The new functionalization strategy adopted for In_2O_3 NWs is to covalently attach antibodies to NW surfaces via the onsite surface synthesis of a succinimidyl linking molecule as shown in Figure 15.6b. In_2O_3 NW devices were first submerged in a solution of 3-phosphonopropionic acid, resulting in binding of the phosphonic acid to the indium oxide surface with the COOH groups available for further reaction. The COOH groups on the nanowire surface were subsequently converted to a carboxylate succinimidyl ester via incubation in *N,N'*-dicyclohexylcarbodiimide (DCC) and *N*-hydroxysuccinimide and treated with a buffered saline solution of PSA-AB at 50 μM concentration.[25] The antibody is thus anchored to the nanowire surface. SWNT devices

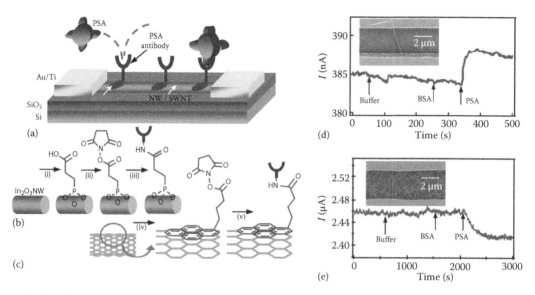

FIGURE 15.6

(a) Schematic diagram of the nanosensor. PSA-ABs are anchored to the NW/SWNT surface and function as specific recognition groups for PSA binding. (b) Reaction sequence for the modification of In_2O_3 NW: (i) deposition of 3-phosphonopropionic acid; (ii) DCC and N-hydroxysuccinimide activation; (iii) PSA-AB incubation (c) Reaction sequence for the modification of SWNT: (iv) deposition of 1-pyrenebutanoic acid succinimidyl ester; (v) PSA-AB incubation. Current recorded over time for an individual In_2O_3 NW device (d) and a SWNT mat device (e) when sequentially exposed buffer, BSA and PSA. Insets: SEM images of respective devices. (Reprinted with permission from Li, C., Curreli, M., Lin, H., Lei, B., Ishikawa, F.N., Datar, R., Cote, R.J., Thompson, M.E., and Zhou, C., Complementary detection of prostate-specific antigen using In2O3 nanowires and carbon nanotubes, *J. Am. Chem. Soc.*, 127, 2005, 12484–12485. Copyright 2005 American Chemical Society.)

were fabricated by a related procedure, illustrated in Figure 15.6c.[25] The SWNT surface is first functionalized with 1-pyrenebutanoic acid succinimidyl ester,[42] followed by treatment with the PSA-AB solution.[25]

After anchoring PSA-AB to the NW and SWNT devices, the chemical gating effect of PSA on the devices was investigated.[25] Devices consisting of both individual NWs and individual semiconducting SWNTs were incubated in a PBS buffered solution containing PSA for 15 h, at a concentration of 1 μg/mL.[25] The device surface was then thoroughly rinsed with deionized water and dried under a stream of nitrogen. The electrical properties of the devices, including both current–voltage ($I–V_{ds}$) and current–gate voltage ($I–V_g$) characteristics, were measured in air before and after the PSA incubation. Increase in conductance for NW devices and reduction in conductance for SWNT devices after PSA incubation were observed.[25] In addition to the complementary change in conductance, the gate dependence of both the NW and SWNT devices also changed. The threshold voltage (V_T) of the NW device shifted from −8 to −14 V, in contrast to a shift from −22 to −25 V for the SWNT device.[25] This complementary response in conductance can be understood as In_2O_3 NWs are *n*-type and SWNTs are *p*-type semiconductors. The origin of the change of the device characteristics is that the chemical gating effect of PSA introduces carriers into In_2O_3 NWs, leading to enhanced conductance, while the PSA binding decreases the carrier concentration in nanotubes, thus reducing the conductance.[25]

The real-time PSA detection was performed in PBS solution with both In_2O_3 NW and SWNT devices. Figure 15.6c and d insets display the device images. SWNT mat devices were used in order to overcome the instability found with individual SWNT devices. The antibody-functionalized nanosensors were submerged in PBS buffer solution. The electrical currents through the NW and the SWNT devices were monitored as several solutions were added to the solution above the nanosensor. The resulting current versus time curves are shown in Figure 15.6d for a single In_2O_3 NW device ($V_{ds} = 100$ mV) and Figure 15.6e for a SWNT mat device ($V_{ds} = 5$ mV). The current readings from both devices displayed little change after the addition of the buffer solution, thus attesting to the sufficiently high stability of the devices. Upon addition of 100 nM BSA in PBS, the readings still did not show any appreciable change, indicating nonspecific binding of BSA was successfully suppressed.[25] In sharp contrast, the current of the nanowire device increased rapidly after being exposed to 0.14 nM (5 ng/mL) PSA, while the current of the SWNT mat device decreased relatively slowly and stabilized at lower values upon exposure to 1.4 nM (50 ng/mL) PSA.[25] The amplitude of the current change was about 1.3% for the NW device and 2% for the nanotube devices.[25] The signal-to-noise ratio is about 20 for the NW device exposed to 5 ng/mL PSA (Figure 15.6d), indicating that the detection limit could approach 250 pg/mL.[25]

15.2.4 Sensing of Severe Acute Respiratory Syndrome Virus Marker with Artificial Antibody

Nanowire sensor technology can benefit immensely from engineered antibodies that are tailored toward specific biomarkers in terms of device cost and detection sensitivity. Engineered antibodies, or antibody mimic proteins (AMPs), are a class of affinity binding agents developed by *in vitro* selection techniques.[50,51] The AMPs can be modified to further improve selectivity and binding affinity over those of antibodies and nucleotide aptamers. In contrast to antibodies, AMPs are usually 2–5 nm in size, less than 10 kDa in molar mass, and stable to a wide range of pH and electrolyte concentrations. Moreover, they can be produced in large quantity at relatively low cost. The combination of these properties makes AMPs particularly attractive for enhancing the performance of nanowire biosensors.

The use of AMPs functionalized on In_2O_3 nanowire biosensors was successfully demonstrated for the detection of the nucleocapsid (N) protein[49], a biomarker for the severe acute respiratory syndrome (SARS) coronavirus.[52] The reported AMP, a fibronectin-based protein (Fn), detects the N protein at sub-nanomolar concentrations, and the NW sensing response was used to accurately determine the N-protein-to-Fn binding constant by applying a conventional Langmuir model.[49]

A schematic of fibronectin-based capture agent anchored to an In_2O_3 nanowire field-effect transistor is shown in Figure 15.7b. The Fn-based AMP was evolved using mRNA display from a large library of potential candidates and possesses a high binding affinity to the N protein ($K_D = 3.3$ nM).[53] The Fn probe was also engineered to have a single cystine residue near the C-terminus of the protein, remote from the binding site (Figure 15.7a). This unique thiol group allows the Fn anchoring to the nanowire to be carried out selectively, since the chosen linker molecule/chemistry (i.e., maleimide groups) gives a nanowire surface that is reactive only toward sulphydryl groups. This conjugation strategy allows every bound Fn to retain full activity,[49] a clear advantage over antibodies, which are often bound to the nanowire surface via amine containing residues randomly distributed on the antibody surface.[25,29,54–57] Moreover, the Fn can also be easily configured with other functional groups, such as azides[46,58] or cyclopentadienes.[59]

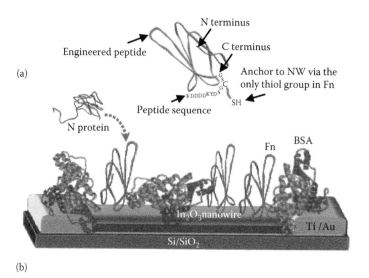

(b)

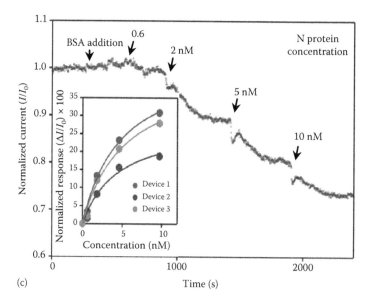

(c)

FIGURE 15.7

(See color insert.) (a) Ribbon structure of the engineered fibronectin (Fn), showing Fn attached to the NWs via the sulphydryl group of a cysteine near the C-terminus, remote from the binding site. (b) Schematic showing Fn immobilized on the surface of an In_2O_3 nanowire FET device. Regions of engineered peptide sequence are in red and are used to capture the target N protein. BSA protein was used to block sites for nonspecific binding. (c) Normalized electrical output (I/I_0) versus time of one sensor. Nonspecific binding is blocked after 40 μM of BSA, and additional BSA produces no response at 300 s. The red arrows indicate the times when the solution was raised to a given concentration of N protein. Inset: Normalized response against N protein concentration from 3 (dots) that are fitted using a Langmuir isotherm model (solid line). (Reprinted with permission from Ishikawa, F.N., Chang, H.K., Curreli, M., Liao, H.I., Olson, C.A., Chen, P.C., Zhang, R. et al., Label-free, electrical detection of the SARS virus N-protein with nanowire biosensors utilizing antibody mimics as capture probes, *ACS Nano*, 3, 2009, 1219–1224. Copyright 2009 American Chemical Society.)

The In_2O_3 nanowires used for this experiment were prepared following a well-established procedure.[24,36,40,60] The NW sensor surface was first functionalized with 6-phosphonohexanoic acid, as prepared in the PSA sensing. Then the carboxylic acid functional groups on the NW surface were activated with 1-Ethyl-3-[3-dimethylaminopropyl] carbodiimide hydrochloride (EDC). The activated COOH groups were allowed to react with N-[β-Maleimidopropionic acid] hydrazide, trifluoroacetic acid salt (BMPH), resulting in a NW surface that's reactive toward the unique thiol group on the Fn probe, which specifically detects SARs N Protein.[49]

The normalized electrical response, I/I_0, of an Fn-modified nanowire device is shown in Figure 15.7c, where I_0 is the I_{ds} response at $t = 0$ s. The experiment was performed in buffer, and I_0 was taken after sufficiently passivating the regions of the sensor that are subject to non-specific binding with the protein bovine serum albumin (BSA). A schematic of BSA passivation on the NW sensor surface is shown in Figure 15.7b. Nonspecific binding is shown to be successfully blocked by BSA, as additional BSA to the sensor surface around 300 s (Figure 15.7c) did not cause a shift in the I/I_0 baseline. The conductance of the device rapidly decreased (4%) upon exposing the nanowire sensor to a solution containing 0.6 nM of N protein in 44 μM BSA. The progressive increase of the N protein concentration induced a consistent decrease in device conductance relative to the baseline. This successful detection of SARS N protein using Fn demonstrated the potential of AMPs in the application of nanobiosensors.[49]

In the inset of Figure 15.7c, three devices were used to perform N protein detection in parallel. All three device responses showed a quantitatively similar concentration dependence (dots), confirming the reproducibility of the results. These plots were fitted using a conventional Langmuir isotherm model[61,62] (solid line) and these fits were used to estimate the binding constant of Fn to the N protein. In applying this model, the response of the sensor was assumed to be proportional to the number of captured molecules on the sensor surface such that $I/I_0 \propto$ Fn surface coverage. Application of this analytical model yields a binding constant of 4.9 ± 0.4 nM[49], which is close to the value of the binding constant ($K_D = 3.3$ nM) obtained from measurements of surface plasmon resonance (SPR).[53] The close match of the binding constant illustrates the validity of the assumption made and the Langmuir isotherm model.

The usage of the NW biosensors for the detection of N protein in the nM range is much quicker and more easily operated than conventional immunological clinical tests. Nanowire sensors with engineered proteins that have elevated affinity toward targets can have potential applications ranging from disease diagnosis to homeland security. This report[49] also demonstrated the potential for nanobiosensors to be used as a convenient and rapid tool to measure the binding constants for biological pairs such as antibody–antigen, protein–ligand, and oligonucleotides.

15.2.5 Development of Calibration Method of Sensor Response

An important challenge holding back the practical application of nanobiosensors to bioanalytical measurements is the device-to-device variation in the device properties such as conductance, threshold voltage, and transconductance. This results in unreliable detection, making quantitative analysis difficult. Efforts have been devoted to both the fabrication front for producing more uniform devices[21,29,64–82] and the analytical front for calibrating device response signals. Such analytical approaches include those based on the Langmuir adsorption theory[83] and the gate dependence (dI_{ds}/dV_g) model.[63] As an example, the dI_{ds}/dV_g method for calibrating In_2O_3 nanowire biosensors will be discussed in detail in this section.

In order to understand how calibrating by dI_{ds}/dV_g suppresses variations in the sensing response between different sensors, it is helpful to revisit the physics of the sensing mechanism in more detail. Ishikawa et al. demonstrated several experiments using biotin/streptavidin binding to pinpoint the most likely cause of NW sensor signal.[63] The In_2O_3 NW sensors in these experiments were fabricated and functionalized following a previously developed procedure,[24,25,84] and biotin was then anchored on the In_2O_3 NW surface. Interdigitated source and drain electrodes were introduced to decrease fabrication cost by increasing yield and scalability.[63] Reported transistor current followed the linear relationship (Equation 15.3) given in the ohmic region,

$$I_{ds} = g_m \times (V_g - V_T) \tag{15.3}$$

where
   V_T is the threshold voltage
   g_m, the transconductance of the device, is influenced by the device mobility, channel dimensions, and dielectric property

Figure 15.8a shows typical I_{ds}–V_g curves from a device before and after exposure to streptavidin. The change of the I_{ds}–V_g after the binding can be described as a parallel shift of the I_{ds}–V_g by ~14 mV. A shift in the I_{ds}–V_g relationship, as opposed to a change in the slope of the curve, indicates that the dominant sensing mechanism can be better attributed to a threshold voltage (V_T) change rather than a change in transconductance (g_m), mobility, or dielectric.[14,54] The V_T shift can be caused by the doping of nanowires from the analytes, and the process can be further classified into two categories: charge transfer[54] and electrostatic interaction.[14] The former depends on the alignment of the chemical potential between the analyte and the sensor[85] as well as on the charge transfer resistance.[86] In contrast, the electrostatic interaction does not require the direct transfer of carriers through the interface, and has a characteristic screening length (Debye length, λ_D) associated with the dielectric properties of the sensing environment (buffer and In_2O_3 nanowire in this case).[15,32] To investigate which type of doping is affecting NW biosensors, buffers with three different electrolyte concentrations, resulting in different Debye lengths, were used in the detection of streptavidin.[63] Figure 15.8b shows I_{ds} versus time plots in 1x PBS ($\lambda_D = 0.7$ nm), 0.01x PBS ($\lambda_D = 7$ nm), and 0.0001x PBS ($\lambda_D = 70$ nm), when the device was exposed to 100 nM streptavidin at $t = 100$ s. The strong dependence of the responses to the ionic concentration indicates that the sensing mechanism is dominant by electrostatic interaction rather than charge transfer. When electrostatic interaction is the dominant sensing mechanism, the change in sensor current after detection (I_2) can be written as

$$I_2 = g_{m1}(V_g - V_{T2}) = g_{m1}\left(V_g - (V_{T1} + \Delta V)\right) \tag{15.4}$$

where ΔV is the equivalent gating voltage (potential) induced by the biomolecules, and the subscripts 1 and 2 indicate before and after analyte detection, respectively. Using this correlation, the normalized response ($\Delta I/I_0$) can be written as

$$\frac{\Delta I}{I_0} = \left(\frac{g_{m1}(V_g - V_{T1}) - g_{m1}\left(V_g - (V_{T1} + \Delta V)\right)}{g_{m1}(V_g - V_{T1})}\right) = \frac{\Delta V}{(V_g - V_{T1})} \tag{15.5}$$

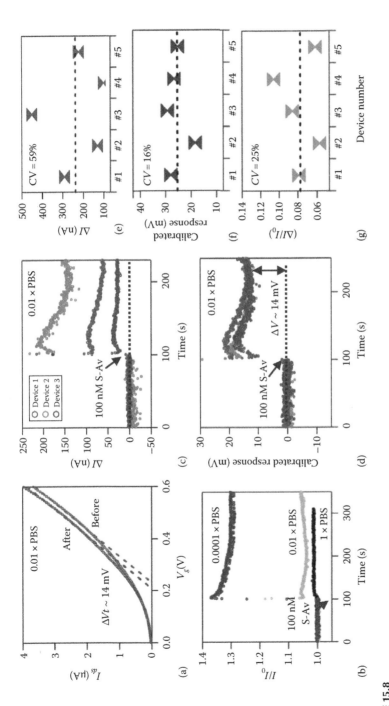

FIGURE 15.8

(See color insert.) (a) I_{ds} versus V_g using the liquid gate before (red) and after (blue) exposure to streptavidin of 100 nM in 0.01× PBS. (b) Plots of current versus time in PBS of different levels of dilution. The devices were exposed to 100 nM streptavidin at $t = 100$ s. Vds of 0.2 V and Vg of 0.6 V were used for the measurement. (c) Typical plots of the change in current versus time for three devices that were exposed to streptavidin (S-Av) of 100 nM at $t = 100$ s in 0.01× PBS. Vds of 0.2 V and Vg of 0.6 V were used for the measurement. (d) Plots of the calibrated response using the data shown in (c). (e) Plots of the absolute responses for five devices versus the device identification number before the calibration. The vertical axis was switched to the calibrated response. (g) Same plots after the calibration. (f) Same plots after the calibration. The vertical axis is the normalized response. (Reprinted with permission from Ishikawa, F.N., Curreli, M., Chang, H.K., Chen, P.C., Zhang, R., Cote, R.J., Thompson, M.E., and Zhou, C., A calibration method for nanowire biosensors to suppress device-to-device variation, *ACS Nano*, 3(12), 2009, 3969–3676. Copyright 2009 American Chemical Society.)

while a calibrated response of the gate dependence $(\Delta I/(dI_{ds}/dV_g))$ can be expressed as follows:

$$\frac{\Delta I}{dI_{ds}/dV_g} = \left(\frac{g_{m1}(V_g - V_{T1}) - g_{m1}\left(V_g - (V_{T1} + \Delta V)\right)}{g_{m1}} \right) = \Delta V \qquad (15.6)$$

As can be seen in Equations 15.5 and 15.6, the normalized response is still affected by V_{T1}, which is subject to device-to-device variation. On the other hand, the calibrated response is no longer a function of the device performance, and it only depends on the equivalent gate potential induced by the biomolecules (ΔV). Therefore, the dI_{ds}/dV_g calibration method is superior to the conventional normalization since it excludes variations in threshold voltage.

Indeed, this has been experimentally confirmed,[63] as shown in Figure 15.8e through g, where the absolute responses, the calibrated responses, and the normalized responses for several sensors were plotted, respectively, against the device identification numbers together with an average of the responses before the calibration. The improvement in device variation was statistically verified by calculating the coefficient of variation (CV) for each set of data, where CV is defined as the standard deviation divided by the mean. CV was reduced from 59% for the absolute response, and 25% for the conventional normalized response, to 16% for the calibrated response, confirming the much reduced device-to-device variation after calibration. The same calibration was also performed on the real-time sensing data,[63] as shown in Figure 15.8b and c. It is clear that the large device-to-device variation observed in Figure 15.8b is significantly reduced in Figure 15.8c after the calibration, confirming the applicability of this method to real-time biosensing. The calibrated responses (change) of ~14 mV for the real-time measurement are consistent with the number observed for the $I_{ds}-V_g$ measurement (~14 mV).

This method is a powerful tool for calibrating the sensor response of biosensors, especially for devices in which it is more challenging to get uniform V_T. Biosensing experiments are usually carried out with small V_{ds} to avoid electrochemical reaction, which may be induced by large V_{ds}; however, the method works as long as I_{ds} is linearly dependent on V_g within small variation. Even for the saturation regime, while I_{ds} is proportional to V_g^2 over a large range, the $I_{ds}-V_g$ within small variation of V_g can still be approximated with a linear curve.

15.2.6 Sensing in Complex Media

Blood is one of the most informative sources for health and disease monitoring in the human body.[88,89] However, the use of whole blood as an input is not typically investigated for biomarker detection, as such complex environments are known to cause problems such as false signal and saturation of receptors. Recently significant progress has been made in biosensing from whole blood using a capture-release microfluidic chip,[90] from desalted serum,[20,87,88] or in diluted serum.[87] Here, the detection of cancer biomarkers in blood serum using the In_2O_3 NW biosensor platform will be used as the example to illustrate the common concerns and possible solutions for nanobiosensing in the complex media.

The general operation of the In_2O_3 NW model system for detection in serum is as follows. The In_2O_3 NW sensors were fabricated and functionalized as in previous reports.[24–25,40,60,63,84] An additional silicon nitride layer was conformally coated on the metal electrodes to ensure the observed signal is from nanowires rather than the electrodes. After blood was collected by a commercially available finger prick device and left to completely clot, it was flowed through a polycarbonate membrane microfilter to remove blood cells. The output of the microfilter directly went to a Teflon mixing cell in order to achieve in-line detection. The filtered whole blood is essentially serum with less than 1% of blood cells remaining, and it is then delivered to the nanosensors attached to the mixing cell for electrical measurement.

The problem of nonspecific binding from serum proteins is first illustrated in Figure 15.9a and b by comparing the performances of nanosensors in buffer and in quasi-serum of the same ionic concentration.[87] In both instances the nanosensors were coated with antibodies for cancer antigen 125 (CA-125), an epithelial ovarian cancer biomarker. In Figure 15.9a, a CA-125 solution with a final concentration of 1 U/mL (5 pM) was introduced to the first sensor in PBS buffer environment. The source-drain current decreased and re-equilibrated to a lower level after being introduced to the CA-125 biomarkers with a 1% change in current. As a comparison, Figure 15.9b is the real-time sensing response for a device submerged in serum and then exposed to CA-125 of 1 U/mL, and there is no noticeable sensing signal. Non-target proteins in serum are known to negatively impact the sensitivity of nanosensors. The loss of sensing response in serum is attributed to the blocking of CA-125 biomarker to binding sites by nonspecific proteins, and the complexity of a medium substantially limits the sensing performance of the nanosensor. In order to overcome the limitation induced by nonspecific binding of non-target proteins, one solution is to use an amphipathic polymer, tween-20, as the passivating agent on the nanowire surface. Tween-20 is often used as a blocking agent in bioanalytical assays. The polymer minimizes nonspecific binding[91] due to its low binding affinity to the abundant proteins present in physiological fluids. Passivation is done by incubating sensors with a tween-20 solution after antibody immobilization to sensor surface. In Figure 15.9c, the tween-20 passivated device is able to successfully detect 1 U/mL of CA-125 in serum with a sensing signal similar to the device in purified buffer (Figure 15.9a). The results clearly suggest that by applying tween-20 passivation to the nanowire surface, we can retain excellent sensing performance, even in a complex medium such as serum.

The effectiveness of tween-20 passivation to sensor performance in serum was further demonstrated using In_2O_3 NW sensors functionalized with biotin, as shown in Figure 15.9d.[87] Detections of streptavidin with 1, 10, and 100 nM were done under the ionic strength of 1.5 mM. The green curve shows the calibrated responses from unpassivated sensors in PBS. The blue curve shows responses from unpassivated sensors in serum, and the sensing response was significantly lower than those in pure buffer (green curve). Furthermore, the detection limit of 10 nM was one order of magnitude worse than that in buffer. Streptavidin sensing was then repeated in serum with tween-20 passivated devices (red curve). In these cases, the response improved to nearly the same level as those done in pure buffer, and the detection limit was recovered. The data suggest that by suppressing the nonspecific binding, the tween-20 passivated biosensors can be as sensitive in serum as in buffer, which is crucial for biosensing applications.

The use of tween-20 to suppress nonspecific serum protein binding has been successfully applied to the concentration-dependent detection of CA-125 and insulin growth factor II (IGF-II), two biomarkers associated with epithelial ovarian cancer, in filtered whole blood collected from a cancer-free person using the aforementioned finger-pricking and filtration technique.[87] Shown in Figure 15.9e is the plot of the normalized current versus time of a tween-20 passivated sensor while the device was exposed to increased concentration of CA-125 consecutively. Here, the Debye screening from the high salt concentration in blood

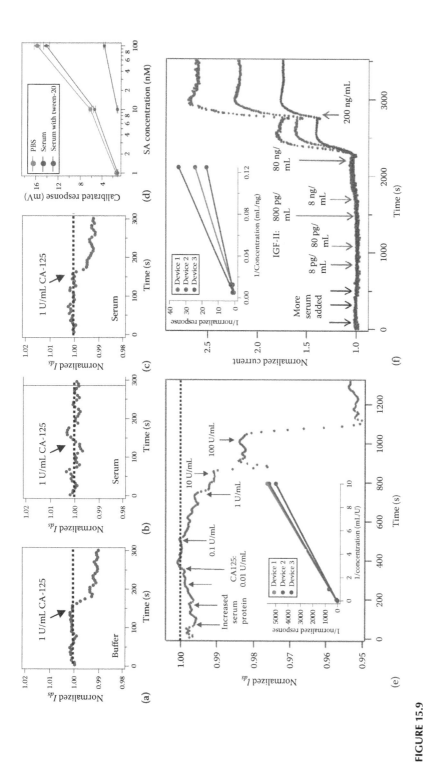

FIGURE 15.9

(See color insert.) Real-time sensing response for (a) unpassivated CA-125 nanosensor in buffer, (b) unpassivated CA-125 nanosensor in serum, and (c) tween-20 passivated nanosensor in serum. (d) Calibrated response versus streptavidin concentration for unpassivated sensors in buffer (green) and serum (blue) and for tween-20 passivated sensors in serum (red). (e) Normalized device current versus time during active CA-125 measurement in whole blood. Inset: 1/normalized response from three CA-125 biosensors versus 1/concentration of CA-125(dots). These plots can be fitted with Langmuir isotherm model (solid line), showing linear fit. (f) Real-time IGF-II sensing response from three nanosensors using integratable gravity desalting column. Inset: 1/normalized response from three IGF-II biosensors versus 1/concentration of IGF-II(dots). These plots can be fitted with Langmuir isotherm model (solid line), showing linear fit. (Reprinted with permission from Chang, H.K., Ishikawa, F.N., Zhang, R., Datar, R., Cote, R.J., Thompson, M.E., and Zhou, C., Rapid, label-free, electrical whole blood bioassay based on nanobiosensor systems, *ACS Nano*, 5(12), 2011, 9883–9891. Copyright 2011 American Chemical Society.)

was reduced by diluting the serum sample 100 times, which reduced the ionic strength to 1.5 mM. The detection limit of 0.1 U/mL corresponds to a concentration of 10 U/mL in non-diluted serum, which is much lower than the clinically relevant level for ovarian cancer diagnosis (100–275 U/mL)[92] and confirmed the feasibility of In_2O_3 NW sensors for clinical usage. Figure 15.9e inset shows that the responses (dots) from three independent devices display consistency. Their linear relationship to biomarker concentration fit the Langmuir isotherm model[61–62] (solid line) and can be used to estimate the CA-125 dissociation constant to 35.7 ± 2.8 U/mL (178.5 ± 14 pM).

The detection of IGF-II has demonstrated a second method for reducing the Debye length in blood or serum.[87] The antibody functionalization technique and device preparation were similar to CA-125 nanosensors. Here the ionic strength was reduced by using a gravity desalting column. As a result, the Debye screening effect was sufficiently reduced without diluting the sample. Figure 15.9f shows that once the devices were stabilized in desalted serum, they showed no response to further addition of serum (and hence increased serum protein concentration). In contrast, all three devices showed positive sensing response to IGF-II at concentrations of 8 ng/mL and beyond. This limit of detection is two orders of magnitude lower than the clinically relevant level for diagnosis.[92] The inset shows consistent sensing behavior (dots) from several devices and again confirms that In_2O_3 NW sensor detection of biomarkers fits the Langmuir isotherm model.

The detection of multiple biomarkers (CA-125 and IGF-II) in serum, with limit of detection much lower than clinically relevant levels, demonstrated that nanowire biosensor systems have great potential as multiplexed diagnosing tool for disease such as cancer. Their rapid, label-free electrical detection of biomarkers has high potential toward cheap and fully portable point-of-care type diagnosis. Furthermore, the promising results thus far represent a significant step forward toward the clinical application of nanobiosensors to drug efficacy monitoring.

15.3 Future Challenges

As has been shown in the earlier chapters, nanowire biosensors have progressed significantly from the proof-of-concept under simple environment to the demonstration of clinically meaningful detection of biomolecules in relatively complex environment. Despite these progresses, there have been a few obstacles that hinder the nanowire biosensors from being commercially available.

First, more reliable and uniform device fabrication must be demonstrated with reasonable price tag, since current fabrication techniques suffer from either nonuniform device property (bottom-up) or high cost (top-down). In these two approaches, top-down method seems more promising in near term to achieve a practical platform with additional research efforts.

Second, integration with complete microfluidic system must be demonstrated, which performs functionalization of devices and delivery of analytes. Such integration would not only enable automated operation of the system but also spatially selective functionalization of the devices within a small footprint. Multiplexed sensory system can thus be accomplished, which is an important goal of the nanowire biosensor community.

Third, packaging the sensor system with reliable insulation from the outer environment must be developed to increase the duration of the system and add portability to the system. Such insulation might enable the use of the sensors *in vivo*, widening the application of the technology.

Fourth, practical consideration, such as the duration of the system and possibility of repeated use of the system, must be taken care to further promote the entry of the technology into commerce.

These considerations might pose the development or use of long-life receptor molecules, such as AMP and aptamers.

As a summary of this chapter, we would like to clarify that in near future, there is a strong possibility for the nanowire biosensors to enter the practical market. Such realization will occur through integration with diverse technologies ranging from microfluidics to biomimetics. Collaborational work among researchers with multiple backgrounds would attain more and more importance for such technological development.

References

1. Chemla, Y. R.; Grossman, H. L.; Lee, T. S.; Clarke, J.; Adamkiewicz, M.; Buchanan, B. B., A new study of bacterial motion: Superconducting quantum interference device microscopy of magnetotactic bacteria. *Biophysical Journal* 1999, 76(6), 3323–3330.
2. Elghanian, R.; Storhoff, J. J.; Mucic, R. C.; Letsinger, R. L.; Mirkin, C. A., Selective colorimetric detection of polynucleotides based on the distance-dependent optical properties of gold nanoparticles. *Science* 1997, 277(5329), 1078–1081.
3. Gerion, D.; Chen, F.; Kannan, B.; Fu, A.; Parak, W. J.; Chen, D. J.; Majumdar, A.; Alivisatos, A. P., Room-temperature single-nucleotide polymorphism and multiallele DNA detection using fluorescent nanocrystals and microarrays. *Analytical Chemistry* 2003, 75(18), 4766–4772.
4. Hu, C. G.; Feng, B.; Xi, Y.; Zhang, Z. W.; Wang, N., Modification of carbon nanotubes and their electrochemical detection. *Diamond and Related Materials* 2007, 16(11), 1988–1991.
5. Kind, H.; Yan, H.; Messer, B.; Law, M.; Yang, P., Nanowire ultraviolet photodetectors and optical switches. *Advanced Materials* 2002, 14(2), 158–160.
6. Kolmakov, A.; Klenov, D. O.; Lilach, Y.; Stemmer, S.; Moskovits, M., Enhanced gas sensing by individual SnO2 nanowires and nanobelts functionalized with Pd catalyst particles. *Nano Letters* 2005, 5(4), 667–673.
7. Kong, J.; Franklin, N. R.; Zhou, C.; Chapline, M. G.; Peng, S.; Cho, K.; Dai, H., Nanotube molecular wires as chemical sensors. *Science* 2000, 287(5453), 622–625.
8. Star, A.; Gabriel, J.-C. P.; Bradley, K.; Grüner, G., Electronic detection of specific protein binding using nanotube FET devices. *Nano Letters* 2003, 3(4), 459–463.
9. Barbaro, A.; Colapicchioni, C.; Davini, E.; Mazzamurro, G.; Piotto, A.; Porcelli, F., CHEMFET devices for biomedical and environmental applications. *Advanced Materials* 1992, 4(6), 402–408.
10. Bergveld, P., Development of an ion-sensitive solid-state device for neurophysiological measurements. *IEEE Transactions on Bio-Medical Engineering* 1970, 17(1), 70–71.
11. Bergveld, P., Development, operation, and application of the ion-sensitive field-effect transistor as a tool for electrophysiology. *IEEE Transactions on Bio-Medical Engineering* 1972, 19(5), 342–351.
12. Colapicchioni, C.; Barbaro, A.; Porcelli, F.; Giannini, I., Immunoenzymatic assay using CHEMFET devices. *Sensors and Actuators B: Chemical* 1991, 4(3–4), 245–250.
13. Schasfoort, R. B. M.; Bergveld, P.; Kooyman, R. P. H.; Greve, J., Possibilities and limitations of direct detection of protein charges by means of an immunological field-effect transistor. *Analytica Chimica Acta* 1990, 238(0), 323–329.
14. Heller, I.; Janssens, A. M.; Mannik, J.; Minot, E. D.; Lemay, S. G.; Dekker, C., Identifying the mechanism of biosensing with carbon nanotube transistors. *Nano Letters* 2008, 8(2), 591–595.

15. Nair, P. R.; Alam, M. A., Screening-limited response of nanobiosensors. *Nano Letters* 2008, 8(5), 1281–1285.

16. Stern, E.; Steenblock, E. R.; Reed, M. A.; Fahmy, T. M., Label-free electronic detection of the antigen-specific T-cell immune response. *Nano Letters* 2008, 8(10), 3310–3314.

17. Tang, X.; Bansaruntip, S.; Nakayama, N.; Yenilmez, E.; Chang, Y. L.; Wang, Q., Carbon nanotube DNA sensor and sensing mechanism. *Nano Letters* 2006, 6(8), 1632–1636.

18. Chen, R. J.; Bangsaruntip, S.; Drouvalakis, K. A.; Kam, N. W.; Shim, M.; Li, Y.; Kim, W.; Utz, P. J.; Dai, H., Noncovalent functionalization of carbon nanotubes for highly specific electronic biosensors. *Proceedings of the National Academy of Sciences of the USA* 2003, 100(9), 4984–4989.

19. Star, A.; Tu, E.; Niemann, J.; Gabriel, J. C.; Joiner, C. S.; Valcke, C., Label-free detection of DNA hybridization using carbon nanotube network field-effect transistors. *Proceedings of the National Academy of Sciences of the USA* 2006, 103(4), 921–926.

20. Zheng, G.; Patolsky, F.; Cui, Y.; Wang, W. U.; Lieber, C. M., Multiplexed electrical detection of cancer markers with nanowire sensor arrays. *Nature Biotechnology* 2005, 23(10), 1294–1301.

21. Bunimovich, Y. L.; Shin, Y. S.; Yeo, W. S.; Amori, M.; Kwong, G.; Heath, J. R., Quantitative real-time measurements of DNA hybridization with alkylated nonoxidized silicon nanowires in electrolyte solution. *Journal of the American Chemical Society* 2006, 128(50), 16323–16331.

22. Byon, H. R.; Choi, H. C., Network single-walled carbon nanotube-field effect transistors (SWNT-FETs) with increased Schottky contact area for highly sensitive biosensor applications. *Journal of the American Chemical Society* 2006, 128(7), 2188–2189.

23. Gui, E. L.; Li, L. J.; Zhang, K.; Xu, Y.; Dong, X.; Ho, X.; Lee, P. S. et al., DNA sensing by field-effect transistors based on networks of carbon nanotubes. *Journal of the American Chemical Society* 2007, 129(46), 14427–14432.

24. Lei, B.; Li, C.; Zhang, D.; Tang, T.; Zhou, C., Tuning electronic properties of In2O3 nanowires by doping control. *Applied Physics A: Material Science and Processing* 2004, 79, 439–442.

25. Li, C.; Curreli, M.; Lin, H.; Lei, B.; Ishikawa, F. N.; Datar, R.; Cote, R. J.; Thompson, M. E.; Zhou, C. W., Complementary detection of prostate-specific antigen using In2O3 nanowires and carbon nanotubes. *Journal of the American Chemical Society* 2005, 127, 12484–12485.

26. Agarwal, A.; Lao, I. K.; Buddharaju, K.; Singh, N.; Balasubramanian, N.; Kwong, D. L. In *Silicon Nanowire Array Bio-Sensor Using Top-Down CMOS Technology, Solid-State Sensors, Actuators and Microsystems Conference, 2007. Transducers 2007. International*, Lyon, France, June 10–14, 2007; 2007; pp. 1051–1054. http://www.proceedings.com/02243.html

27. Gao, A.; Lu, N.; Dai, P.; Li, T.; Pei, H.; Gao, X.; Gong, Y.; Wang, Y.; Fan, C., Silicon-nanowire-based CMOS-compatible field-effect transistor nanosensors for ultrasensitive electrical detection of nucleic acids. *Nano Letters* 2011, 11(9), 3974–3978.

28. Hakim, M. M.; Lombardini, M.; Sun, K.; Giustiniano, F.; Roach, P. L.; Davies, D. E.; Howarth, P. H.; de Planque, M. R.; Morgan, H.; Ashburn, P., Thin film polycrystalline silicon nanowire biosensors. *Nano Letters* 2012, 12(4), 1868–1872.

29. Stern, E.; Klemic, J. F.; Routenberg, D. A.; Wyrembak, P. N.; Turner-Evans, D. B.; Hamilton, A. D.; LaVan, D. A.; Fahmy, T. M.; Reed, M. A., Label-free immunodetection with CMOS-compatible semiconducting nanowires. *Nature* 2007, 445(7127), 519–522.

30. Patolsky, F.; Zheng, G.; Hayden, O.; Lakadamyali, M.; Zhuang, X.; Lieber, C. M., Electrical detection of single viruses. *Proceedings of the National Academy of Sciences of the USA* 2004, 101(39), 14017–14022.

31. Kulkarni, G. S.; Zhong, Z., Detection beyond the Debye screening length in a high-frequency nanoelectronic biosensor. *Nano Letters* 2012, 12(2), 719–723.

32. Stern, E.; Wagner, R.; Sigworth, F. J.; Breaker, R.; Fahmy, T. M.; Reed, M. A., Importance of the Debye screening length on nanowire field effect transistor sensors. *Nano Letters* 2007, 7(11), 3405–3409.

33. Zhang, G.-J.; Zhang, G.; Chua, J. H.; Chee, R.-E.; Wong, E. H.; Agarwal, A.; Buddharaju, K. D.; Singh, N.; Gao, Z.; Balasubramanian, N., DNA sensing by silicon nanowire: Charge layer distance dependence. *Nano Letters* 2008, 8(4), 1066–1070.

34. Liu, Y.; Sauer, J.; Dutton, R. W., Effect of electrodiffusion current flow on electrostatic screening in aqueous pores. *Journal of Applied Physics* 2008, 103(8), 084701–084704.

35. Minot, E. D.; Janssens, A. M.; Heller, I.; Heering, H. A.; Dekker, C.; Lemay, S. G., Carbon nanotube biosensors: The critical role of the reference electrode. *Applied Physics Letters* 2007, 91(9), 93507.

36. Li, C.; Lei, B.; Zhang, D.; Liu, X.; Han, S.; Tang, T.; Rouhanizadeh, M.; Hsiai, T.; Zhou, C., Chemical gating of In_2O_3 nanowires by organic and biomolecules. *Applied Physics Letters* 2003, 83(19), 4014–4016.

37. Li, C.; Zhang, D.; Han, S.; Liu, X.; Tang, T.; Zhou, C., Diameter-controlled growth of single-crystalline In2O3 nanowires and their electronic properties. *Advanced Materials* 2003, 15(2), 143–146.

38. Zhang, D.; Li, C.; Liu, X.; Han, S.; Tang, T.; Zhou, C., Doping dependent NH[sub 3] sensing of indium oxide nanowires. *Applied Physics Letters* 2003, 83(9), 1845–1847.

39. Sevanian, A.; Asatryan, L.; Ziouzenkova, O., Low Density Lipoprotein (LDL) modification: Basic concepts and relationship to atherosclerosis. *Blood Purification* 1999, 17(2–3), 66–78.

40. Curreli, M.; Li, C.; Sun, Y. H.; Lei, B.; Gundersen, M. A.; Thompson, M. E.; Zhou, C. W., Selective functionalization of In2O3 nanowire mat devices for biosensing applications. *Journal of the American Chemical Society* 2005, 127(19), 6922–6923.

41. Chan, E. W. L.; Yousaf, M. N.; Mrksich, M., Understanding the role of adsorption in the reaction of cyclopentadiene with an immobilized dienophile. *The Journal of Physical Chemistry A* 2000, 104(41), 9315–9320.

42. Chen, R. J.; Zhang, Y.; Wang, D.; Dai, H., Noncovalent sidewall functionalization of single-walled carbon nanotubes for protein immobilization. *Journal of the American Chemical Society* 2001, 123(16), 3838–3839.

43. Nguyen, C. V.; Delzeit, L.; Cassell, A. M.; Li, J.; Han, J.; Meyyappan, M., Preparation of nucleic acid functionalized carbon nanotube arrays. *Nano Letters* 2002, 2(10), 1079–1081.

44. Koehne, J. E.; Chen, H.; Cassell, A. M.; Ye, Q.; Han, J.; Meyyappan, M.; Li, J., Miniaturized multiplex label-free electronic chip for rapid nucleic acid analysis based on carbon nanotube nanoelectrode arrays. *Clinical Chemistry* 2004, 50(10), 1886–1893.

45. Patolsky, F.; Lieber, C. M., Nanowire nanosensors. *Materials Today* 2005, 8(4), 20–28.

46. Bunimovich, Y. L.; Ge, G.; Beverly, K. C.; Ries, R. S.; Hood, L.; Heath, J. R., Electrochemically programmed, spatially selective biofunctionalization of silicon wires. *Langmuir* 2004, 20(24), 10630–10638.

47. Li, X.; Zhang, Y. P.; Kim, H. S.; Bae, K. H.; Stantz, K. M.; Lee, S. J.; Jung, C. et al., Gene therapy for prostate cancer by controlling adenovirus E1a and E4 gene expression with PSES enhancer. *Cancer Research* 2005, 65(5), 1941–1951.

48. Kelloff, G. J.; Coffey, D. S.; Chabner, B. A.; Dicker, A. P.; Guyton, K. Z.; Nisen, P. D.; Soule, H. R.; D'Amico, A. V., Prostate-specific antigen doubling time as a surrogate marker for evaluation of oncologic drugs to treat prostate cancer. *Clinical Cancer Research: An Official Journal of the American Association for Cancer Research* 2004, 10(11), 3927–3933.

49. Ishikawa, F. N.; Chang, H. K.; Curreli, M.; Liao, H. I.; Olson, C. A.; Chen, P. C.; Zhang, R. et al., Label-free, electrical detection of the SARS virus N-protein with nanowire biosensors utilizing antibody mimics as capture probes. *ACS Nano* 2009, 3, 1219–1224.

50. Binz, H. K.; Amstutz, P.; Pluckthun, A., Engineering novel binding proteins from nonimmunoglobulin domains. *Nature Biotechnology* 2005, 23(10), 1257–1268.

51. Binz, H. K.; Pluckthun, A., Engineered proteins as specific binding reagents. *Current Opinion in Biotechnology* 2005, 16(4), 459–469.

52. Zakhartchouk, A. N.; Viswanathan, S.; Mahony, J. B.; Gauldie, J.; Babiuk, L. A., Severe acute respiratory syndrome coronavirus nucleocapsid protein expressed by an adenovirus vector is phosphorylated and immunogenic in mice. *Journal of General Virology* 2005, 86, 211–215.

53. Liao, H. I.; Olson, C. A.; Ishikawa, F. N.; Curreli, M.; Chang, H.-K.; Thompson, M. E.; Zhou, C.; Roberts, R. W.; Sun, R., *Manuscript in Preparation* 2009.

54. Gruner, G., Carbon nanotube transistors for biosensing applications. *Analytical and Bioanalytical Chemistry* 2006, 384(2), 322–335.

55. Patolsky, F.; Zheng, G.; Lieber, C. M., Nanowire sensors for medicine and the life sciences. *Nanomedicine* 2006, 1(1), 51–65.

56. Allen, B. L.; Kichambare, P. D.; Star, A., Carbon nanotube field-effect-transistor-based biosensors. *Advanced Materials* 2007, 19(11), 1439–1451.

57. Curreli, M.; Zhang, R.; Ishikawa, F. N.; Chang, H.-K.; Cote, R. J.; Zhou, C.; Thompson, M. E., Real-time, label-free detection of biological entities using nanowire-based FETs. *IEEE Transactions on Nanotechnology* 2008, 7(6), 651–667.

58. Rohde, R. D.; Agnew, H. D.; Yeo, W. S.; Bailey, R. C.; Heath, J. R., A non-oxidative approach toward chemically and electrochemically functionalizing Si(111). *Journal of the American Chemical Society* 2006, 128(29), 9518–9525.

59. Yousaf, M. N.; Houseman, B. T.; Mrksich, M., Using electroactive substrates to pattern the attachment of two different cell populations. *Proceedings of the National Academy of Sciences of the United States of America* 2001, 98(11), 5992–5996.

60. Liu, F. B., M.; Wang, K. L.; Li, C.; Lei, B.; Zhou, C., One- dimensional transport of In2O3 nanowires. *Applied Physics Letters* 2005, 86, 213101–213103.

61. Langmuir, I., The constitution and fundamental properties of solids and liquids Part I Solids. *Journal of the American Chemical Society* 1916, 38, 2221–2295.

62. Halperin, A.; Buhot, A.; Zhulina, E. B., On the hybridization isotherms of DNA microarrays: the Langmuir model and its extensions. *Journal of Physics-Condensed Matter* 2006, 18(18), S463–S490.

63. Ishikawa, F. N.; Curreli, M.; Chang, H. K.; Chen, P. C.; Zhang, R.; Cote, R. J.; Thompson, M. E.; Zhou, C., A calibration method for nanowire biosensors to suppress device-to-device variation. *ACS Nano* 2009, 3(12), 3969–3676.

64. Smith, P. A.; Nordquist, C. D.; Jackson, T. N.; Mayer, T. S.; Martin, B. R.; Mbindyo, J.; Mallouk, T. E., Electric-field assisted assembly and alignment of metallic nanowires. *Applied Physics Letters* 2000, 77(9), 1399–1401.

65. Huang, Y.; Duan, X. F.; Wei, Q. Q.; Lieber, C. M., Directed assembly of one-dimensional nanostructures into functional networks. *Science* 2001, 291(5504), 630–633.

66. Tao, A.; Kim, F.; Hess, C.; Goldberger, J.; He, R. R.; Sun, Y. G.; Xia, Y. N.; Yang, P. D., Langmuir-Blodgett silver nanowire monolayers for molecular sensing using surface-enhanced Raman spectroscopy. *Nano Letters* 2003, 3(9), 1229–1233.

67. Rao, S. G.; Huang, L.; Setyawan, W.; Hong, S. H., Large-scale assembly of carbon nanotubes. *Nature* 2003, 425(6953), 36–37.

68. Kim, Y.; Minami, N.; Zhu, W. H.; Kazaoui, S.; Azumi, R.; Matsumoto, M., Langmuir-Blodgett films of single-wall carbon nanotubes: Layer-by-layer deposition and in-plane orientation of tubes. *Japanese Journal of Applied Physics Part 1-Regular Papers Short Notes & Review Papers* 2003, 42(12), 7629–7634.

69. Tsukruk, V. V.; Ko, H.; Peleshanko, S., Nanotube surface arrays: Weaving, bending, and assembling on patterned silicon. *Physical Review Letters* 2004, 92(6), 065502.

70. Han, S.; Liu, X. L.; Zhou, C. W., Template-free directional growth of single-walled carbon nanotubes on a- and r-plane sapphire. *Journal of the American Chemical Society* 2005, 127(15), 5294–5295.

71. Kocabas, C.; Hur, S. H.; Gaur, A.; Meitl, M. A.; Shim, M.; Rogers, J. A., Guided growth of large-scale, horizontally aligned arrays of single-walled carbon nanotubes and their use in thin-film transistors. *Small* 2005, 1(11), 1110–1116.

72. Wang, Y. H.; Maspoch, D.; Zou, S. L.; Schatz, G. C.; Smalley, R. E.; Mirkin, C. A., Controlling the shape, orientation, and linkage of carbon nanotube features with nano affinity templates. *Proceedings of the National Academy of Sciences of the United States of America* 2006, 103(7), 2026–2031.

73. Lee, M.; Im, J.; Lee, B. Y.; Myung, S.; Kang, J.; Huang, L.; Kwon, Y. K.; Hong, S., Linker-free directed assembly of high-performance integrated devices based on nanotubes and nanowires. *Nature Nanotechnology* 2006, 1(1), 66–71.

74. Liu, X. L.; Han, S.; Zhou, C. W., Novel nanotube-on-insulator (NOI) approach toward single-walled carbon nanotube devices. *Nano Letters* 2006, 6(1), 34–39.

75. Yu, G. H.; Cao, A. Y.; Lieber, C. M., Large-area blown bubble films of aligned nanowires and carbon nanotubes. *Nature Nanotechnology* 2007, 2(6), 372–377.

76. Li, X. L.; Zhang, L.; Wang, X. R.; Shimoyama, I.; Sun, X. M.; Seo, W. S.; Dai, H. J., Langmuir-Blodgett assembly of densely aligned single-walled carbon nanotubes from bulk materials. *Journal of the American Chemical Society* 2007, 129(16), 4890–4891.

77. Fan, Z. Y.; Ho, J. C.; Jacobson, Z. A.; Razavi, H.; Javey, A., Large-scale, heterogeneous integration of nanowire arrays for image sensor circuitry. *Proceedings of the National Academy of Sciences of the United States of America* 2008, 105(32), 11066–11070.

78. Heo, K.; Cho, E.; Yang, J. E.; Kim, M. H.; Lee, M.; Lee, B. Y.; Kwon, S. G. et al., Large-scale assembly of silicon nanowire network-based devices using conventional microfabrication facilities. *Nano Letters* 2008, 8(12), 4523–4527.

79. Li, M. W.; Bhiladvala, R. B.; Morrow, T. J.; Sioss, J. A.; Lew, K. K.; Redwing, J. M.; Keating, C. D.; Mayer, T. S., Bottom-up assembly of large-area nanowire resonator arrays. *Nature Nanotechnology* 2008, 3(2), 88–92.

80. Fan, Z. Y.; Ho, J. C.; Jacobson, Z. A.; Yerushalmi, R.; Alley, R. L.; Razavi, H.; Javey, A., Wafer-scale assembly of highly ordered semiconductor nanowire arrays by contact printing. *Nano Letters* 2008, 8(1), 20–25.

81. Monica, A. H.; Papadakis, S. J.; Osiander, R.; Paranjape, M., Wafer-level assembly of carbon nanotube networks using dielectrophoresis. *Nanotechnology* 2008, 19(8), (Manuscript in preparation).

82. Agarwal, A.; Buddharaju, K.; Lao, I. K.; Singh, N.; Balasubramanian, N.; Kwong, D. L., Silicon nanowire sensor array using top-down CMOS technology. *Sensors and Actuators a-Physical* 2008, 145, 207–213.

83. Abe, M.; Murata, K.; Ataka, T.; Matsumoto, K., Calibration method for a carbon nanotube field-effect transistor biosensor. *Nanotechnology* 2008, 19(4), 045505.

84. Li, C. Z., D.; Han, S.; Liu, X.; Tang, T.; Lei, B.; Liu, Z.; Zhou, C., Synthesis, electronic properties, and applications of indium oxide nanowires. *In Molecular Electronics III; New York Academy of Sciences: New York* 2003, 1006, 104–121.

85. Li, C.; Zhang, D. H.; Lei, B.; Han, S.; Liu, X. L.; Zhou, C. W., Surface treatment and doping dependence of In2O3 nanowires as ammonia sensors. *Journal of Physical Chemistry B* 2003, 107(45), 12451–12455.

86. Chidsey, C. E. D., Free-energy and temperature-dependence of electron-transfer at the metal-electrolyte interface. *Science* 1991, 251(4996), 919–922.

87. Chang, H. K.; Ishikawa, F. N.; Zhang, R.; Datar, R.; Cote, R. J.; Thompson, M. E.; Zhou, C., Rapid, label-free, electrical whole blood bioassay based on nanobiosensor systems. *ACS Nano* 2011, 5(12), 9883–9891.

88. Lathrop, J. T.; Anderson, N. L.; Anderson, N. G.; Hammond, D. J., Therapeutic potential of the plasma proteome. *Current Opinion in Molecular Therapeutics* 2003, 5(3), 250–257.

89. Fujii, K.; Nakano, T.; Kanazawa, M.; Akimoto, S.; Hirano, T.; Kato, H.; Nishimura, T., Clinical-scale high-throughput human plasma proteome clinical analysis: Lung adenocarcinoma. *Proteomics* 2005, 5(4), 1150–1159.

90. Stern, E.; Vacic, A.; Rajan, N. K.; Criscione, J. M.; Park, J.; Ilic, B. R.; Mooney, D. J.; Reed, M. A.; Fahmy, T. M., Label-free biomarker detection from whole blood. *Nature Nanotechnology* 2010, 5(2), 138–142.

91. Steinitz, M., Quantitation of the blocking effect of tween 20 and bovine serum albumin in ELISA microwells. *Analytical Biochemistry* 2000, 282(2), 232–238.

92. Visintin, I.; Feng, Z.; Longton, G.; Ward, D. C.; Alvero, A. B.; Lai, Y.; Tenthorey, J. et al., Diagnostic markers for early detection of ovarian cancer. *Clinical Cancer Research: An Official Journal of the American Association for Cancer Research* 2008, 14(4), 1065–1072.

Section III

Magnetic Nanoparticles for Biosensing and Cancer Treatment

16

Biosensing and Cancer Treatment with Magnetic Nanoparticles

Stefan Bossmann, Viktor Chikan, and Raj Kumar Dani

CONTENTS

16.1 Introduction to Magnetic Nanomaterials: Why Nano?

The term "nano" stands for dwarf in Greek. Quantitatively, it is a prefix for one billionth. For length, 1 nm means one billionth of a meter. By comparison, 1 nm is approximately 1/50,000–1/100,000 as thick as a human hair, or 3.5 atoms of gold lined up in a row equal 1 nm. All particles with at least one dimension between 1 and 100 nm fall in the category of nanoparticles (NPs). NPs have attracted great attention of scientists as they bridge bulk materials with atomic or molecular structures. The history of artificial NPs by humans dates back to Roman times when they used noble metal NPs for decorative purposes.[1] A good example is the "Lycurgus Cup" containing silver and gold bimetallic NPs of around 50–100 nm size. This cup is red in color with transmitted light and is green in color with reflected light.[2] In the Middle Ages, a gold colloid that contained metallic gold with slightly pink color was known as "drinkable gold." This "drinkable gold" was described as "a solution where solid is present in such a degree of communication that it is not visible to the human eye" and was largely used to cure some diseases like dysentery, epilepsy, and tumors and for the diagnosis of syphilis.[3] Later in 1857, Michael Faraday discovered the first metallic gold colloidal solution while he was conducting research on the optical properties of gold. He described the various colors of gold particles by using different preparation methods.[4] However, the modern history of nanotechnology starts with a physicist, Richard P. Feynman. He shared his vision of "what very small things are and how they would behave" at the annual meeting of the American Physical Society (December 26, 1959) in his talk titled "There's Plenty of Room at the Bottom" and suggested to start from bottom or nano-level, which is the key of the advancement of nanotechnology.[5]

NPs have been utilized in the biomedical area because the size of NPs is smaller than cells (10–100 µm) and comparable with viruses (20–450 nm), proteins (5–50 nm), and genes (2 nm wide by 10–100 nm long).[6] It means that NPs can communicate closely with biomolecules and they can cross biological membranes and deliver genes. Figure 16.1 shows the comparison of different NPs, cells, and biological entities.

The properties of NPs are interesting and sometimes exceptionally different from their counterpart atomic or bulk properties. In an average NP, the number of atoms ranges from a few hundreds up to approximately a million.[7] This is a size regime where quantum chemistry and solid state physics meet. In the nano size, the material can exhibit properties from both phase regions. Quantum chemistry investigates chemical systems where the charge carriers are confined in the electrostatic potential of nuclei. On the other hand, solid state physics discusses infinitely large systems where these charged carriers could move as quasi free particles. Regardless of size, bulk materials always have the same physical properties. The properties of NPs including optical, magnetic, specific heat, melting point, and surface activities are size dependent, which make the NPs unique. At the nano-level, the fundamental electronic, optical, magnetic, chemical, and biological properties of a material are changed. NPs have very high surface area to volume ratio. This is because the surface area is the function of square of radius ($4\pi r^2$) while volume the function of cube of radius (($4/3)\pi r^3$). For a typical NP, half or more of the atoms will be in the bulk phase,

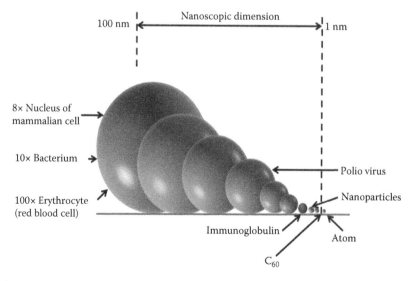

FIGURE 16.1
Comparison of sizes of atoms, nanoparticles, and biological entities.

only a relatively small fraction of atoms will be near the surface. These atoms provide more coordination sites and hence more probability to be easily manipulated so that they can achieve the required conditions to make them very reactive. Therefore, the surface plays a crucial role in determining the properties of the material. Overall, the following properties are the reasons that NPs are being used in biomedical applications:

- Exhibit intermediate properties of both atomic/molecular and bulk regions
- Easy to prepare with controllable sizes in nanometer range
- Tunable physical properties by adjusting composition, size, and shape
- Suitable size to communicate closely with biomolecules and facilitate intimate interactions with cells and molecular constituents
- Easy to manipulate their surface property through surface modification and functionalization to make them biocompatible and detectable
- Magnetic property of NPs: superparamagnetism in magnetic materials for drug delivery, imaging, and releasing heat (hyperthermia treatment)
- Plasmonic property of NPs: dielectric confinement in plasmonic materials for detection and thermal ablation

16.2 Physics of Magnetic Nanomaterials

16.2.1 Magnetism at Nanoscale

NPs that show magnetic behavior are defined as magnetic NPs. Magnetic NPs are abundant in nature, in the human brain, in bacteria, algae, birds, ants, and bees[8] and are also found in many other biological objects.[9] Interestingly, some vertebrates use NP-assisted natural navigation system for their long distance migration.[10] Nanoscale magnetic NPs are of interest for applications in ferrofluids, high-density magnetic storage, high-frequency electronics, high-performance permanent magnets, magnetic refrigerants, etc.[11] The intrinsic magnetic properties of bulk magnetic materials like saturation magnetization (M_S), coercive force (H_C), and Curie temperature (T_C) depend only on chemical and crystallographic structures. The shape and the size of the bulk materials are not crucial to determine the magnetic property. On the other hand, the properties of magnetic NPs not only depend on size and shape but also depend on chemical composition, type and degree of defects of the crystal lattice, interaction of the particles with the surrounding materials, and the neighbor particles.[12] Magnetic NPs show different properties from atoms and bulk materials, because these NPs have very high magnetic anisotropy with different Néel (T_N) and Curie (T_C) temperatures. By tuning all the properties mentioned earlier, properties of the magnetic NPs can be manipulated. These properties of the magnetic materials determine their classification. Diamagnetic materials have negative susceptibility and show weak repulsion with the external magnetic field while in paramagnetic materials, the magnetic moments are randomly orientated due to thermal fluctuations. When a magnetic field is applied, these randomly orientated magnetic moments start to align parallel to the field. Hence, paramagnetic materials are weakly attracted to the external magnetic field. They exhibit small and positive susceptibility. Ferromagnetic materials such as iron, cobalt, and nickel, have a higher tendency to align with the applied magnetic field and they are highly attracted toward the applied external magnetic field. They have very high positive magnetic susceptibility and show hysteresis. Diamagnetic and paramagnetic materials do not show any magnetic properties when the applied external magnetic field is removed. They show a linear response with the applied magnetic field. Ferromagnetic materials remain magnetized even after the removal of the external magnetic field.

When the size of the ferromagnetic materials decreases to a limit, they are no longer able to show ferromagnetic properties. This transition introduces another property known as superparamagnetism. A superparamagnetic material consists of small particles of ferromagnetic material and is able to flip the direction of its spin due to thermal fluctuations. As a result, superparamagnetic materials show magnetic properties only in the presence of a magnetic field. When the magnetic field is removed, thermal energy disrupts the magnetic moment of the material. For superparamagnetic particles, the net magnetic moment is zero in the absence of a magnetic field. When a magnetic field is applied, there will be a net statistical alignment of magnetic moments, which is analogous to paramagnetism. However, the magnetic moment is not that of a single atom, but of a single domain and a single domain contains thousands to millions of atoms. Hence, the term superparamagnetism is used, which denotes a much higher susceptibility value than that for simple paramagnetism.

Superparamagnetism can be understood considering single-domain particles. The magnetic anisotropy energy of a particle is responsible for holding the magnetic moments along a certain direction and is given by $E(\theta) = KV \sin^2\theta$ where K is the anisotropy constant, V is the volume of the particle, and θ is the angle between the direction of magnetization and the easy axis. The energy barrier KV separates the two energetically equivalent directions of magnetization.[13] With decreasing particle size, the thermal energy $k_B T$ exceeds the energy barrier KV (as shown in Figure 16.2), and the magnetization is easily flipped in direction. This is the hallmark of superparamagentic behavior.

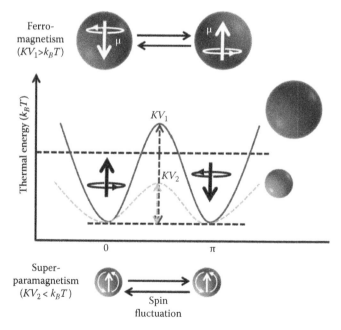

FIGURE 16.2
Energy diagram of magnetic nanoparticles with different magnetic spin alignment, showing ferromagnetism in a large particle and superparamagnetic in a small nanoparticle.

The size at which magnetic materials exhibit superparamagnetic behavior is called critical size (D_c). The critical size is a strong function of the saturation magnetization of the particles, anisotropy energy, and exchange interactions between individual spins.[14] Typical ferromagnetic materials contain a number of small magnetic regions called magnetic domains. The boundaries between the domains in these materials are called domain walls. In larger NPs, energetic considerations favor the formation of a domain wall but when the size decreases below a certain level, the formation of domain walls becomes unfavorable. The multi-domain state is energetically favorable if the energy consumption for the formation of domain walls is lower than the difference between the magnetostatic energies (ΔE_{MS}) of the single-domain and multi-domain states. When an external magnetic field is applied, creation, extinction, and growth of domain size may take place.[15] The creation of domain depends on the magnetostatic energy and the domain wall energy (E_{dw}). When the size of the materials decreases, the number of domain walls per unit area increases, which is energetically unstable and forces the material into a single domain configuration. The size below which the materials exist in a single domain is determined by the aforementioned two energies. ΔE_{MS} increases with volume of the material and increases with the interfacial area between domains. When these two energies become equal, then the following relation holds for critical size D_c:[13a]

$$D_c \approx 18 \frac{\sqrt{AK}}{\mu_0 M_s^2} \tag{16.1}$$

where
  A is the exchange constant
  K is the anisotropy constant
  μ_0 is the vacuum permeability
  M_s is the saturation magnetization

Typical values of D_c for some important magnetic materials[15] are listed in Table 16.1. Figure 16.3 summarizes the magnetization behavior of the single- and multi-domain magnetic NPs in relation to common diamagnetic and paramagnetic materials.

Magnetization is reversed by the movement of domain wall in ferromagnetic materials, but in superparamagnetic materials the reversal is due to the spin rotation of the magnetic

TABLE 16.1

Estimated Single-Domain Size for Different Spherical Magnetic Particles

Materials	M_s (emu/g)	D_{cr} (nm)
Iron (α-Fe)	217.9	7–11
Nickel	57.5	110
Cobalt	162.7	60
Magnetite, Fe_3O_4	91.6	20–30
$CoFe_2O_4$	80.8	40
Hematite, α-Fe_2O_3	1	13
NdFeB	171	300
$SmCo_5$	164	750
$BaFe_{12}O_{19}$	72	900

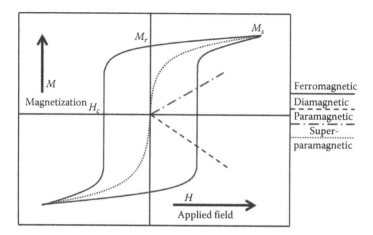

FIGURE 16.3

Hysteresis of different magnetic materials. H_c is coercive force, M_r is magnetization remanence, M_s is saturation magnetization. (From Arruebo, M. et al., *Nano Today*, 2, 22, 2007.)

moment. Superparamagnetism is useful in biomedical applications because as the applied magnetic field is removed, magnetization disappears then there will be no agglomeration of NPs. The superparamagnetic behavior can be characterized in terms of a relaxation time, τ, which is the time it takes for the system to achieve zero magnetization after the removal of the external magnetic field. The relaxation time, τ, for a particle is given by the Néel expression:[17]

$$\tau = \tau_0 \exp\left(\frac{\Delta E}{k_B T}\right) \tag{16.2}$$

where τ_0 is the characteristic time of the order 10^{-10} to 10^{-12} s for non-reacting particles and weakly depends on temperature, $\Delta E\ (= KV)$ is the energy barrier to moment reversal, and $k_B T$ is the thermal energy. If the particle magnetic moment reverses at times shorter than the experimental time scales, the system is in superparamagnetic state, if not, it is in the so-called blocked state. The temperature that separates these two states is the so-called blocking temperature, T_B.[13a]

16.2.2 Heating of Magnetic Nanomaterials in AC Magnetic Fields

In general, the energy of the rapidly changing electromagnetic field can be converted into heat energy. Both the electric field (E) and the magnetic field strength (H) are able to generate heat. The most common conversion takes place through resistive heating, capacitive heating, and induction heating.[18] Resistive and capacitive heating are possible through the electric component (E) of the alternating electromagnetic field. In resistive heating, heat energy is produced when an electric current flows through a resistive material. The heat energy produced depends on the current flow and the resistance of the material and is calculated as square of current multiplied by the resistance (I^2R). This is the principle of the electric heater. As the frequency of alternating electromagnetic field increases, the amount of internal atomic distortion also increases. This increasing internal atomic distortion produces a large amount of heat in the medium,[18] which is known as capacitive or dielectric heating. Capacitive heating is the working principle of household microwaves. Capacitive heating takes place at higher frequencies (10 MHz) and is able to heat water and even insulators as well. Therefore, higher frequencies cannot be used in clinical applications for humans since a human being consists of more than 75% water. Moreover, there is one more mechanism that can convert an alternating magnetic field into heat. The mechanism is known as inductive heating, which occurs at low frequencies. At low frequencies, the effect of electric component is insignificant and the heat is mainly due to the magnetic component (H).[19] In inductive heating, heat is produced in a magnetic material when the material is exposed to an AC field. Current is induced in the material heated by electromagnetic induction.[18] Inductive heating can be used in clinical applications such as magnetic hyperthermia treatment (MHT). Tolerable limits of inductive heating of tissues restrict the safe range of magnetic field amplitude and frequency that can be employed for MHT. It has been shown that any combination of field strength (H) and frequency (f) will be biologically noninvasive when $H \times f \leq 4.85 \times 10^8$ Hz-A m^{-1}.[20]

MHT is a technique where magnetic fluid is exposed to an alternating magnetic field; then the magnetic particles can act as an effective source of heat,[21] which could be used to destroy the cancer cells. Cell death occurs either due to the protein denaturation or the dissolution of parts of the cell membrane.[22] The fundamental basis of magnetic hyperthermia is that cells show signs of apoptosis and necrosis when heated around 46°C.[23] At this temperature, the function of many structural and enzymatic proteins within cells is modified, which in turn alters cell growth and differentiation and can induce apoptosis. Magnetic hyperthermia leads to more desirable apoptosis cell destroying method rather than necrosis. Unfortunately, the temperature at which the apoptosis of cancer cells takes place is too close to that of normal cells. Therefore, precise temperature control would be necessary.[24] The first experimental investigation of the magnetic hyperthermia was suggested by Gilchrist et al. in 1957 by heating various tissue samples using 20–100 nm of γ-Fe$_2$O$_3$ NPs with 1.2 MHz magnetic fields.[25] Nowadays, magnetic hyperthermia is becoming a promising tool in treating various types of cancer. This is because tumor cells are more susceptible to heat than normal tissue cells.[26] Thermal resistance of cancer cells is lower than the normal cells because the flow of blood is insufficient in tumors and the inadequate blood flow makes tumors more acidic due to the lactic acid buildup (higher rates of metabolism) in the tumor tissues from lack of oxygen (hypoxic) while the normal cells are well oxygenated (euoxic). Acidic nature increases the temperature sensitivity of the cells and temperature will rise easily when the blood flow is insufficient and cancer cells can be eliminated selectively by raising the local temperature of the tumor sites.[27]

The heating effect of the magnetic fluid is a result of absorbing energy from an alternating magnetic field and converting it into heat by the eddy current losses and relaxation losses.[28] Essentially the origin of heat, when magnetic particles are exposed in an alternating magnetic field, depends on the size of the particles and hence their magnetic properties.[6a] When the magnetic particle size is larger than 1 µm, generation of the eddy currents in the particles is responsible for heat generation. For multi-domain magnetic particles, the heating is mainly due to hysteresis loss. Larger particles have a number of sub-domains with well-defined magnetization direction. When such particles are exposed to the alternating magnetic field, the domain with the magnetization direction along the magnetic field axis grows and the others shrink. This phenomenon is called domain wall displacement.[29] When the magnetization curves with increasing and decreasing magnetic field amplitudes do not coincide, then the material is said to exhibit a hysteresis behavior and generates heat under the influence of the alternating magnetic field. The amount of heat that is generated during hysteresis loss can be calculated by determining the area of the hysteresis loop.

When the size of NPs decreases to single-domain particle regime (super-paramagnetic NPs), generation of heat due to hysteresis loss is not possible since there are no domain walls and the domain wall displacement is not possible. Even then, these NPs can produce heat under the influence of the alternating magnetic field. The generation of heat by single-domain magnetic particles is due to the relaxation loss. There are two distinct relaxation loss mechanisms by which the magnetization of magnetic NPs can relax back to their equilibrium position after the applied magnetic field is removed.

The first relaxation mechanism is the Néel relaxation where rotation of magnetic moment within the particles takes place to reverse magnetization direction. This process needs to overcome an energy barrier given by $E = KV$ (for uniaxial anisotropy), where K is the anisotropy constant of the material and V is the volume of the particles. An external alternating magnetic field supplies energy and assists magnetic moments to overcome the energy barrier. This energy is dissipated when the particle moment relaxes to its equilibrium orientation. The relationship between the characteristic time of thermal fluctuation of the magnetic moment of a single-domain particle with uniaxial anisotropy is obtained by the Néel relaxation time, τ_N, as[30]

$$\tau_N = \tau_0 \, e^{(\Delta E / k_B T)} \tag{16.3}$$

where
k_B is the Boltzmann constant and the pre-exponential factor
τ_0 is an expression of the anisotropy energy and depends on several parameters, including temperature, gyromagnetic ratio, saturation magnetization, anisotropy constants, and the height of barrier.

However, for the sake of simplicity, the value of τ_0 is often considered to be a constant[31] in the range of 10^{-9} to 10^{-13} s, and T is the temperature. In summary, Néel relaxation time represents the time required to achieve zero magnetization after the external magnetic field is removed.

The second relaxation mechanism is the Brownian relaxation. If particles move freely within the suspension, the entire particle can rotate to align along the external magnetic field. This mechanism generates heat due to the viscous friction between the rotating particle and the surrounding medium. The Brownian relaxation time is given by[32]

$$\tau_B = \frac{3 \eta V_H}{k_B T} \tag{16.4}$$

where
η is the dynamic viscosity of the carrier liquid
V_H is the hydrodynamic volume of the particle

Hydrodynamic volume (particle + ligand layer) characterizes how a particle moves through the fluid in which it is suspended and may be different from the magnetic volume due to agglomeration, coating, or interactions between the fluid and the NP surface.

The two relaxation mechanisms are shown in Figure 16.4.

In summary, of these two mechanisms, the faster relaxation mechanism is dominant in the heat dissipation process. The Néel relaxation depends exponentially on magnetic anisotropy and particle volume. The Brownian relaxation depends linearly on the particle volume and viscosity of carrier liquid. Due to different size dependence of Néel and Brownian relaxation, there is a boundary for these two relaxations where the crossover of relaxation

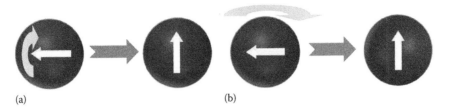

(a) (b)

FIGURE 16.4
Schematic depiction of (a) Néel and (b) Brownian relaxation.

takes place. The crossover between Néel and Brownian relaxation takes place when $\tau_N = \tau_B$. The dominant relaxation times of the maghemite/water system are shown in Figure 16.5. In general, Néel relaxation prevails at higher frequency combined with smaller particle size, and vice versa for Brownian relaxation.[33] The boundary frequency (f_c) and the corresponding particle diameter (D_c) of some of the selected ferrofluids are given in Table 16.2.[33]

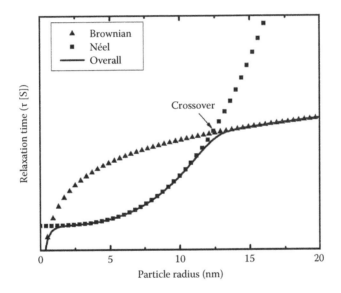

FIGURE 16.5
Relaxation times of maghemite/water system.

TABLE 16.2

Estimated Critical Nanoparticle Size Separating Néel and Brownian Relaxation Regimes

Ferrofluid	D_c nm	f_c kHz
Maghemite/water	25	8
Maghemite/ester oil	24	0.1
Ba-hexaferrite/water	11	50
Co-ferrite/water	7	10,000
Co-ferrite/glycerin	9	0.1
Co, hexag./water	6	2,500

In most cases, both relaxation mechanisms work together and the effective relaxation time is given by

$$\frac{1}{\tau} = \frac{1}{\tau_N} + \frac{1}{\tau_B} \tag{16.5}$$

Rosensweig[34] developed the analytical relationships for the power dissipation of ferrofluids in alternating magnetic fields. Briefly, magnetization of ferrofluids cannot follow the applied time varying magnetic field. The phase lag between the applied magnetic field and the magnetization of the ferrofluid results in the conversion of magnetic work into internal energy. It is convenient to express the magnetization in terms of the complex ferrofluid susceptibility as $\chi = \chi' - i\chi''$, where χ' is the in-phase component and χ'' is the out-of-phase component of susceptibility. The change in internal energy is given by

$$\Delta U = 2\mu_0 H_0^2 \chi'' \int_0^{2\pi/\omega} \sin^2 \omega t \; dT \tag{16.6}$$

Here, only the out-of-phase component χ'' survives, hence it is also known as loss component of susceptibility. Integrating and multiplying the result by cyclic frequency ($f = \omega/2\pi$) gives the mean volumetric power dissipation (loss power density, Wm^{-3}):

$$P = f\Delta U = \mu_0 \pi \chi'' f H_0^2 \tag{16.7}$$

The susceptibility components are given by

$$\chi' = \frac{1}{1 + (\omega\tau)^2} \chi_0 \tag{16.8}$$

$$\chi'' = \frac{\omega\tau}{1 + (\omega\tau)^2} \chi_0 \tag{16.9}$$

Then the Equations 6.5 and 6.7 give the power dissipation for a monodispersed ferrofluid, which is expressed as

$$P = \pi\mu_0 \chi_0 H_0^2 f \frac{2\pi f \tau}{1 + (2\pi f \tau)^2} \tag{16.10}$$

For polydispersed ferrofluid, the volumetric heat dissipation rate is given by

$$P = \int_0^\infty P g(R) dR \tag{16.11}$$

where $g(R)$ is the log normal size distribution, which is given by

$$g(R) = \frac{1}{\sqrt{2\pi}\sigma R} \exp\left[\frac{-(\ln R/R_0)^2}{2\sigma^2}\right] \qquad (16.12)$$

where
  $\ln R_0$ is the median radius
  σ is the standard deviation of $\ln R$

The loss power density P (Wm^{-3}) is related to the specific loss power, SLP (Wg^{-1}), by the mean mass density of the particles.[35] The maximum loss power could be reached with small particles and high frequencies. Here, a typical example for γ-Fe$_2$O$_3$ NP is shown in Figure 16.6.

Independent of the heating mechanism, the heating efficiency of the particles is quantified in terms of the power of heating of a magnetic material per gram (specific loss power, SLP), which is also called the specific absorption rate (SAR).[37] SAR is defined by the following expression

$$SAR = C\frac{dT}{dt} \qquad (16.13)$$

where
  C is the specific heat capacity of the system (Jg^{-1}K^{-1})
  dT is the change in temperature
  dt is the change in time

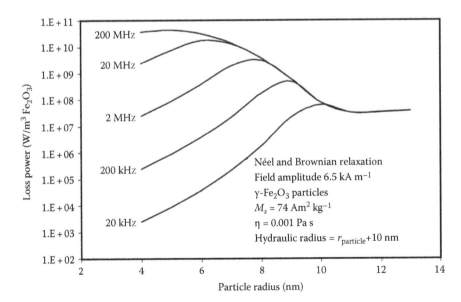

FIGURE 16.6
Loss power of γ-Fe$_2$O$_3$ with its size and frequency of applied alternating magnetic field. (From Hofmann-Amtenbrink, M. and Rechberg, B.V., In *Nanostructured for Biomedical Applications*, Tan, M.C., Ed., Transword Research Network, Trivandrum, India. Copyright 2009.)

16.2.3 Effect of Magnetic Nanoparticles on Spin Relaxation

Many nuclei are NMR-active; they feature a nuclear spin and thus a permanent magnetic dipole moment. The most important spin for medical and biosensing applications is the hydrogen nucleus (^{1}H) in water molecules. The human tissue contains various amounts of water, in average 55%–60% in adults.[41] In a static magnetic field (B_0), the spins are directed either in the direction of the field (lower energy state) or in the opposite direction of the field (higher energy state). The two states are populated according to a Boltzmann distribution:[42]

$$N_n = N_0 e^{- \frac{E_n}{kT}}$$ (16.14)

where
N_0 is the lower energy state
N_n is the higher energy state
E_n is the energy difference between the lower and higher state
k is the Boltzmann constant ($1.3806503 \times 10^{-23}$ m^2 kg s^{-2} K^{-1})
T is the temperature (309.8 K (healthy) to 316 K in humans)

The difference in population of both, the lower and higher states, leads to a small but measurable net magnetization M_0. The difference in occupation of the lower and higher states is small (usually in the range of 1:0.999995 at $B_0 = 3$ T), because the thermal energy that is available in a human is large compared to the energy difference between both states, which scales linearly with the strengths of the external magnetic field B_0:

$$\Delta E = \frac{\mu B_0}{I}$$ (16.15)

where
ΔE is the energy difference between lower and higher energy state
μ (^{1}H) = 2.7927 nuclear magnetons (5.05078×10^{-17} J T^{-1})
I is the spin (1/2 for ^{1}H)

Transitions between the two states can be triggered by applying an oscillating magnetic field perpendicular to the main magnetic field B_0. The frequency of the second magnetic field is $\omega = 1/4\, \gamma\, B_0$. γ is the gyromagnetic ratio, which is dependent on the nature of the nucleus. For ^{1}H the gyromagnetic ratio is 42.6 MHz T^{-1}. Therefore, in a typical MRI with a B_0 field of 3 T, the radiofrequency required to promote spins from the lower to the higher state is 127.8 MHz. Nuclear resonance imaging devices used for small samples are commercially available up to field strengths of more than 20 T, resulting in a radiofrequency of more than 900 MHz.[43]

Nanoparticles as Contrast Agents for Magnetic Resonance Imaging (MRI): Suspensions of paramagnetic and superparamagnetic NPs are potentially very good contrast agents for the *in vivo* detection of numerous pathologies. The optimization of their efficiency requires the understanding of the relationships between the process of proton relaxation and the physical properties of the NPs. The latter are highly influenced by the size, shape, and crystallinity of the NPs, and, of course, by their chemical composition (Figure 16.7).

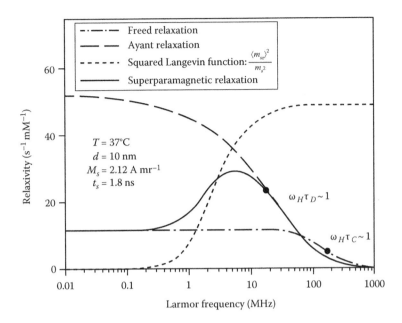

FIGURE 16.7
Different contributions to proton relaxation in the simplified model for crystals with large anisotropy. (From Dias, M.H.M. and Lauterbur, P.C.: *Magn. Reson. Med.* 1986. 3. 328. Copyright Wiley-VCH Verlag GmbH & Co. KGaA. Reprinted with permission.)

The nuclear magnetic relaxation properties of a NP are obtained by studying its nuclear magnetic resonance dispersion profile (NMRD). "Relaxivity" is defined as the increase of the relaxation rate of water (or aqueous buffer) induced by mmol L^{-1} of active ion. For an iron oxide (e.g., Fe_3O_4), the relaxivity is the relaxation rate enhancement observed for an aqueous solution containing mmol L^{-1} of Fe per liter. Note that the total concentration of iron is used, disregarding whether it exists as Fe(0), Fe^{2+}, Fe^{3+}, or mixtures thereof. It is also not of importance whether the contrast agent is molecularly dissolved or in a (nano) particle (Figure 16.8):[44]

$$R_{i(obs)} = \frac{1}{T_{i(obs)}} = \frac{1}{T_{i(diam)}} + r_i C \quad i = 1 \text{ or } 2 \tag{16.16}$$

where
$R_{i(obs)}$ is the global relaxation rate (s^{-1})
$T_{i(diam)}$ is the relaxation time of the system in the absence of the contrast agent (mmol L^{-1})
r_i is the relaxivity (s^{-1} mmol^{-1} L).

Paramagnetic Relaxation: There are two contributions to proton relaxation in paramagnetic systems: inner- and outersphere relaxations. Innersphere relaxation is caused by the direct exchange of energy between the protons and electrons located in the first hydration sphere of the paramagnetic ion or particle. This mechanism is dominated by dipolar and scalar coupling of the spins. Important parameters in paramagnetic relaxation are the rotation of the paramagnetic center τ_R, the residence time of water molecules in the first hydration sphere τ_M, and the electron relaxation of the electronic spin

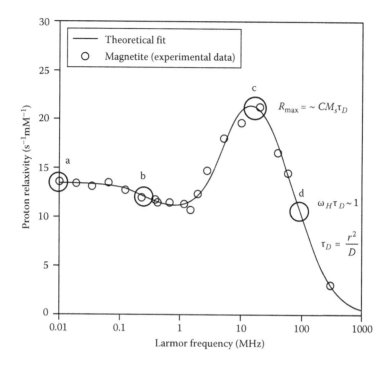

FIGURE 16.8
NMRD profile of magnetite particles in colloidal solution: fitted parameters: $r = 4$ nm, $M_s = 53$ m^{2}kg^{-1}; (a) the low field relaxation rate depends on the anisotropy energy of the magnetic NPs; (b) low field dispersion is another indicator of the anisotropy energy of the magnetic NPs; (c) The maximum of proton relaxivity is dependent on M_s and τ_D; (d) ω_H can be calculated from the inflection point if proton relaxivity at high field. (From Dias, M.H.M. and Lauterbur, P.C.: *Magn. Reson. Med.* 1986. 3. 328. Copyright Wiley-VCH Verlag GmbH & Co. KGaA. Reprinted with permission.)

associated with the paramagnetic ion τ_S. The correlation time τ_C is used to define the modulation of the dipolar coupling: [45]

$$\frac{1}{\tau_C} = \frac{1}{\tau_R} + \frac{1}{\tau_M} + \frac{1}{\tau_S} \tag{16.17}$$

Innersphere relaxation is a field-dependent phenomenon that can be quantitatively described by the Solomon–Bloembergen equation

$$\frac{1}{\tau_M} = \frac{2}{15}\left(\frac{\mu_0}{4\pi}\right)^2 \gamma_H^2 \gamma_E^2 \, \bar{h} S(S+1)\frac{1}{r^6}\left[\frac{7\tau_{C2}}{1+(\omega_E \tau_{C2})^2} + \frac{3\tau_{C1}}{1+(\omega_H \tau_{C1})^2}\right] \tag{16.18}$$

$$\frac{1}{\tau_{S1}} = \frac{1}{5\tau_{S0}}\left[\frac{1}{1+\omega_E^2 \tau_V^2} + \frac{4}{1+4\omega_E^2 \tau_V^2}\right] \tag{16.19}$$

$$\frac{1}{\tau_{S2}} = \frac{1}{10\tau_{S0}}\left[3 + \frac{1}{1+\omega_E^2 \tau_V^2} + \frac{2}{1+4\omega_E^2 \tau_V^2}\right] \tag{16.20}$$

where
  γ_E and γ_H are the gyromagnetic ratios of an electron (E) and a proton (H)
  ω_E and ω_H are the angular frequencies of electron and proton
  r is the distance between the water protons and the unpaired spin
  τ_{S1} and τ_{S2} are the longitudinal and transverse relaxation times of the electron
  τ_{S0} is the correlation time at zero field
  τ_V is the correlation time for electronic relaxation

The outersphere relaxation is described in the model by Freed:[46]

$$R_1^{OS} = \frac{6400\pi}{81}\left(\frac{\mu_0}{4\pi}\right)^2 \gamma_H^2\gamma_E^2\bar{h}^2 S(S+1)N_A\frac{[C]}{dD}\left[7j(\omega_E\tau_D)+3j(\omega_H\tau_D)\right] \tag{16.21}$$

with

$$j(\omega\tau_D)=Re\left[\frac{1+\frac{1}{4}\left(i\omega\tau_D+\dfrac{\tau_D}{\tau_{S1}}\right)^{\frac{1}{2}}}{1+\left(i\omega\tau_D+\dfrac{\tau_D}{\tau_{S1}}\right)^{\frac{1}{2}}+\left(i\omega\tau_D+\dfrac{\tau_D}{\tau_{S1}}\right)+\left(i\omega\tau_D+\dfrac{\tau_D}{\tau_{S1}}\right)^{\frac{3}{2}}}\right] \tag{16.22}$$

where
  $[C]$ is the molar concentration of the paramagnetic ion
  $\tau_D = d^6D^{-1}$ is the translational correlation time
  N_A is the Avogadro number

Superparamagnetic Relaxation: It is noteworthy that the contribution by innersphere relaxation processes to the superparamagnetic relaxation is very small. Therefore, superparamagnetic relaxation can be adequately described by Freed's model (see earlier).[38] We will discuss the case next when the translational diffusion time is significantly shorter than the Néel relaxation time.[39]

In general, the efficiency of superparamagnetic relaxation depends on whether its correlation time τ_C is shorter or longer than the precession period of the ^{1}H spins within the external magnetic field B_0: if the global correlation time τ_C ($\tau_C^{-1}=\tau_D^{-1}+\tau_N^{-1}$) is longer than the precession period of the spins, the fluctuation is averaged by spin precession and, therefore, inefficient. However, if it is shorter, superparamagnetic relaxation becomes an efficient process. Equation 23 defines the boundary separating the conditions, where the fluctuation characterized by a correlation time τ_C induces relaxation ($\omega_H\tau_C >1$), and where it does not (($\omega_H\tau_C<1$):

$$\omega_H\tau_C = 1 \tag{16.23}$$

It is noteworthy that the relaxation induced by superparamagnetic crystals is dependent on their magnetic moment, which is modulated by the Néel relaxation. The latter depends on the anisotropy of the NP. For large and/or very anisotropic superparamagnetic crystals, the anisotropy energy is larger than the thermal energy. Consequently, the direction of the nanocrystal's magnetic moment has practically the same orientation as the NP's anisotropy axes. In this well-defined case, the use of a simplified model is justified. On the contrary, in very small and spherical NPs, the anisotropy energy is comparable to the thermal energy. Therefore, the magnetic moment can point virtually in any direction. Therefore, electron precession becomes allowed and has to be accounted for.

There are two main contributions to the overall spin relaxation: (1) Curie relaxation, which is diffusion into the inhomogeneous nonfluctuating magnetic field created by the mean crystal moment, aligned in the direction of B_0; (2) Néel relaxation (fluctuations of the electronic magnetic moment). Principally, the Curie relaxation accounts for the high field part of the longitudinal relaxation rate profiles (NMRD), where B_0 is larger than 0.02 T, because the mean magnetization increases linearly with B_0, as described by the Langevin function.

High anisotropy model: If the anisotropy energy barrier is sufficiently high, any precession of the magnetic moment of superparamagnetic NPs is forbidden. Therefore, magnetic fluctuations are caused only by jumps of the magnetic moments between the principal directions of magnetization. At low field, the electron Larmor frequency is set to zero and the proton longitudinal relaxation rate is described by the Freed equations (see Equation 16.21). The spectral density function is then characterized by a global correlation time depending on τ_N and τ_D (Equations 16.24 and 16.25).[40] Figure 16.9 shows the dispersion of this density spectra function (Freed function [38,39b]), which is centered around $\omega_H = \tau_C^{-1}$:

$$\frac{1}{T_1} = 10c\mu^2 J_F(\omega_H, \tau_D, \tau_N) \tag{16.24}$$

$$\frac{1}{T_2} = c\mu^2 \left[8J_F(\omega_H, \tau_D, \tau_N) + 2J_F(0, \tau_D, \tau_N) \right] \tag{16.25}$$

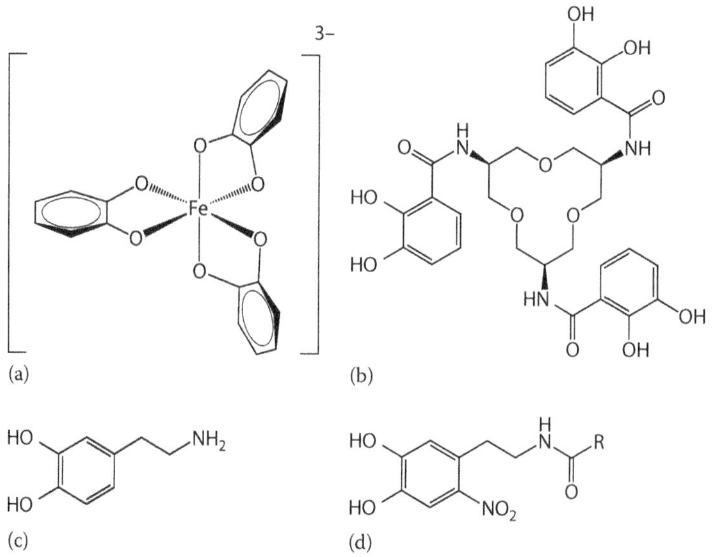

FIGURE 16.9
(a) Iron(III)-tris-cathecholate [Fe(cat)$_3$]$^{3-}$ [45], (b) the structure of the siderophore enterobactin[53], (c) dopamine[45], and (d) 5-nitrodopamine with amide-linked side group.[56] This can either be oligo/polyethylene glycol or a positively or negatively charged side chain. (From Simo, F. and Sima, J., *Chem. Pap.*, 65, 730, 2011.)

where

$$c = \left(\frac{32\pi}{40} 5000 \right) \gamma^2 N_A \frac{[M]}{r^3} \tag{16.26}$$

where

r is the NP radius
N_A is the Avogadro number
μ is the magnetic moment of the NP
γ is the proton gyromagnetic ratio
J_F is Freed's density spectral function:

$$J_F(\omega_H, \tau_D, \tau_N) = Re \left(\frac{1 + \frac{1}{4}\left(i\omega_H\tau_D + \frac{\tau_D}{\tau_N}\right)^2}{1 + \left(i\omega_H\tau_D + \frac{\tau_D}{\tau_N}\right)^{\frac{1}{2}} + \frac{4}{9}\left(i\omega_H\tau_D + \frac{\tau_D}{\tau_N}\right) + \frac{1}{9}\left(i\omega_H\tau_D + \frac{\tau_D}{\tau_N}\right)^{\frac{3}{2}}} \right) \tag{16.27}$$

Ayant's model[39c] predicts the relaxation rates occurring at high field when the magnetic vector is essentially locked in the B_0 direction. Therefore, Curie relaxation is the dominating process:[39c]

$$R_2 = c\mu^2 \left[4.5 J_A (2\omega_H\tau_D)^{1/2} + 6 J_A(0) \right] \tag{16.28}$$

$$\frac{1}{T_1} = c\mu^2 \left[9L^2(x) J_A (2\omega_H\tau_D)^{\frac{1}{2}} \right] \tag{16.29}$$

J_A is Ayant's density spectral function:

$$J_A(z) = \frac{1 + \frac{5z}{8} + \frac{z^2}{8}}{1 + z + \frac{z^2}{2} + \frac{z^3}{6} + \frac{4z^4}{81} + \frac{z^5}{81} + \frac{z^6}{648}} \tag{16.30}$$

The dispersion of spectral density under high field conditions occurs at $\omega_H\tau_D \sim 1$.

The quantitative understanding of the relationship between proton relaxivity and the chemical and physical properties of magnetic NPs provides a tool for controlling the reproducibility of NP synthesis. It also has the power to suggest pathways for the further optimization of nanoscale MRI contrast agents.[44]

Notes:

Average radius (r): At high magnetic fields, the relaxation rate only depends on τ_D. The inflection point is defined as $\omega_H\tau_D \sim 1$. Measuring τ_D will yield the NP radius r, because $\tau_D = r^2 D^{-1}$.

Specific magnetization (M$_s$): At high field condition, M_s can be calculated from $M_s \sim (R_{max} C^{-1} \tau_D^{-1})^{1/2}$. C is a constant and R_{max} is the maximal relaxation rate.

Néel relaxation time (τ_N): At very low field, the relaxation rate R_0 is determined by a "zero magnetic field" correlation time τ_{C0}, which is equal to τ_N if the condition $\tau_N \ll \tau_D$ is met.

16.3 Synthesis and Characterization of Magnetic Nanoparticles

16.3.1 Colloidal Synthesis of Magnetic Nanoparticles

The vast majority of the synthetic techniques to produce NPs apply colloidal synthesis. The colloidal synthesis of magnetic NPs provides a fast and economical way to produce particles in the 1–100 nm size range via co-precipitation method, hydrothermal synthesis, microemulsion, sol-gel synthesis, and sonochemical synthesis in aqueous medium. In addition to the aqueous syntheses, non-aqueous synthetic methods are also utilized that allow synthesis of magnetic particles at temperatures above the boiling point of water and in the absence of oxygen, therefore, improving crystallinity. The non-aqueous synthetic methods may include thermal decomposition, polyol/solvothermal process, and laser or spray pyrolysis. The basic aim of all of these synthetic techniques is to control the nucleation of growth steps during synthesis to create particles, with well-defined size, crystallinity, and magnetic properties. For example, in the thermal decomposition approach, the nucleation step of the NPs is achieved by rapidly injecting precursor molecules into a hot solution heated above the decomposition temperature of the precursor. The solution contains coordinating ligands for stabilizing the particles, reducing the reactivity of the monomers, thereby allowing the slow incorporation of the monomers into the particles with reduced defect density and high crystallinity. The high temperature is needed to accelerate the growth of the magnetic NPs and increase the annealing rate of the NPs at those temperatures. This general strategy can be further modified to adapt to the material properties of the magnetic material. Many of the magnetic NPs are in a reduced state and may require a reducing agent to grow the magnetic NPs.

Fe_3O_4 along with the Fe_2O_3 magnetic NPs are is of the most common magnetic nanomaterials produced for biosensing and hyperthermia applications. Monodispersed Fe_3O_4 NPs are produced through the reaction of $Fe(acac)_3$ and a long-chain alcohol (Figure 16.10). The reaction results in magnetic NP with controllable size in the 5–20 nm range. The particles exhibit high crystallinity as well as uniform size distribution.

16.3.2 Gas Phase Synthesis of Magnetic Nanoparticles

Alternatively, magnetic nanomaterials can be prepared via gas phase synthesis.[42] There are several reasons why gas phase synthesis may be desirable over solution-based synthetic routes. The gas phase synthetic techniques are inherently purer than their condensed phase counterpart. Typically, every liquid solution contains trace amount of minerals or organic contaminants that are either detrimental to the engineering approach used during synthesis or produce side effects (cytotoxicity) in biological systems. The droplets formed during aerosol synthesis do not permit phase segregation. The synthetic process can be easily scaled up and is very economical since it does not require expensive reactors. Arguably, the crystallinity, particle size, and composition can be also controlled reasonably well. From the fundamental growth kinetics, the nucleation is homogeneous resulting in very narrow size distribution. From the technical standpoint, the magnetic NPs in the gas phase can be produced in a furnace flow reactor, a laser reactor, a flame reactor, a plasma reactor, via laser

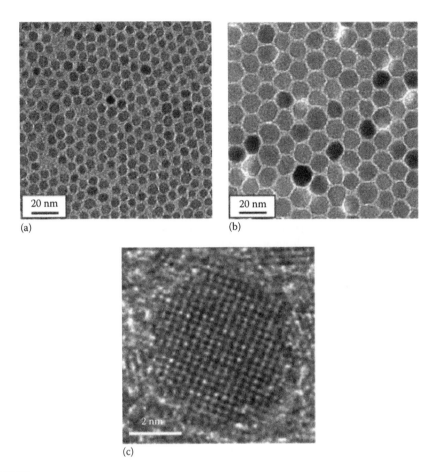

FIGURE 16.10
TEM bright field images of (a) 6 nm and (b) 12 nm Fe$_3$O$_4$ nanoparticles deposited from their hexane dispersion on an amorphous carbon-coated copper grid and dried at room temperature. (c) High-resolution TEM image of a single 6 nm Fe$_3$O$_4$ nanoparticle. (Reprinted with permission from Sun, S.H., Zeng, H., Robinson, D.B., Raoux, S., Rice, P.M., Wang, S.X., and Li, G.X., *J. Am. Chem. Soc.*, 126, 2004, 273. Copyright 2004 American Chemical Society.)

vaporization of solids, exploding wire or spark synthesis, sputtering, inert gas condensation, expansion cooling, and homogeneous aerosol reaction. The gas phase synthesis allows coating the particles with carbon, which allows the isolation of the magnetic material from leaching out to the biological medium. The example given next (Figure 16.11) shows the carbon-coated iron particle from a reaction in arc discharge in a flowing helium reactor.

16.3.3 Surface Functionalization of Magnetic Nanoparticles

Surface functionalization of NPs has several functions: First, NPs have to be soluble for *in vitro* and *in vivo* sensing and diagnostics applications. However, many synthetic procedures do lead to NPs that are not soluble in aqueous buffers. It is noteworthy that this problem is increased in the presence of dissolved salts and proteins, which form adducts with NPs and consequently precipitate them. Second, NPs have to be protected against magnetically induced precipitation once a magnetic field is applied. Aggregation will lead to significant changes in their magnetic properties and, therefore, their performance. Although

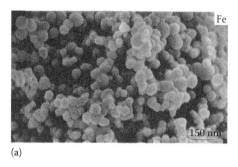
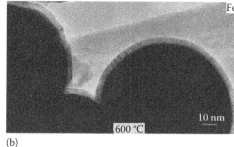

FIGURE 16.11
(a) FE-SEM overview of the morphology of carbon-coated metal particles: iron particles. (b) Internal structure of as-made carbon-coated metal particles revealed by high resolution. TEM: iron particles covered by amorphous carbon. (Reprinted with permission from Jiao, J., Seraphin, S., Wang, X.K., and Withers, J.C., *J. Appl. Phys.*, 80, 2004, 103. Copyright 2004 American Chemical Society.)

aggregation is a welcome effect for some applications, such as *in vivo* MRI sensing, it has to be prevented for all medicinal applications that involve NPs circulating in the bloodstream.[43]

In general, the stability of a dispersion of magnetic NPs is a result of the equilibrium between attractive and repulsive forces. In magnetic suspensions dipolar forces between the NPs lead to overall attractive forces that have to be counterbalanced if precipitation is to be avoided. Two strategies for stabilizing magnetic NPs have emerged: electrostatic and steric repulsion.[39a]

Whereas electrostatic repulsion can be monitored by measuring their diffusion potential, which is essentially equal to their zeta potential (zeta), steric repulsion is not easily quantifiable for monomeric ligands. Steric repulsion is better understood when polymers are used as ligands. Critical parameters are the molecular weight of the polymer and its density in aqueous solution.[44] In all iron oxides the surface iron ions act as Lewis acids and coordinate with functional groups that are Lewis bases (e.g., they donate lone-pair electrons).[44] All iron(0) NPs are covered with either an amorphous or crystalline layer of Fe_3O_4 (magnetite). Therefore, they can be stabilized by the same surface chemistry as iron oxide NPs. In the absence of a ligand sphere, the isoelectric point of magnetite occurs at pH = 6.8. At this pH, Fe_3O_4 has its PZC (point of zero charge) and is no longer stable in water.[44] In the presence of (usually hydrophobic) ligands, such as organic amines, thiols, or dopamines, resulting from the synthesis of the NPs,[44] these ligands have to be replaced by water-soluble ligands. In this procedure, a competitive ligand exchange has to be performed in a solvent, in which both ligands are soluble (e.g., an alcohol). Although Fe(II) and Fe(III) are known to form adducts with organic ligands that are—thermodynamically—very stable, they nevertheless show fast exchange kinetics.[45] This kinetic instability enables gradual ligand exchange procedures. However, it is difficult to avoid cluster formation due to inefficient ligand exchange by any of the known exchange procedures (see Figure 16.12).

Monomeric Stabilizers: Carboxylates, organic phosphates, and sulfates, as well as dopamine-anchored ligands exhibit strong binding to iron oxide surfaces. Surface binding ligands are known to influence the morphology of the NPs if they are present during growth. VSOP C184 is an iron oxide (currently in its preclinical stage) for angiography that is characterized by the adsorption of citric acid at its surface.[46] Other examples for monomeric stabilizers are gluconic acid[47], dimercaptosuccinic acid[48], and phosphoryl-choline.[49] Dopamine-based ligands are ofspecial importance, because bidentate catechol (1,2-dihydroxybenzene) ligands form extremely stable complexes with Fe(III). A stability

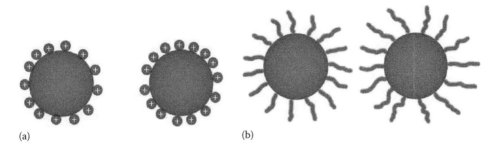

(a)   (b)

FIGURE 16.12
(a) Particles stabilized by the electrostatic layer. (b) Particles stabilized by steric repulsion.

constant $K_{stab} = 10^{44.9}$ has been determined for the octahedral complex between three cat-echol units and Fe(III).[50] Interestingly, catecholate groups are found in siderophores (iron-transporting proteins, e.g., enterobactin,[51]) and in adhesive mussel proteins.[52]

Dopamine is chemically not stable when bound to Fe_2O_3 or Fe_3O_4. It slowly undergoes oxidation. Fe(III) acts as electron acceptor and reacts to Fe(II), which then leaves the nano-crystal and forms $Fe(OH)_2$ under physiological conditions. This reaction slows down sig-nificantly, if the amine group of dopamine is converted into an amide, thus preventing the formation of cyclic redox products, such as dopaminochrome.[53] According to Reimhult and coworkers, 5-nitro-dopamine possesses the highest NP-binding affinities and the low-est oxidation tendencies.[54]

Inorganic Materials as Nanoparticle Stabilizers: A silica coating of iron and iron/oxide NPs prevents their aggregation in aqueous buffers, improves their chemical stability, and reduces their acute toxicity because of the resulting slower bio-corrosion processes. Principally, three processes have been successfully utilized to synthesize silica shells around iron oxide NPs. First of all, the Stöber process deposits silica through the hydrolysis of suitable sol-gel precursors, such as tetraeythyl orthosilicate (TEOS).[55] The second approach relies on the condensation of silicic acid in solution. This method is especially suited to form thick silica layers.[56] In the third method, micelles or inverse micelles are used to confine and control the silica coating. This method usually requires a greater effort to separate the core-shell NPs from the large amount of surfactants associated with the emulsion system.[57]

Ferumoxsil (AMI-121, $d = 300$ nm) has been tested in clinical trials.[58] Fe_3O_4 NPs are coated with a layer of inert silicon ([3-(2-amino-ethylamino)propyl] trimethoxysilane). After oral administration, it improves the definition of organ boundaries, such as the uterus and lymph nodes.

In some cases, it is desirable to coat the magnetic NP with metal such as gold (Figure 16.13). The gold coating of the particles introduces additional fine control over the particles' phys-ical properties. The ligand chemistry can be precisely controlled on the surface of gold via the manipulation of gold thiol bond.[59] In addition, the gold shell can enhance both the magnetic and plasmonic properties of the particles. The plasmonic shell allows eva-nescent wave excitation of nearby molecules to the particles,[60] enhancing processes that require the interaction of multiple photons, such as surface enhanced Raman signal[61] or multi-photon excitation of fluorophores. These properties can be effectively utilized for cancer cell detection as well.[62] The gold shell also enhances the magnetic properties of the particles such as the strength of Faraday rotation of the particles.[63]

Polymer Stabilizers: Three main strategies exist for coating magnetic NPs with poly-meric stabilizers. (1) In the first approach, the NPs are coated during their synthesis.[64]

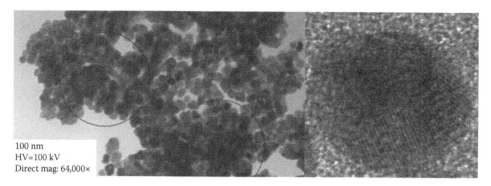

FIGURE 16.13
Left: Cluster formation during the exchange oleylamine vs. dopamine at Fe/Fe_3O_4 NPs (Wang and Bossmann unpublished, clustering is marked with circles). Right: HRTEM of a single gold-coated Fe_2O_3 NPs (Dani and Chikan, unpublished).

(2) The post-synthesis method consists of grafting the polymer on the magnetic NPs after synthesis.[65] (3) In the third strategy, the polymer will be synthesized in the presence of the NPs, which have been synthesized earlier.[66] To date, the most common polymer coatings are dextran, carboxymethylated dextran, carboxydextran, starch, chitosan, arabinogalactan, glycosaminoglycan, sulfonated styrene-divinylbenzene, polyethylene glycol (PEG), polyvinyl alcohol (PVA), poloxamers, and polyoxamines.[53]

16.3.4 Characterization of Magnetic Nanoparticles

The magnetic NPs are characterized to understand their properties in relation to their structure and composition. Typical characterization techniques obtain parameters such as magnetic moment, saturation magnetization, remnant magnetization, and coercivity. Understanding the hysteretic behavior of the magnetic NPs is critical and absolutely necessary if their properties are to be exploited for application purposes. Vibrating sample magnetometer (VBS) represents one of the simplest measurements to extract this information of the magnetic NPs. The sample is placed in a homogenous magnetic field between poles of a large variable electromagnet. The sample is vibrated in the presence of a magnetic field, and via the changing magnetic flux it induces voltage in the nearby pick up coil. The voltage is proportional to the magnetic moment of the sample and able to detect the magnetic hysteresis of the sample as well. Figure 16.14 shows the variation of the magnetization curve and hysteresis of e-cobalt NPs[67] as a function of size taken by VBS. These data vary significantly with the physical state of magnetic NPs. The saturation magnetization, the remnant magnetization, and the coercivity field gradually increase as the magnetic NPs are separated from each other, thereby decreasing the influence of the nearby magnetic NPs.

Variation of the important magnetic parameters depending on the physical state shows that in order to effectively apply these magnetic NPs under physiological conditions one requires techniques that can shed some light on how the aggregation states can affect magnetic properties. Faraday rotation has been found to be greatly enhanced in magnetic NPs, even compared to traditional Faraday rotor materials such as terbium gallium garnet. As will be shown next, Faraday rotation can be very sensitive to the aggregation state of the magnetic NPs and can provide a characterization tool to describe the dynamics of magnetic moments in these aggregates. Typically, magneto-optical effects provide physical information on the electronic and spin structure of materials. Faraday rotation is the rotation of

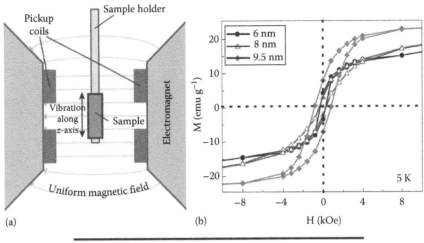

Physical state	M_s (emu g^{-1})	M_r (emu g^{-1})	$M_r M_s$	H_c (Oe)
Powder in a capsule	14.0	1.5	0.11	163
Diluted particles with wax	59.6	7.3	0.12	600
On HOPG substrate	61.6	12.6	0.20	790

(c)

FIGURE 16.14
(a) Schematics of vibrating sample magneto meter.[67] (b) Magnetization versus field (M vs. H) hysteresis loops at 5 K for 6.5, 8, and 9.5 nm ε-Co nanoparticles samples. The coercive field Hc for 6.5, 8.0, and 9.5 nm Co nanoparticles is 247, 386, and 838 Oe, respectively. (c) Magnetic properties of cobalt nanoparticles in different physical states. (Reprinted with permission from Yang, H.T., Su, Y.K., Shen, C.M., Yang, T. Z., and Gao, H.J., *Surf. Interface Anal.*, 36, 2011, 155. Copyright 2011 American Chemical Society.)

the plane of polarization of polarized light as it propagates through a dielectric medium in a magnetic field. The rotation is due to magnetic-field-induced circular birefringence in a material. In a nonabsorbing or weakly absorbing medium, a linearly polarized monochromatic light beam passing through the material along the direction of the applied magnetic field experiences circular birefringence, which results in the rotation of the plane of polarization of the incident light beam. The angle of rotation is proportional to both applied magnetic field and optical path length. So, the angle of rotation (φ) can be expressed as

$$\varphi = \nu BL = \frac{\pi \Delta n L}{\lambda} \qquad (16.31)$$

where
Δn is the magnitude of the circular birefringence (a difference in refractive index of the left and the right circularly polarized light in the medium)
L is the optical path length
λ is the wavelength of light
B is the applied magnetic field
ν is a constant and known as the Verdet constant

The rotation of the plane of polarization of linearly polarized light can be measured by changing the amplitudes of two orthogonally linear polarized components. The measurement of

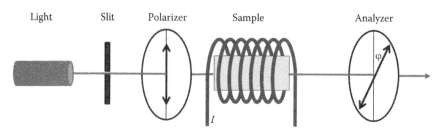

FIGURE 16.15
Simple experimental scheme of Faraday rotation measurement.

change in intensity of linearly polarized light by means of an analyzer is the fundamental basis of the Faraday rotation measurement. A simple Faraday rotation measurement setup is shown in Figure 16.15. It consists of a light source, a pair of polarizers (polarizer and analyzer), and a photodiode as a detector. The polarizer makes the light beam from the source polarized and that polarized light travels through the sample and reaches the analyzer and then the photodiode. If the sample is not magnetized, the plane of polarization of the light beam is not affected and the amount of light energy that reaches the photodiode depends on the angle between polarizer and analyzer. When the sample is magnetized, the polarization of the transmitted light rotates slightly. The direction of rotation depends on the direction of magnetization. The effect of the magnetization variation is the same as the rotation of the analyzer and the current of the photodiodes is changed accordingly. The magneto-optic effect is the difference in rotation angle for two opposite magnetization directions and the rotation is calculated from the current or voltage of photodiodes.

Figure 16.16 shows the relationship between the phase lag of the Faraday signal and the magnetic field of gold coated magnetic NPs in aqueous solution.[63b] Phase lag of the Faraday rotation of bare Fe_2O_3 is relatively high. After the addition of gold solution that produces a gold shell around the magnetic core, the phase lag is reduced. The cluster size of the magnetic NPs from dynamic light scattering experiments with the gold concentration is also shown in Figure 16.16. Similarly, the cluster size decreases with the addition of the gold solution for the first three additions and remains almost constant for other additions. This effect shows that on the time scale of the experiment, the NPs show a dynamic alignment effect as a result of the rearrangement of the magnetic spins in a cluster consisting of many magnetic NPs. The estimated times of the full alignment of the magnetic spins are 0.65 and 0.17 μs for the bare vs. coated NPs, respectively. These data show that increasing cluster size results in slower relaxation in a cluster consisting of small magnetic NPs.

16.3.5 Toxicology of Iron and Iron Oxide Nanoparticles

Iron toxicity in humans becomes noticeable at doses above 10–20 mg kg^{-2} of iron. Ingestions of more than 50 mg kg^{-2} of iron are associated with severe toxicity. Typical symptoms of iron poisoning are metabolic acidosis and organ damage (particularly brain and liver). Iron(II/III) leads to a higher concentration of reactive oxygen species (ROS) and therefore free radicals in the cells, causing oxidative stress, inflammation, and finally damage to proteins, membranes, and DNA.[68] Liver failure and massive shock syndrome occur frequently in cases of iron poisoning. It is noteworthy that right after the injection of a contrast agent the patient has received an overdose of iron![69] Iron and iron oxide NPs possessing a hydrodynamic radius smaller than 5 nm can be excreted via the renal pathway.[70] Excess iron can also be excreted from the liver as bile.[71] The most important factors determining the

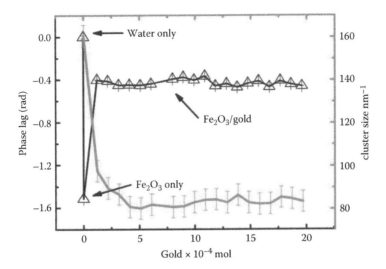

FIGURE 16.16

Phase lag between the signal of Faraday rotation and the magnetic field of gold- coated Fe_2O_3 nanoparticles as a function of gold concentration. The cluster size of nanoparticles from dynamic light scattering is also shown in the figure. (Reprinted with permission from Dani, R.K., Wang, H.W., Bossmann, S.H., Wysin, G., and Chikan, V., *J. Chem. Phys.*, 135. Copyright 2011, American Institute of Physics.)

toxicity of iron-containing NPs are their size and their surface coating. Without an effective surface coating, iron-containing NPs bio-corrode within 24 h within the human body, thus releasing their iron content. The surface coating of (magnetic) NPs has a great influence on their pharmacokinetics. Macrophages and proliferating cells are able to internalize NPs when they are smaller than 200 nm.[72] The uptake mechanism in macrophages is receptor-mediated endocytosis. In proliferating cells, e.g., tumor cells, active internalization takes place, where the uptake occurs by fluid phase endocytosis in the G1 cell cycle phase.[68] The dependence of cellular uptake on NP size is somewhat counterintuitive: NPs that are smaller than 50 nm have the tendency to cluster on the cells' surfaces. The resulting structures are big enough to trigger endocytosis, whereas NPs that are larger than 100 nm are bound as single NPs and, therefore, are not taken up as fast, because the signal cascade leading to the wrapping of the cell membrane around the NP cluster will not occur.[73] NPs with a size of 10 to 180 nm are taken up by phagocytotic cells such as Kupffer cells in the liver and macrophages but also microglia in the brain. Their primary elimination from the blood circulation occurs in the reticuloendothelial system.[74]

16.4 Application of Magnetic Nanoparticles for Bioseparation, Biosensing, Drug Delivery, and Cancer Therapy

16.4.1 Magnetoseparation

Magnetic NPs have proven to be very useful practical tools to manipulate biological materials at the molecular level. Several of the applications below are already being commercialized and some others are still under development. Early on, it was realized that

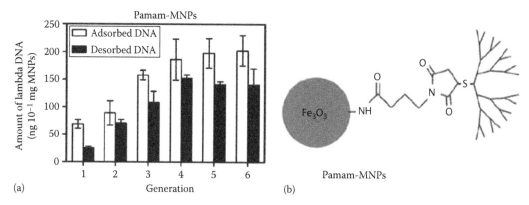

FIGURE 16.17

(a) Amount of adsorbed and desorbed kDNA from PAMAM–MNPs as a function of dendrimer generation. (b) PAMAM magnetic nanoparticles for DNA capture. (Reprinted from *J. Colloid Interface Sci.*, 377, Tanaka, T., Shibata, K., Hosokawa, M., Hatakeyama, K., Arakaki, A., Gomyo, H., Mogi, T., Taguchi, T., Wake, H., Tanaami, T., and Matsunaga, T., 469, Copyright 2012, with permission from Elsevier.)

superparamagnetic NPs can attract each other when placed in external magnetic field gradient while they could form stable colloids in the absence of the field. The large surface area of the magnetic NPs provides an excellent platform to interact with molecules in solution. After the reaction on the surface, the magnetic NPs can be separated exposing them to magnetic field gradients. Tagging the magnetic NPs is possible via chemical modification of the surface of the magnetic NPs. There are a number of specific magnetic separation techniques used depending on the purpose of the magnetic separation. The simple example is shown next how Fe_3O_4 magnetic NPs from magnetotactic bacterium can be utilized for efficient DNA purification. The particles are coated with a thiol functionalized polyamidoamine (PAMAM) dendron.[75] As Figure 16.17 shows, the larger dendrons become more efficient to recover the lambda DNA in the test reactions.

Magnetic Tweezers: Remotely controlling cell function and understanding how cellular properties can be probed with magnetic beads (Figure 16.18)[76] has been proposed and demonstrated as a potential tool, not only to regulate cross membrane molecular transport, but to probe mechanical properties of living cell membranes (magnetic twisting cytometry). In that methodology, several hundred nm large magnetic beads are attached to the surface of the cell membrane to actively control cellular functions.[76] In another interesting approach,[77] 200 nm-sized magnetic beads are attached to chiral colloidal propellers and controlled by homogeneous magnetic fields. The technique has already demonstrated the possibility of carrying out targeted drug delivery and microsurgery.

16.4.2 Drug Delivery Using Magnetoliposomes

Magnetic NPs can be effectively used in drug delivery systems, such as liposomes. Liposomes were first described in 1961 (published 1964[78]) by Alec Bangham. Liposomes (and the payload that they have trapped inside during formation), can be separated from smaller molecules simply by gel filtration or dialysis, making them very useful delivery agents.[79] Liposomes are stable in blood, not releasing their contents,[79a,80] and when incubated with plasma constituents, they retain their spherical shape.[79b,81] Liposomes made

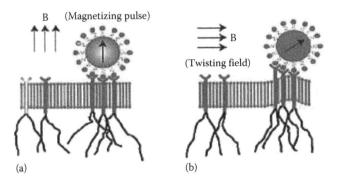

FIGURE 16.18

Magnetic twisting cytometry: large (micrometer-sized) magnetic particles coated with RGD molecules attach to integrin receptors on the cell membrane. The receptors are linked to actin filaments (black lines). A magnetizing pulse is applied (a), which gives the particle a remnant magnetization (B = magnetic field vector). A torque is then applied (b) to the particle via a "twisting field." The force required to twist the particle is related to the mechanical properties of the actin filaments. (Reproduced with permission from Macmillan Publishers Ltd. *Nat. Nanotechnol.*, Dobson, J., 3, 139, Copyright 2008.)

from L,α-dipalmitoylphosphatidylcholine (DPPC) are widely used for the intravenous delivery of drugs, because they are not prohibitively expensive and feature suitable biophysical properties. To date, several liposomal drug delivery systems have been developed (e.g., Nicoderm and others)[82] that rely on the slow release of their payload. However, for the treatment of cancer or infectious diseases, it is certainly desirable to deliver the payload (drug) at once after the target has been reached. Several research groups have used AC-magnetic hyperthermia to trigger the release of magnetoliposomes' payload by heating magnetic NPs within the supramolecular nanostructure until they either burst or (partially) dissolve in the surrounding aqueous medium.[22] Although this approach appears to work, it has the disadvantage that the liposomes' payload may be damaged by the heat. To eliminate this, instead of using AC magnetic fields, short magnetic pulses could be used to reduce the temperature increase. Figure 16.19 shows a scheme of magnetic NPs at

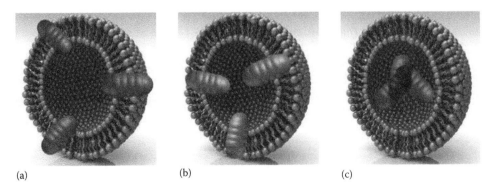

FIGURE 16.19

(a) Unilamellar liposome featuring double-layer embedded hydrophobic nanorods. (b) Unilamellar liposome featuring amphiphilic nanorods at the bilayer/core interface. (c) Unilamellar liposome featuring hydrophilic nanorods in its inner core.

different locations in the liposomes for efficient liposome burst triggering. It is anticipated that magnetic NPs placed within or in close proximity of the bilayer of the lipid will be more effective in drug delivery allowing the reduction of the concentration of magnetic NPs that are needed for successful triggering of the liposomes.

16.4.3 A/C-Magnetic Hyperthermia

Localized hyperthermia is a powerful therapeutic modality. When administered with high selectivity, *hyperthermia* treatment can become a very potent approach against many types of cancer, because it is not based on the intake of drugs by cancer cells, but on the application of heat. When heated to 45°C, vital proteins of the cancer cell become damaged (e.g., misfolded) and/or the cell membrane partially dissolves in the surrounding aqueous medium.[22] A multitude of heat-induced deviations from the "normal" metabolism of a cancer cell can eventually lead to apoptosis (programmed cell death). Although many cancer types are slightly more susceptible to hyperthermia than healthy cells, the latter principally share the same fate when heated.[22] Therefore, the development of methods to target hyperthermia in cancer cells remains one of the challenges in this field. This is equally important when attempting to treat solid tumors within the human body, as well as for the treatment of metastasizing cancers. A/C-magnetic hyperthermia has the potential to treat tumors that are inoperable. Using magnetic NPs to absorb alternating magnetic field energy as a method of generating localized hyperthermia has been shown to be a potential cancer treatment (see earlier). Tumor-homing cells have the potential to take up NPs and to migrate to tumors and metastases (Figure 16.20).[22] Among the numerous cell types that could potentially be used, neural progenitor cells[22] and monocyte/macrophage-like cells (Mo/Ma cells)[97] have been especially successful. Both cell types were able to take up dopamine- and silica-stabilized Fe/Fe_3O_4 NPs[22] and carry the NPs to the tumors.

Pancreatic cancer is known to be one of the most lethal forms of cancer with 5 year survival rates of less than 5%. Patients diagnosed with pancreatic cancer typically have a poor prognosis, partly because the cancer usually causes no symptoms early on, leading to locally advanced or metastatic disease at the time of diagnosis. A murine model of disseminated peritoneal pancreatic cancer was then generated by intraperitoneal (i.p.) injection of Pan02 cells. After tumor development, monocyte/macrophage-like cells loaded with iron/iron oxide NPs were injected i.p. and allowed to migrate into the tumor. Three days after injection, mice were exposed to an alternating magnetic field for 20 min to cause the cell-delivered NPs to generate heat. This treatment regimen was repeated three times. A survival study demonstrated that this system (Figure 16.21) can significantly increase survival in a murine pancreatic cancer model, with an av. post-tumor insertion life expectancy increase of 31%. This system has the potential to become a useful method for specifically and actively delivering NPs for local hyperthermia treatment of cancer.[97]

16.4.4 Magnetic Nanoparticles for Diagnostic Magnetic Resonance

Magnetic NPs should possess the following characteristics to be a viable tool in diagnostic magnetic resonance: (1) they should exhibit superparamagnetic properties; (2) they have to have high stability in aqueous media to avoid spontaneous aggregation, which could mimic target-induced or spontaneous dissolution, that would lead to rapid iron poisoning and loss of the detection system.

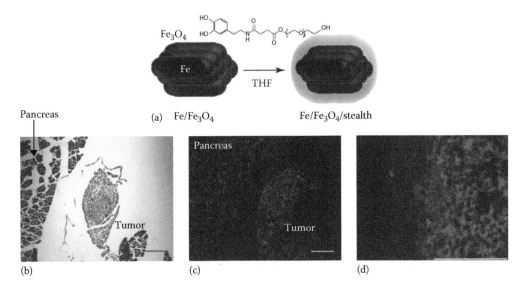

FIGURE 16.20
(See color insert.) (a) Core/shell iron/iron oxide nanoparticles were synthesized and then coated in a dopamine-based stealth ligand. (b and c): Mo/Ma loaded with PKH26 were injected into mice bearing intraperitoneal Pan02 tumors. Six days later mice were euthanized and tumors were harvested. Hoechst nuclear counterstained section shows Mo/Ma labeled with PKH26 in tumor. Hematoxylin and eosin staining of serial sections shows irregular morphology demonstrating that the targeted area is a tumor. Scale bars = 100 µm. (d) Mo/Ma labeled with Hoechst before injection was injected into mice bearing Pan02 expressing firefly luciferase tumors. Five days later mice were euthanized and tumors were harvested. Sections were stained with rabbit α-firefly luciferase and DyLight® 650-goat α-rabbit (Abcam, Cambridge, MA) (sections were not counterstained with Hoechst). Immunohistochemistry verifies that the Mo/Ma infiltrate pancreatic tumors. Abbreviations: Fe, iron; Fe_3O_4, iron oxide; THF, tetrahydrofuran. Scale bar = 100 µm.

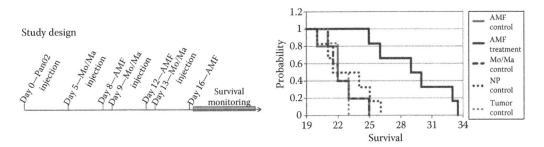

FIGURE 16.21
Duration to clinical symptoms ("survival"). Mice were euthanized when they displayed clinical signs of cancer and the day/time was recorded ($n = 5$ or 6 for each group). $P < 0.005$ for alternating magnetic field treatment versus all other groups. Abbreviations: AMF, alternating magnetic field; Mo/Ma, monocyte/macrophage-like cells; NP, nanoparticle.

Cross-linked iron oxide (CLIO) NPs have been widely used for DMR applications because they fulfill the requirements discussed earlier.[83] CLIO NPs consist of a superparamagnetic iron oxide core (3–5 nm monocrystalline iron oxide) composed of ferromagnetic magnetite (Fe_3O_4) and/or maghemite (γ-Fe_2O_3). The magnetic inorganic core is coated with dextran after NP synthesis and then cross-linked with epichlorohydrin and activated by ammonia to provide primary amine group functionality. Bioconjugation is achieved by linking various spacers to the amine groups. Since these systems can be assembled following a LEGO approach by using the same NP system and various spacers and different linkers, it is very versatile.[83]

Amine-terminated CLIO NPs have an average hydrodynamic diameter of 25–40 nm, approximately 40–80 amines per NP for bioconjugation, and a r_2 relaxation time of ~50 s^{-1}mM^{-1} [Fe].[83] Clustering of individual CLIOs leads to a substantial decrease in r_2 and can be, therefore, detected *in vitro* and *in vivo*. Typical applications of this technique comprise the detection of DNA telomeres, antibody activities of various kinds, enzyme activities (especially proteases and caspase-3), as well as pathogens (Figure 16.22).[83]

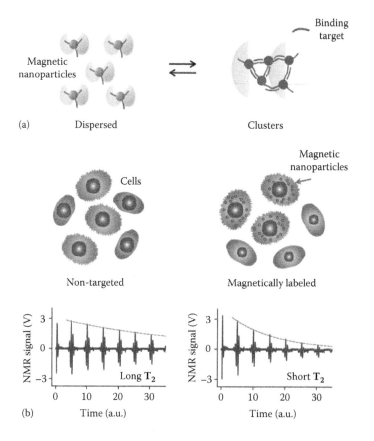

FIGURE 16.22
(See color insert.) DMR assay configurations with magnetic nanoparticles (MNPs). (a) Magnetic relaxation switching (MRSw) assays detect the clustering of MNPs (forward switching), using a small target biomarker as a cross-linker, or the disassembly of pre-formed clusters (reverse switching) using an enzyme or competitive binding. When dispersed MNPs aggregate upon binding to targets, the self-assembled magnetic clusters become more efficient at dephasing nuclear spins of surrounding water protons, leading to a decrease in T_2 relaxation time. The reverse is true upon cluster disassembly. (b) Magnetic tagging assays detect the presence of bound MNPs on larger biological entities. Tagging of cell surface markers via targeted MNPs imparts a magnetic moment to cells, leading to a decrease in T_2 relaxation time. Note that unbound MNPs must be removed to ensure detection sensitivity of this assay mode. (Reprinted with permission from Macmillan Publishers Ltd. *Nat. Biotech.*, Perez, J.M., Josephson, L., O'Loughlin, T., Hogemann, D., and Weissleder, R., 20, 816, Copyright 2002.)

16.5 Future Outlook and Challenges

Magnetic NPs have become viable nanotools for diagnostics and treatment of many diseases. This is especially true for cancer. Cancer is not just one disease but many diseases. According to the National Cancer Institute, there are more than 100 different types of cancer.[83] Magnetic diagnostics and treatment techniques of the future will allow a high degree of versatility and adaptability, which will greatly help to find not "the cure," but "many cures" for cancer. Magnetic NPs have shown their ability to function in many conceptually different nanosystems, as described in this book's chapters. The physics behind these magnetic nanomachines is well understood. The greatest challenge is to develop synthetic methodologies that permit not only the reproducible synthesis of NPs with precisely defined size, but also with precisely defined shape. Designing future magnetic nanomachines will depend on the close collaboration of synthetic and physical chemists, physicists, biologists, and physicians. It is our observation that communication between these groups is not always optimal. This translational effort will strongly depend on the successful exchange of data and mechanistic hypotheses/paradigms/theories between all groups involved.

References

1. Giljohann, D.; Seferos, D.; Daniel, W.; Massich, M.; Patel, P.; Miskin, C. 2010. *Angewandte Chemie* (International ed. in English), 49, 3280.
2. Freestone, I.; Meeks, S.; Higgitt, C. *Gold Bull.* 2007, 40, 270.
3. Daniel, M. C.; Astruc, D. *Chem. Rev.* (Washington, DC) 2004, 104, 293.
4. Tweney, R. D. *Perspect. Sci.* 2006, 14, 97.
5. Feynman, R. P. *J. Microelectromech. Syst.* 1992, 1, 60.
6. (a) Duguet, E.; Vasseur, S.; Mornet, S.; Devoisselle, J.-M. *Nanomedicine* 2006, 1, 157; (b) Wu, A.; Ou, P.; Zeng, L. *NANO* 05, 245.
7. Klabunde, K. *J. Nanoscale Materials in* Chemistry; John Wiley & Sons, New York, 2001.
8. (a) Wiltschko, R.; Wilschko, W. *Magnetic Orientation in Animals*; Springer, Berlin, Germany, 1995; (b) Kirschvink, J. L. *Bioelectromagnetics* 1989, 10, 239; (c) Stokroos, I; Litinetsky, L.; Ishay, J. S. *Nature* 2001, 411, 654.
9. Frankel, R. B.; Blakemore, R. P.; Wolfe, R. S. *Science* 1979, 203, 1355.
10. Walker, M. M.; Diebel, C. E.; Haugh, C. V.; Pankhurst, P. M.; Montgomery, J. C. *Nature* 1997, 390, 371.
11. Koksharov, Y. A. In *Magnetic Nanoparticles*, Gubin, S. P., Ed.; Willey-VCH, Weinheim, Germany, 2007.
12. Gubin, S. P.; Koksharov, Y. A.; Khomutov, G. B.; Yurkov, G. Y. *Russ. Chem. Rev.* 2005, 74, 489.
13. (a) Lu, A.-H.; Salabas, E. L.; Schueth, F. *Angewandte Chemie* (International ed. in English) 2007, 46, 1222; (b) Jun, Y. W.; Seo, J. W.; Cheon, J. *Acc. Chem. Res.* 2007, 41, 179.
14. Batlle, X.; Labarta, A. *J. Phys. D-Appl. Phys.* 2002, 35, R15.
15. Goya, G. F.; Grazu, V.; Ibarra, M. R. *Curr. Nanosci.* 2008, 4, 1.
16. Arruebo, M.; Fernandez Pacheco, R.; Ibarra, M. R.; Santamaria, J. *Nano Today* 2007, 2, 22.
17. Pankhurst, Q. A.; Connolly, J.; Jones, S. K.; Dobson, J. *J. Phys. D, Appl. Phys.* 2003, 36, R167.
18. Patrick, D. R.; Fardo, S. W. *Electrical Distribution Systems*; The Fairmont Press, Lilburn, GA, 2009.
19. Nikiforov, V. N. *Russ. Phys. J.* 2007, 50, 913.
20. Ondeck, C. L.; Habib, A. H.; Ohodnicki, P.; Miller, K.; Sawyer, C. A. *J. Appl. Phys.* 2009, 105, 07B324.

21. Jordan, A.; Wust, P.; Scholz, R.; Tesche, B.; Fahling, H. *Int. J. Hypertherm.* 1996, 12, 705.
22. Bossmann, S. H. In *Fabrication and Bio-application of Functionalized Nanomaterials*, Wang, X., Katz, E., Eds.; Research Signpost: Trivandrum, India, 2009.
23. Tran, N.; Webster, T. *J. Mater. Chem.* 2010, 20, 8760.
24. Mornet, S.; Vasseur, S.; Grasset, F.; Duguet, E. *J. Mater. Chem.* 2004, 14, 2161.
25. Gilchrist, R. K.; Medal, R.; Shorey, W. D.; Hanselman, R. C.; Parrott, J. C. *Ann. Surg.* 1957, 146, 596.
26. Nedelcu, G. *Dig. J. Nanomater. Biostruct.* 2008, 3, 103.
27. Maenosono, S.; Saita, S. *IEEE Trans. Magn.* 2006, 42, 1638.
28. Bekovic, M.; Hamler, A. *IEEE Trans. Magn.* 2010, 46, 552.
29. Mornet, S.; Vasseur, S.; Grasset, F.; Veverka, P.; Goglio, G. *Prog. Solid State Chem.* 2006, 34, 237.
30. Laurent, S.; Dutz, S.; Haefeli, U.; Mahmoudi, M. *Adv. Colloid Interface Sci.* 2011, 166, 8.
31. LesliePelecky, D. L.; Rieke, R. D. *Chem. Mater.* 1996, 8, 1770.
32. Leslie-Pelecky, D. L.; Labhasetwar, v.; Kraus, R. H. In *Advanced Magnetic Nanostructures*, Sellmyer, D. J., Skomski, R., Eds.; Springer: New York, 2006.
33. Hergt, R.; Dutz, S.; Zeisberger, M. *Nanotechnology* 2009, 21, 015706.
34. Rosensweig, R. E. *J. Magn. Magn. Mater.* 2002, 252, 370.
35. Hergt, R.; Dutz, S.; Mueller, R.; Zeisberger, M. *J. Phys. Conden. Matter.* 2006, 18, S2919.
36. Hofmann-Amtenbrink, M.; Rechberg, B. V. In *Nanostructured for Biomedical Applications*; Tan, M. C., Ed.; Transword Research Network: Trivandrum, India, 2009.
37. Fortin, J.-P.; Wilhelm, C.; Servais, J.; Menager, C.; Bacri, J.-C. *J. Am. Chem. Soc.* 2007, 129, 2628.
38. Freed, J. H. *J. Chem. Phys.* 1978, 68, 4034.
39. (a) Laurent, S.; Forge, D.; Port, M.; Roch, A.; Robic, C.; Elst, L. V.; Muller, R. N. *Chem. Rev.* (Washington, DC, U. S.) 2008, 108, 2064; (b) Hwang, L.-P.; Freed, J. H. *J. Chem. Phys.* 1975, 63, 118(c) Ayant, Y.; Belorizky, E.; Alizon, J.; Gallice, J. *J. De Physique* 1975, 36, 991.
40. Dias, M. H. M.; Lauterbur, P. C. *Magn. Reson. Med.* 1986, 3, 328.
41. Sun, S. H.; Zeng, H.; Robinson, D. B.; Raoux, S.; Rice, P. M.; Wang, S. X.; Li, G. X. *J. Am. Chem. Soc.* 2004, 126, 273.
42. Jiao, J.; Seraphin, S.; Wang, X. K.; Withers, J. C. *J. Appl. Phys.* 1996, 80, 103.
43. Levy, M.; Wilhelm, C.; Luciani, N.; Deveaux, V.; Gendron, F.; Luciani, A.; Devaud, M.; Gazeau, F. *Nanoscale* 2011, 3, 4402.
44. Cornell, R. M.; Schertmann, U. *Iron Oxides in the Laboratory: Preparation and Characterization*; VCH: Weinheim, Germany, 1991.
45. Simo, F.; Sima, J. *Chem. Pap.* 2011, 65, 730.
46. Wagner, S.; Schnorr, J.; Pilgrimm, H.; Hamm, B.; Taupitz, M. *Invest. Radiol.* 2002, 37, 167.
47. Fauconnier, N.; Bee, A.; Roger, J.; Pons, J. N. *Prog. Colloid Polym. Sci.* 1996, 100, 212.
48. Fauconnier, N.; Pons, J. N.; Roger, J.; Bee, A. *J. Colloid Interface Sci.* 1997, 194, 427.
49. Denizot, B.; Tanguy, G.; Hindre, F.; Rump, E.; Le, J. J. J.; Jallet, P. *J. Colloid Interface Sci.* 1999, 209, 66.
50. Yuen, A. K.; Hutton, G. A.; Masters, A. F.; Maschmeyer, T. *Dalton Trans.* 2012, 41, 2545.
51. Raymond, K. N.; Dertz, E. A.; Kim, S. S. *Proc. Natl. Acad. Sci. USA* 2003, 100, 3584.
52. Lee, H.; Dellatore, S. M.; Miller, W. M.; Messersmith, P. B. *Science* (Washington, DC, U. S.) 2007, 318, 426.
53. El-Ayaan, U.; Herlinger, E.; Jameson, R. F.; Linert, W. *J. Chem. Soc., Dalton Trans.* 1997, 2813.
54. Amstad, E.; Gillich, T.; Bilecka, I.; Textor, M.; Reimhult, E. *Nano Lett.* 2009, 9, 4042.
55. Ni, X.; Zheng, Z.; Xiao, X.; Huang, L.; He, L. *Mater. Chem. Phys.* 2010, 120, 206.
56. Kang, S. M.; Kim, W.-J.; Choi, I. S. *J. Nanosci. Nanotechnol.* 2008, 8, 5347.
57. Tartaj, P.; Serna, C. *J. J. Am. Chem. Soc.* 2003, 125, 15754.
58. Johnson, W. K.; Stoupis, C.; Torres, G. M.; Rosenberg, E. B.; Ros, P. R. *Magn. Reson. Imaging* 1996, 14, 43.
59. Paciotti, G. F.; Myer, L.; Weinreich, D.; Goia, D.; Pavel, N.; McLaughlin, R. E.; Tamarkin, L. *Drug Deliv.* 2004, 11, 169.
60. Kelly, K. L.; Coronado, E.; Zhao, L. L.; Schatz, G. C. *J. Phys. Chem. B* 2003, 107, 668.

61. Kneipp, K.; Wang, Y.; Kneipp, H.; Perelman, L. T.; Itzkan, I.; Dasari, R.; Feld, M. S. *Phys. Rev. Lett.* 1997, 78, 1667.
62. Durr, N. J.; Larson, T.; Smith, D. K.; Korgel, B. A.; Sokolov, K.; Ben-Yakar, A. *Nano Lett.* 2007, 7, 941.
63. (a) Jain, P.; Xiao, Y.; Walsworth, R.; Cohen, A. *Nano Lett.* 2009, 9, 1644; (b) Dani, R. K.; Wang, H. W.; Bossmann, S. H.; Wysin, G.; Chikan, V. *J. Chem. Phys.* 2011, 135.
64. Wahajuddin; Arora, S. *Int. J. Nanomed.* 2012, 7, 3445.
65. Ngaboni, O. L.; Marchais, H.; Douziech-Eyrolles, L.; Cohen-Jonathan, S.; Souce, M.; Dubois, P.; Chourpa, I. *Int. J. Pharm.* 2005, 302, 187.
66. Ouyang, R.; Lei, J.; Ju, H. *Nanotechnology* 2010, 21, 185502/1.
67. Yang, H. T.; Su, Y. K.; Shen, C. M.; Yang, T. Z.; Gao, H. *J. Surf. Interface Anal.* 2004, 36, 155.
68. Mahmoudi, M.; Azadmanesh, K.; Shokrgozar, M. A.; Journeay, W. S.; Laurent, S. *Chem. Rev. (Washington, DC, U. S.)* 2011, 111, 3407.
69. Levy, M.; Lagarde, F.; Maraloiu, V.-A.; Blanchin, M.-G.; Gendron, F.; Wilhelm, C.; Gazeau, F. *Nanotechnology* 2010, 21, 395103/1.
70. Choi, H. S.; Liu, W.; Misra, P.; Tanaka, E.; Zimmer, J. P.; Ipe, B. I.; Bawendi, M. G.; Frangioni, J. V. *Nat. Biotechnol.* 2007, 25, 1165.
71. Adams, P. C.; Lin, E.; Barber, K. R.; Grant, C. W. M. *Hepatology (St. Louis)* 1991, 14, 1230.
72. Chomoucka, J.; Drbohlavova, J.; Huska, D.; Adam, V.; Kizek, R.; Hubalek, J. *Pharmacol. Res.* 2010, 62, 144.
73. Chithrani, B. D.; Chan, W. C. W. *Nano Lett.* 2007, 7, 1542.
74. Weinstein, J. S.; Varallyay, C. G.; Dosa, E.; Gahramanov, S.; Hamilton, B.; Rooney, W. D.; Muldoon, L. L.; Neuwelt, E. A. *J. Cereb. Blood Flow Metab.* 2010, 30, 15.
75. Tanaka, T.; Shibata, K.; Hosokawa, M.; Hatakeyama, K.; Arakaki, A.; Gomyo, H.; Mogi, T.; Taguchi, T.; Wake, H.; Tanaami, T.; Matsunaga, T. *J. Colloid Interface Sci.* 2012, 377, 469.
76. Dobson, J. *Nat. Nanotechnol.* 2008, 3, 139.
77. (a) Ghosh, A.; Fischer, P. *Nano Letts.* 2009, 9, 2243; (b) Zhang, L.; Abbott, J. J.; Dong, L. X.; Peyer, K. E.; Kratochvil, B. E.; Zhang, H. X.; Bergeles, C.; Nelson, B. J. *Nano Lett.* 2009, 9, 3663; (c) Wang, Y.; Fei, S. T.; Byun, Y. M.; Lammert, P. E.; Crespi, V. H.; Sen, A.; Mallouk, T. E. *J. Am. Chem. Soc.* 2009, 131, 9926.
78. Bangham, A. D.; Horne, R. W. *J. Molecul. Biol.* 1964, 8, 660.
79. (a) Gregoriadis, G. In *Enzyme Replacement Therapy of Lysosomal Storage Diseases*; J.M. Tager, G.J.M. Hooghwinkel, Daems, W. T., Eds.; North Holland Publishing Company, 1974; (b) Bangham, A. D.; Hill, M. W.; Miller, N. G. A. In *Methods in Membrane Biology*; E.D. Korn, E. P., Ed.; Plenium Press: New York, 1974.
80. (a) Gregoriadis, G.; Ryman, B. E. *Euro. J. Biochem.* 1972, 24, 485; (b) Gregoriadis, G.; Putman, D.; Louis, L.; Neerunjun, D. *Biochem. J.* 1974, 140, 323; (c) Gabizon, A. A. *Nanotechnol. Cancer Ther.* 2007, 595.
81. Fenske, D. B.; Cullis, P. R. *Methods Enzymol.* 2005, 391, 7.
82. (a) Moses, M. A.; Brem, H.; Langer, R. *Cancer Cell* 2003, 4, 337; (b) Allen, T. M.; Cullis, P. R. *Science* 2004, 303, 1818.
83. Perez, J. M.; Josephson, L.; O'Loughlin, T.; Hogemann, D.; Weissleder, R. *Nat. Biotech.* 2002, 20, 816.

Section IV

Biosensors Based on Thermal Properties

17

Solid–Liquid Phase Change Nanoparticles as Thermally Addressable Biosensors

Chaoming Wang, Yan Hong, Liyuan Ma, and Ming Su

CONTENTS

17.1 Introduction

A challenge of turning molecular biology knowledge into advance in disease detection to benefit patients is that most of available biomarkers are not powerful, lacking either sensitivity or specificity. Parallel to the effort of finding more specific biomarkers, one feasible way of providing better predictive value is to detect multiple low specificity biomarkers, and collectively analyze the response of multiple biomarkers contained in a sample.[1–5] The multiplexed detection can enhance the reliability and reduce the number of invasive and painful biopsies. In addition, the concentrations of biomarkers can vary several orders of magnitude.[6,7] Thereby an ideal detection should be able to detect biomarkers with high sensitivity and high multiplicity.

Although microarray is powerful in identifying biomarkers, it is not well-suited to detect multiple biomarkers, whose concentrations may span several orders of magnitude due to intrinsic heterogeneity of biomarkers at various stages of disease, and identical feature size and capacity within an array to bind biomarkers. The biomarker concentration may be too low to be detected, or too high that causes signal saturation.[8–10] In this aspect, systematic sample dilution or enrichment does not help, since concentration of each species will be changed at the same ratio. Microarray cannot be used readily to detect proteins due to difficulty of pattern generation. Enzyme-linked immunosorbent assay (ELISA) has high sensitivity, but is limited by signal saturation at high enzyme concentrations or after long incubation; polymerase chain reaction (PCR) can generate errors due to non-discriminative amplification of all DNA fragments.[11–14] Although multiple protein and genetic biomarkers exist in samples, DNA microarray, PCR, or ELISA can only detect genetic or protein biomarkers, and cannot detect both protein and genetic biomarkers at the same time and conditions.

Nanoparticle-based detections achieve extremely high sensitivity at pico- or femto-mole/liter levels by converting biorecognition events into measurable physical signals that can be amplified. But the multiplicities are limited due to narrow detection range and broad peak: only one or few types of biomarkers can be detected at one time, and screening a sample for multiple biomarkers will take a long time and a lot of agents and efforts.[15–19]

All metals exhibit solid–liquid phase transitions at their melting points. During melting, metals can absorb heat without temperature rise according to the Gibbs phase rule. If the dimension of a metal is small enough that the melting time can be negligible, a sharp melting peak will appear during a liner thermal scan owing to high thermal conductivity of the metal. Although a miscible solid can be formed when metals of the same crystal structures are mixed (such as gold–silver), most alloys have eutectic compositions. Eutectic alloys go directly from solid to liquid states without pasty stage, and have sharp melting peaks as metals. The melting temperature depends on atomic number (metal) or composition (alloy), provided the size of the material is larger than the critical size (10 nm), below which surface atoms will contribute more and cause reduction of melting temperature. The fusion enthalpy depends on the mass (composition) and latent heat of fusion of metal or alloy and larger fusion enthalpy provides higher sensitivity. Compared to paraffin, metal and alloy have higher volumetric latent heat of fusion, and thus can provide higher sensitivity. Differential scanning calorimetry (DSC) is normally used to obtain the melting point and fusion enthalpy of solids. A variety of eutectic alloys with two or multiple metal components and sharp melting points can be designed based on phase diagram knowledge and made into nanoparticles using colloid methods.

17.2 Thermal Biosensing

Instead of relying on existing optical, electric, magnetic, or mechanical methods for signal transductions, we have developed a new biosensing method, that is, thermal biosensing, in which nanoparticles of solid-to-liquid phase change materials (nano-PCMs) are used to detect multiple biomarkers (proteins and oligonucleotides) (Figure 17.1).[20–22] The nanoparticles are first modified with ligands that can bind to biomarkers, and then incubated in buffer or body fluid that contains biomarkers. After incubation, a high thermal conductivity solid substrate (silicon and aluminum) modified with multiple ligands is immersed into the solution to capture nanoparticles by forming sandwich complexes. After washing away unbounded nanoparticles, those attached on the substrate are read out using differential scanning calorimetry (DSC), where the peak position and area reflect the nature and amount of biomarker, respectively. A series of alloy nanoparticles with composition-encoded melting temperatures are used to detect multiple protein and DNA biomarkers after establishing a one-to-one correspondence between one type of nanoparticle and one type of biomarker.

High multiplicity: By using normal DSC equipment, the peak widths at half maximum of metal nanoparticles and eutectic alloy nanoparticles can be < 1°C (0.6°C) at ramp rate of 1°C/min. If thermal scan range is from 100°C to 700°C, the maximal number of melting peaks that can be resolved will be 1000 according to Rayleigh's criterion on spectral resolution, which means that about 1000 different types of biomarkers can be detected in one thermal scan by detecting nanoparticles.

Composition-encoded nanoparticles: Although metal nanoparticles have sharp melting peaks, only a small number of metals in the periodic table can be used to produce

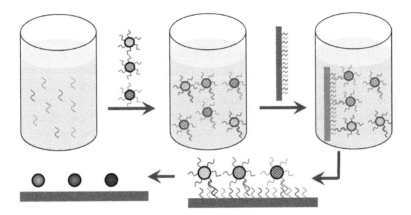

FIGURE 17.1
Nanoparticle-based three-stranded (left) and sandwiched (right) configuration for DNA and protein detection, respectively.

```
0                            1                        1     0
1                         1     1                     2     1
2                      1     2     1                  4     3
3                   1     3     3     1               8     7
4                1     4     6     4     1            16    15
5             1     5    10    10    5     1          32    31
6          1     6    15    20    15    6     1       64    63
7       1     7    21    35    35    21    7     1    128   127
8    1     8    28    56    70    56    28    8    1  256   255
9  1   9    36    84   126   126   84    36   9   1   512   511
10 1  10   45   120   210   252   210  120   45   10  1  1024  1023
n                                                    2ⁿ    2ⁿ−1
```

FIGURE 17.2
Pascal's triangle and number of possible combinations enabled by phase change nanoparticles.

nanoparticles due to availability and safety issues. Alloy nanoparticles with eutectic compositions have single sharp melting peaks, where the melting points are determined by compositions (provided that their sizes are larger than critical ones). According to combination rule, if any two of three metals can form binary eutectic alloys, the three metals will form one ternary eutectic alloy, and three binary eutectic alloys (Figure 17.2); and the total number of metals and alloys will be seven. For a given number of metals that form binary eutectic alloys among any two of them, the numbers of binary alloys, ternary alloys, and so on can be derived graphically from the Pascal's triangle (1653), and the total number of metals and eutectic alloys is

$$\sum_{k=1}^{n} C_n^k - 1 = \sum_{k=1}^{n} \frac{n!}{k!(n-k)!} - 1 = 2^n - 1$$

where
n is the total number of metals
k is the number of metals inside one nanoparticle

We have identified 10 different metals that can form binary eutectic alloys among any two of them from the periodic table. These metals include aluminum, bismuth, cadmium, copper, gadillium, indium, lead, magnesium, palladium, and silver. These metals will be able to form 10 types of metal nanoparticles, 45 types of binary alloy nanoparticles, 120 types of ternary eutectic alloy nanoparticles, 210 types of quaternary eutectic alloy nanoparticles, and so on. The total number of metals and eutectic alloys will be 1023. Note that the combination corresponding to no metal (n is 0) is removed. Nanoparticles of these metals and eutectic alloys have sharp and discrete melting peaks that can be resolved by DSC with high peak resolution (0.01°C).

Theoretical detection limit: Taking root mean square (RMS) noise of a commercial DSC instrument (DSC 7, Perkin Elmer) as 0.2 µW, the minimal detectable heat flow will be 0.2 µJ for a 1°C wide peak at ramp rate of 1°C/s. If 30 nm diameter copper nanoparticles (latent heat of 205 J/g, density of 13.6 g/cm^3) were used, the number of nanoparticles that absorb 0.2 µJ heat during phase change is 2.6×10^6. Provided that one antibody is attached on each nanoparticle, the antigen concentration in a 1 mL solution will be 4.3×10^{-15} M or 4.3 fM, which is lower than that available using most of available detection techniques. In addition, by using large nanoparticles or materials with high latent heat, the detection sensitivity can be increased.

Uniqueness: The unique features of thermal biosensing using phase change nanoparticles include (1) high multiplicity owing to sharp melting peak, large scan range and wide material choice; (2) high sensitivity and adjustable detection range using nanoparticles with varied size, composition, and ligand grafting density; (3) minimal sample preparation by detecting biomarker contained in body fluid; and (4) simultaneous detection of different biomarkers (i.e., proteins and oligonucleotides) at the same time and under the same conditions. Although an enzyme thermistor can detect heat absorption and evolution of biochemical reactions associated with analytes, the multiplicity of detection is low, and only one species can be detected each time. Nanoparticles of low melting temperature metals and alloys have been made as solder materials or as heat transfer additives, but there is no attempt to use them for biomarker detection due to lack of awareness on their unique thermal properties and on critical need for multiplexed detection of biomarkers.

17.3 Multiplexed Protein Detection

This method has been used to detect proteins using nanoparticles of indium and lead–tin alloy. The nanoparticles are made with colloid method and modified to have amine groups. The aluminum surface with native oxide is also modified to have amine groups. The nanoparticles and aluminum surface are conjugated with biotin by incubating with amine reactive biotinylation reagent (NHS-LC-biotins), which is followed by washing with dimethyl sulfoxide (DMSO) and phosphate buffer saline (PBS). Figure 17.3a shows DSC curves of indium nanoparticles attached on aluminum surfaces at different avidin concentrations, where thermal scan is carried out from 50°C to 300°C at a thermal ramp rate of 10°C/min. The melting peaks at 156°C confirm that indium nanoparticles have been immobilized on aluminum surfaces. The measured heat fluxes decrease as the concentrations of avidin decrease (Figure 17.3b). Similarly, lead–tin alloy nanoparticles have been used to detect rabbit IgG, where heat flow is proportional to the concentration of rabbit IgG.

The multiplicity of thermal detection is reflected in simultaneous detection of rabbit IgG and human IgG, where lead–tin nanoparticles and tin nanoparticles are modified with

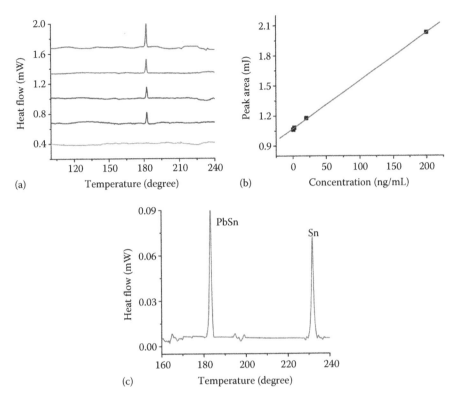

FIGURE 17.3
DSC curves (a) and concentration-dependent heat flows (b) of indium nanoparticles that are immobilized on aluminum surfaces through biotin-avidin interaction, where the curves from up to down are at avidin concentrations of 20, 2, and 0.05 ng/mL, respectively; (c) DSC curve of the multiplexed detection of 2 ng/mL of human IgG and 2 ng/mL of rabbit IgG using tin nanoparticles and lead–tin nanoparticles, respectively.

anti-IgGs of the rabbit and human, respectively. In order to modify aluminum surfaces, both anti-IgGs of rabbit and human are mixed at the same molar ratio and immobilized on amine-ended aluminum surfaces. The multiplexed detection is done by incubating the modified aluminum surface in a mixture containing 2 ng/mL rabbit IgG and 2 ng/mL human IgG in PBS (pH 7.4). After washing, the surface is incubated in a mixture of two types of surface-modified nanoparticles. After second washing, the aluminum surface is tested by DSC. Figure 17.3c shows two melting peaks of tin and lead–tin nanoparticles at 183°C and 230°C, respectively. The difference in heat flows of two peaks may be induced by the differences in latent heats of indium and lead–tin alloy with sizes of two types of nanoparticles or grafting densities of anti-IgGs on nanoparticles.

17.4 Multiplexed DNA Detection

Thermal detection does not rely on optical transparency, and is immune to inference from colored species. This method has been used to detect single strand oligonucleotides (ssDNAs) in body fluids. The target ssDNAs are added in fresh milk to make samples

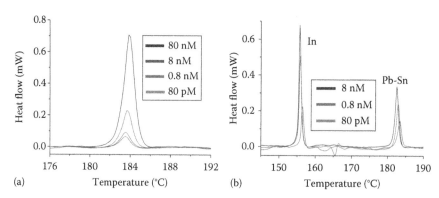

FIGURE 17.4
(See color insert.) (a) DSC curves of indium nanoparticles captured by target ssDNA at different concentrations in buffer solutions, where the concentration of target ssDNA is from 80 nM to 80 pM; (b) target ssDNA detection in cell lysate using indium and lead–tin nanoparticles as probes, the concentrations of target ssDNA are at 8 nM, 0.8 nM, and 80 pM, respectively.

that are not transparent. The probe ssDNA-modified nanoparticles and capture ssDNA-modified aluminum surface are added in the milk for hybridization. After hybridizing for 3 h, the aluminum surface is taken out, washed with phosphate buffer and tested by DSC. The pH values and ion concentrations of milk are adjusted to 10 mM Tris-HCl at pH 7.5, 100 mM NaCl, and 1 mM EDTA. Figure 17.4a shows the DSC curves of lead–tin nanoparticles collected at different concentrations of target ssDNA, where the melting peaks are attributed to immobilized lead–tin nanoparticles. The method has been used to detect two types of ssDNA by modifying capture and probe ssDNA on aluminum surface, and two types of nanoparticles (i.e., indium and lead–tin alloy). Meanwhile, two target ssDNAs are dispersed in PBS at pH of 7.5 and 1M NaCl. The probe ssDNA-modified indium and lead–tin nanoparticles and the capture ssDNA-modified aluminum surfaces are immersed into PBS that contains two types of target ssDNAs for 3 h. After DNA hybridization, the aluminum surface is washed with a phosphate buffer and tested by DSC. Figure 17.4b shows the melting peaks of indium and alloy nanoparticles covalently bonded on aluminum surfaces, thus confirming the existence of two types of target ssDNA in the solution.

17.5 Enhanced Detection Sensitivity with Nanostructured Substrate

The detection sensitivity is dependent on the mass and the latent heat of fusion of phase change nanoparticles immobilized on substrates. By increasing the surface area of the substrate, the detection sensitivity can be enhanced. Silicon surfaces with vertically aligned high-aspect-ratio nanopillars have been made by combining nanosphere lithography and gold nanoparticle enhanced etching of silicon.[23] The SEM image shows (Figure 17.5a) that the nanopillar is about 200 nm in diameter and 2 μm in height. The silicon nanopillars are modified by 3-aminopropyl-triethoxysilane (APTES) and activated by disuccinimidyl suberate (DSS). After reacting with aptamer with a sequence of 5′-AmMC6-TTT TTT TTT TTT TTT GGT TGG TGT GGT TGG-3′ that is specific to thrombin for 2 h, the substrate

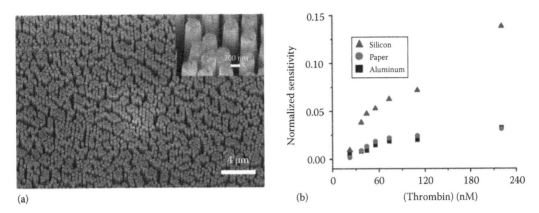

(a)   (b)   (Thrombin) (nM)

FIGURE 17.5
SEM image of silicon nanopillars, and the inset is a tilt-angle magnified SEM image (a); normalized sensitivity (melting peak area/mm^2) on different substrates (nanostructured silicon, filter paper, and aluminum surfaces) versus the concentration of thrombin (22–220 nM) (b).

is immersed in a buffer solution containing different concentrations of thrombin. The aptamer functionalized surface is incubated with aptamer-functionalized nanoparticles in a buffer solution containing thrombin for 1 h. The surface area of a substrate with an array of nanopillars (200 nm in diameter, and 2 μm in height) is about 10 times larger than that of a flat surface with the same size. Figure 17.5b shows the normalized sensitivity (peak area/mm^2) at different thrombin concentrations (22–220 nM) with different substrates, where the sensitivity of the nanostructured silicon surface is enhanced by four times at a thrombin concentration of 55 nM compared to filter paper and aluminum surfaces.

17.6 Thermal Barcodes

The composition-dependent melting point and sharp melting peak of nanoparticles allow creation of a large number of microspheres that have a distinguishable pattern of melting behavior. The melting temperatures of nanoparticles of Field's alloy, indium, lead–tin alloy, and tin are 62°C, 156°C, 183°C, and 232°C, respectively. A panel of these phase change nanoparticles is selected and embedded in silica microsphere. The melting enthalpies (peak areas) are proportional to mass and latent heat of fusion of nanoparticles. The number of thermal probes formed by four types of nanoparticles is 15. Figure 17.6 shows the DSC curves collected from 16 different types of silica microspheres, where each curve is flattened to remove slope and smoothed to remove fluctuation. Each melting peak can be denoted as one or zero depending on whether there is detectable heat flux or not. 16 combinations of four elements are 0000, 1000, 0100, 0010, 0001, 1100, 1010, 1001, 0110, 0101, 0011, 1110, 1101, 1011, 0111, and 1111. The height (or area) of each peak corresponds to the amount of certain particles in microspheres. The information in each microsphere can be decoded by counting melting peaks in DSC curves. One scan from 0°C to 300°C with ramp rate of 10°C/min takes 30 min, and the decoding time can be reduced by increasing ramp rates.

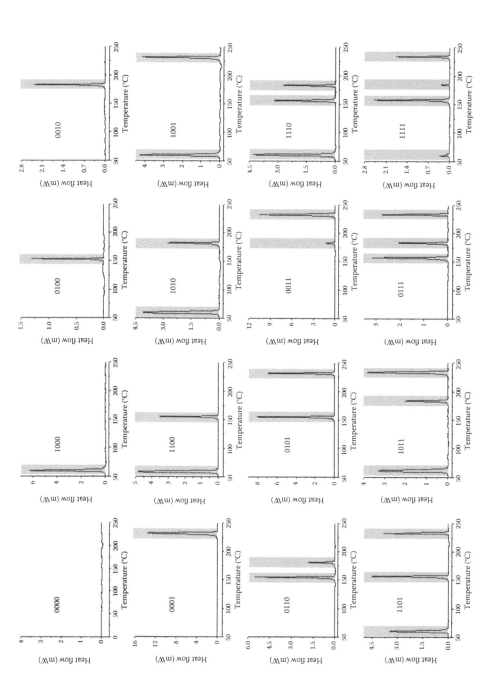

FIGURE 17.6

Panel of DSC curves collected from a series of silica microspheres that contain different ratios of nanoparticles of Field's metal, indium, lead–tin, and tin at melting points of 62°C, 156°C, 183°C, and 231°C, respectively.

17.7 Summary

Thermal biosensing is based on nanoparticles of solid–liquid nano-PCMs, where each type of nanoparticles is conjugated with ligands of protein and DNA biomarkers, and immobilized on ligand-modified substrates by forming double helix DNA chain or sandwiched antibody–antigen complex. The type and concentration of biomarkers are reflected in melting temperature and fusion enthalpy of nanoparticles in differential scanning calorimetry (DSC). Owing to sharp melting peaks and large thermal scan range, thermal biosensing allows detection of multiple biomarkers at the same time.

References

1. Makarov, D. V., Loeb, S., Getzenberg, R. H., Partin, A. W., Biomarkers for prostate cancer. *Annu. Rev. Med.* 2009, *60*, 139.
2. Rhodes, D. R., Sanda, M. G., Otte, A. P., Chinnaiyan, A. M., Rubin, M. A., Multiplex biomarker approach for determining risk of prostate-specific antigen-defined recurrence of prostate cancer. *J. Natl. Cancer Inst.* 2003, *95*, 661.
3. Smith, M. Q., Staley, C. A., Kooby, D. A., Styblo, T., Wood, W. C., Yang, L., Multiplexed fluorescence imaging of tumor biomarkers in gene expression and protein levels for personalized and predictive medicine. *Curr. Mol. Med.* 2009, *9*, 1017.
4. Medintz, I. L., Uyeda, H. T., Goldman, E. R., Mattoussi, H., Quantum dot bioconjugates for imaging, labelling and sensing. *Nat. Mater.* 2005, *4*, 435.
5. Jaiswal, J. K., Mattoussi, H., Mauro, J. M., Simon, S. M., Long-term multiple color imaging of live cells using quantum dot bioconjugates. *Nat. Biotechnol.* 2003, *21*, 47.
6. Etzioni, R., Urban, N., Ramsey, S., McIntosh, M., Schwartz, S., Reid, B., Radich, J., Anderson, G., Hartwell, L., The case for early detection. *Nat. Rev. Cancer* 2003, *3*, 243.
7. Nagrath, S., Sequist, L. V., Maheswaran, S., Bell, D. W., Irimia, D., Ulkus, L., Smith, M. R. et al. Isolation of rare circulating tumour cells in cancer patients by microchip technology. *Nature* 2007, *450*, 1235.
8. Skvortsov, D., Abdueva, D., Curtis, C., Schaub, B., Tavare, S., Explaining differences in saturation levels for Affymetrix GeneChip arrays. *Nucl. Acids. Res.* 2007, *35*, 4154.
9. Dudley, A. E. M., Aach, J., Steffen, M. A., Church, G. M., Measuring absolute expression with microarrays with a calibrated reference sample and an extended signal intensity range. *Proc. Natl. Acad. Sci.* 2002, *99*, 7554.
10. Hart, T., Zhao, A., Garg, A., Bolusani, S., Marcotte, E. M., Human cell chips: Adapting DNA microarray spotting technology to cell-based imaging assays. *PLoS ONE* 2009, *4*, e7088.
11. Sanchez, F. G., Diaz, A. N., Diaz, A. F. G., Eremin, S. A., Quantification of 2,4,5-trichlorophenoxyacetic acid by fluorescence enzyme-linked immunosorbent assay with secondary antibody. *Anal. Chim. Acta* 1999, *378*, 219.
12. High, K., Meng, Y., Washabaugh, M. W., Zhao, Q. J., Determination of picomolar equilibrium dissociation constants in solution by enzyme-linked immunosorbent assay with fluorescence detection. *Anal. Biochem.* 2005, *347*, 159.
13. Toriello, N. M., Liu, C. N., Mathies, R. A., Multichannel reverse transcription-polymerase chain reaction microdevice for rapid gene expression and biomarker analysis. *Anal. Chem.* 2006, *78*, 7997.
14. Parks, S. B., Popovich, B. W., Press, R. D., Real-time polymerase chain reaction with fluorescent hybridization probes for the detection of prevalent mutations causing common thrombophilic and iron overload phenotypes. *Am. J. Clin. Pathol.* 2001, *115*, 439.

15. Bao, Y. P., Wei, T.-F., Lefebvre, P. A., An, H., He, L., Kunkel, G. T., Müller, U. R., Detection of protein analytes via nanoparticle-based bio bar code technology. *Anal. Chem.* 2006, *78*, 2055.
16. Rosi, N. L., Mirkin, C. A., Nanostructures in biodiagnostics. *Chem. Rev.* 2005, *105*, 1547.
17. Han, M., Gao, X., Su, J. Z., Nie, S., Quantum-dot-tagged microbeads for multiplexed optical coding of biomolecules. *Nat Biotechnol.* 2001, *19*, 631.
18. Zimmer, J. P., Kim, S.-W., Ohnishi, S., Tanaka, E., Frangioni, J. V., Bawendi, M. G., Size series of small indium arsenide–zinc selenide core–shell nanocrystals and their application to in vivo imaging. *J. Am. Chem. Soc.* 2006, *128*, 2526.
19. Josephson, L., Perez, J. M., Weissleder, R., Magnetic nanosensors for the detection of oligonucle-otide sequences. *Angew. Chem. Int. Ed.* 2001, *40*, 3204.
20. Ma, L., Wang, C., Hong, Y., Zhang, M., Su, M., Thermally addressed immunosorbent assay for multiplexed protein detections using phase change nanoparticles. *Anal. Chem.* 2010, *82*, 1186.
21. Wang, C., Ma, L., Chen, L.-M., Chai, K. X., Su, M., Scanning calorimetric detections of multiple DNA Biomarkers contained in complex fluids. *Anal. Chem.* 2010, *82*, 1838.
22. Wang, C., Sun, Z., Ma, L., Su, M., Simultaneous detection of multiple biomarkers with over three orders of concentration difference using phase change nanoparticles. *Anal. Chem.* 2011, *83*, 2215.
23. Wang, C., Hossain, M., Ma, L., Ma, Z., Hickman, J. J., Su, M., Highly sensitive thermal detection of thrombin using aptamer-functionalized phase change nanoparticles. *Biosens. Bioelectron.* 2010, *26*, 437.

18

Microfluidic and Lab-on-Chip Technologies for Biosensors

Yuxin Liu and Xiang Li

CONTENTS

18.1 Introduction and Overview of Microfluidics and Sensor Integration

Biological or biochemical sensing and quantification are of critical importance for medical, biological, chemical, and biotechnological applications. Biosensor represents a device that can detect and measure a specific biological organism (i.e., cells, proteins, enzymes, or nucleic acids) in a biological or biochemical process with a large variety of samples including body fluids, food samples, cell cultures, and environmental samples. The sensing ability relies on one or more sensing mechanisms that produce signals that indicate the presence and quantity of the specific biological organism. Typically, a biosensor consists of (1) bioreceptors that can specifically bind to the analytes, (2) an interface architecture where a specific biological or biochemical signal generated from, (3) the transducer element converting the signal to another form of signals for detection, and (4) detectors to amplify and detect the transduced signals [1].

The fabrication and measurement of biosensors and micro- and nanostructures have seen an explosive growth based on the advancement in microfluidic and Lab-on-Chip (LOC) technologies, which allow the handling of bioanalysis at extremely low volumes in an integrated platform that would not be possible using the conventional systems. Some significant benefits of using microfluidics and LOC as a miniaturized research tool include the following:

1. *Scaling of the dimensions*: Sizes of the biological organisms are in the range of nanoscale to microscale. For example, bacterial Escherichia coli (*E. coli*) cells are typically rod-shaped and are about 2.0 μm long and 0.5 μm in diameter with a cell volume of 0.6–0.7 μm³ [2,3], most plant and animal cells are between 1 and 100 μm [4], and proteins are in the range of a few nanometers with molecular masses varying from 5 to 500 kDa [5]. Microfluidic systems typically manipulate and process small volumes of fluids (picoliters to nanoliters) using channels with dimensions of a few to hundreds of micrometers [6]. The development of tools and processes used to detect analyte molecules or cells by microfluidic technologies can lead to creation of biosensors that can interact with extremely small numbers of organisms with a very low concentration detection and high specificity.

2. *Rapid bioanalysis*: Compared to conventional assays, the surface to volume ratios of micro-channels are significantly increased and can significantly enhance chemical reactions and reduce reaction time. For example, different groups of researchers investigated protein digestion in the field of proteomics using microfluidic chips [7–10]. Their results showed that the protein digestion time was significantly reduced (50–720 fold) depending on the surface properties and dimensions of micro-channels.

3. *Low costs in materials and chemical reagents*: The manufacturing of microfluidic devices has benefited from employing polymer/plastic materials, which reduce cost and simplify manufacturing procedures, particularly when compared to glass and silicon. In addition, the wide range of available polymer materials allows the manufacturer to choose material properties suitable for their specific applications [11]. For example, polydimethylsiloxane (PDMS) is the primary material and commonly used for microfluidic device fabrication. PDMS has many advantages, such as being chemically inert, non-toxic, transparent, gas permeable, and biocompatible. The soft lithographic micro-molding processes are simple and rapid compared with conventional microfabrication procedures (i.e., etching, deposition, and bonding approaches). On the other hand, nanoliter volumes of different chemical solutions can be controlled and pumped through the micro-scale channels for complex chemical reactions.

4. *Highly integrated and parallel processing potential for in situ monitoring and/or point-of-care (POC) analysis*: POC, which is a different model from the historic central laboratory, is performed close to or at the patient's location, and often by non-laboratorians and is considered one of the main driving forces for the future of the *in vitro* diagnostic market [12]. The significant strength of microfluidic systems lies in their integration ability, which leads to the development of LOC systems. The integrated LOC devices incorporate sample preparation, handling,

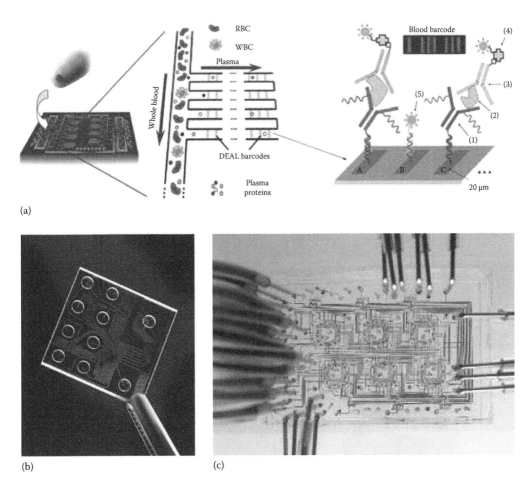

FIGURE 18.1
(See color insert.) (a) An integrated blood barcode chip (IBBC) using DNA-encoded antibody library (DEAL) barcode arrays. (Reprinted from Fan, R. et al., *Nat. Biotechnol.*, 26(12), 1373, 2008. With permission.) (b) An Agilent lab-on-chip cartridge shows the microfluidic channels. (Reprinted from Thilmany, J., *EMBO Rep.*, 6, 913, 2005. With permission.) (c) The microfluidic chip houses bioreactors, where bacteria can be cultured and observed. (Reprinted from El-Ali, J. et al., *Nature*, 442, 403, 2006. With permission.)

detection, and analysis, enable high-throughput screening studies, and strive for simple incorporation in a user-friendly automated system [13–15]. An integrated microfluidic LOC system was applied for blood analysis for biomarkers [16] (Figure 18.1a). A commercially available LOC system has been used for analysis of biological molecules (Figure 18.1b). This technology replaces slab gel electrophoresis in nucleic acid and protein analysis applications, generating more precise data, improving reproducibility, shortening analysis time, using smaller quantities of precious samples, and facilitating automated workflows. Other applications include pharmaceutical quality-control and environmental analysis [17]. In addition, an integrated microfluidic bioreactor chip (Figure 18.1c) was investigated for bacteria culture and observation [18]. Stanford researchers made the chips using optical lithography to etch the circuit pattern into silicon. The etched silicon acts as a mold. PDMS was poured into the mold and then removed. By stacking several layers of molded PDMS layers and then encasing them in glass, an integrated circuit of channels, microvalves, and chambers for chemicals and cells were created.

Microfluidic and LOC technologies enable the fabrication of highly integrated, parallel, and automatic chip-based platforms, which are revolutionizing biological and chemical assays with the advantages of short reaction time, reduced reagent volumes, reduced energy consumption, low unit cost, and high throughput. This technology would ultimately provide biosensors for environmental monitoring and POC medical applications.

In this chapter, we focus on the state-of-the-art technological development in microfluidics-based biosensor integration, including the past achievements, current status, and future development and potentials of microfluidics and LOC integration technologies in the applications of biosensors and biomedical devices. We start with the introduction of microfluidics and its fabrication techniques, followed by the introduction of microfluidic components, fluid control, biosensor integration, and their applications. Most current state-of-the-art accomplishments are presented as examples following the introduction of each section.

18.2 Microfluidic Technology

Microfluidics is the science and technology of handling and analyzing fluids in the micrometer scale. Because of scaling, shrinking existing large devices and expecting them to function well at the microscale is often counterproductive [19]. It is critical for researchers who design new devices to understand microfluidic physics and physical phenomena including laminar flow, diffusion, fluidic resistance, surface area to volume ratio, and surface tension that dominate at the microscale. The physics of microfluidics in biology has been reviewed [20]. Later, a more comprehensive review of the physics of small volumes (nanoliters) of fluids underlying microfluidic devices was published with the emphasis on the variety of physical phenomena and the manner in which they have been exploited [21]. A series of dimensionless numbers (i.e., Reynolds number, Péclet number, capillary number, etc.) expressing the relative importance of various physical phenomena in microfluidic systems was discussed. Recently, a review of theory, fabrication, and applications of microfluidic and nanofluidic biosensors was published [22]. Here, we will focus on the introduction of the state-of-the-art microfluidic fabrication technologies and important microfluidic components and fluidic control by presenting the most recent research accomplishments.

18.3 Microfluidic Fabrication

Significant growth in the development of new microfluidic applications in recent years requires quick, simple, and inexpensive fabrication approaches to rapid prototyping of microfluidic devices. Various microfluidic fabrication approaches have been investigated based on the applied materials and device applications. Among different microfabrication materials, fabrication in polymers is easily compared with the conventional microfabrication materials (i.e., glass and silicon). The polymers commonly used in micro-fabrication include PDMS, poly (methyl methacrylate) (PMMA), polyurethane, polyimide, and polystyrene (PS). Compared with conventional microfabrication materials, polymers are inexpensive, flexible, and transparent to visible/UV lights, with easily molded, easily modified surface properties and improved biocompatibility or bioactivity. The uses of polymers in the fabrication processes reduce the time and the cost, avoid complexity in fabricated steps and sophisticated requirements for the facilities, and provide fast prototyping and manufacturing [23,24]. However, there are still several limitations that need to be kept in mind when choosing a specific polymer because of low thermal stability, low thermal and electrical conductivity, techniques for polymer fabrication on micro/nanoscale not as well developed, and the interface connection and integration with other microfabricated components (i.e., electrodes, tubing).

In the following sections, we introduce the most common methods for the fabrication of polymer microfluidic devices and describe each method with its fabrication processes, specific characteristics, advantages, and disadvantages. For the choice of method for actual device fabrication one needs to consider several factors, such as available technologies and equipment, cost, the desired feature size and profile, the preferred material substrate, operation requirement and applications, reagents, and throughput.

18.3.1 Polymer Replica Molding

PDMS has been one of the most actively developed polymers for microfluidics [25]. Fabrication of systems and channels in PDMS is particularly straightforward since it can be cast against a suitable mold with sub-0.1-μm fidelity. PDMS is also more than a structural material; its chemical and physical properties make it possible for fabrication of devices with useful functionality [26]. Currently, the most commonly used approach for microfluidic fabrication is the combination of photolithography and soft lithography techniques using PDMS as a material for microfluidic fabrication [27,28]. As shown in Figure 18.2, a layer of photoresist, typically using negative tone (i.e., SU-8 [Microchem]) or positive tone photoresists (i.e., AZ series of photoresists) is exposed to UV light through a mask layer to generate master patterns on a silicon substrate. PDMS (Sylgard 184, Dow Corning, ML) with a mixing ratio (i.e., 10:1) is cast onto the master mold to replicate the master patterns. Then the cured PDMS is peeled from the master mold, and the inlets and outlets for the chemical fluids and biological organisms are cut out using a sharpened puncher. The surfaces of both the channel-side of the PDMS and a clean glass cover slide are treated with oxygen plasma (i.e., for 20 s) and bonded together to form an irreversible seal. Except for glass as a substrate material, PDMS can also bond to other materials, such as another plain PDMS layer or PDMS layer with patterns, or other polymer materials (i.e., polystyrene) after appropriate surface treatments or coatings or using an intermediate adhesive layer [29].

Figure 18.2 shows a typical fabrication procedure for soft lithography-based micromolding. In addition, there are other soft lithography molding techniques for directly patterning polymer structures or biological organisms in two or three dimensions. Other soft lithography methods include microcontact printing, microtransfer molding, replica molding, micromolding in capillaries, and solvent-assisted micromolding [30]. For example, the microcontact printing has proven to be a useful technique in the patterned functionalization of certain chemicals onto surfaces. It has been particularly valuable in the patterning of biological materials with nanoscale resolutions through patterning of molecules that form self-assembled monolayers (SAMs) [31].

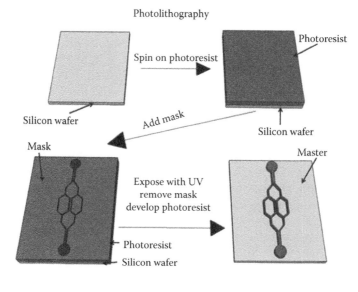

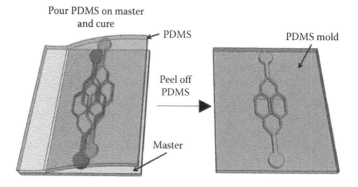

FIGURE 18.2
Schematic process for PDMS microfluidic fabrication by the combination of photolithography and soft lithography processes. A mask for microfluidic channels is designed in a CAD (i.e., AutoCAD, L-Edit) program. A commercial printer uses the CAD file to produce a high-resolution transparency mask, which is used as a photomask in contact photolithography to produce a master mold. The master mold consists of a positive relief of photoresist on a silicon wafer and serves as a mold for PDMS. During the micromolding soft lithographic process, liquid PDMS pre-polymer is poured over the master mold and cured for 1 h at 70°C. Then the PDMS replica is peeled from the master mold, and the replica is sealed to a flat surface substrate (i.e., glass, another PDMS layer, or other polymers with appropriate surface treatment for bonding to PDMS).

In addition to soft lithography approaches, other polymer fabrication techniques for microfluidic devices include hot embossing, micro-injection molding, laser ablation and micromachining, and shrinky-dink microfluidics.

18.3.2 Hot Embossing

Hot embossing of polymers is a very versatile replication method to transfer structures from a master mold into the thermal polymer under high pressures and elevated temperatures, and it is an alternative approach to traditional silicon processing and promising for

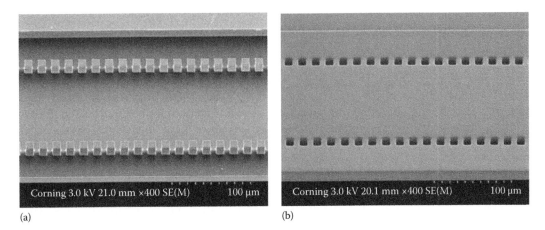

(a)   (b)

FIGURE 18.3
(a) SEM image of PDMS mold with a 10 μm × 10 μm square and 15 μm tall micropillar array; (b) SEM image of polystyrene slide replicas from the PDMS mold. (Reprinted from Goral, V.N., *J. Micromech. Microeng.*, 21, 017002, 2001, doi: 10.1088/0960-1317/21/1/017002. With permission.)

microfluidic fabrication. Hot embossing is essentially the pressing of patterns into a polymer by raising the temperature above the polymer's glass transition temperature (T_g). The whole part is cooled and the polymer is removed from the pattern mold after a period of time under high pressures and elevated temperatures. It fulfills the demands as a low-cost method for mass production of microcomponents and microsystems, and addresses a wide range of applications, such as polymer-based LOC systems, where imprinting is done on thick polymer substrates to the fabrication of sub 50 nm features for bio-sensing or data recording applications. For example, hot embossing has been applied to the fabrication of microfluidic devices on PMMA substrates for analytical chemistry and biomedical applications such as micro-total analysis systems (μ-TAS) or LOC devices [32,33]. Polymer microfabrication by hot embossing is also becoming increasingly important as a low-cost alternative to silicon- or glass-based MicroElectroMechanical Systems (MEMS) technologies [34,35].

Hot embossing as a standard method has been used in industry for high throughput production of polymer devices. However, it requires expensive machining and mold fabrication, and is unsuitable for quick prototyping in a laboratory setting. For example, the commercial process uses expensive electroplated nickel molds [36], while the hot embossing process in a laboratory uses silicon [33] or silicon anodic bonded on glass [37]. A soft PDMS mold has been investigated as a hot embossing mold as shown in Figure 18.3 [38]. This PDMS-based hot embossing process simplifies the existing hot embossing process and can be used in regular laboratory settings. Elastic properties of PDMS result in several advantages for the hot embossing process, such as lower operational pressure required for structure replication and ease of mold separation without special model designs [38]. In addition, soft molds can be used multiple times and for large area replication, achieve high resolution replicated features for biosensing applications (<50 nm) as well as micro fluidic channels, and largely reduce the fabrication costs.

18.3.3 Microinjection Molding

Micromolding is another standard method of mass production used in the fabrication of commercial products. Several micromolding techniques, including microinjection molding, reaction injection molding, hot embossing, and thermoforming, are available for the manufacturing of microfluidic devices from polymers. Of these, microinjection molding is one technique that offers mass-production capabilities with relatively low costs. Microinjection molding is the process of transferring a thermoplastic material in the form of granules from a hopper into a heated barrel so that it becomes molten and soft. The material is then forced under pressure inside a mold cavity where it is subjected to hold pressure for a specific time to compensate for material shrinkage. The material solidifies as the mold temperature is decreased below the glass-transition temperature of the polymer. After sufficient time, the material freezes into the mold shape and gets ejected; the cycle is then repeated. A typical cycle lasts between few seconds to few minutes [39]. In addition, microinjection molding offers advantages of short cycle time, the potential for full automation, accurate replication and dimensional control, as well as the existence of considerable know-how, and is transferable from conventional injection molding [39]. This set of advantages make microinjection molding commercially applicable with potential for further developments in the future.

For microfluidics and LOC applications in medical diagnostics, chemical analysis, and environmental safety, different components are required to be integrated together, such as micropumps, microvalves, sample inlets and outlets, separation of solutions, reagents mixing, signal detection, and waste collection. Microinjection molding, one of the main fabrication techniques, is more convenient to produce and integrate polymeric microfluidic functional units when compared with other techniques for microfluidic device manufacturing (i.e., hot embossing and PDMS casting). Figure 18.4 shows the fabrication process of microinjection molding for a microfluidic biochip [40]. In this biochip, flow splitting microchannels, chaotic micromixers, reaction microchambers, and detection microfilters were fully integrated. Figure 18.5 shows the final microfluidic biochip after thermal bonding. This low-cost, compact-size microchip for blood typing requires a very small sample blood volume of the order of 1 μL. In addition, this integrated microchip could be capable of automated diagnosis with further development and suitable for the level of hospitals in function and capacity.

There are several other commercially available microfluidics-based disposable medical devices that are produced by microinjection molding. For example, ThinXXS produces an integrated microfluidic optical blood analysis system for POC cardiac risk diagnostics [41]. It includes functional units for metering, mixing, and detection. Each trial only requires a 10 min processing time. This processing includes the application of the blood sample, the centrifugation of the erythrocytes, the dosing and aqueous dilution of the remaining plasma, and the dissolution of the freeze-dried reagents with the homogenized sample.

Microinjection molding is a technology for fabricating disposable microfluidic devices in terms of mass-production, variety of polymer materials, and accurate replication of micro-scaled features. In addition, for an integrated microfluidic system with complex requirements for functional units, microinjection molding is capable of developing in-line integration techniques to allow the mass-fabrication of polymeric microfluidic devices that are economically feasible for commercial use.

18.3.4 Shrinky-Dink Microfluidics

Shrinky-Dink approach for microfluidic fabrication is different than the traditional fabrication approaches, which normally use either microfabricated molds by lithographic processes in clean-room facilities or complicated equipment (i.e., hot embossing or micromolding). In the 1980s, Shrinky Dinks® were popular children's toys or activity kits which

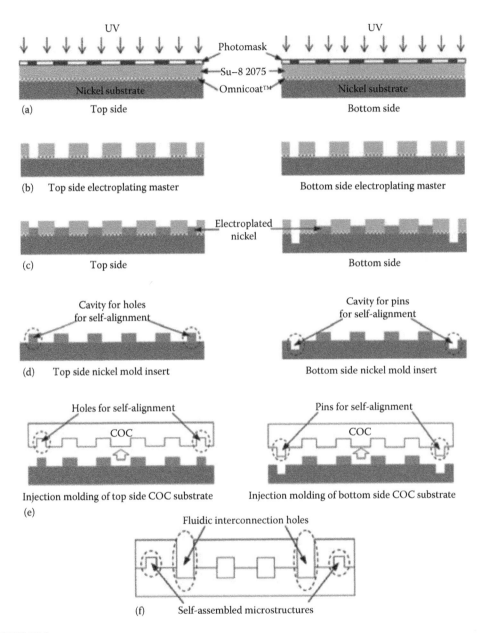

FIGURE 18.4

Schematic fabrication process for micro-injection molding of a blood typing integrated microfluidic biochip: (a) UV photolithography, (b) SU-8 and OmniCoat™ layers patterned on the nickel substrates as masters for electroplating, (c) electroplated nickel in the masters, (d) nickel mold inserts after removing SU-8 and OmniCoat™ layers, (e) injection molding of cyclic olefin copolymer (COC) substrates, and (f) final microfluidic biochip after thermal bonding. (Reprinted from Kim, D.S. et al., *Lab Chip*, 6, 794, 2006. With permission.)

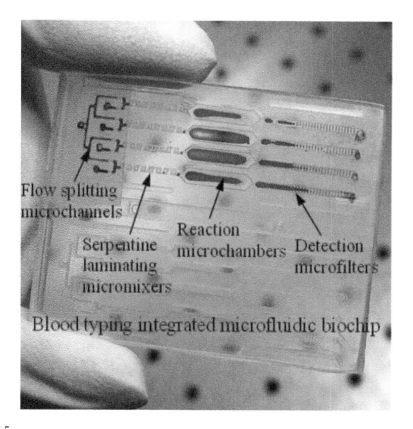

FIGURE 18.5
A blood typing microfluidic biochip integrated flow splitting microchannels, serpentine laminating micromixers, reaction chambers, and detection microfilters. (Reprinted with permission from Kim, D.S. et al., *Lab Chip*, 6, 794, 2006.)

consisted of flexible thermoplastic PS sheets, which had been preheated and stretched. When the sheets are reheated in an oven or with a heat gun, they shrink to their original size, and anything drawn on them shrinks without altering the color and shape. The drawn features become narrower and more raised as the ink lines are compressed. Shrinky-Dink microfluidics was developed by Professor Michelle Khine at the University of California, Merced (currently at Irvine) for printing microfluidic mold patterns onto Shrinky Dinks. She used the shrunken mold to make patterns of channels by PDMS replication for mixing fluids and moving cells. This technique allows the whole process from device design conception to working device to be completed with very simple tools (only a laser jet printer and a toaster oven) within minutes [42–44]. This novel approach yields channels deep enough for mammalian cell assays, with the channel heights easily fabricated up to 80 µm. In addition, the replica channels can easily achieve rounded cross sections, multi-height channels, and channels as thin as 65 µm in width [42]. Shrinky-Dink microfluidic fabrication represents a rapid, non-photolithographic approach, ultralow cost for microfluidic pattern generation. The company, Shrink Nanotechnologies, was developed based on this technique for affordable and disposable microfluidic devices applied in molecular detection, rapid prototyping, and stem-cell research. They may make microfluidic devices more accessible to scientists and speed important research.

18.3.5 Laser Ablation and Micromachining

Laser ablation involves the use of a high-powered pulsed laser to remove material from a sheet of thermoplastic [45] and is an ubiquitous technology with numerous existing applications such as laser surgery, cutting, and micromachining [46]. Common thermoplastics used in laser ablation include poly(ethylene terephthalate glycol) (PETG), polycarbonate (PC), poly(vinyl chloride) (PVC), polyimide, and poly(methyl methacrylate) (PMMA). Figure 18.6a shows the process of the creation of patterns in polymer substrates using the technique of UV excimer laser photoablation [47]. A metal mask (lithographic mask) can be used to designate areas to be protected and areas to be exposed to the laser for ablation. Alternatively, a direct-write process can be used for pattern transfer, which typically involves the use of a programmable high-resolution and high-stability translation stage on which the plastic substrate rests [45]. Figure 18.6b shows an integrated parallel microfluidic channel fixture fabricated using laser ablated plastic laminates for electrochemical and chemiluminescent biodetection of DNA [48]. This multilayer device was produced by laser machining of plastic PMMA and PET laminates by ablation. The fixture consisted of an array of nine individually addressable gold or gold/ITO working electrodes and a resistive platinum heating element. Laser machining of the fluidic pathways in the plastic laminates and the stencil masks for thermal evaporation to form electrode regions on the plastic laminates enabled rapid and inexpensive implementation of design changes. Electrochemiluminescence reactions in the fixture were achieved and monitored through ITO electrodes for electrochemical multianalyte DNA detection from double stranded DNA (dsDNA) samples. This versatile and simple method of laser machining for prototyping devices shows potential for further development of highly integrated, multi-functional bioanalytical devices.

Laser ablation, as a direct-write process, is advantageous for the fabrication of polymer microfluidic devices for prototyping applications. In addition, the unique feature of

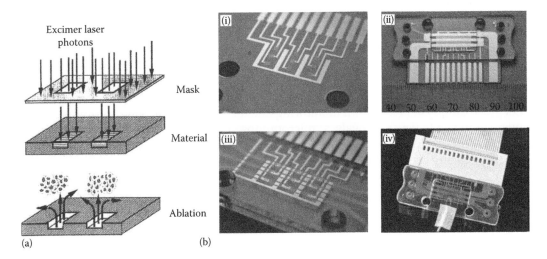

FIGURE 18.6
(a) Schematic diagram of UV laser micromachining process. UV excimer laser pulse rapidly breaks chemical bonds within a restricted volume to cause a mini-explosion and ejection of ablated material. (Reprinted from Roberts, M.A., *Anal. Chem.* 69(11), 2035, 1997. With permission.). (b) An integrated parallel microfluidic channel fixture fabricated using laser ablated plastic laminates for electrochemical and chemiluminescent biodetection of DNA. (Reprinted from Edwards, T.L., *Biomicrofluidics*, 5(4), 044115, 2011. With permission.)

laser ablation provides the capability of surface modification of channel walls concurrent with microchannel formation because many reactive species can be formed both at the polymer surface and in the gas phase during the laser ablation process [49–50]. The incorporation or reaction of these ablation products at the nascent channel walls can result in surface chemical functionality that is significantly different from that in the bulk of the polymer [51]. For example, incorporation of nitrogen or oxygen can give rise to amino, hydroxyl, carboxylic, or phenolic functional groups at the surface [47]. These types of surface functionalities are thought to play an important role in electroosmotic flow (EOF), a commonly used means to pump solution through microchannels [52,53]. With these capabilities, polymer-based microfluidic devices fabricated by laser ablation have the potential to replace traditional EOF microfluidic platforms fabricated in silicon and glass by micromachining. Micromachining of silicon and glass involves the use of photolithography, electron beam lithography, wet and dry etching, and deposition or sputtering techniques, all of which require the use of clean-room facilities and equipment. The high cost involved in these fabrication processes could possibly limit the uses of silicon and glass for disposable devices.

Although laser ablation and micromachining provide advantages for fast microfluidic device prototyping and surface modification and characterization for biological and biochemical analysis, the disadvantage of direct-write laser ablation process is its inherent serial nature, which severely limits its throughput compared with previously introduced methods for fabricating polymer microfluidic devices.

18.4 Microfluidic Components

Microfluidics is promising to be a big commercial success in the field of life sciences. The microfluidic systems have shown to be powerful tools for handling biomolecules and have been successfully implemented in a variety of biological applications, including DNA analysis and sequencing, polymerase chain reaction (PCR), protein separation and analysis, immunoassays, cell sorting and manipulation, and novel *in vitro* organ-level models, ranging from disposable LOCs to high throughput microfluidic systems.

A major goal for LOC microfluidic biosensors is to develop a highly integrated and parallel processing system for *in situ* monitoring and/or POC analysis. Various fluid manipulation components (i.e., microvalves, micropumps, and mixers) have been developed to integrate different functional units (i.e., analytical separation and detection techniques) for complete on-chip control of the fluids and analysis.

18.4.1 On-Chip Microvalves

Microvalves are critical in the operation of integrated microfluidic chips for a wide range of applications. Ideally a microvalve exhibits no leakage, no power consumption, no dead volumes, infinite differential pressure capability, very rapid response time, insensitivity to particulate contamination, ability to operate with any fluids, and reliability and biocompatibility. During the last 20 years, many microvalve structures have been developed using MEMS-based bulk or surface micromachining techniques. Silicon is one of the most commonly used fabrication materials for these microvalves. Microvalves can be classified as active microvalves or passive microvalves. Each can be further classified into mechanical microvalves and non-mechanical microvalves based on the operating mechanisms. Typically in active microvalves, a flexible membrane, actuated by magnetic, electric, piezoelectric, thermal, or pneumatic methods, is operated and functioned as a switch to control the fluid flows. The switching time of these microvalves varies dramatically, ranging from 0.1 ms to 25 s. In addition, these valves were fabricated through a series of micromanufacturing procedures and had complicated structures, which could result in difficulties of the microvalve interfacing with other fluid units and limit these valves' application for an integration system. Non-mechanical active microvalves are operated by using smart or intelligent materials (i.e., hydrogel, sol–gel, and paraffin) through the phase change processes under different chemical (i.e., pH) or thermal (i.e., temperature) conditions [54]. The switching time of non-mechanical microvalves ranges from a few seconds to 30 min and is much slower compared to mechanical-based ones. In addition, some of these microvalves are irreversible and only designed for a single use, such as using paraffin as the valve's material [55,56]. Because of the slow response time, compatibility of the valve materials, and phase changing relying on specific conditions, the applications of these non-mechanical microvalves are limited.

With the development of multilayer soft lithography methods, the microfluidic channels with pneumatic microvalves were fabricated together through replication molding of soft elastomeric materials [57,58]. Figure 18.7a shows the fabrication assembly process for a double layer microvalve. The membrane of polymer between the channels is engineered to be relatively thin (typically 30 μm). Either the lower layer or the upper layer can work as the flow channel or the control channel respectively. For example, when the pressure was applied to the lower channel ("control channel"), the membrane deflected upward. A sufficient pressure closed the upper channel ("flow channel"). As shown in Figure 18.7b, the DI water with fluorescent dye was run through the top flow channel, and the positive pressure (8 psi) was applied and released through the bottom control channel. As indicated in the figure, the valve completely sealed the flow channel. This type of microvalve can quickly respond to the pressure applying (valve ON and channel CLOSE) and releasing (valve OFF and channel OPEN) in a few milliseconds. The elastomer is a soft material (PDMS) with Young's modulus of ~750 kPa that allows large deflections with small actuation forces in small area devices [59]. In addition, the use of the PDMS and the multilayer soft lithography method provides a number of advantages over conventional micromachining [57], such as rapid prototyping, ease of fabrication, and low cost. The multilayer fabrication avoids the problems of interlayer adhesion and thermal stress buildup that are endemic to conventional micromachining, making the construction of complex multilayer microfabricated structures more convenient. The PDMS is transparent to visible light, making optical interrogation of microfluidic devices simple. The pneumatically actuated valves have shown to be very useful for a wide variety of fluidic manipulation for LOC applications. For example, the Dynamic Array® integrated fluidic circuits (IFCs) from Fluidigm (California, USA) deliver a new level of efficiency and throughput for real-time PCR and genotyping applications. Dynamic Array IFCs have an on-chip network of microfluidic channels, chambers, and microvalves that automatically assemble individual PCR reactions, decreasing the number of pipetting steps required by up to 100-fold. Reusable chip formats have also been developed to dramatically decrease costs and increase throughput [60].

Although there are several benefits from aforementioned microvavles, the configuration of the microvalve requires the fluidic microchannels to be fabricated with a rounded cross-section because a square cross-section microchannel cannot be completely sealed. In addition, the aspect ratio (height:width) of the fluidic channels is limited to 1:10 for a complete seal. Folch's group at the University of Washington has demonstrated parallel mixing of subnanoliter volumes via two integrated PDMS microvalve arrays (Figure 18.7c–d). The main advantages of their microvalve design are (1) no extra energy source is required to close the fluidic path, hence the loaded device is highly portable; and (2) the device can be built by PDMS replicas from photolithographically patterned SU-8 molds, allowing for microfabricating of deep channels (up to 1 mm) with vertical sidewalls and resulting in very precise features [61,62].

Because of the swelling of PDMS after the channels undergo prolonged exposure to fluid, the multilayer valves can cause inter-layer misalignment that affects the proper functioning of the entire microfluidic device, especially in microarray devices [63]. Recently pneumatically controlled rigid thermoplastic polymer (PMMA) microvalves have been developed by Ng's group for the fabrication of microfluidic devices due to PMMA's low susceptibility to swelling and high biocompatibility. The principle of valve actuation is based on pressurizing/depressurizing an air chamber that supports a moving elastomeric

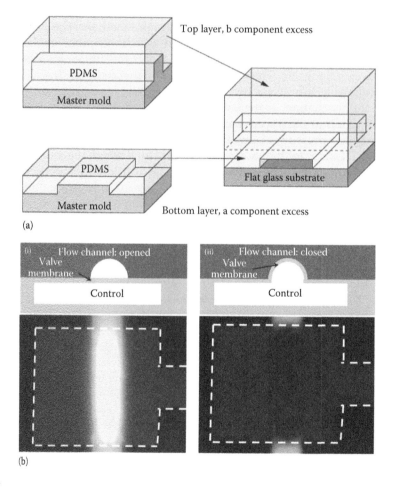

FIGURE 18.7
(a) Multilayer soft lithography assembly. (Reprinted from Pandolfi, A. and Ortiz, M., *J. Micromech. Microeng.*, 17, 1487, 2007. With permission.) (b) On-chip pneumatic push up valve (i) Fluidic channel was open. (ii) Fluidic channel was close. The DI water with fluorescent dye was used to indicate a completely seal of the flow channel. (Reprinted from Li, N. et al., *Electrophoresis*, 26(19), 3758, 2005. With permission.)

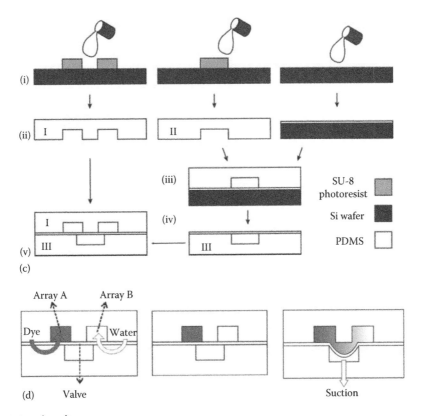

FIGURE 18.7 (continued)
(c) Schematic diagram of fabrication procedures to fabricate the fluidic layer (I), control layer (II), and the thin PDMS membrane. (d) Initial filling of microchambers, isolation of each fluidic chamber, and diffusive mixing between each A–B pairs after suction is applied to the bottom pneumatic lines. (Reprinted from Li, N. et al., *Electrophoresis*, 26(19), 3758, 2005. With permission.)

membrane located below a PMMA fluidic channel. The microvalves are capable of actuation at low pressures [59].

In addition, other groups have been working on improving the pneumatically controlled microvalve design embedded in the PDMS multilayer structure [64–67]. Similar double layer microvalve has been further developed with different polymer materials, mainly to overcome the swelling problem of PDMS within a solvent environment [68].

Except for applying pneumatic forces to operate the microvalves, other actuation mechanisms, such as electrokinetical force and capillary force, have been investigated in polymer microfluidic devices. For example, an oil droplet trapped inside the microchannel was utilized as a sequence valve driven by electrokinetical force as shown in Figure 18.8a [69]. The core design of the microfluidic chip is a pair of electrokinetically controlled oil-droplet sequence valves (ECODSVs). EOF was used to control the ECODSVs and hence the sequential fluidic operation on the chip. In a recently developed capillary soft valve (CSV) shown in Figure 18.8b, a liquid was prevented from filling into a capillary-driven network until the CSV was deformed by gently pressing on the top of it at the inlet of the valve by creating a capillary barrier. The capillary barrier was achieved by abruptly expanding the cross-section of a wettable microchannel (i.e., the inlet of the valve). The CSVs are easy to fabricate, implement, monitor, and actuate.

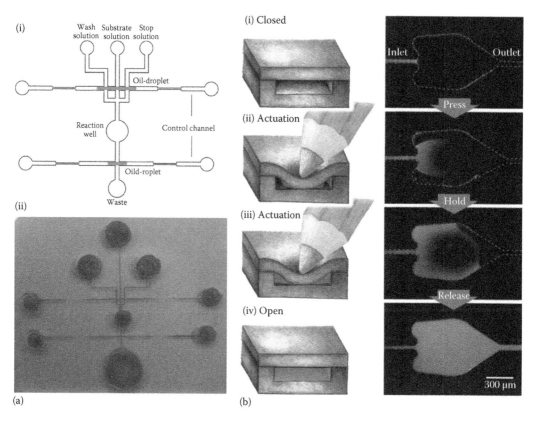

FIGURE 18.8
(a) Schematic illustration of microchip using oil droplet as sequence valves, and a picture of an actual chip. The channel was filled with Rhodamine B for visualization. (Reprinted from Weng, X. et al., *J. Biotechnol.*, 155, 330, 2011. With permission.) (b) Working principle of a capillary soft valve (CSV). A liquid (green) filling a capillary-driven microfluidic network stopped at the inlet of the CSV because of a capillary pressure barrier. Pressing the CSV reduced the dimension of the valve, which pulled the liquid into the valve by capillarity. The fluorescence micrographs show an aqueous solution containing fluorescent nanoparticles that passed the valve upon actuation. The valve was assembled by sealing a 2 mm thick PDMS layer on a plastic microfluidic chip having 60 μm deep structures. (Reprinted from Hitzbleck, M., *Lab Chip*, 12, 1972, 2012. With permission.)

They allow various reaction time and temperature conditions to be applied by using capillary-driven networks. The authors also illustrated how these valves work in the context of detecting DNA analytes using DNA probes, dyes, and receptors that were integrated into a microfluidic chip [70].

18.4.2 On-Chip Micropumps

Several different actuation mechanisms have been applied to drive the solution flow through the microfluidic devices, including pressure driven by syringe pumps [27,71] or by gravity [72], electrokinetically driven [73], capillary driven [74], electrowetting-based and droplet-based driven platform [75], and centrifuge-driven [76] devices. Micropumps are the most essential devices for controlling the transport of fluids in these devices. A micropump needs to precisely deliver micro-level volumes of fluidic samples to a targeted location in an analysis system. The factors to be considered to develop microfluidics-based micropumps include (1) Precise control of delivering fluidic volumes because many applications require high accuracy delivery of sample solutions and precise cycling time of pumping; (2) The ability to control and maintain instantaneous flow and flow changes and/or reversals; (3) The ability to recirculate and combine flow sources; (4) Good connectivity with other microfluidic components and devices (i.e., mixers and sensing elements); (5) Miniaturization and cost-effective fabrication; (6) Minimal leakage; (7) Maximal pump head pressure and zero-head flow rate; and (8) The accessories and drivers [77,78].

Based on multilayer on-chip microvalve design [57], a peristaltic on-chip micropump from three valves or four valves arranged on a single channel has been developed by the similar pneumatically controlled PDMS double layer structure as shown in Figure 18.9a. The valves and pumps were quite durable and no wear or fatigue was observed after more than 4 million actuations as reported by the authors. A maximum pumping rate, which

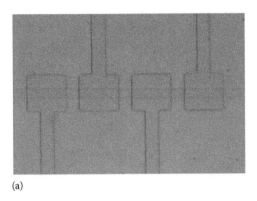

(a)

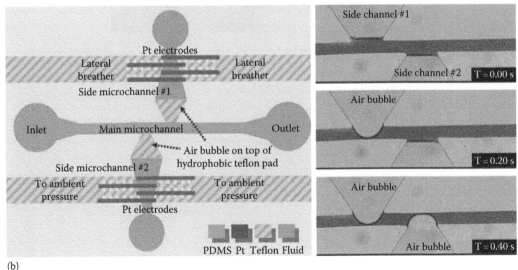

(b)

FIGURE 18.9
(a) Double-layer pneumatically controlled peristaltic pump. (b) Illustration of the design and the pumping principle of the air bubble operated micropump. Schematic top view of the micropump, and the time-sequential pictures show the processes of pumping flow in one pumping cycle. (Reprinted from Chiu, S.H. and Liu, C.-H., *Lab Chip*, 9, 1524, 2009. With permission.)

(*continued*)

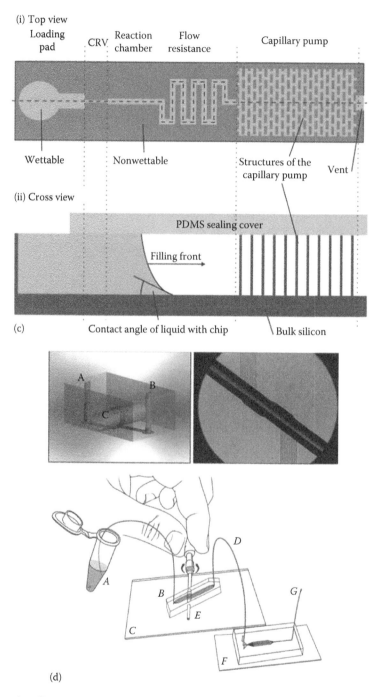

FIGURE 18.9 (continued)
(c) (i) A capillary system. (ii) The pumping power of a capillary pump depends on the contact angles of the filling liquid with its walls and the characteristic dimensions of its structures. (Reprinted from Zimmermann, M. et al., *Lab Chip*, 7, 119, 2007. With permission.) (d) Metering rotary nanopump. Top left: 3-D rendering showing the input channel A: output channel B: connected by four microfluidic channels wrapped around a camshaft C: Rotation of an eccentric cam in the camshaft pumps compresses the channels and moves fluid from A to B; counter-rotation moves fluid from B to A. (Reprinted from Darby, S.G., *Lab Chip*, 10, 3218, 2010. With permission.)

was attained at ~75 Hz, was achieved at 2.35 nL/s with 100 μm ×100 μm × 10 μm microvalves. The pumping rate was nearly constant until above 200 Hz and fell off slowly until 300 Hz. Increasing numbers of pump cycles resulted in incomplete valve opening and closing when the response time of the PDMS membrane's deflection and recovering could not follow the frequencies.

The bubble-driven micropumps have been developed to use the pressure of a gas generated by different methods such as electrolysis, thermal bubble generation, injection, or chemical reaction to drive a liquid through a microfluidic platform [79,80]. The surface tension of the bubble can be used as an actuation force for driving solutions in microfluidic devices. In addition, the surface tension on the bubble decreases as the temperature increases. Thus, low temperature, low power consumption, and large actuation force electrolytic bubble pumping was developed [81–83]. As shown in Figure 18.9, an electrolysis-based micropump using air bubbles to achieve indirect actuation for blood transportation was demonstrated [83]. The electrolytic bubbles used to pump the fluids were isolated from the main channel by utilizing the hydrophobic trapeziform pattern located at the junction of the T-shaped microchannel. With an applied voltage of 2.5 V, the maximum pumping rates for DI water and whole blood were 121 and 88 nL/min, respectively, with a channel cross-section of 100×50 μm. The micropump can drive microfluids without inducing the pH value variation in the main channel and the choking/sticking phenomena of electrolytic bubbles. The on-chip micropump was operated at room temperature with low driving voltage and low power consumption, and could generate large actuation force. In addition, a micro direct methanol fuel cell–based micropump was reported to regenerate CO_2 gas pushing liquid sample [84].

Currently, most of the pumping systems require integration with external power sources for actuation. For disposable microfluidics-based biochips or biochemical detection systems, however, the active micropumps should be integrated with disposable batteries, which increases the cost and also involves many technical difficulties [85].

Autonomous capillary systems (CSs), where liquids are displaced by means of capillarity, are efficient, fast, and convenient platforms for many bioanalytical applications [86]. Delamarche's group developed passive microfluidics driven by capillary forces for bioanalytics and patterning biomolecules on surfaces [87–89]. As shown in Figure 18.9c, their CSs were microfabricated into silicon chips and sealed with PDMS. The CSs comprise a loading pad, a capillary retention valve (CRV), and a reaction chamber, in which an immunoassay can be performed, as well as a flow resistance and a capillary pump with a vent. In addition, passive microfluidics has been used for micromolding in capillaries to study the dynamics of the wetting of liquid pre-polymers in rectangular capillaries or to locally deposit enzymes within capillaries [90,91].

Wikswo's group demonstrated a microfabricated metering rotary nanopump, which was composed of a set of microfluidic channels wrapped in a helix around a central camshaft in which a non-cylindrical cam rotates as shown in Figure 18.9d [78]. The cam compressed the helical channels to induce peristaltic flow as it was rotated. The nanopump was able to produce intermittent delivery or removal of several nanoliters of fluid as well as consistent continuous flow rates ranging from as low as 15 nL/min to above 1.0 μL/min. The nanopump would be useful for a wide variety of biological experiments and POC devices with several advantages, including durability, biocompatibility, ease of fabrication, a simple rotary motor, no power consumption or fluidic conductance in the resting state, low cost, and versatile implementation.

Built-in micropumps have the potential to integrate in portable devices for investigating various chemistry and biochemistry problems that are usually difficult, if at all possible, to be studied using conventional methods [92]. The actuation forces, used for the development of micropumps, have been investigated. These forces include evaporation [93], gravitation [94,95], osmosis [96,97], capillary flow [86], electrostatics [98], piezoelectrics [99], electrical wetting [100], surface tension [101,102], and thermal actuation [103,104]. The chosen actuation mechanisms and methods are determined by the type of driven solutions, materials used for device fabrication, the cost consideration, the necessary pumping speed and volumes, and system integration. A novel macro-to-micro adaptor has also been developed to provide a reversible and reliable interconnect [105]. A pulsed laser was used to generate vapor bubbles which could trigger a high speed liquid jet [106].

18.4.3 Microfluidic Mixers

One of the typical physical features of microfluidic channel is the laminar flow with low Reynolds number (*Re*). The spontaneous fluctuations of velocity that tend to homogenize fluids in turbulent flows are absent, and molecular diffusion across the channels is slow. The low *Re* makes it difficult to mix solutions and thus prolongs the reaction time required in micro-channels. To quicken the process of solution mixing and chemical reactions, there must be transverse components of flow that stretch and fold volumes of fluid over the cross-section of the channel. Thus, in microfluidic devices, micromixer structures are commonly used when the rapid reaction time or detection of fast decay signal is desired in biochemistry analysis and biological processes, such as drug delivery, sequencing or synthesis of nucleic acids, cell activation, enzyme reactions, and protein folding. Mixing is also necessary in LOC platforms for complex chemical reactions [107].

Similar to other microfluidic components, such as microvalves and micropumps, micromixers can be categorized as passive micromixers and active micromixers depending on whether an external energy is applied or not. No external energy is required for passive micromixers, thus the mixing process relies entirely on diffusion or chaotic advection. Additionally, passive structures are robust, stable in operation, and easily integrated in a more complex system. For example, chaotic advection has been reported to improve microscale mixing significantly [108]. This staggered herringbone micromixer was fabricated with two steps of photolithography to fabricate the microchannel and the patterns of grooves on the floor of the channel. Then soft lithography was used to make the actual channels in PDMS. These grooves and ridges presented an anisotropic resistance to viscous flows. There was less resistance to flow in the direction parallel to the peaks and valleys of the ridges than in the orthogonal direction [108]. Some other similar micromixer designs showed that two different solutions can completely mix a few millimeters away from their entrance in a 200 µm wide micro-channel [109,110]. Some other common mixer designs (Figure 18.10a) have been developed for mixing different fluids within continuous flows and the *Re* was also needed to be considered for the designs of the devices [108,111–116]. The general philosophy behind those designs is to increase the total channel length, enhance the particle–surface interaction [117], and create more chaotic flows. In addition, computational models have been developed to investigate the dimensional optimization of such designs [110,118–121].

In active micromixers, the disturbance generated by an external field is applied for the mixing process. The actuation mechanisms based on different external fields can be categorized as pressure, thermal effects, electrohydrodynamics, dielectrophoretics, electrokinetics, magnetohydrodynamics, EOF, and acoustics as shown in Figure 18.10b

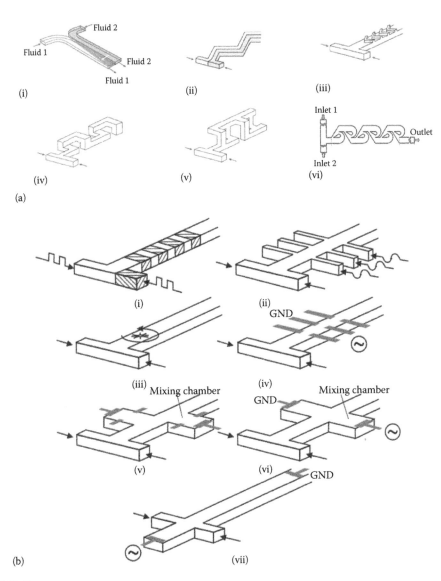

FIGURE 18.10
(a) Mixing of the fluid streams under laminar flow conditions. (i) The component streams mix only by diffusion, creating a dynamic diffusive interface with predictable geometry. (Reprinted from deMello, A.J., *Nature*, 442, 394, 2006. With permission.) (ii) Zigzag-shaped channel for chaotic mixing at high *Re* numbers. (Reprinted from deMello, A.J., *Nature*, 442, 394, 2006. With permission.) (iii) Three-dimensional L-shaped channel for chaotic mixing at intermediate *Re* numbers. (Reprinted from deMello, A.J., *Nature*, 442, 394, 2006. With permission.) (iv) Three-dimensional, connected out-of-plane channel for chaotic mixing at intermediate *Re* numbers. (Reprinted from deMello, A.J., *Nature*, 442, 394, 2006. With permission.) (v) Staggered-herringbone grooves for chaotic mixing at low *Re* numbers. (Reprinted from deMello, A.J., *Nature*, 442, 394, 2006. With permission.) (vi) A modified Tesla structure at relatively high flow rate (Reprinted from Hossain, S. et al., *Chem. Eng. J.*, 158(2), 305, 2010. With permission.) (b) Active micromixers. (i) serial segmentation, (ii) pressure disturbance along the mixing channel, (iii) integrated microstirrer in the mixing channel, (iv) electrohydrodynamic disturbance, (v) dielectrophoretic disturbance, (vi) electrokinetic disturbance in the mixing chamber, (vii) electrokinetic disturbance in the mixing channel. (Reprinted from Nguyen, N.-T., and Wu, Z., *J. Micromech. Microeng.*, 15, R1, 2005. With permission.)

(continued)

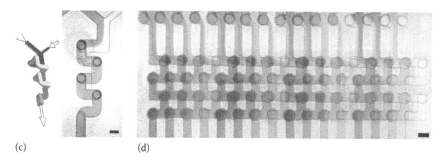

(c)   (d)

FIGURE 18.10 (continued)
(c) A single unit of the combinatorial mixer showed that yellow solution was mixed with the clear solution in a smaller serpentine mixer. (d) Homogeneous combinatorial mixtures were generated after the yellow dye solutions and the blue dye solutions passed through an array of serpentine mixers. Scale bars were 1 mm. (Reprinted from D: Neils, C. et al., *Lab chip*, 4, 342, 2004. With permission.)

[107,122]. Folch's group developed a combinatorial microfluidic mixing device for multiple combinations of multiple dilutions as shown in Figure 18.10c and d [123]. The device is capable of creating all the desired combinations of mixtures from small amounts of the input solutions, and avoids manually mixing and dispensing solutions, as well as the cost of robotic equipment and biochemical reagents. The microfluidic combinatorial mixer showed to continuously produce 16 chemically unique outputs from two dye solutions and two diluent inputs. The mixers can be paired with cell patterning techniques and biosensors to increase the complexity and throughput of biochemical analyses, and can potentially be used for drug testing or biological assays. Compared with conventional large-scale testing approaches based on robotic fluid handling and multi-well plates, this mixing approach provides a low cost, short time, practical, and feasible solution for LOC integration system.

In summary, passive micromixers primarily rely on the microchannel geometry for fluid mixing by folding fluids to increase the interfacial area over which diffusion occurs. As there is no external force applied, mixing in these devices is achieved solely based on diffusion between the two fluid streams. The mixing length is generally of the order of tens of centimeters, which is not practical for most LOC devices [109]. In general, parallel passive micromixers work well at low Re numbers ($Re < 10$) and low Péclet numbers. For intermediate ($10 < Re < 100$) and high ($Re > 100$) Re numbers, structures for introducing chaotic advection have been investigated for micromixers. In addition, effective passive micromixers have been mostly applied in analytical chemistry because of simple designs, easy fabrication, and low cost using polymer materials. Compared with passive mixing, active perturbation requires an external energy input to achieve mixing, which often leads to higher cost and complex systems and manufacturing process as well as challenges in integrating with other microfluidic components.

18.4.4 Microfluidic Assembly Units

It has been widely recognized that microfluidic systems provide advantageous platforms for biological assays, including reduced requirements for expensive reagents, short analysis times, and portability. Currently because of a lack of standardization of activities, the microfluidic devices are more customized systems, which require significant time and expertise and result in high cost and high level of expertise to work with microfluidic systems. There is a critical gap that exists between the technology developers mostly in engineering and chemistry and potential users especially in the life sciences [124]. Thus, such customized systems incur substantial initial costs and delays due to low volume production and are less suited for prototyping or test setups. To address this limitation, an assembly approach for microdevice construction was demonstrated to facilitate the use of microfluidic systems by non-experts [124]. The approach involved fabrication of microfluidic assembly blocks (MABs) in PDMS followed by the construction of a full functioning microfluidic system by assembling the blocks as shown in Figure 18.11. Each MAB has its own unique function, such as inlet/outlet, microvalves, straight/curved/bifurcated channels, and chambers. Once the MABs are fabricated, non-expert users can assemble microfluidic devices with the blocks in minutes without going through the complicated training process and using expensive clean-room facilities. Figure 18.11a shows the microfluidic assembly process using basic functional units, and an array of PCR chambers is shown in Figure 18.11b. The MAB system provides a simple way for non-fluidic researchers to construct custom, complex microfluidic devices. Most importantly, the idea of MABs may provide a novel approach for microfluidic applications and standardization.

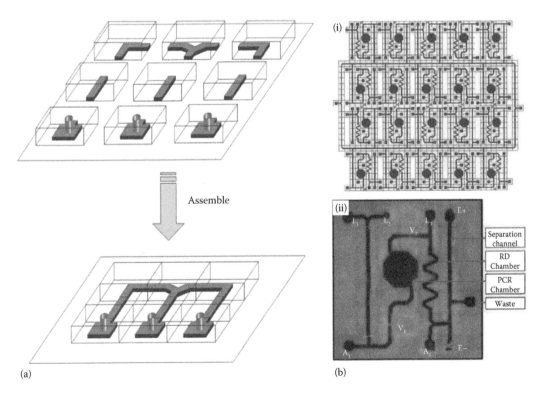

FIGURE 18.11

(a) A schematic of the basic concept of the MAB approach. Users build a custom device by assembling MABs on a glass slide. (b) (i) A conceptualization of a large-scale integration of a complex system that can perform 20 independent assays simultaneously from one sample. (ii) Visual demonstration of an independent assay unit. Each unit device can perform reagent mixing, PCR, restriction digest reaction, and a separation. (Reprinted from Rhee, M. and Burns, M.A., *Lab Chip*, 8, 1365, 2008. With permission.)

18.4.5 Nonspecific Adsorption

Nonspecific adsorption (NSA) of biomolecules is a persistent challenge in microfluidic biosensors. Microfluidic biosensors often have immobilized bioreceptors such as antibodies, enzymes, and DNAs [125]. Microfluidic devices have been routinely fabricated using PDMS for a wide range of assay developments. PDMS is prone to NSA of organic and biomolecules due to its high hydrophobicity [126,127]. Thus therapeutic and fluorescent molecules tend to diffuse into the PDMS walls of the microfluidic devices that reduce their concentrations in solution and consequently affect the accuracy and reliability of these assays [128]. Results showed that the adsorption of a given solute into PDMS depends on the hydrophilic/hydrophobic balance defined by its partition coefficient (log P) value. This value is defined as the ratio between a molecule's concentration in a hydrophobic solvent and concentration in a hydrophilic solvent upon dissolution and reaching equilibrium in a biphasic solvent system [129]. As reported by the authors, different molecules and their absorption into PDMS microfluidic channels, including [3H]-dexamethasone, [3H]-diazepam, [14C]-mannitol, [3H]-phenytoin, and rhodamine 6G, were investigated and it was shown that the molecules with log P less than 2.47 exhibit minimal absorption (<10%) into PDMS channels whereas molecules with log P larger than 2.62 exhibit extensive absorption (>90%) into PDMS channels. Furthermore, they tested the devices coated with TiO_2 and glass and found that they reduced absorption of hydrophobic molecules (log $P > 2.62$) by 2- and 4.5-fold, respectively.

Additionally, other groups have reported to prevent from the NSA of PDMS microfluidic channels and electrode surfaces by surface-functionalization with polyethylene glycol (PEG) following the simple "click" chemistry-based grafting procedure [130,131]. Other researchers investigated reducing the NSA of alkanethiol self-assembled monolayers (SAMs), which are popular linker molecules used to enhance immobilization in microfluidic biosensors [125]. Their results showed that optimizing three parameters (SAM incubation time, gold surface roughness, and gold crystal orientation) can improve SAM sensitivity for fibrinogen–anti-fibrinogen conjugates by a factor of 5, suggesting that the methods are effective for reducing NSA in microfluidic biosensors.

18.5 Lab-on-Chip Biosensor Systems

Since the introduction of soft lithography in the late 1990s, microfluidics and LOC technologies have given rise to an enormous number of scientific and technological developments. Microfluidic devices provide platforms to meet specific needs, such as single cell manipulating and cell trapping [132,133], blood separation [134], chemical reaction [135], and integration with various sensing/detecting components including optics sensing [136–138], electrochemical signal sensing (impedance [139] and current–voltage [$I–V$] curve) [140,141], polymerase chain reaction (PCR) [142], fluorescence sensing [143], field effect transistor (FET) [144], nuclear magnetic resonance (NMR) [145], and surface enhanced Raman spectroscopy (SERS) [146]. In recent years, more papers have been published focusing on fabricating LOC type systems for specific applications. Research groups are not only introducing certain concepts or single functional devices, but are working forward to developing practical platforms that have the potential for commercialization. With those developments, it is time to provide cheap and robust miniaturized platforms to integrate those functions previously realized by macro-scale devices, such as sample preparations transferring, mixing, reaction, sensing, and monitoring. The miniaturized systems require small volumes of samples and reagents, achieve shorter analyzing time and high sensitivity, and provide advantages of low cost and simplicity.

18.5.1 Multiplex Protein Diagnostic Assays and Sensors

A recent and growing trend for biosensing is to assess the low levels of molecular bio-markers from small blood samples or tissue specimens for increasingly large panels. Protein biomarkers are the most informative measurement for monitoring evolving health conditions such as the response of a patient to a drug, assessing immune system status, or for monitoring evolving disease within a patient [147]. An integrated microflu-idic system, called the integrated blood barcode chip (IBBC) shown in Figure 18.1a, was developed for on-chip blood separation and the *in situ* rapid measurement of a panel of plasma proteins from small quantities of blood samples including a fingerprick of whole blood [16]. The device was integrated with human whole blood plasma separa-tion, plasma skimming channel, barcode immunoassay array, and florescence sensing. As reported by the authors, a PDMS mold containing 13–20 parallel microfluidic chan-nels, with each channel conveying a different DNA oligomer as DNA-encoded antibody library (DEAL) code, was fabricated by soft lithography. The PDMS mold was bonded to a polylysine-coated glass slide via thermal treatment at 80°C for 2 h. The polyamine surfaces permit significantly higher DNA loading than do more traditional aminated surfaces. The plasma separation was achieved by exploiting the Zweifach–Fung effect of highly polarized blood cell flow at branch points of small blood vessels. About 15% of the plasma was skimmed into the plasma skimming channels, which was pre-patterned with a dense barcode-like array of ssDNA oligomers. The pre-patterned ssDNA barcode microarray was then converted to an antibody microarray by the DEAL technique. This barcode immunoassay was further confirmed by detecting human chorionic gonado-tropin (hCG) from human serum from 22 cancer patients. Finally, the integrated micro-fluidic IBBC was utilized to assay a blood protein biomarker panel from whole human blood within 10 min of fingerprick blood collection (Figure 18.12). This platform holds potetial for inexpensive, noninvasive, and informative clinical diagnoses, particularly for POC applications.

18.5.2 Marketable Diagnostics Lab-on-Chip System

New trends in biomedicine lead to a new way of diagnostics with a higher degree of com-plexity because more parameters are being measured. In the context of personalized medi-cine, diagnostics can further be used as a tool for screening and monitoring of patients, leading to a customized therapy and subsequently to therapy control [148–150]. The LOC systems hold the potential for being a key technology in future *in vitro* diagnostics for more cost-effective and POC needs. A LOC system called "Fraunhofer ivD-platform" has been reported as a novel innovative approach toward marketable POC diagnostics [150]. As shown in Figure 18.13, the Fraunhofer ivD-platform meets three requirements for the establishment of a LOC system, including open platform for all kinds of common biomedi-cal assays, high degree of integration, and possibility for serial production. The essential part of the LOC system is a cartridge, which contains 8 reservoirs with volumes of 150 μL (reservoir 1–4) and 75 μL (reservoir 5–8), one sample reservoir (up to 45 μL), a sensor area,

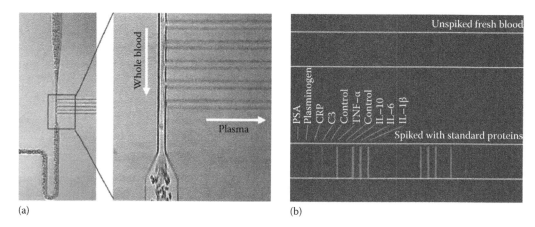

(a)   (b)

FIGURE 18.12
(a) Optical micrographs show the effective separation of plasma from fresh whole blood. (b) IBBC for the rapid measurement of a panel of serum biomarkers from a fingerprick of whole blood. (Reprinted from Fan, R. et al., *Nat. Biotechnol.*, 26(12), 1373, 2008. With permission.)

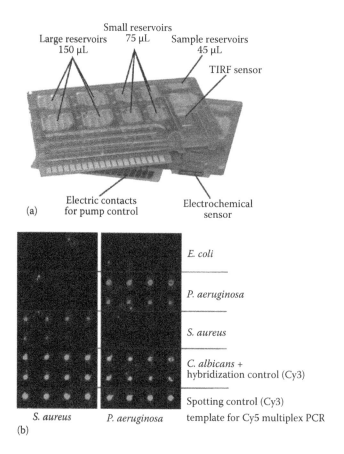

FIGURE 18.13
(a) Pictures of the ivD-cartridges. (b) False-color fluorescence image of spotted and hybridized cyclic olefin polymer (COP) slides. (Reprinted from Dixit, C.K. and Kaushik, A., *Biochem. Biophys. Res. Commun.*, 419, 316, 2012. With permission.)

and a waste reservoir. The fluid pumping was achieved by the unidirectional deflection of a membrane due to electrolytic gas generation inside a hydrogel. The measuring principle of the transducer is total internal reflectance fluorescence (TIRF). The authors have demonstrated the assays used for nucleic acids (detection of different pathogens) and protein markers (such as CRP and PSA) by an electrochemical readout based on redox cycling or an optical readout based on TIRF. In combination with a fully automated instrumentation, the assay can be performed in about 15 min. The miniaturized assay covers the whole value chain ranging from microfluidics, material and polymer sciences, assay and sensor development to the production, and assembly design as reported [150].

18.5.3 Nanostructured Arrays for Multiplex Analyses

Nanotechnology provides new structured materials with amazing properties, which can be applied to develop advanced instrumentation for biomedical diagnostics and personalized therapy, as well as biosensing in the environment [151]. It is critical to develop rapid and efficient biomolecular identification technologies for applications in genomics, proteomics, and biosensing because of the high diversity and complexity of bio-samples. An on-chip silicon nanowire (SiNW) filtering, selective separation, desalting, and pre-concentration platform has been demonstrated for the direct analysis of whole blood and other complex bio-samples (Figure 18.14) [152]. The separation of required protein analytes from raw bio-samples on a single chip was first performed using an antibody-modified roughness controlled SiNW forest of ultra-large binding surface area, followed by the release of target proteins in a controlled liquid medium, and their subsequent detection by supersensitive SiNW-based FET arrays fabricated on the same chip platform. Furthermore, the authors demonstrated the use of a nanowire forest-based separation device to integrate with downstream SiNW-based sensor arrays for the real-time ultrasensitive detection of protein biomarkers directly from blood samples in less than 10 min. In addition, nanostructured arrays (NAs) have recently been reported to incorporate with a customized microfluidic system to demonstrate its applicability as an alternative easy and efficient platform for multiplex analysis and LOC applications [153].

18.5.4 Ultralow Cost Microfluidic Diagnostics

Microfluidic paper-based analytical devices (μPADs) have been reported as a new class of POC diagnostic devices, which are inexpensive, easy to use, and designed specifically for use in developing countries (Figure 18.15a) [154]. The approaches and devices are aiming to provide effective technologies in health-related diagnostics for developing countries and coupling these technologies to existing communication infrastructures and healthcare in areas where trained medical personnel, reliable power, refrigeration, and modestly expensive tests could possibly not be available. These paper-based devices were patterned and fabricated by photolithography [155,156]. To use the devices, the users first dip the entrance channel into a drop of the sample, which is then driven by the capillary force into the test zones, and the results are shown in different colors around 30 min. Glucose and protein in artificial urine were tested on a simple μPAD with a central channel for sample introduction, which branched into three test zones into which the reagents for each assay had been spotted and dried during fabrication of the device (Figure 18.15b). Additionally, the ultralow cost μPADs have the potential to be alternatives to current diagnostic technologies, not only for developing countries, but also for militaries in harsh environments, clinical laboratories, and home healthcare.

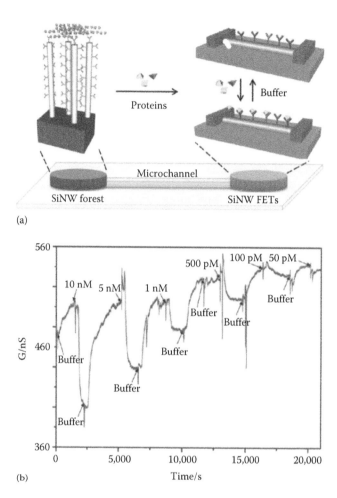

FIGURE 18.14

(a) Schematic representation of the operation of a whole SiNW selective filtering and sensing device on a single chip platform. (b) Real-time calibration sensing experiments using anti-troponin T modified SiNW FETs at different concentrations of the antigen. (Reprinted from Krivitsky, V. et al., *Nano Lett.*, 12(9), 4748, 2012, doi: 10.1021/nl3021889. With permission.)

18.6 Future Directions

Researchers are now moving their focus to the application of microfluidic systems that incorporate strategic biosensor integration to address high impact clinical needs. Today, many different types of microfluidic devices, such as microvalves, micropumps, and mixers have been investigated and developed by researchers. The field of microfluidics is maturing slowly but steadily and new products are entering the market. In academic areas, many different kinds of customized microfluidic devices are also developed, showing a bewildering number of technologies and formats [157]. For future development and commercialization of the microfluidic LOC products for biomedicine, biosensor, diagnostics, and POC, standardization is expected to lay a solid foundation upon which future

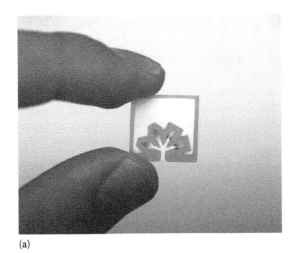

(Glucose) /mM		(BSA) /μM
0		0
2.5		0.38
5.0		0.75
10		1.5
50		7.5
500		75

(a)   (b)

FIGURE 18.15
(a) Microfluidic paper-based analytical device (μPAD). (b) Results of paper-based glucose and protein assays using a range of concentrations of glucose and BSA in artificial urine. (Reprinted from Martinez, A.W. et al., *Anal. Chem.*, 82(1), 3, 2010. With permission.)

new products will be developed. Microfluidic interconnections will become a major consideration because interconnections should enable users to make a number of fluidic connections easily, as well as be fast and reliable. No intensive training should be needed so that there is no need to change the existing infrastructure or acquire expensive devices. Only modification of the design rules is needed [158]. The future of microfluidics is a platform that provides easy combination of reliable components and is universally integrated using well-defined low cost fabrication technology. Rapid, highly multiplex, and robust products will be developed driven by the needs of POC and companion diagnostics, high throughput screening, cell-based assays, environmental sensing, forensics, genomics, artificial organs, stem cell handling, and circulating tumor cells.

References

1. Grieshaber, D., MacKenzie, R., Vörös, J., and Reimhult, E. 2008. Electrochemical biosensors—Sensor principles and architectures. *Sensors* 8: 1400–1458.
2. Britannica.com 2011. Facts about *E. coli*: Dimensions, as discussed in bacteria: Diversity of structure of bacteria: Britannica Online Encyclopedia. http://www.britannica.com/facts/5/463522/E-coli-as-discussed-in-bacteria.
3. Kubitschek, H.E. 1990. Cell volume increase in Escherichia coli after shifts to richer media. *J. Bacteriol.* 172(1): 94–101.
4. Campbell, N.A., Brad, W., and Robin, J.H. 2006. *Biology: Exploring Life*. Boston, MA: Pearson Prentice Hall.
5. Erickson, H.P. 2009. Size and shape of protein molecules at the nanometer level determined by sedimentation, gel filtration, and electron microscopy. *Biol. Proc. Online* 11(1): 32–51.
6. Whitesides, G.M. 2006. The origins and the future of microfluidics. *Nature* 442: 368–373.
7. Lazar, I.M., Ramsey, R.S., and Ramsey, J.M. 2001. On-chip proteolytic digestion and analysis using "wrong-way-round" electrospray time-of-flight mass spectrometry. *Anal. Chem.* 73(8): 1733–1739.

8. Peterson, D.S., Rohr, T., Svec, F., and Frechet, J.M.J. 2002. High-throughput peptide mass mapping using a microdevice containing trypsin immobilized on a porous polymer monolith coupled to MALDI TOF and ESI TOF mass spectrometers. *J. Proteome Res.* 1(6): 563–568.

9. Throckmorton, D.J., Shepodd, T.J., and Singh, A.K. 2002. Electrochromatography in microchips: Reversed-phase separation of peptides and amino acids using photopatterned rigid polymer monoliths. *Anal. Chem.* 74(4): 784–789.

10. Wang, C., Oleschuk, R., Ouchen, F., Li, J.J., Thibault, P., and Harrison, D.J. 2000. Integration of immobilized trypsin bead beds for protein digestion within a microfluidic chip incorporating capillary electrophoresis separations and an electrospray mass spectrometry interface. *Rapid Commun. Mass Spectrom.* 14(15): 1377–1383.

11. Becker, H. and Locascio, L.E. 2002. Polymer microfluidic devices. *Talanta* 56(2): 267–287.

12. Dutse, S.W. and Yusof, N.A. 2011. Microfluidics-based lab-on-chip systems in DNA-based biosensing: An overview. *Sensors* 11(6): 5754–5768.

13. Livak-Dahl, E., Sinn, I., and Burns, M. 2011. Microfluidic chemical analysis systems. *Annu. Rev. Chem. Biomol. Eng.* 2: 325–353.

14. Reyes, D.R., Iossifidis, D., Auroux P-A., and Manz, A. 2002. Micro total analysis systems. 1. Introduction, theory, and technology. *Anal. Chem.* 74(12): 2623–2636.

15. Sundberg, S.A. 2000. High-throughput and ultra-high-throughput screening: Solution- and cell-based approaches. *Curr. Opin. Biotechnol.* 11(1): 47–53.

16. Fan, R., Vermesh, O., Srivastava, A., Yen, B.K.H., Qin, L., Ahmad, H., Kwong, G.A., Liu, C.-C., Gould, J., Hood, L., and Heath, J.R. 2008. Integrated barcode chips for rapid, multiplexed analysis of proteins in microliter quantities of blood. *Nat. Biotechnol.* 26(12): 1373–1378.

17. Thilmany, J. 2005. Think small. *EMBO Rep.* 6: 913–916.

18. El-Ali, J., Sorger, P.K., and Jensen, K.F. 2006. Cells on chips. *Nature* 442: 403–411.

19. Purcell, E. 1977. Life at low Reynolds number. *Am. J. Phys.* 45: 3–11.

20. Beebe, D.J., Mensing, G.A., and Walker, G.M. 2002. Physics and applications of microfluidics in biology. *Annu. Rev. Biomed. Eng.* 4: 261–286.

21. Squires, T.M. and Quake, S.R. 2005. Microfluidics: Fluid physics at the nanoliter scale. *Rev. Mod. Phys.* 77: 977–1026.

22. Prakash, S., Pinti, M., and Bhushan, B. 2012. Theory, fabrication and applications of microfluidic and nanofluidic biosensors. *Phil. Trans. R. Soc. A.* 370(1967): 2269–2303.

23. Soper, S.A., Ford, S.M., Qi, S., McCarley, R.L., Kelly, K., and Murphy, M.C. 2000. Polymeric microelectromechanical systems. *Anal. Chem.* 72(19): 642A–651A.

24. Becker, H. and Gartner, C. 2000. Polymer microfabrication methods for microfluidic analytical applications. *Electrophoresis* 21(1): 12–26.

25. McDonald, J.C., Duffy, D.C., Anderson, J.R., Chiu, D.T., Wu, H., Schueller, O.J.A., and Whitesides, G.M. 2000. Fabrication of microfluidic systems in poly(dimethylsiloxane). *Electrophoresis* 21: 27–40.

26. McDonald, J.C. and Whitesides, G.M. 2002. Poly(dimethylsiloxane) as a material for fabricating microfluidic devices. *Acc. Chem. Res.* 35(7): 491–499.

27. Liu, Y., Sai, J., Richmond, A., and Wikswo, J.P. 2008. Microfluidic switching system for analyzing wortmannin-inhibited HL-60 cells. *Biomed. Microdevice* 10: 499–507.

28. Huang, Z., Li, X., Martins-Green, M., and Liu, Y. 2012. Microfabrication cylindrical microfluidic channel networks for microvascular research. *Biomed. Microdevice* 14(5): 873–883. Online publication first. doi: 10.1007/s10544-012-9667-2.

29. Schlautmann, S., Besselink, G.A.J., Radhakrishna Prabhu G., and Schasfoort, R.B.M. 2003. Fabrication of a microfluidic chip by UV bonding at room temperature for integration of temperature-sensitive layers. *J. Micromech. Microeng.* 13(4): 81–84.

30. Xia, Y. and Whitesides, G.M. 1998. Soft lithography. *Annu. Rev. Mater. Sci.* 28: 153–184.

31. Ruiz, S.A. and Chen, C.S. 2007. Microcontact printing: A tool to pattern. *Soft Matter* 3: 168–177.

32. Lee, G.B., Chen, S.H., Huang, G.R., Sung, W.C., and Lin, Y.H. 2001. Microfabricated plastic chips by hot embossing methods and their applications for DNA separation and detection. *Sens. Actuat. B* 75: 142–148.

33. Liu, Y., Cady, N., and Batt, C. 2007. A plastic microchip for nucleic acid purification. *Biomed. Microdevice.* 9(5): 769–776.

34. Becker, H. and Heim, U. 2000. Hot embossing as a method for fabrication of polymer high aspect ratio structures. *Sens. Actuat. A* 83: 130–135.

35. Rötting, O., Köhler, B., Reuther, F., Blum, H., and Bacher, W. 1999. Production of movable metallic microstructures by aligned hot embossing and reactive ion etching, *Proc. SPIE* 3680(2): 1038–1045.

36. Lin, L., Cheng, Y.T., and Chiu, C.J. 1998. Comparative study of hot embossed micro structures fabricated by laboratory and commercial environments. *Microsyst. Technol.* 4(3): 113–116.

37. Zhao, Y. and Cui, T. 2003. Fabrication of high-aspect-ratio polymer-based electrostatic comb drives using the hot embossing technique. *J. Micromech. Microeng.* 13: 430–435.

38. Goral, V.N., Hsieh, Y.-H., Petzold, O.N., Faris, R.A., and Yuen, P.K. 2011. Hot embossing of plastic microfluidic devices using poly(dimethylsiloxane) molds. *J. Micromech. Microeng.* 21: 017002. doi: 10.1088/0960-1317/21/1/017002.

39. Attia U.M., Marson, S., and Alcock, J.R. 2009. Micro-injection moulding of polymer microfluidic devices, *Microfluid. Nanofluid.* 7(1): 1–28.

40. Kim, D.S., Lee, S.H., Ahn, C.H., Lee, J.Y., and Kwon, T.H. 2006. Disposable integrated microfluidic biochip for blood typing by plastic microinjection moulding. *Lab Chip* 6: 794–802.

41. Rohlder, D., Winclker-Desprez, V., and Klaunick, C. 2012. Optical blood analyses for cardiac risk diagnostic at the Point-of-Care. ThinXXS Microtechnology AG. http://www.thinxxs.com/fileadmin/website/pdf/Cardiac-PoC-Disk.pdf (accessed Aug 2012).

42. Grimes, A., Breslauer, D.N., Long, M., Pegan, J., Lee, L.P., and Khine, M. 2008. Shrinky-Dink microfluidics: Rapid generation of deep and rounded patterns. *Lab Chip* 8(1): 170–172.

43. Chen, C.S., Breslauer, D.N., Luna, J.I., Grimes, A., Chin, W.C., Lee, L.P., and Khine, M. 2008. Shrinky-Dink microfluidics: 3D polystyrene chips. *Lab Chip* 8(4): 622–624.

44. Chen, C.S., Pegan, J., Luna, J.I., Xia, B., McCloskey, K., Chin, W.C., and Khine, M. 2008. Shrinky-Dink hanging drops: A simple way to form and culture embryoid bodies. *JoVE* 13, http://www.jove.com/index/Details.stp?ID=692. doi: 10.3791/692.

45. Fiorini, G.S. and Chiu, D.T. 2005 Disposable microfluidic devices: fabrication, function, and application. *BioTechniques* 38: 429–446.

46. Jalali, B., Goda, K., Shiong, P.S., and Tsia, K.K.M. 2010. Time-stretch imaging and its applications to high-throughput microscopy and microsurgery. *IEEE Photon. Soc. Newsl.* 11–15.

47. Roberts, M.A., Rossier, J.S., Bercier, P., and Girault, H. 1997. UV laser machined polymer substrates for the development of microdiagnostic systems. *Anal. Chem.* 69(11): 2035–2042.

48. Edwards, T.L., Harper, J.C., Polsky, R., Lopez, D.A.M., Wheeler, D.R., Allen, A.C., and Brozik, S.M. 2011. A parallel microfluidic channel fixture fabricated using laser ablated plastic laminates for electrochemical and chemiluminescent biodetection of DNA. *Biomicrofluidics* 5(4): 044115.

49. Johnson, T.J., Ross, D., Gaitan, M., and Locascio, L.E. 2001. Laser modification of performed polymer microchannels: Application to reduce band broaden round turns subject to electrokinetic flow. *Anal. Chem.* 73: 3656–3661.

50. Pugmire, D.L., Waddell, E.A., Haasch, R., Tarlov, M.J., and Locascio, L.E. 2002. Surface characterization of laser-ablated polymers used for microfluidics. *Anal. Chem.* 74(4): 871–878.

51. Chtaib, M., Roberfroid, E.M., Novis, Y., Pireaux, J.J., Caudano, R., Lutgen, P., and Feyder, G.J. 1989. Polymer surface reactivity enhancement by ultraviolet ArF laser irradiation: An x-ray photoelectron spectroscopy study of polytetrafluoroethylene and polyethyleneterepthalate ultraviolet treated surfaces. *Vac. Sci. Technol. A* 7: 3233–3237.

52. Barker, S.L.R., Ross, D., Tarlov, M.J., Gaitan, M., and Locascio, L.E. 2000. Control of flow direction in microfluidic devices with polyelectrolyte multilayers. *Anal. Chem.* 72(24): 5925–5929.

53. Culbertson, C.T., Jacobson, S.C., and Ramsey, J.M. 2000. Microchip devices for high-efficiency separations. *Anal. Chem.* 72(23): 5814–5819.

54. Oh, K.W. and Ahn, C.H. 2006. A review of microvalves. *J. Micromech. Microeng.* 16: R13–R39.

55. Liu, R.H., Bonanno, J., Yang, J., Lenigk, R., and Grodzinski, P. 2004. Single-use, thermally actuated paraffin valves for microfluidic applications. *Sens. Actuat. B* 98: 328–336.

56. Liu, R.H., Yang, J., Lenigk, R., Bonanno, J., and Grodzinski, P. 2004. Self-contained, fully integrated biochip for sample preparation, polymerase chain reaction amplification, and DNA microarray detection. *Anal. Chem.* 76(7): 1824–1831.

57. Unger, M.A., Chou, H.-P., Thorsen, T., Scherer, A., and Quake, S.R. 2000. Monolithic microfabricated valves and pumps by multilayer soft lithography. *Science* 288: 113–116.

58. Pandolfi, A. and Ortiz, M. 2007. Improved design of low-pressure fluidic microvalves. *J. Micromech. Microeng.* 17: 1487–1493.

59. Toh, A.G.G., Wang, Z.F., and Ng, S.H. 2008. Fabrication of embedded microvalve on PMMA microfluidic devices through surface functionalization. *DTIP of MEMS & MOEMS*, pp. 267–272.

60. Fluidigm Corporation. http://www.fluidigm.com/ (accessed August 2012).

61. Li, N., Hsu, C.H., and Folch, A. 2005. Parallel mixing of photolithographically defined nanoliter volumes using elastomeric microvalve arrays. *Electrophoresis* 26(19): 3758–3764.

62. Au, A.K., Lai, H., Utela, B.R., and Folch, A. 2011. Microvalves and micropumps for BioMEMS. *Micromachines* 2: 179–220.

63. Lee, J.N., Park C., and Whitesides, G.M. 2003. Solvent compatibility of poly(dimethylsiloxane)-based microfluidic devices. *Anal. Chem.* 75(23): 6544–6554.

64. Hosokawa, K. and Maeda, R. 2000. A pneumatically-actuated three-way microvalve fabricated with polydimethylsiloxane using the membrane transfer technique. *J. Micromech. Microeng.* 10: 415–420.

65. Go, J.S. and Shoji, S. 2004. A disposable, dead volume-free and leak-free in-plane PDMS microvalve. *Sens. Actuat. A* 114: 438–444.

66. Zheng, C., Wang, J., Pang, Y., Wang, J., Li, W., Ge, Z., and Huang, Y. 2012. High-through put immunoassay through in-channel microfluidic patterning. *Lab chip* 12: 2487–2490. doi: 10.1039/c2lc40145b.

67. Kim, J., Kang, M., Jensen, E.C., and Mathies, R.A. 2012. Lifting gate polydimethylsiloxane microvalves and pumps for microfluidic control. *Anal. Chem.* 84(4): 2067–2071.

68. Rolland, J.P., Van Dam, R.M., Schorzman, D.A., Quake, S.R., and DeSimone, J.M. 2004. Solvent-resistant photocurable "Liquid Teflon" for microfluidic device fabrication. *J. Am. Chem. Soc.* 126(8): 2322–2323.

69. Weng, X., Jiang, H., Chon, C.H., Chen, S., Cao, H., and Li, D. 2011. An RNA–DNA hybridization assay chip with electrokinetically controlled oil droplet valves for sequential microfluidic operations. *J. Biotechnol.* 155: 330–337.

70. Hitzbleck, M., Avrain L., Smekens, V., Lovchik, R.D., Mertens, P., and Delamarche E. 2012. Capillary soft valves for microfluidics. *Lab Chip* 12: 1972–1978.

71. Sai, J., Raman, D., Liu, Y., Wikswo, J., and Richmond, R. 2008. Parallel phosphatidylinositol 3-kinase(PI3K)-dependent and Src-dependent pathways lead to CXCL8-mediated Rac2 activation and chemotaxis. *J. Biol. Chem.* 283(39): 26538–26547.

72. Huh, D., Bahng, J.H., Ling, Y., Wei, H.H., Kripfgans, O.D., Fowlkes, J.B., Grotberg, J.B., and Takayama, S. 2007. Gravity-driven microfluidic particle sorting device with hydrodynamic separation amplification. *Anal. Chem.* 79(4): 1369–1376.

73. Chang, H.-C. and Leslie, Y.Y. 2010. *Electrokinetically Driven Microfluidics and Nanofluidics*. New York: Cambridge University Press.

74. Hitzbleck, M., Gervais, L., and Delamarche, E. 2011. Controlled release of reagents in capillary-driven microfluidics using reagent integrators. *Lab Chip* 11: 2680–2685.

75. Teh, S.-Y., Lin, R., Hung, L.-H., and Lee, A.P. 2008. Droplet microfluidics. *Lab Chip* 8: 198–220.

76. Gorkin, R., Park, J., Siegrist, J., Amasia, M., Lee, B.S., Park, J.-M., Kim, J., Kim, H., Madou, M., and Cho, Y.-K., 2010. Centrifugal microfluidics for biomedical applications. *Lab Chip* 10: 1758–1773.

77. Lee, D.E. 2006. Development of micropump for microfluidic applications. PhD dissertation, Louisiana State University, Baton, Rouge, LA.

78. Darby, S.G., Moore, M.R., Friedlander, T.A., Schaffer, D.K., Reiserer, R.S., Wikswo, J.P., and Seale, K.T. 2010. A metering rotary nanopump for microfluidic systems. *Lab Chip* 10: 3218–3226.

79. Erickson, D. and Li, D. 2004. Integrated microfluidic devices. *Anal. Chim. Acta.* 507(1): 11–26.
80. Lui, C., Stelick, S., Cady, N., and Batt, C. 2010. Low-power microfluidic electro-hydraulic pump (EHP). *Lab Chip* 10: 74–79.
81. Boöhm, S., Olthuis, W., and Bergveld, P. 2000. A bi-directional electrochemically driven micro liquid dosing system with integrated sensor/actuator electrodes. *Proceedings of IEEE Thirteenth Annual International Conference on Micro Electro Mechanical Systems (MEMS)*, 2000, pp. 92–95.
82. Papavasiliu, A.P., Liepmann D., and Pisano, A.P. 2001. High-speed and bi-stable electrolysis-bubble actuated gate valves. *The 11th International Conference on Solid-State Sensors and Actuators.* Munich, Germany, vol. 2. Berlin, Germany: Springer, pp. 940–943.
83. Chiu, S.H. and Liu, C.-H. 2009. An air-bubble-actuated micropump for on-chip blood transportation. *Lab Chip* 9: 1524–1533.
84. Esquivel, J.P., Castellarnau, M., Senn, T., Löchel, B., Samitier, J., and Sabaté, N. 2012. Fuel cell-powered microfluidic platform for lab-on-a-chip applications. *Lab Chip* 12: 74–79.
85. Hong, C.C., Choi, J.W., and Ahn, C.H. 2007. An on-chip air-bursting detonator for driving fluids on disposable lab-on-a-chip systems. *J. Micromech. Microeng.* 17: 410–417.
86. Zimmermann, M., Schmid, H., Hunziker, P., and Delamarche, E. 2007. Capillary pumps for autonomous capillary systems. *Lab Chip* 7: 119–125.
87. Delamarche, E., Juncker, D., and Schmid, H. 2005. Microfluidics for processing surfaces and miniaturizing biological assays. *Adv. Mater.* 17(24): 2911–2933.
88. Juncker, D., Schmid, H., Drechsler, U., Wolf, H., Wolf, M., Michel, B., de Rooij, N., and Delamarche, E. 2002. Autonomous microfluidic capillary system. *Anal. Chem.* 74(24): 6139–6144.
89. Zimmermann, M., Bentley, S., Schmid, H., Hunziker, P., and Delamarche, E. 2005. Continuous flow in open microfluidics using controlled evaporation. *Lab Chip* 5: 1355–1359.
90. Kim, E., Xia Y., and Whitesides, G.M. 1995. Polymer microstructures formed by moulding in capillaries. *Nature* 376: 581–584.
91. Tseng, F.G., Lin, K., Hsu, H., and Chieng, C. 2004. A surface-tension-driven fluidic network for precise enzyme batch-dispensing and glucose detection. *Sens. Actuat. A* 111: 107–117.
92. Li, W., Chen, T., Chen, Z., Fei, P., Yu, Z., Pang, Y., and Huang, Y. 2012. Squeeze-chip: A finger-controlled microfluidic flow network device and its application to biochemical assays. *Lab Chip* 12: 1587–1590.
93. Lynn, N.S. and Dandy, D.S. 2009. Passive microfluidic pumping using coupled capillary/evaporation effects. *Lab Chip* 9: 3422–3429.
94. Walker, G.M. and Beebe, D.J. 2002. A passive pumping method for microfluidic devices. *Lab Chip* 2: 131–134.
95. Zhu, X., Chu, L.Y., Chueh, B., Shen, M., Hazarika, B., Phadke N., and Takayama, S. 2004. Arrays of horizontally-oriented mini-reservoirs generate steady microfluidic flows for continuous perfusion cell culture and gradient generation. *Analyst* 129: 1026–1031.
96. Xu, Z., Yang, C., Liu, C., Zhou, Z., Fang, J., and Wang, J. 2010. An osmotic micro-pump integrated on a microfluidic chip for perfusion cell culture. *Talanta* 80(3): 1088–1093.
97. Jen, C.-P., Amstislavskaya, T.G., Liu, Y.-H., Hsiao J.-H., and Chen, Y.-H. 2012. Single-cell electric lysis on an electroosmotic-driven microfluidic chip with arrays of microwells. *Sensors* 12: 6967–6977.
98. Xie, J., Shih, J., Lin, Q., Yang, B., and Tai, Y.C. 2004. Surface micromachined electrostatically actuated micro peristaltic pump. *Lab Chip* 4: 495–501.
99. Smits, J.G. 1990. Piezoelectric micro pump with three valves working peristaltically. *Sens. Actuat. A* 21: 203–206.
100. Noh, J.H., Noh, J., Kreit, E., Heikenfeld, J., and Rack, P.D. 2012. Toward active-matrix lab-on-a-chip: Programmable electrofluidic control enabled by arrayed oxide thin film transistors. *Lab Chip* 12: 353–360.
101. Swickrath, M.J., Burns, S.D., and Wnek, G.E. 2009. Modulating passive micromixing in 2-D microfluidic devices via discontinuities in surface energy. *Sens. Actuat. B* 140: 656–662.
102. Resto, P.J., Berthier, E., Beebe, D.J., and Williams, J.C. 2012 An inertia enhanced passive pumping mechanism for fluid flow in microfluidic devices. *Lab Chip* 12: 2221–2228.

103. Hong, C.-C., Tsai, C.-H., Chen, S.-Y., and Chen C.-P. 2011. Disposable microfluidic vacuum modules using inductively-triggered transformative polymers for point-of-care diagnostics. *Transducers' 11*, Beijing, China, June 5–9.

104. Weinert, F.M., Kraus, J.A., Franosch, T., and Braun, D. 2008. Microscale fluid flow induced by thermoviscous expansion along a traveling wave. *Phys. Rev. Lett.* 100: 164501.

105. Chen, A. and Pan, T. 2010. Fit-to-Flow (F2F) interconnects: Universal reversible adhesive-free microfluidic adaptors for lab-on-a-chip systems. *Lab Chip* 11: 727–732.

106. Wu, T.-H., Chen, Yue., Park, S-Y., Hong, J., Teslaa, T., Zhong, J.F., Carlo, D.D., Teitell, M.A., and Chiou P.-Y. 2012. Pulsed laser triggered high speed microfluidic fluorescence activated cell sorter. *Lab Chip* 12: 1378–1383.

107. Nguyen, N.-T. and Wu, Z. 2005. Micromixers—A review. *J. Micromech. Microeng.* 15: R1–R16.

108. Stroock, A., Dertinger, S.K.W., Ajdari, A., Mezic, I., Stone, H.A., and Whitesides, GM. 2002. Chaotic mixer for microchannels. *Science* 295: 647–651.

109. Bhagat, A.A.S., Peterson, E.T.K., and Papautsky, I. 2007. A passive planar micromixer with obstructions for mixing at low Reynolds numbers. *J. Micromech. Microeng.* 17(5): 1017–1024. doi: 10.1088/0960-1317/17/5/023.

110. Wang, H., Iovenitti, P., Harvey, E., and Masood, S. 2002. Optimizing layout of obstacles for enhanced mixing in microchannels. *Smart Mater. Struct.* 11: 662–667.

111. deMello, A.J. 2006. Control and detection of chemical reactions in microfluidic systems. *Nature* 442: 394–402.

112. Hong, C.-C., Choi, J.-W., and Ahn, C.H. 2004. A novel in-plane passive microfluidic mixer with modified Tesla structures. *Lab Chip* 4: 109–113.

113. Hossain, S., Ansari, M.A., Husain, A., and Kim, K.-Y. 2010. Analysis and optimization of a micromixer with a modified Tesla structure. *Chem. Eng. J.* 158 (2): 305–314.

114. Mengeaud, V., Josserand, J., and Girault, H.H. 2002. Mixing processes in a zigzag microchannel: finite element simulation and optical study. *Anal. Chem.* 74(16): 4279–4286.

115. Liu, R.H., Stremler, M.A., Sharp, K.V., Olsen, M.G., Santiago, J.G., Adrian, R.J., Aref, H., and Beebe, D.J. 2000. Passive mixing in a three-dimensional serpentine microchannel. *J. Microelectromech. Syst.* 9(2): 190–197.

116. Vijayendran, R.A., Motsegood, K.M., Beebe, D.J., and Leckband, D.E. 2003. Evaluation of a three-dimensional micromixer in a surface-based biosensor. *Langmuir* 19: 1824–1828.

117. Melin, J., Giménez, G., Roxhed, N., van der Wijngaart, W., and Stemme, G. 2004. A fast passive and planar liquid sample micromixer. *Lab Chip* 4: 214–219.

118. Walker, G.M., Ozers, M.S., and Beebe, D.J. 2003. Cell infection within a microfluidic device using virus gradients. *Sens. Actuat. B* 98: 347–355.

119. Maeng, J.-S., Yoo, K., Song, S., and Heu, S. 2006. Modeling for fluid mixing in passive micromixers using the vortex index. *J. Korean Phys. Soc.* 48(5): 902–907.

120. Munson, M.S. and Yager, P. 2004. Simple quantitative optical method for monitoring the extent of mixing applied to a novel microfluidic mixer. *Anal. Chim. Acta* 507: 63–71.

121. Forbes, T.P. and Kralj, J.G. 2012. Engineering and analysis of surface interactions in a microfluidic herringbone micromixer. *Lab Chip* 12: 2634–2637.

122. Sasaki, N., Kitamori, T., and Kim, H.-B. 2006. AC electroosmotic micromixer for chemical processing in a microchannel. *Lab Chip* 6: 550–554.

123. Neils, C., Tyree, Z., Finlayson, B., and Folch, A. 2004. Combinatorial mixing of microfluidic streams. *Lab chip* 4: 342–350.

124. Rhee, M. and Burns, M.A. 2008. Microfluidic assembly blocks. *Lab Chip* 8: 1365–1373.

125. Choi, S. and Chae, J. 2010. Methods of reducing non-specific adsorption in microfluidic biosensors. *J. Micromech. Microeng.* 20(7): 075015. doi: 10.1088/0960-1317/20/7/075015.

126. Shao, G., Wang, W., Wang, J., and Lin, Y. 2010. Design and fabrication of a PDMS microchip based immunoassay. *Proc. SPIE.* 7593: 75930Q. doi: 10.1117/12.847138.

127. Zhou, J.W. 2010. Recent developments in PDMS surface modification for microfluidic devices. *Electrophoresis* 31: 2–16.

128. Wang, J.D., Douville, N.J., Takayama, S., and ElSayed, M. 2012. Quantitative analysis of molecular absorption into PDMS microfluidic channels. *Ann. Biomed. Eng.* 40(9): 1862–1873.

129. Leo, A., Hansch, C., and Elkins, D. 1971. Partition coefficients and their uses. *Chem. Rev.* 71(6): 525–616.

130. Zhang, Z.W., Feng, X.J., Xu, F., Liu, X., and Liu, B.-F. 2010. "Click" chemistry-based surface modification of poly(dimethylsiloxane) for protein separation in a microfluidic chip. *Electrophoresis* 31(18): 3129–3136.

131. Harbers, G.M., Emoto, K., Greef, C., Metzger, S.W., Woodward, H.N., Mascali, J.J., Grainger, D.W., and Lochhead, M.J. 2007. Functionalized poly(ethylene glycol) bioassay surface chemistry facilitates bio-immobilization and inhibits non-specific protein, bacterial, and mammalian cell adhesion. *Chem. Mater.* 19(18): 4405–4414.

132. Salehi-Reyhani, A., Kaplinsky, J., Burgin, E., Novakova, M., deMello, A.J., Templer, R.H., Parker, P., Neil, M.A.A., Ces, O., French, P., Willison, K.R., and Klug, D. 2011. A first step towards practical single cell proteomics: A microfluidic antibody capture chip with TIRF detection. *Lab Chip* 11: 1256–1261.

133. Zhu, Z., Frey, O., Ottoz, D.S., Rudolf, F., and Hierlemann, A. 2012. Microfluidic single-cell cultivation chip with controllable immobilization and selective release of yeast cells. *Lab Chip* 12: 906–915.

134. Browne, A.W., Ramasamy, L., Cripe, T.P., and Ahn, C.H. 2011. A lab-on-a-chip for rapid blood separation and quantification of hematocrit and serum analytes. *Lab Chip* 11: 2440–2446.

135. Ryu, G., Huang, J., Hofmann, O., Walshe, C.A., Sze, J.Y.Y., McClean, G.D., Mosley, A., Rattle, S.J., deMello, J.C., deMello, A.J., and Bradley, D.D.C. 2011. Highly sensitive fluorescence detection system for microfluidic lab-on-a-chip. *Lab Chip* 11: 1664–1670.

136. Yokokawa, R., Kitazawa, Y., Terao, K., Okonogi, A., Kanno, I., and Kotera, H. 2012. A perfusable microfluidic device with on-chip total internal reflection fluorescence microscopy (TIRFM) for in situ and real-time monitoring of live cells. *Biomed. Microdevices* 14(4): 791–797. doi 10.1007/s10544-012-9656-5.

137. Harazim, S.M., Quiñones, V.A.B., Kiravittaya, S., Sanchez., S., and Schmidt, O.G. 2012. Lab-in-a-Tube: On-chip integration of glass optofluidic ring resonators for label-free sensing applications. *Lab Chip* 12(15): 2587–2750. doi: 10.1039/c0xx00000x.

138. Lee, S.S., Vizcarra, I.A., Huberts, D.H.E.W., Lee, L.P., and Heinemann, M. 2012. Whole lifespan microscopic observation of budding yeast aging through a microfluidic dissection platform. *PNAS* 109(13): 4916–4920.

139. Meissner, R., Joris, P., Eker, B., Bertsch, A., and Renaud, P. 2012. A microfluidic-based frequency-multiplexing impedance sensor (FMIS). *Lab Chip* 12: 2712–2718. doi: 10.1039/C2LC40236J.

140. Jung, W., Jang, A., Bishop, P.L., and Ahn, C.H. 2011. A polymer lab chip sensor with microfabricated planar silver electrode for continuous and on-site heavy metal measurement. *Sens. Actuat. B* 155: 145–153.

141. Moraes, F.C., Lima, R.S., Segato, T.P., Cesarino, I., Cetino, J.L.M., Machado, S.A.S., Gomez, F., and Carrilho, E. 2012. Glass/PDMS hybrid microfluidic device integrating vertically aligned SWCNTs to ultrasensitive electrochemical determinations. *Lab Chip* 12: 1959–1962.

142. Cooney, C.G., Sipes, D., Thakora, N., Holmberg, R., and Belgrader, P. 2012. A plastic, disposable microfluidic flow cell for coupled on-chip PCR and microarray detection of infectious agents. *Biomed. Microdevices* 14: 45–53.

143. Lefèvre, F., Chalifour, A., Yu, L., Chodavarapu, V., Juneau, P., and Izquierdo, R. 2012. Algal fluorescence sensor integrated into a microfluidic chip for water pollutant detection. *Lab Chip* 12: 787–793.

144. Choi, K., Kim, J.-Y., Ahn, J.-H., Choi, J.-M., Im, M., and Choi, Y.-K. 2012. Integration of field effect transistor-based biosensors with a digital microfluidic device for a lab-on-a-chip application. *Lab Chip* 12: 1533–1539.

145. Ahola, S., Telkki, V.-V., and Stapf, S. 2012. Velocity distributions in a micromixer measured by NMR imaging. *Lab Chip* 12: 1823–1830. doi: 10.1039/c2lc21214e.

146. Walter, A., März, A., Schumacher, W., Rösch, P., and Popp, J. 2011. Towards a fast, high specific and reliable discrimination of bacteria on strain level by means of SERS in a microfluidic device. *Lab Chip* 11: 1013–1021.
147. Heath, J.R. 2010. In vitro multiplex protein assays and sensors for cancer research and clinical applications. *Cancer Nanotechnol. Plan* 9–11.
148. Blair, E.D. 2010. Molecular diagnostics and personalized medicine: Value-assessed opportunities for multiple stakeholders. *Pers. Med.* 7(2): 143–161.
149. Dalton, W.S., Sullivan, D.M., Yeatman, T.J., and Fenstermacher, D.A. 2010. The 2010 health care reform act: A potential opportunity to advance cancer research by taking cancer personally. *Clin. Cancer Res.* 16: 5987–5996. doi: 10.1158/1078-0432.CCR-10-1216.
150. Schumacher, S., Nestler, J., Otto, T., Wegener, M., Ehrentreich-Förster, E., Michel, D., Wunderlich, K., Palzer, S., Sohn, K., Weber, A., Burgard, M., Grzesiak, A., Teichert, A., Brandenburg, A., Koger, B., Albers, J., Nebling, E., and Bier, F.F. 2012. Highly-integrated lab-on-chip system for point-of-care multiparameter analysis. *Lab Chip* 12(3): 464–473.
151. Carrara, S. 2010. *Nano-Bio-Sensing*, 1st edn. New York: Springer.
152. Krivitsky,V., Hsiung, L.-C., Lichtenstein, A., Brudnik, B., Kantaev, R., Elnathan, R., Pevzner, A., Khatchtourints, A., and Patolsky, F. 2012. Si nanowires forest-based on-chip biomolecular filtering, separation and preconcentration devices: Nanowires do it all. *Nano Lett.* 12(9): 4748–4756. doi: 10.1021/nl3021889.
153. Dixit, C.K. and Kaushik, A. 2012. Nano-structured arrays for multiplex analyses and Lab-on-a-Chip applications. *Biochem. Biophys. Res. Commun.* 419: 316–320.
154. Martinez, A.W., Phillips, S.T., Carrilho, E., and Whitesides, G.M. 2010. Diagnostics for the developing world: Microfluidic paper-based analytical devices. *Anal. Chem.* 82(1): 3–10.
155. Martinez, A.W., Phillips, S.T., Butte, M.J., and Whitesides, G.M. 2007. Patterned paper as a platform for inexpensive, low-volume, portable bioassays. *Angew. Chem. Int. Ed.* 46(8): 1318–1320.
156. Martinez, A.W., Phillips, S.T., Wiley, B.J., Gupta, M., and Whitesides, G.M. 2008. FLASH: A rapid method for prototyping paper-based microfluidic devices. *Lab Chip* 8: 2146–2150.
157. van Heeren, H. 2012. Standards for connecting microfluidic devices? *Lab Chip* 12: 1022–1025.
158. The Microfluidic Consortium. www.cfbi.com/index_files/microfluidics.htm (accessed Aug 2012).

Index